Obesity

Science to Practice

Obesity

Science to Practice

Gareth Williams
Faculty of Medicine and Dentistry,
University of Bristol, Bristol, UK

Gema Frühbeck
Department of Endocrinology, Clínica Universitaria,
University of Navarra, Pamplona

⟨JW⟩WILEY-BLACKWELL

A John Wiley & Sons, Ltd., Publication

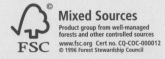

Mixed Sources
Product group from well-managed
forests and other controlled sources
www.fsc.org Cert no. CQ-COC-000012
© 1996 Forest Stewardship Council

This edition first published 2009, © 2009 John Wiley & Sons, Ltd

Wiley-Blackwell is an imprint of John Wiley & Sons, formed by the merger of Wiley's global Scientific, Technical and Medical business with Blackwell Publishing.

Registered office: John Wiley & Sons Ltd, The Atrium, Southern Gate, Chichester, West Sussex, PO19 8SQ, UK

Other Editorial Offices:
9600 Garsington Road, Oxford, OX4 2DQ, UK

111 River Street, Hoboken, NJ 07030-5774, USA

For details of our global editorial offices, for customer services and for information about how to apply for permission to reuse the copyright material in this book please see our website at www.wiley.com/wiley-blackwell

Library of Congress Cataloguing-in-Publication Data

Obesity : science to practice / [edited by] Gareth Williams, Gema Frühbeck.
  p. ; cm.
 Includes bibliographical references and index.
 ISBN 978-0-470-01911-5 (cloth)
 1. Obesity–Textbooks. I. Williams, Gareth. II. Frühbeck, Gema.
 [DNLM: 1. Obesity. WD 210 012583 2008]
 RC628.O296 2008
 616.85'26–dc22

                                        2008041508

ISBN: 978-0-470-01911-5

A catalogue record for this book is available from the British Library.

Typeset in 9/11 pt ITC Officina Sans by Thomson Digital, Noida, India
Printed in Italy by Printer Trento S.r.l., Trento, Italy

First Impression 2009
Cover Image reproduced courtesy of Robert Partridge, The Ancient Egypt Picture Library.

Contents

Preface

For many scientists and clinicians, obesity has at last come of age. When the editors were going through medical school and even specialist training in diabetes and endocrinology, obesity was a nonentity that fell out of the mainstream of 'real' diseases and was notable for being dull and unrewarding to treat. Admittedly, this was in a previous century – although not quite, we hasten to point out, a whole century ago.

Over the last 20 years, obesity has moved steadily in from the wings to centre stage and is now acknowledged by a wide range of players – health-care professionals, governments, the media and even the general public – to be one of the most challenging threats to global health for the foreseeable future. We prefer to avoid using that cliched expression 'an explosion of knowledge', but this is a reasonable description of the rapid and accelerating growth in the scientific and medical literature on obesity during the last decade or so. At the same time, the mismatch between what we know and what we can usefully do with that knowledge has become ever more striking. In an age when many other diseases have been conquered, or at least beaten into submission, obesity stands out as a condition whose prevalence continues to rise, often at rates that exceed the most pessimistic predictions of a few years ago. Obesity is still waiting for a therapeutic breakthrough; although the focus is inevitably on novel drugs and surgical procedures, the most important advance will be in finding new, effective and affordable measures to make whole populations change the ways in which they have become accustomed to live. So obesity is here to stay, and an ever-increasing number of people will need to know about it.

Visit any good medical bookshop or its e-counterpart and you will find a metre or so of shelf space occupied by books about obesity, some of which are very good. So why have we decided to invest the time and energy in bringing another textbook into an already crowded field? Indeed, isn't the relentless advance of electronic publishing pushing big medical books towards the brink of extinction?

Perhaps predictably, we don't subscribe to the view that medical textbooks are about to join 35-mm film and tape cassettes in the dustbin of defunct technologies. Also, we believe that there is room for a book on obesity with the qualities that we have aimed for here – namely, comprehensive but balanced coverage of the field, with the scientific background, clinical practice and wider societal aspects all well integrated with each other. Any voyage of discovery should be enjoyable, and we also set out to produce an attractive book that will be a pleasure to read and to look at.

A book of this size can never be as up to date as a speed-of-light electronic tour of the current literature, but it serves an entirely different purpose. A good textbook should provide expert guidance through the field, building understanding while laying the ground for new knowledge; it should also highlight areas that remain uncertain, and explain why. In this book, we have attempted to capture not only the essential facts, but also to show how these fit into the wider landscape of the science and clinical practice of obesity. Each chapter stands alone as a self-contained overview of the topic – with the key points summarised succinctly at the start – and can be read as such. Throughout the book, links and cross-references indicate the important portals of entry into other relevant areas. We have tried to make this book accessible and of interest to a wide readership, primarily doctors, dietitians, specialist nurses and other health-care professionals as well as scientists working in the many disciplines touched by obesity. We hope that it will also be valuable to those in public health and economics, and to policy makers at national and international level.

If we have succeeded in our aims, it is mainly because of the outstanding team of contributors that we have been fortunate to assemble. It will be immediately obvious from reading their chapters that they are world-class experts in their fields; we are also deeply grateful to them for having written for us – in an age when books command a lower priority than papers and reviews – and for their good nature and generous tolerance of editorial interference. It has been a great pleasure and a privilege to have worked with them on this book, and we hope that they are as happy with the end-product as we are.

We are similarly indebted to another world-class team, who are essentially invisible to the reader – namely, our friends and colleagues at Wiley. The relationship between editor and publisher is absolutely crucial for a healthy gestation and the safe delivery of a book; in real life, it can lie anywhere on the broad spectrum that extends from blessing to curse. In this instance, we have been blessed throughout all our dealings with the editorial and production teams, ever since the idea for the book first emerged from a meeting with Joan Marsh. She and her colleagues – notably Fiona Woods, Robert Hambrook, Ruth Graham, Andrew Finch and Poirei Sanaman – have been inspiring, wise and great fun to work with throughout this project. We've continually benefitted from their expertise and encouragement, and it's been exciting to see the book taking shape under their guidance.

On the home front, numerous people in Bristol and Pamplona have served (and suffered) far beyond any reasonable call of duty, while grappling heroically with various generations of editorial intervention, let alone the editors' handwriting. We believe it to be a coincidence that several have now left these cities (and in some instances are untraceable). We are particularly grateful to Jane Stevens, Jenny Russe, Carys Solman, Laura Heaney, Susanna Simm, Javier Gómez Ambrosi and Javier Salvador. We would also like to record our thanks to Anna Smith (Wellcome Trust History of Medicine Museum and Archives, London), Veronika Hölzer (Natural History Museum, Vienna), Robert Partridge (The Ancient Egypt Picture Library), Eric Delcommenne (Belgian Post Office), Cameron Kennedy, Julian Kabala, Josanne Vassala, Gauden Galea, David Savage, Nicola Moon, Jimmy Bell, María Angela Burrell, Pilar Sesma, Secundino Fernández, María José García Velloso and Alfonso Macías for their invaluable help in unearthing various of the illustrations. In addition, Colin Gardner deserves much gratitude for helping to maintain editorial well-being and good cheer at various critical moments.

Finally, and only partly to ensure that it is safe to go home, we owe a heartfelt thank you to our families, for their understanding, support and ability to keep a straight face each time we told them that it was nearly finished.

You'll gather that we've had great fun in putting this book together; we hope you will enjoy it too.

Gareth Williams

Gema Frühbeck
Bristol and Pamplona
November, 2008

Contributors

Nimantha de Alwis
Faculty of Medical Sciences Medical School
Framlington Place
Newcastle upon Tyne
NE2 4HH
UK

Robert Andrews
Dorothy Hodgkin Building
Whitson Street
Bristol BS1 3NY
UK

Ellen Blaak
Department of Human Biology
Nutrition Research Centre
Maastricht University
P.O. Box 616
6200 MD Maastricht
The Netherlands

Les Bluck
MRC Human Nutrition Research
Elsie Widdowson Laboratory
Fulbourn Road,
Cambridge
CB1 9NL
UK

George Bray
Pennington Centre
6400 Perkins Road
Baton Rouge
LA 70808
USA

Susan Byrne
School of Psychology
Mailbag M304
The University of Western Australia
35 Stirling Highway
CRAWLEY WA 6009
Australia

Juliana Chan
Department of Medicine and Therapeutics
Chinese University of Hong Kong
The Prince of Wales Hospital Shatin
N.T.
Hong Kong

Mimi Chen
Diabetes and Metabolism
    Research Group,
University of Bristol,
Department of Clinical Sciences at
    North Bristol,
Southmead Hospital,
Bristol BS10 8NB.
UK

Chris Day
Clinical Medical Sciences
4th Floor William Leech Building
Medical School
Framlington Place
University of Newcastle upon
Tyne NE2 4HH
UK

Mervyn Deitel
Obesity Surgery
5863 Leslie Street
Box 1002
Toronto, ON M2H
Canada

Emma Dove
Health and Human Sciences
University of Essex
Wivenhoe Park
Colchester
Essex, CO4 3SQ
UK

Keith Frayn
Oxford Centre for Diabetes, Endocrinology and
    Metabolism
University of Oxford Radcliffe
    Infirmary
Oxford OX2 6HE
UK

Gema Frühbeck
Dept. of Endocrinology
Clínica Universitaria
    de Navarra
Avda. Pío XII, 36
31008 - Pamplona
Spain

Luc Van Gaal
Antwerp University Hospital
Dept. Diabetology
Metabolism and Clinical Nutrition
Wilrijkstraat 10
B-2650 Edegem (Antwerp)
Belgium

Nori Geary
Institute of Animal Sciences
Swiss Federal Institute of Technology
Zurich Schwerzenbach 8603
Switzerland

Gail Goldberg
MRC Human Nutrition Research
Elsie Widdowson Laboratory
Fulbourn Road,
Cambridge
CB1 9NL
UK

Joanne Harrold
Department of Psychology
The University of Liverpool
Eleanor Rathbone Building
Bedford Street South
Liverpool L69 7ZA
UK

Andrew Hill
Academic Unit of Psychiatry
    and Behavioural Sciences
Leeds Institute of Health Sciences
Charles Thackrah Building
University of Leeds
101 Clarendon
Road Leeds, LS2 9LJ
UK

Rachel Huxley
Nutrition and Lifestyle Division
Faculty of Medicine, University of Sydney
NSW 2006
Australia

Gianluca Iacobellis
Gianluca Iacobellis:
Cardiovascular Obesity Research & Management
    School of Medicine, McMaster University
    Hamilton Medical Hospital
237 Barton Street East,
Hamilton, ON, L8L 2X2
Canada

Susan Jebb
Head of Nutrition and Health Research
MRC Human Nutrition Research
Elsie Widdowson Laboratory
Fulbourn Road,
Cambridge CB1 9NL
UK

Alexandra Johnstone
The Rowett Institute of Nutrition
    and Health
University of Aberdeen
Greenburn Road, Bucksburn,
Aberdeen AB21 9SB
UK

Jens Jordan
Institut für Klinische Pharmakologie
Medizinische Hochschule Hannover
Carl-Neuberg-Straße 1
30625 Hannover
Germany

Gary Ko
Department of Medicine and Therapeutics
Chinese University of Hong Kong
The Prince of Wales Hospital Shatin
N.T.
Hong Kong

Shiriki Kumanyika
Department of Biostatistics and
    Epidemiology,
School of Medicine, University of Pennsylvania
3451 Walnut Street,
Philadelphia, PA 19104
USA

Max Lafontan
Max Lafontan:
INSERM Unité 317
Institut Louis Bugnard
Faculté de Médecine, Hôpital Rangueil
31 403 Toulouse Cedex 4
France

Wolfgang Langhans
ETH Zürich Wolfgang Langhans
Institut für Nutztierwissenschaften Physiologie
    und Tierhaltung
SLA C 3
Schorenstrasse 16
8603 Schwerzenbach
Switzerland

Dominique Langin
Unité de recherches sur les obésités
INSERM UPS U586, IFR31
Institut Louis Bugnard, Toulouse
France

Rachel Leach
IASO
231 North Gower Street
London
NW1 2NR
UK

David Levitsky
Division of Nutritional Sciences
Cornell University,
Ithaca, New York
NY 14853
USA

Tim Lobstein
The Food Commission
94 White Lion Street
London N1 9PF
UK

Ronald Ma
Department of Medicine and Therapeutics
Chinese University of Hong Kong
The Prince of Wales Hospital Shatin
N.T.
Hong Kong

Ilse Mertens
Dept. Endocrinology, Diabetology & Metabolism
Metabolic Unit
Antwerp University Hospital
Antwerp
Belgium

Neville Rigby
(Formerly)
IASO
231 North Gower Street
London NW1 2NR
UK

Arya Sharma
Professor of Medicine
Chair for Obesity Research & Management
University of Alberta
Royal Alexandra Hospital
10240 Kingsway Avenue
Edmonton, AB T5H 3V9
Canada

Julian Shield
JP Hamilton-Shield
Institute of Child Life & Health
UBHT Education Centre
Upper Maudlin Street
Bristol BS2 8AE
UK

John Speakman
Zoology Building
Tillydrone Avenue
University of Aberdeen
Aberdeen AB24 2TZ
UK

Carolyn Summerbell
School of Health & Social Care
Centuria Building
University of Teesside
Middlesbrough
Tees Valley TS1 3BA
UK

Janet Warren
MRC Human Nutrition Research
Elsie Widdowson Laboratory
Fulbourn Road,
Cambridge
CB1 9NL
UK

Susanne Wiesner
Obesity Center
Lindberg Clinic
Schickstrasse 11
CH-8400 Winterthur
Switzerland

John Wilding
School of Clinical Sciences
Clinical Sciences Centre
University Hospital Aintree
Liverpool L9 7AL
UK

History of Obesity

Chapter 1

Chapter 1   History of Obesity

George A. Bray

Obesity has been evident in the human record for over 20 000 years and affected numerous aspects of human life and society (Bray, 2007a; Bray, 2007b). This introductory chapter describes the early history of human obesity, and then reviews how understanding has developed in the basic biology of obesity, its definitions and measurement, the complications of the disease, and finally its management. Some of the major scientific and medical milestones in the history of obesity are shown in Table 1.1.

Early human history

Prehistory

Human obesity is clearly depicted in Stone Age artefacts, notably numerous figurines that have been found within a 2000-kilometre band crossing Europe from South-Western France to Southern Russia. Palaeolithic (Old Stone Age) statuettes, produced some 23 000–25 000 years ago, were made of ivory, limestone or terracotta. Most famous is the 'Venus of Willendorf', an 11-centimetre figurine found in Austria (Figure 1.1). Typical of many such figurines, the Venus shows marked abdominal obesity and pendulous breasts. Anne Scott Beller (1977) has suggested that 'obesity was already a fact of life' for Palaeolithic humans, although one can only speculate about the purpose or significance of these artefacts.

The New Stone Age (Neolithic) period, spanning the interval between 8000 and 5500 B.C., saw the introduction of agriculture and the establishment of human settlements. This era also yielded numerous statuettes depicting obesity, notably the 'Mother Goddess' artefacts found especially in Anatolia (modern Turkey). Similar figures from this period have been found in many other sites in Europe and other continents. Anthropological studies indicate that hunter-gatherers are typically lean and that overt overweight is unusual (Prentice, Rayco-Solon and Moore, 2005) – although the enhanced ability to store energy as fat would have clear survival advantages. This fact makes these representations of severe obesity all the more striking.

The ancient period

Obesity and its sequelae have long figured in the medical traditions of many diverse cultures. Ancient Egyptian stone reliefs show occasional obese people, such as a cook in Ankh-ma-Hor's tomb (Sixth Dynasty; 2340–2180 B.C.), and a fat man enjoying food presented to him by his lean servant, in Mereruka's tomb (Figure 1.2). Studies of the reconstructed skin folds of royal mummies suggest that some were fat, including Queen Inhapy, Hatshepsut and King Rameses III (Reeves, 1992). Overall, it appears that stout people were not uncommon in ancient Egypt, at least among the higher classes; interestingly, Darby et al. (1977) were led to conclude that obesity 'was regarded as objectionable'.

Elsewhere in the world, corpulent human figures are depicted in artefacts from the ancient Mesopotamian civilization in the basin of the Rivers Tigris and Euphrates, and from the Meso-American cultures of the Incas, Mayans and Aztecs.

Ancient Greece and Rome

The health hazards associated with obesity were well known to the Ancient Greek physician Hippocrates, who stated that 'sudden death is more common in those who are naturally fat than in the lean' (Littré, 1839). Greek physicians also noted that obesity was a cause of infrequent menses and infertility in women.

Obesity: Science to Practice   Edited by Gareth Williams and Gema Frühbeck
© 2009 John Wiley & Sons, Ltd

Table 1.1   Some landmarks in the history of obesity since the seventeenth century

Seventeenth Century

1614	Santorio	Uses beam balance to measure metabolism
1628	Harvey	Discovers circulation of the blood
1679	Bonet	First dissections of obese cadavers

Eighteenth Century

1727	Short	First English language monograph on obesity
1760	Flemyng	Monograph on the treatment of obesity
1780	Cullen	Disease classification that includes obesity
1780s	Lavoisier	First measurements of heat production by living animals; formulated the 'oxygen theory' (which replaced 'phlogiston' of the Ancients)

Nineteenth Century

1810	Wadd	*Treatise on Corpulence*
1826	Brillat-Savarin	Diet-based method for weight loss
1835	Quételet	Obesity quantified as weight/(height squared)
1848	Helmholtz	Published Law of the Conservation of Energy (First Law of Thermodynamics)
1849	Hassall	Described structure and growth of fat cells
1863	W. Banting	*Letter on Corpulence Addressed to the Public* (first widely popular diet book)
1866	Russell	Sleep apnoea described as a complication of obesity
1879	Hoggan	Described growth of fat cells
1896	Atwater	First human calorimeter constructed

Twentieth Century

1900	Babinski	Described syndrome of hypothalamic obesity
1901	Fröhlich	
1912	Cushing	Described obesity caused by basophil pituitary tumour
1916	Cannon & Carlson	Proposed gastric mechanism for hunger
1921	F. Banting, Best, Macleod & Collip	Insulin isolated from pancreas and used to treat human diabetes
1927	Various	Dinitrophenol used to treat obesity (poor outcome)
1936	Himsworth	Insulin-insensitive diabetic patients identified
1937	Abramson	Amphetamine used to treat obesity
1944	Behnke	Underwater weighing used to estimate body density and composition
1947	Vague	'Android' (central) obesity predisposes to diabetes and cardiovascular risk
1949	Fawcett	Described brown adipose tissue (BAT)
1954	Stellar	Formulated 'dual centre' hypothesis to explain control of feeding
1955	Lifson	Doubly-labelled water used to measure energy expenditure
1959	Berson & Yalow	Discovered radioimmunoassay technique to measure insulin concentrations
1962	Neel	'Thrifty gene' hypothesis
1963	Randle	Glucose-fatty acid (Randle) cycle described
1967	Stewart	First use of behavioural therapy to treat obesity
1968	Various	Association for the Study of Obesity founded in UK
1968	Mason	Performed first gastric bypass operations to treat obesity
1973	Gibb	Cholecystokinin (CCK) found to induce satiety in rats
1979	DeFronzo	Insulin-glucose clamp developed to measure insulin sensitivity
1982	Nedergaard *et al.*	Thermogenin (later renamed UCP1) identified as source of heat production in BAT
1986	Various	International Association for the Study of Obesity founded
1988	Reaven	Described 'Syndrome X' (the insulin resistance or metabolic syndrome)

1989	Strosberg *et al.*	Identified β_3-adrenoceptor
1994	Friedman *et al.*	Discovered leptin
1997	O'Rahilly *et al.*	Described leptin and melanocortin 4 receptor mutations as causes of human obesity
1998	WHO	International classification of obesity and identifies Global Epidemic of Obesity
Twenty-first Century		
2007	Sjöström *et al.*	Demonstrated that bariatric surgery prolongs life

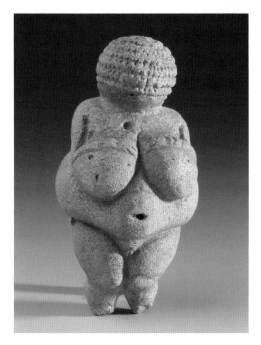

Figure 1.1 Venus of Willendorf, a Palaeolithic figurine carved out of fine-grained limestone, was found near Willendorf in the Wachau region of Lower Austria in 1908. It can be seen in the Natural History Museum, Vienna. Image reproduced courtesy of the Natural History Museum, Vienna.

Some 500 years after Hippocrates, the leading Roman physician Galen distinguished 'moderate' and 'immoderate' forms of obesity, the latter perhaps anticipating the 'morbid' category of current classifications.

Obesity was also familiar to Abu Ali Ibn Sina (Avicenna in the westernized version of his name), one of the most prominent figures of the Arabic medical tradition. Avicenna was a prolific and influential author who published over 40 medical works and 145 treatises on philosophy, logic and theology. In his medical encyclopaedia, written in the early twelfth century, Avicenna described the sweet taste of diabetic urine, and also referred to obesity and its dangers to health.

Eastern medical traditions

The Hindu physicians, Sushrut (Susrata) and Charak (500–400 B.C.) are credited with very early recognition of the sugary taste of diabetic urine, and also observed that the disease often affected indolent, overweight people who ate excessively, especially sweet and fatty foods.

The seventeenth century Tibetan medical treatise entitled *The Blue Beryl* recognized obesity as a condition that required treatment through

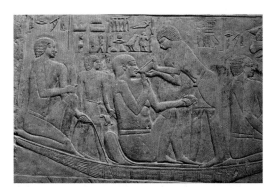

Figure 1.2 Stone relief from the tomb of the nobleman Mereruka at Saqqara, Egypt (c. 2350 B.C.), showing Mereruka in a boat, being fed by one of his servants. Image reproduced courtesy of Robert Partridge, The Ancient Egypt Picture Library.

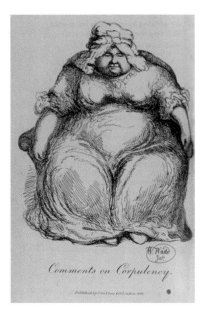

Figure 1.3 Illustration from William Wadd's monograph, *Comments on Corpulency* (1829). Image reproduced courtesy of the Wellcome Trust's History of Medicine Archive.

weight loss. The author, Sangye Gyamtso, noted scholar and Regent of Tibet, also wrote that 'overeating … causes illness and shortens lifespan'. He made two suggestions for treating obesity, namely the vigorous massage of the body with pea flour, and eating the gullet, hair and flesh of a wolf (which was also recommended to treat goitre and oedematous states).

History of the biology of obesity

Adipose tissue: structure and function

Vesalius laid the foundations of modern anatomy with his famous treatise, *De humani corporis fabrica* (1543), which was based on his own dissections. The first dissections of specifically obese individuals are attributed to Bonetus (1679), followed in the eighteenth century by descriptions from Morgagni and from Haller, and in the early nineteenth century by the notable monograph, *Comments on Corpulency, Lineaments of Leanness,* of Wadd (1829). Wadd presented 12 cases, two of whom had been examined *post mortem* and were found to have extensive accumulations of fat (Figure 1.3).

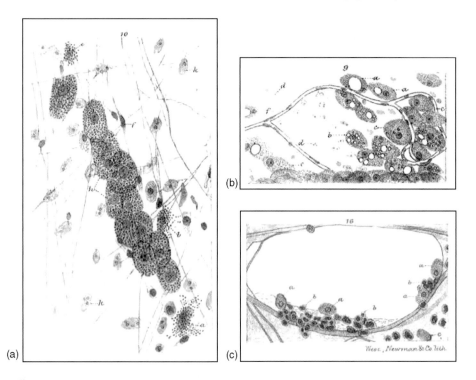

(a)　　(b)　　(c)

Figure 1.4 Microscopic studies of adipose tissue and its development. Illustration from Hoggan and Hoggan (1879), reproduced courtesy of the Royal Microscopical Society, London.

The adipocyte was recognized as a specific cell-type when the first substantive text books of microscopic anatomy were published in the 1850s, and the growth and development of fat cells were described by Hassall (1849) and by Hoggan and Hoggan (1879) (Figure 1.4). In his early observations on the development of the 'fat vesicle' (adipocyte), Hassall suggested that certain types of obesity might result from an increased number of fat cells – the precursor of the concept of 'hyperplastic' obesity that twentieth-century workers such as Bjurulf, Hirsch and Björntorp would later elaborate.

Much work was conducted on digestion during the seventeenth and eighteenth centuries, leading in the early twentieth century to the seminal and long-lasting theory that hunger resulted from gastric contractions; this was based on direct measurement of gastric motility, and its association with hunger by Washburn and Cannon, and independently by Carlson.

Descriptions and measurements of obesity

The first monographs devoted to obesity appeared during the eighteenth century, notably two works published in English by Short (1727) and Flemyng (1760). Short's work (Figure 1.5) opens with the statement: 'I believe no age did ever afford more instances of corpulency than our own'. He believed that the treatment of obesity required restoration of the body's natural balance and removal of secondary causes, ideally by living where the air was not too moist or soggy and avoiding flat, wet countries, cities and woodlands. Short considered that exercise was important and that the diet should be 'moderate, spare and of the more detergent kind'.

Flemyng listed four causes of corpulency, beginning with 'the taking in of too large a quantity of food, especially of the rich and oily kind' – although he went on to note that not all obese people were big eaters. His second cause of obesity was 'too lax a texture of the cellular or fatty membrane ... whereby its cells or vesicles are liable to be too easily distended', and the third an abnormal state of the blood that facilitated the storage of fat in the vesicles. The fourth cause was 'defective evacuation'; Flemyng believed that sweat, urine and faeces all contained 'oil', and therefore that obesity could be treated by eliminating this oil through the administration of laxatives, diaphoretics or diuretics.

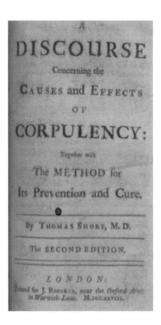

Figure 1.5 Frontispiece from Thomas Short's monograph, *A Discourse Concerning the Causes and Effects of Corpulency* (1727). Image reproduced courtesy of the Wellcome Trust History of Medicine Archive.

As already mentioned, observations made in antiquity by Roman and Indian physicians hinted at attempts to distinguish different types of obesity and diabetes. Many classifications of diseases have been proposed, with an early approach by the seventeenth century English physician, Thomas Sydenham (1624–1689). Perhaps the two best-known systematic classifications of diseases were those of William Cullen (1710–1790), a physician who became professor of chemistry in Edinburgh, and the French doctor Sauvages (1706–1767). Both referred to 'polysarcia', from the Greek for 'much flesh'. In Cullen's work, polysarcia falls in the 'Order II' ('Intumescentiae', or swellings) of 'Class III' (Cachexiae), with the generic name of *Corporis pinguedinosa intumescentia molesta* ('harmful swelling of the body's fat'). During the nineteenth century, 'obesity' (from the Latin *obesitas* meaning fatness) gradually came to replace polysarcia and other terms such as 'corpulence' and 'embonpoint'.

There have been numerous attempts to quantify excess weight in ways that are appropriate to clinical practice, research and epidemiology; of particular interest has been the relationship between the severity of obesity and the various diseases to which it predisposes (see Chapters 3 and 9). The Belgian statistician

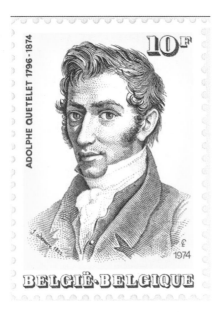

Figure 1.6 Adolphe Quételet (1796–1874), Belgian statistician. Image reproduced courtesy of the Belgian Postal Service.

Adolphe Quételet (1796–1874) was one of the early leaders in developing and validating mathematical measures of obesity (Figure 1.6). Quételet was responsible for the concept of the 'average man' and suggested that the ratio of the subject's weight divided by the square of the height could be used as a measure of fatness that corrected for differences in height. This unit, the Body Mass Index (BMI), is still known as the 'Quételet Index' (QI) in some European countries; BMI has been shown to correlate with body fat content, and to predict risk for several of the comorbidities of obesity.

The twentieth century witnessed the application of a wide range of techniques to measure fatness with increasing sophistication, and to define the content and distribution of fat throughout the body, as well as its impact on metabolism. Body density (and thus body fat content) was first calculated by applying Archimedes' Principle to the reduction in body weight when the subject was reweighed under water; the technique has been successfully adapted to the displacement of air rather than water, in the plethysmograpic devices in use today (see Chapter 3).

The widespread clinical use of ultrasound, computerized tomographic (CT) scanning, dual-energy X-ray absorptiometry (DEXA) and magnetic resonance (MR) imaging has shown that all these techniques are useful in measuring aspects of body composition, and the distribution and volume of specific fat depots. In addition, the metabolic impact of obesity, notably the insulin resistance that it induces (see below), has been clarified using a variety of techniques, including the insulin clamp invented by Ralph DeFronzo during the 1970s, the minimal model intravenous glucose tolerance test devised by Richard Bergman, and the homeostatic modelling (HOMA) developed by David Matthews during the 1980s (see Chapter 3).

Metabolism and energy balance

The importance of oxygen in metabolism and indeed life itself was first revealed by the work of Robert Boyle (1627–1691), who established the concept of the chemical elements (Figure 1.7). Crucially, Boyle demonstrated that when a lighted candle went out in a closed chamber, a mouse confined to the same chamber rapidly died.

This theme was developed a century later by the French chemist, Antoine Lavoisier (1743–1794), whose research culminated in the Oxygen

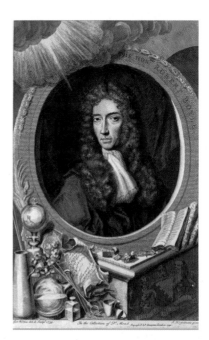

Figure 1.7 Robert Boyle (1627–1691), English chemist. Image reproduced courtesy of the Wellcome Trust History of Medicine Archive.

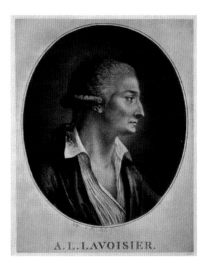

A. L. LAVOISIER.

Figure 1.8 Antoine Lavoisier (1743–1794), French chemist. Image reproduced courtesy of the Wellcome Trust History of Medicine Archive.

Theory that was to prove fundamental to the science of energy balance and obesity (Figure 1.8). Lavoisier, who died at the guillotine during the French Revolution, recognized that oxidation and combustion both entailed combination with oxygen. He conducted the first measurements of heat production (calorimetry) – calculated from the weight of ice melted by a guinea pig's respiration – and inferred that metabolism was analogous to slow combustion. Helmholtz went on to develop the Laws of the Conservation of Mass and of the Elements. His work ultimately formed the basis for the Law of Surface Area, formulated by the German Max Rubner (1854–1932). Rubner adapted the bomb calorimeter method developed by Pettenkofer and Voit to determine expired carbon dioxide, and went on to measure energy expenditure in human subjects and experimental animals. He also observed a consistent linear relationship between energy expenditure and surface area among mammals of diverse species and sizes.

Interest in the Law of Conservation of Energy, and whether it also applied to humans, stimulated Wilbur Olin Atwater and Edward Bennett Rosa to construct the first human calorimeter at the Wesleyan College in Middletown, Connecticut in 1896. By measuring the oxygen consumed by a subject in a sealed chamber, they proved that humans, like all other animals, obey the first Law of Thermodynamics, namely that the energy expenditure of an individual in steady state equals their energy intake. Their basic concept is perpetuated in the human calorimeters in use today, albeit with much more sophisticated measurements of oxygen consumption and carbon dioxide production that can yield detailed information about minute-by-minute energy expenditure and the utilization of specific macro-nutrients (see Chapter 3).

Other modern refinements in the measurement of energy expenditure in humans have included portable hoods suitable for use at the bedside, and the ingenious 'doubly-labelled water' technique. The latter exploits differences in the ways that the hydrogen and oxygen atoms of the water molecule are metabolized in the body, and from the elimination rates of ^{2}H (deuterium) and ^{18}O after administration of a known dose of ^{2}H$_2$^{18}O, energy expenditure can be calculated (see Chapter 3).

Application of these techniques has helped to unravel the complicated physiology of human energy balance, and has confirmed the fundamental principle that obese people in general expend more energy than the lean, and must therefore consume more energy in order to maintain their higher body weight. Interestingly, it has also been demonstrated that overweight people underestimate their food intake to a greater degree than do lean people. This finding has challenged the validity of a large body of research based on conventional dietary records, and has important implications for the practical management of obesity.

The organs and tissues that are most metabolically active and responsible for energy expenditure have attracted interest, including as potential sites of defects in energy expenditure that could contribute or lead to obesity. During the latter half of the twentieth century, much research focused on brown adipose tissue (BAT), or brown fat (Figure 1.9). This interesting tissue, first described in 1949 by Fawcett and Jones, is extremely rich in mitochondria and owes its brown colour to mitochondrial cytochromes. BAT is metabolically highly active and, in lower mammals, is an important physiological defence against cold (and in waking animals from hibernation). It has been shown that reductions in the thermogenic activity of BAT contribute to obesity in certain genetic obesity syndromes, such as the *ob/ob* mouse and *fa/fa* rat (see below). In humans, BAT is present in the neonate but soon atrophies and is now known to play no important role in common human obesity.

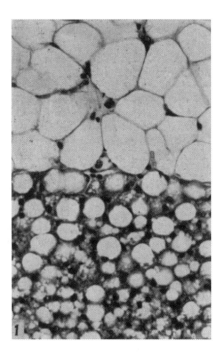

Figure 1.9 Histological appearance of brown fat (lower part of field) compared with white adipose tissue (upper field). From Fawcett and Jones (1949), with kind permission of the Endocrine Society.

BAT oxidizes fatty acids to generate heat rather than adenosine triphosphate (ATP), a property finally explained in the early 1980s when Jens Nedergaard and colleagues discovered a protein that they named 'thermogenin' (Cannon, Hedin and Nedergaard, 1982). Thermogenin was shown the following year by Daniel Ricquier and colleagues in Paris to be a specific uncoupling protein, now termed UCP-1 (Ricquier *et al.*, 1983). UCP-1 was shown to 'uncouple' fatty oxidation from ATP production by short-circuiting the proton electrochemical gradient across the inner mitochonndrial membrane, thus producing heat. The mechanism of heat production in other tissues, which do not express UCP-1, was further clarified by the finding of other related uncoupling proteins, UCP-2 and UCP-3, by Ricquier's group in France (Fleury *et al.*, 1997), Lowell's group in Boston (Vidal-Puig *et al.*, 1997) and Boss and colleagues in Geneva (Boss *et al.*, 1997).

During the nineteenth century, the prevailing concept was that only macronutrients – carbohydrates, proteins and fat – were needed to sustain human life. The discovery of vitamins in the early twentieth century overthrew this theory, and gave birth to the broader discipline of nutrition. Subsequently, the impact of macronutrients on human health and the development of obesity has returned to centre stage through the recognition of the role of dietary fats and simple sugars (for example in carbonated drinks) as causes of obesity and contributors to cardiovascular and other obesity-related diseases.

Health hazards of obesity

Ancient clinical observations, mentioned above, suggest that obesity was already recognized in association with both diabetes and sudden death, although the significance of the morbidity and excess mortality conferred by overweight and obesity has only been fully appreciated much more recently.

Interestingly, the life insurance industry can claim credit for having drawn attention to the relationship between obesity and premature death. As early as 1901, actuarial data showed that excess weight, especially around the abdomen, was associated with a shortened life expectancy. This risk has been confirmed by large numbers of systematic studies in numerous populations, and these led to the World Health Organization (WHO) classification of obesity which stratifies increasing degrees of risk according to rising BMI. This classification was first formulated in 1995 and has subsequently been modified to make allowance for the increased susceptibility of Asian populations to the adverse effects of obesity (see Chapter 9).

A particular relationship between abdominal obesity and early death could be discerned from the early life-insurance data, but it was the thorough studies of Jean Vague (1947) (Figure 1.10), working in Marseille, which clearly established the overriding importance of abdominal (central) obesity in conferring excess mortality. Vague's conclusions were clear, but the 'adipo-muscular ratio' that he used to distinguish 'android' obesity (in the abdominal distribution typical of males) from 'gynoid' (gluteofemoral) adiposity characteristic of women was cumbersome. Simpler measures of abdominal obesity – the ratio of waist circumference to hip circumference, and even waist circumference alone – are now widely used in clinical practice and in research settings. Indeed, cut-off values of waist circumference that indicate increased cardiovascular risk and premature death have been proposed and these appear to be more powerfully predictive than BMI (see Chapter 9).

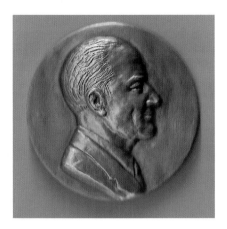

Figure 1.10 Jean Vague (born 1912), French endocrinologist. The image is from a medal, designed by his wife, and struck in 1981.

Obesity predisposes to type 2 (non-insulin dependent) diabetes, and is largely responsible for the current pandemic of the disease, which is predicted to double the number of diabetic people worldwide in just 30 years, from 150 million in 1995 to over 300 million in 2025 (see Chapters 2 and 10). The association between obesity and type 2 diabetes was highlighted in classical studies of isolated ethnic groups which, after centuries of active and frugal existence, had suddenly become sedentary and overfed. Notable examples were the Pima Indians living near the Gila river in Arizona and the inhabitants of the Pacific island of Nauru (Figure 1.11).

Such studies led to the 'thrifty gene' hypothesis proposed by Neel in the early 1960s. This postulated that 'thrifty' genes whose products promoted the storage of fat and ultimately diabetes might favour survival and therefore be selected in populations subject to periodic famine; however, in a westernized setting of inactivity and over-abundant food, obesity and type 2 diabetes might then emerge (Neel, 1962).

No 'thrifty' genes have yet been convincingly identified, but much progress has been made in elucidating the functional links between obesity and type 2 diabetes. Many of the metabolic consequences of obesity have been attributed to decreased sensitivity of various tissues and organs to insulin action ('insulin resistance'). The concept of insulin resistance can be traced back to the English diabetologist, Harold Himsworth, who in 1936, classified diabetic patients as either insulin-sensitive or insulin-insensitive, according to whether or not their blood glucose level fell after the co-administration of oral glucose and intravenous insulin (Figure 1.12). The American diabetologist, Gerald Reaven coined the phrase 'insulin resistance syndrome' or 'syndrome X' (now generally known as the 'metabolic syndrome') in the late 1980s. However, this concept had been anticipated by Vague some 40 years earlier, who recognized that central obesity was associated with, and predisposed to, diabetes, atherosclerosis and gout – all core features of the metabolic syndrome. Indeed, the Swedish physician Eskil Kylin (1889–1975)

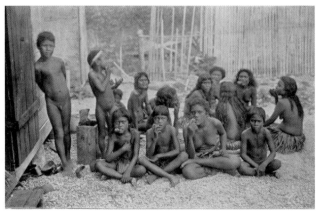

Tafel 17 (siehe Seite 446). Eingeborene von Nauru.

Figure 1.11 A group of Nauruan Islanders, photographed in 1896. At this time, this population was generally lean and diabetes was a rare disease. Following the advent of a Westernised lifestyle, the prevalences of obesity and type 2 diabetes have risen progressively and are now among the highest in the world. From Krämer, A (1906). *Hawaii, Ostmikronesien und Samoa.* Stuttgart: Schweizerbartsche Verlagsbuchhandlung, page 449.

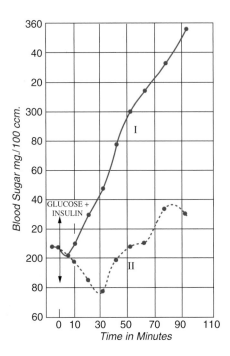

Figure 1.12 The 'insulin–glucose challenge' test devised
by Harold Himsworth (1936). This contrasts the typical
responses in an 'insulin-insensitive' subject (Patient I)
and an 'insulin-sensitive' subject (Patient II). Reproduced by kind permission of the editor of the *Lancet*.

had described the association of hypertension,
diabetes and gout during the 1920s (Kylin, 1923).
Other notable contributions include the demonstration in 1963 by Philip Randle, Nick Hales
and colleagues in Oxford that high free fatty
acid levels could interfere with glucose utilization (thus effectively counteracting the action
of insulin) through the Randle or glucose-fatty
acid cycle (Randle *et al.*, 1963).

Other comorbidities of obesity have been recognized since antiquity. Associated respiratory
problems – possibly reminiscent of the obesity
hypoventilation syndrome – were described as
long ago as the Greco-Roman era (Kryger, 1983).
The first clear medical report of sleep apnoea
was apparently that of Russell in 1866. The latter was published some 30 years after Charles
Dickens' novel *Pickwick Papers*, which features a
fat boy, Joe, who frequently falls asleep – hence
the alternative name of 'Pickwickian' syndrome
that William Osler applied to the obesity hypoventilation syndrome. Fatty liver, long recognized as a consequence of overfeeding in geese
(*foie gras*) and a feature of human obesity, was

only identified in 1980 by Ludwig as a significant comorbidity that can lead to progressive
liver damage.

Causes of obesity

The importance of overeating and inactivity was
recognized by the Ancients and has continued
to be assumed to the present day. In addition,
many diseases that cause obesity have been identified, and during the last two decades attention has shifted to the nature of the inherited
predisposition to obesity and the specific
genetic defects that underlie this susceptibility. Striking genetic obesity syndromes in other
species (especially rodents) have yielded valuable information about the normal regulation of
energy homeostasis, and some of these 'lessons
of nature' have helped to clarify the aetiology
of certain subsets of human obesity.

The role of the brain in controlling body
weight, initially highlighted by clinical cases,
has been extensively explored. Obesity has
long been recognized in association with hypothalamic damage (mostly caused by tumours),
notably in the 'adiposogenital syndrome'
(obesity with sexual infantilism) described by
Joseph Babinski (1857–1932) in Paris, and by
A. Fröhlich (1871–1953) in Vienna (Figure 1.13)
(Fröhlich, 1901). The co-occurrence of truncal
obesity with hypertension and other characteristic features in subjects with a basophil (ACTH-
secreting) tumour of the pituitary was described
in 1912 by the American neurosurgeon Harvey
Cushing (1869–1939), and the syndrome of
glucocorticoid excess now bears his name.

These and other clinical observations stimulated interest in the central nervous system
(CNS) and especially the hypothalamus, which in
turn heralded the development of experimental
techniques to produce localized brain damage
in animals in order to identify the regions that
controlled eating and body weight. These methods were made possible by the precise targeting
of specific brain regions using the 'stereotactic' frame apparatus originally designed by the
English neurosurgeon V.A.H. Horsley (1857–1916).
Damage was induced by microinjection of toxins
such as chromic oxide, or by localized heating or
electrolysis produced by special probes. Classical
findings included the dramatic hyperphagia and
obesity induced by bilateral lesions of the ventromedial hypothalamus, in striking contrast to

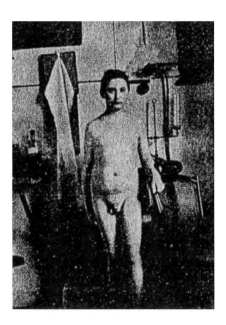

Figure 1.13 The 'adiposogenital syndrome' of obesity with sexual infantilism, due to hypothalamic damage. The illustration shows Fröhlich's original patient. Reproduced courtesy of the editor of *Endocrinology*.

the loss of appetite and wasting that followed destruction of the lateral hypothalamus. These observations led to Eliot Stellar, in the early 1950s, to advance the 'dual centre' hypothesis (Stellar, 1954). This proposed that feeding and weight were controlled by the balance between a ventromedial 'satiety centre' and a lateral hypothalamic 'appetite centre'; the hypothesis shaped thinking about hunger and satiety for over two decades, although it is now recognized to be over-simplistic.

Knowledge about the CNS has advanced in waves, driven by technological innovations. During the 1970s–1980s, refinements in methods such as radioimmunoassay and immunocytochemistry and the tracing of neuroanatomical tracts helped to identify the neurotransmitters that control energy balance; subsequent research, including advanced molecular and transgenic techniques, has clarified their sites of production and action, the factors regulating their activity, and the receptors that mediate their effects. These transmitters include classical monoamines such as norepinephrine-serotonin (whose potent appetite-suppressing action has been exploited in several anti-obesity drugs), peptides including the potent orexigen (appetite-stimulator) neuropeptide Y (NPY) and the

anorectic melanocortin, α-MSH, and the endocannabinoids that stimulate feeding. Landmark studies include the demonstration by James Gibbs and colleagues in 1973 that injection of cholecystokinin (CCK), the gut peptide named for its ability to stimulate gall-bladder contraction, powerfully inhibited feeding in rats (Gibbs, Young and Smith, 1973); this indicated that the gut could communicate through secreted peptides with the CNS to control feeding (see Chapter 6). Subsequent research has shown that the hypothalamus and other regulatory regions of the brain are surprisingly accessible to circulatory hormones that are now known to signal fat mass and energy needs, such as insulin, leptin and ghrelin.

The first of the animal obesity syndromes to be understood at a molecular genetic level was the yellow obese (A^y) mouse, whose striking coat colour had been prized in Ancient China. The cause, discovered in 1994 by Bultman *et al.*, (1992) was 'ectopic' over-expression of a peptide termed 'agouti' in tissues where it does not normally occur. Agouti is an endogenous antagonist of α-MSH at its melanocortin receptors, leading to hyperphagia and obesity from inhibition of the appetite-suppressing effect of α-MSH in the hypothalamus, and lightening of the fur because agouti also blocks the melanocortin-mediated production of melanin in the hair follicle. Interestingly, mutations of the human proopiomelanocortin have now been identified as rare causes of obesity; some subjects have red hair, the counterpart of the yellow fur in the A^y mouse.

Other genetic obesity syndromes in rodents were soon to cast new light on the regulation of energy balance. Notable were the *ob/ob* (obese) and *db/db* (diabetes) mice, and the *fa/fa* (fatty) Zucker rat (Chapter 6). These mutants had been identified during the 1950s and 1960s as autosomal recessive traits that conferred hyperphagia and obesity. The causes were unknown, but meticulous cross-circulation 'parabiosis' studies by Coleman during the 1970s suggested that the *ob/ob* syndrome was due to deficiency of an appetite-suppressing hormone, whereas the *db* mutation apparently disabled the receptor that normally recognized this hormone (Coleman, 1973) (Figure 1.14). The hypothetical appetite-suppressing hormone would function as an 'adipostat', whose existence had previously been postulated by Kennedy (1953) to explain how eating and energy expenditure were modulated

Diabetologia 9, 294—298 (1973)
© by Springer-Verlag 1973

Effects of Parabiosis of Obese with Diabetes and Normal Mice*

D.L. Coleman

The Jackson Laboratory** Bar Harbor, Maine 04609, USA

Received: March 1, 1973, accepted: April 10, 1973

Summary. Parabiosis of obese (*ob/ob*) with diabetes (*db²ᴶ/db²ᴶ*) mice caused the obese partner to become hypoglycemic, to lose weight and to die of starvation, while no abnormal changes were observed in the diabetes partner. The striking similarity of this response to that observed in normal mice in parabiosis with diabetes mice suggests that obese mice are like normal mice in having normal satiety centers sensitive to the satiety factor produced by the diabetes partner. In contrast, parabiosis of obese with normal mice is a fully viable combination suggesting that the obese partner does not produce sufficient satiety factor to turn off the normal partner's eating drive. However, obese mice in parabiosis with normal mice gain weight less rapidly and eat less than obese mice in parabiosis with obese mice. These observations suggest that some humoral factor is provided by the normal partner that regulates food consumption in the obese partner. To explain the identical obese-hyperglycemic syndromes produced by these two unrelated and separate genes when on identical genetic backgrounds, it is postulated that the obese mouse is unable to produce sufficient satiety factor to regulate its food consumption, whereas the diabetes mouse produces satiety factor, but cannot respond to it because of a defective satiety center.

Key words: Parabiosis, obese mice, diabetes mice, satiety factor, satiety center.

Figure 1.14 The paper by Coleman (1973), in which he concluded from cross-circulation (parabiosis) experiments that obesity in the obese (*ob/ob*) mouse was due to absence of an endogenous satiety factor, whereas that in the diabetes (*db/db*) mouse was caused by failure of the satiety factor to exert its normal action. Reproduced courtesy of the editor of *Diabetologia*.

appropriately under conditions of under- or over-nutrition so as to keep fat mass constant.

An important breakthrough in obesity research was the discovery by Jeffrey Friedman's team in 1994 of the *ob* gene by positional cloning, and the characterization of its protein product (Zhang *et al.*, 1994) (Figure 1.15). This cytokine-like protein, which Friedman named 'leptin' (from the Greek leptos, meaning 'thin'), was secreted by adipocytes and circulated at concentrations proportional to total fat mass. Leptin was found to act in the hypothalamus to inhibit feeding and cause weight loss and therefore fulfilled the criteria for an adipostat, by signalling adiposity to the brain and effecting appropriate responses to maintain a constant fat mass. Hyperphagia and obesity were explained in the *ob/ob* mouse by the *ob* mutation deleting bioactive leptin, whereas the *db/db* and *fa/fa* syndromes were subsequently shown to be due to various mutations affecting the leptin receptor.

Very rare cases of human obesity are due to mutations of leptin or its receptors, causing a striking phenotype of severe hyperphagia and morbid obesity that develops in early childhood. The first case, who subsequently showed a dramatic response to treatment with recombinant human leptin, was reported by Stephen O'Rahilly's group in Cambridge

(Montague *et al.*, 1997). However, the vast majority of obese people have raised leptin concentrations, roughly in proportion to their increased fat mass, suggesting that leptin is

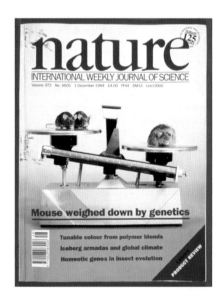

Figure 1.15 Cover of the issue of *Nature* that contained the paper by Friedman's group reporting their discovery of leptin (Zhang *et al.*, 1994). Reproduced by kind permission of the editor of *Nature*.

irrelevant to human energy balance as long as basal levels are present.

Research into the genetic susceptibility to 'common' human obesity has also benefited from advances in molecular genetics. Earlier observational and epidemiological studies included those of Charles Davenport in 1923 on the inheritance of BMI in families, and the work of Verscheuer in the 1920s, Newman *et al.* in the 1930s and Stunkard *et al.* in the 1980s on identical twins raised together or separately, with the aim of determining the contribution of genetic versus environmental factors. Studies by Claude Bouchard and others have suggested that genetic susceptibility is determined by multiple genes that individually have only minor effects. A large and growing number of candidate genes have been explored and several have been shown to make a significant but limited contribution.

Treatment of obesity

Restricting food intake and increasing physical activity have been the main stays of managing obesity since antiquity. Many dietary regimes have been tried, ranging from total starvation to unlimited quantities of various foods. Success has generally been limited, and only achieved if a significant fall in energy intake can be sustained in the long term.

Numerous drugs have been used in an attempt to treat obesity, mostly acting by reducing appetite. During the eighteenth century, and perhaps following the lead of Flemyng (see above), various laxatives were employed, sometimes together with hydrotherapy. In the 1890s, the newly-discovered thyroid extract was given to treat obesity in euthyroid subjects, although inappropriate and potentially dangerous thyroid hormones were still being used in this context until recently. The notion of stimulating an underactive endocrine system has been repeatedly invoked, ranging from various proprietary drugs (see Figure 1.16) to the more recent use of human growth hormone and human chorionic gonadotrophin.

In the late nineteenth century, the synthetic organic chemistry industry yielded various compounds with weight-reducing properties such as derivatives of aniline, which was used to make dyes for fabrics. One such product was dinitrophenol, which was found to induce marked weight loss in workers who handled

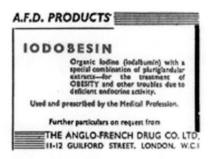

Figure 1.16 Advertisement in medical journals from the 1950s, for a product that was supposed to induce weight loss by stimulating endocrine function.

the compound; much later, the mechanism was shown to be an uncoupling of oxidative phosphorylation to produce heat instead of ATP, mimicking the action of UCP-1 in brown fat. Dinitrophenol was used to treat obesity during the 1930s, but was abandoned when it was shown to cause cataracts and peripheral neuropathy. This early therapeutic tragedy emphasizes the need for careful evaluation of the efficacy and safety of new drugs before their introduction into clinical practice.

Another early product of the organic chemical industry was D-amphetamine, synthesized in 1887. It was used during the 1930s as a stimulant to treat narcolepsy, when it was found to induce weight loss. Amphetamine was approved in the USA for the treatment of obesity in 1947, but was soon shown to be addictive, and its use declined markedly during the 1970s. Phentermine and diethylpropion, structurally related to amphetamine, were introduced into clinical practice during the 1950s and were widely promoted (see Chapter 17). All these drugs are sympathomimetic agents that enhance the action of noradrenaline in the CNS and thus reduce appetite. Another structurally-related compound, fenfluramine – which increases the release of the anorectic neurotransmitter, serotonin – was also shown to reduce appetite and weight. Fenfluramine and its dextroisomer, D-fenfluramine, were prescribed widely during the 1980s and 1990s, sometimes given together with phentermine. Fenfluramine was withdrawn in 1997 when it was shown that, it caused cardiac valvular disease and primary pulmonary hypertension – which had previously been recognized as a rare complication of anti-obesity drugs.

Other drugs that have been used to treat obesity, often without a specific licence, have included phenylpropanolamine and ephedrine (both sympathomimetic agents), the latter in combination with caffeine. Phenylpropanolamine was withdrawn because it was shown to cause stroke, and the safety and efficacy of ephedrine/caffeine remains uncertain. Various compounds designed to stimulate thermogenesis have been developed, and many have shown promising properties in animals. During the 1980s and 1990s, there was much interest in agonists at the β_3-adrenoceptor, responsible for activating heat production in brown fat and other thermogenic tissues including skeletal muscle. These compounds proved highly effective and relatively selective in animals, but because of differences between the rodent and human β_3-adrenoceptor proved to be ineffective or plagued by sympathetic side effects when tried in humans.

The three anti-obesity drugs in current use are described in Chapter 17. These are sibutramine, an inhibitor of the neuronal reuptake of serotonin and noradrenaline, which was found to induce weight loss in rodents when tested as an antidepressant; orlistat, an inhibitor of the gastrointestinal lipases that hydrolyse dietary triglyceride, thus decreasing lipid absorption; and rimonabant, an antagonist at the cannabinoid CB-1 receptor that mediates the orexigenic effects of the endocannabinoids.

A brief trawl of Internet sites will reveal the huge range of substances being sold as treatments for obesity. These include amphetamines and other compounds that have been withdrawn because of safety concerns; herbal, homeopathic and traditional remedies with no hard evidence of efficacy; diuretics and laxatives; and powerful endocrine agents such as anabolic steroids. The main motivation would appear to be cosmetic rather than health-related.

Bariatric (weight-reducing) surgery began in the mid-1950s with the Norwegian surgeon Hendrikson, who removed much of the small bowel to reduce nutrient absorption. This irreversible operation caused intractable losses of nutrients and electrolytes and was replaced in the 1950s by the jejuno-ileal bypass operation developed by Payne and DeWind and others. The jejuno-ileal bypass causes major side effects, notably the 'blind-loop' syndrome, and is now little performed. As described in Chapter 18, gastric bypass operation (developed during the 1980s by Edward Mason in Iowa) and various forms of

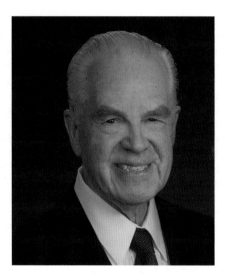

Figure 1.17 Edward E. Mason (born 1912), American bariatric surgeon. Image reproduced courtesy of Mervyn Deitel MD, past President of the American Society for Metabolic and Bariatric Surgery.

gastroplasty (initiated by Mason in the 1970s) have now become popular (Figure 1.17). Recent innovations include the sleeve gastrectomy, gastric banding using an inflatable implanted band whose tension can be varied by injecting saline into a subcutaneously-buried port, and the adaptation of many bariatric techniques to be performed laparascopically. In striking contrast to the poor outcomes of the early bariatric procedures, those in current use have proved effective, and the substantial weight loss that results can often improve or even reverse established type 2 diabetes. Modern bariatric procedures also have low rates of morbidity and mortality.

Numerous other forms of treatment for obesity have been attempted. One notable example was the use, for a brief period during the 1960s, of stereotactic lesioning of the lateral hypothalamus in an attempt to mimic the hypophagia and weight loss induced in rodents by this procedure. This approach was soon abandoned because of poor outcomes and anxieties about its safety.

Growth of the scientific community

It was not until the 1960s that concerted attempts were made to bring together those interested in the science and clinical management of obesity. An early initiative, following the example of the long-established specialist societies in diabetes, endocrinology and other disciplines, was the formation of various national associations to promote research into obesity. The first, the Association for the Study of Obesity (ASO) in the UK, held its inaugural meeting in London in 1968. This was followed in 1973 by an American conference organized by the National Institutes of Health, in recognition of the important health problems posed by obesity, and in 1974 by the first International Congress on Obesity (ICO) in London. The North American Association for the Study of Obesity (NAASO) first met at Poughkeepsie, New York, in 1982, and the International Association for the Study of Obesity (IASO) was formed in 1986 under the leadership of Barbara Hansen.

Following the first ICO, it was clear that a specialist journal devoted to obesity was required, and the *International Journal of Obesity* began publication in 1976 under the joint editorship of Alan Howard and George Bray. Other journals have followed: *Obesity Surgery* in 1991, and *Obesity Research* (now renamed *Obesity*), published by NAASO, in 1993.

References

Anne Scott Beller, A. (1977) *Fat and Thin: A Natural History of Obesity*, Farrar, Straus, and Giroux, New York.

Boss, O., Samec, S., Paoloni-Giacobino, A. *et al.* (1977) Uncoupling protein-3: a new member of the mitochondrial carrier family with tissue-specific expression. *FEBS Letters*, **408**, 39–42.

Bray, G. (2007a) *The Battle of the Bulge*, Dorrance Publishing, Pittsburgh, PA.

Bray, G. (2007b) *Obesity and the Metabolic Syndrome*, Humana Press, Totowa, NJ.

Bultman, S.J., Michaud, E.J., Woychik, R.P. (1992) Molecular characterization of the mouse agouti locus. Cell, **71** (7), 1195–1204.

Cannon, B., Hedin, A. and Nedergaard, J. (1982) Exclusive occurrence of thermogenin antigen in brown adipose tissue. *FEBS Letters*, **150**, 129–32.

Coleman, D.L. (1973) Effects of parabiosis of obese with diabetes and normal mice. *Diabetologia*, **9**, 294–8.

Darby, W.J., Ghalioungui, P. and Grevetti, L. (1977) *Food: the Gift of Osiris*, Academic Press, London, p. 60.

Fawcett, D.W. and Jones, I.C. (1949) The effects of hypophysectomy, adrenalectomy and of thiouracil feeding on the cytology of brown adipose tissue. *Endocrinology*, **45**, 609–21.

Flemyng, M. (1760) *A Discourse on the Nature, Causes and Cure of Corpulency*, L Davis and C Reymers, London.

Fleury, C., Neverova, M., Collins, S. *et al.* (1997) Uncoupling protein-2: a novel gene linked to obesity and hyperinsulinemia. *Nature Genetics*, **15**, 269–72.

Fröhlich, A. (1901) Ein Fall von Tumor der Hypophysis cerebri ohne Akromegalie. *Wiener Klinische Rundschau*, **75**, 883–86 and 906–8.

Gibbs, J., Young, R.C. and Smith, G.P. (1973) Cholecystokinin elicits satiety in rats with open gastric fistulas. *Nature*, **245**, 323–5.

Hassall, A. (1849) Observations on the development of the fat vesicle. Lancet, **1**, 63–4.

Himsworth, H.P. (1936) Diabetes mellitus: its differentiation into insulin-sensitive and insulin-insensitive types. *Lancet*, **i**, 127–30.

Hoggan, G. and Hoggan, F.E. (1879) On the development and retrogression of the fat cell. *Journal of the Royal Microscopical Society*, **2**, 353.

Kennedy, G.C. (1953) The role of depot fat in the hypothalamic control of food intake in the rat. *Proceedings of the Royal Society of London. Series B, Biological Sciences*, **140**, 578–92.

Kryger, M.H. (1983) Sleep apnea. From the needles of Dionysius to continuous positive airway pressure. *Archives of Internal Medicine*, **143**, 2301–3.

Kylin, E. (1923) Studien über das hypertonie-hyperglykemie-hyperurikemie syndrom. *Zentralblatt für Innere Medizin*, **44**, 105–12.

Littré, E. (1839) *Hippocrates. Oeuvres Complètes d'Hippocrate. Traduction nouvelle avec le texte grec*, JB Baillière, Paris.

Montague, C.T., Farooqi, I.S., Whitehead, J.P. *et al.* (1997) Congenital leptin deficiency is associated with severe early-onset obesity in humans. *Nature*, **307**, 903–9.

Neel, J.V. (1962) Diabetes mellitus: a thrifty genotype rendered detrimental by 'progress'? *American Journal of Human Genetics*, **14**, 353–62.

Prentice, A.M., Rayco-Solon, P. and Moore, S.E. (2005) Insights from the developing world: thrifty genotypes and thrifty phenotypes. *Proceedings of the Nutrition Society*, **64**, 153–61.

Randle, P.J., Garland, P.B., Hales, C.N., Newsholme, E.A. (1963) The glucose fatty-acid cycle. Its role in insulin sensitivity and the metabolic disturbances of diabetes mellitus. Lancet, **1** (7285), 785–9.

Reeves, C. (1992) *Egyptian Medicine*, Shire Publications, London.

Ricquier, D., Barlet, J.P., Garel, J.M. *et al.* (1983) An immunological study of the uncoupling protein of brown adipose tissue mitochondria. *The Biochemical Journal*, **210**, 859–66.

Short, T. (1727) *A Discourse Concerning the Causes and Effects of Corpulency Together with the Method for Its Prevention and Cure*, J. Robert, London.

Stellar, E. (1954) The physiology of motivation. *Psychological Review*, **61**, 5–22.

Vague, J. (1947) La differenciation sexuelle facteur determinant des formes de l'obésité. Presse Medicale. **55**, 339–40.

Vidal-Puig, A., Solanes, G., Grujic, D. *et al.* (1997) UCP3: an uncoupling protein homologue expressed preferentially and abundantly in skeletal muscle and brown adipose tissue. *Biochemical and Biophysical Research Communications*, **235**, 79–82.

Wadd, W. (1829) *Comments on Corpulency, Lineaments of Leanness: Mems On Diet and Dietetics*, John Ebers, London.

Zhang, Y., Proenca, R., Maffei, M. *et al.* (1994) Positional cloning of the mouse *obese* gene and its human homologue. *Nature*, **372**, 425–32.

Epidemiology and Social Impact of Obesity

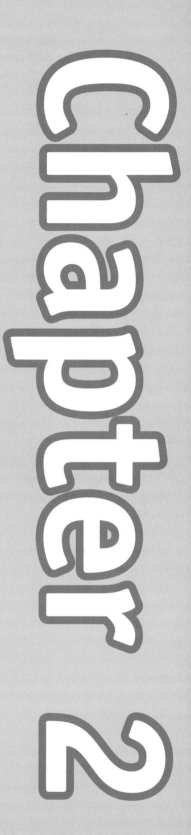

Key points

- In 2005, 800 million people were overweight (BMI 25.0–29.9 kg/m^2) and 400 million were obese (BMI $\geq$30 kg/m^2). Obesity is most prevalent in westernized countries (with up to one-third of adults affected), but is increasing in the developing world, especially in urban populations. The highest prevalence worldwide is 80%, among certain Pacific Islanders.

- Most countries show progressive increases in the prevalences of overweight and obesity, including the USA, Europe (notably the UK), the Middle East and Asia. Obesity is less common in sub-Saharan Africa (except for South Africa) and is increasingly prevalent among urban populations in India and especially China.

- Childhood obesity is already common in westernized countries and is rapidly increasing in the USA, Latin America, Europe, Middle East and affluent Asian populations. In 2004, it was estimated that 10% of children worldwide were overweight and that 2–3% were obese.

- Factors contributing to the global spread of obesity include the westernized lifestyle, with increased energy intake and declining levels of physical activity. Overall, socio-economic status and educational status are inversely related to the prevalence of obesity, but the relationship is complex.

- It is predicted that, by 2015, 1.6 billion people will be overweight including 700 million obese. The greatest increases are forecast in the USA (with 75% of adults overweight or obese), South America, Europe, Central Asia and the Pacific Rim. The combined prevalence of overweight and obesity among children could exceed 40% in the Americas, Middle East and North Africa.

- Obesity predisposes to type 2 diabetes, cardiovascular disease, some cancers and numerous other disorders, including osteoarthritis. It is thought to account for almost 60% of the risk for developing type 2 diabetes, over 20% of that for hypertension and coronary-heart disease, and between 10% and 30% for various cancers.

- Markers of central obesity are more robust indices of obesity-associated health risk than BMI. In Caucasians, a waist circumference of $\geq$94 cm in men or $\geq$80 cm in women indicates increased risk, while values of $\geq$102 cm (men) and $\geq$88 cm (women) indicate substantially increased risk.

- Relationships between obesity and health risks vary between populations, with Asians being more susceptible. Accordingly, BMI risk thresholds are lower than in other populations, with an action point for overweight defined at 23 kg/m^2.

- In 2000, obesity was estimated to cause 2.5 million deaths and over 30 million disability-adjusted life years (DALYs), mainly due to ischaemic heart disease and diabetes. In England, obesity is estimated to shorten life on average by 9 years.

- The costs related to obesity account for 6% of direct health expenditure in Europe and >1% of the gross domestic product (GDP) in many countries. The psychological and social costs of obesity to individuals and society are also considerable.

- The obesity pandemic is driving up the prevalence of type 2 diabetes, and is likely to render the forecast of 366 million cases by 2030 an underestimate. Increases in the prevalences of cardiovascular disease and several cancers are similarly anticipated.

Chapter 2 **Epidemiology and Social Impact of Obesity**

Neville Rigby, Rachel Leach, Tim Lobstein, Rachel Huxley, and Shiriki Kumanyika

The global epidemic of obesity is now recognized as one of the most important public health problems facing the world today. Epidemiological surveys from many countries show that the mean weight of the population is increasing and that the prevalences of clinically-significant overweight and obesity are rising rapidly in adults and, of particular concern, in children and adolescents. Up to one-third of the adults in some westernized countries are obese and over two-thirds in certain smaller populations such as Pacific Islanders; very few countries remain unaffected by obesity (WHO/NUT/NCD, 2000).

The World Health Organization (WHO) has estimated that 200 million people worldwide were obese in 1995, rising to 300 million in 2000 (WHO, 2007). Revised estimates suggest that 400 million people aged ≥15 years were obese in 2005, with almost 800 million overweight (BMI 25.0–29.9 kg/m²). By 2015, the WHO predicts that these numbers will increase to 2.3 billion overweight and 700 million obese (WHO, 2006a) (see Figure 2.1).

Obesity is a major risk factor for several common and important diseases, notably type 2 diabetes, cardiovascular disease and certain cancers and is thought to contribute to many more (see Chapters 9–13). It also inflicts large direct and indirect costs that drain healthcare and social resources. Overall it is an important cause of morbidity, disability and premature death (WHO, 2004).

This chapter reviews the epidemiological data defining the prevalence and spread of obesity across the world, including evidence that has led to the revision of criteria for obesity in certain populations who are particularly susceptible to its comorbidities. The impact on children and future projections of the obesity pandemic is also discussed, as well as the social and financial impact of the disease.

Definitions of obesity

Most epidemiological surveys have used the BMI thresholds proposed by WHO expert reports (WHO/NUT/NCD, 2000; WHO Expert Committee, 1997). As originally stated, a BMI of 25.0–29.9 kg/m² represented pre-obesity, with BMI >30 kg/m² defining obesity; the 'overweight' cut-off of a BMI exceeding 25 kg/m² covered all categories of overweight, including obesity. However, the term 'overweight' is commonly used to refer to a BMI in the range 25–29.9 kg/m² alone, and this convention is followed throughout this book (Table 2.1).

Across populations, BMI is closely associated with whole-body adiposity, and the cut-off levels for overweight and obesity reflect the increasing risk of metabolic, cardiovascular and other complications of obesity as BMI increases above an optimal range of 21–23 kg/m² – which remains the recommended median goal for adult Caucasian populations (WHO/NUT/NCD, 2000). These thresholds also provide convenient benchmarks for public health actions, proportionate to the degree of risk (see Chapter 22).

However, some important caveats qualify the common use of BMI to predict risk and define obesity. For instance, the distribution and content of body fat are crucial determinants of some important obesity-associated risks. Visceral and especially abdominal fat are strongly associated with type 2 diabetes and cardiovascular disease, and indeed more significantly

Obesity: Science to Practice Edited by Gareth Williams and Gema Frühbeck
© 2009 John Wiley & Sons, Ltd

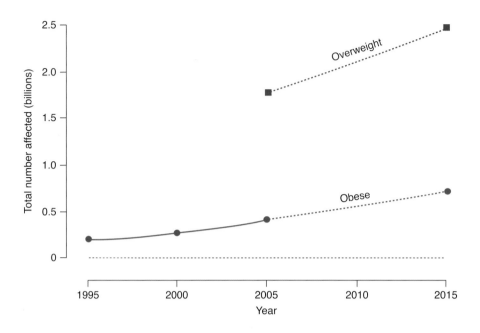

Figure 2.1 Worldwide prevalences of obesity and overweight up to 2005, with predictions up to 2015. Global data for overweight were not available before 2005. From (WHO, 2004).

Table 2.1   The World Health Organization (WHO) international classification according to body mass index.

	Body Mass Index (kg/m²)	
Classification	**Principal cut-off points**	**Additional cut-off points**
Underweight	<18.50	<18.50
• Severe thinness	<16.00	<16.00
• Moderate thinness	16.00–16.99	16.00–16.99
• Mild thinness	17.00–18.49	17.00–18.49
Normal range	18.50–24.99	18.50–22.99
		23.00–24.99
Overweight	≥25.00	≥25.00
• Pre-obese	25.00–29.99	25.00–27.49
		27.50–29.99
Obese	≥30.00	≥30.00
• Obese class I	30.00–34.99	30.00–32.49
		32.50–34.99
• Obese class II	35.00–39.99	35.00–37.49
		37.50–39.99
• Obese class III	≥40.00	>40

Source: WHO web site (http://www.who.int/bmi).

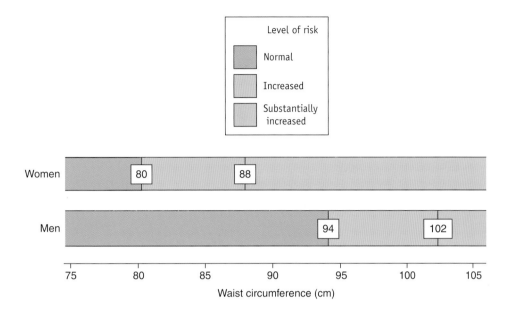

Figure 2.2 Stratification of obesity-associated health risk according to waist circumference, in men and women. Note that thresholds may be lower in Asian populations.

than BMI (see Chapters 9 and 12). Accordingly, markers of central obesity, such as waist:hip ratio and waist circumference, provide more robust indices of overall obesity-related risk than BMI alone. In Caucasians, a waist:hip ratio of >1.0 in men and >0.85 in women is considered to indicate clinically significant abdominal obesity, while the simpler measurement of waist circumference is correlated with intra-abdominal fat mass and reflects metabolic and cardiovascular risk. In Caucasian populations, a waist circumference of ≥94 cm in men or ≥80 cm in women indicates increased risk, while values of ≥102 and ≥88 cm, respectively, indicate substantially increased risk (see Figure 2.2). A recent proposal, taking greater account of the risk of diabetes, has suggested that the thresholds for substantially increased risk should be reduced to 99 cm in men and 85 cm in women (Huxley *et al.*, 2008).

In addition, the relationships between risk and adiposity – whether measured as BMI or waist circumference – vary among certain populations and ethnic groups, because they have differing susceptibilities to the complications of obesity. For example, Asians are at greater risk of type 2 diabetes and cardiovascular disease when compared with Caucasians at equivalent BMI values. The reasons

are not fully understood, but may relate partly to the relatively higher body fat content of Asian subjects across all levels of BMI (James, Chunming and Inoue, 2002; WHO/IASO/IOTF, 2000; see Chapter 9). Accordingly, a WHO expert group (WHO Expert Consultation, 2004) recommended that the BMI threshold for risk in Asian populations should be lowered to 23 kg/m². It has also been suggested that the waist circumference thresholds for substantially increased risk should be lower than in Caucasians, namely 80 cm in women and 85 cm in men (Huxley *et al.*, 2008). The WHO intends to review waist circumference data before making further formal recommendations.

It should be noted that current WHO estimates of global prevalence rates of obesity, and of obesity-related morbidity and mortality, are based on the conventional BMI thresholds. This may underestimate the total burden of obesity because it neglects the impact on Asian populations who are susceptible to risk, but whose BMI falls below the Caucasian-derived thresholds. As Asians contribute 60% of the world's total population (6.5 billion), this underestimate is potentially significant. The additional cut-off levels proposed for BMI (Table 2.1) will enable consistent reporting and facilitate international comparisons, thus producing clearer pictures of both the prevalence of overweight and obesity and their impacts on health across the world.

Difficulties in estimating obesity prevalence

Some surveys yield less robust results because they are based on subjective rather than objective data. In particular, self-reported data on height and weight – used in several influential reports – have been shown by systematic analyses to underestimate the prevalence of overweight and obesity. This is because respondents tend to over-report their own height and underestimate weight, to an extent that varies considerably between different ethnic and age groups (Connor Gorber et al., 2007; Gillum and Sempos, 2005). The unreliability of self-reported data is clearly shown

Table 2.2   Reported prevalences of overweight and obesity in the European Union.

Country	Year of data collection	Males			Females		
		% BMI 25–29.9	%BMI ≥30	Total BMI ≥25	% BMI 25–29.9	%BMI ≥30	Total BMI >25
Austria	2005/2006	42.3	23.3	65.6	32.4	20.8	53.2
Belgium	1994–1997	49	14	63	28	13	41
Cyprus	1999–2000	46	26.6	72.6	34.3	23.7	58
Czech Republic	1997/1998	48.5	24.7	73.2	31.4	26.2	57.6
Denmark	*2001*	*40.1*	*11.8*	*51.9*	*26.9*	*12.5*	*39.4*
England	2005	43.4	23.1	66.5	32.1	24.3	56.4
Estonia	*2004*	*32*	*13.7*	*45.7*	*28.4*	*14.4*	*42.8*
Finland	1997	48	19.8	67.8	33	19.4	52.4
France	*2006*	*35.6*	*11.8*	*47.4*	*23.3*	*13*	*36.3*
Germany	*2002/2003*	*52.9*	*22.5*	*75.4*	*35.6*	*23.3*	*58.9*
Greece (ATTICA)	2001/2002	53	20	73	31	15	46
Hungary	1992–1994	41.9	21	62.9	27.9	21.2	49.1
Ireland	1997–1999	46.3	20.1	66.4	32.5	15.9	48.4
Italy	2003	42.1	9.3	51.4	25.8	8.7	34.5
Latvia	1997	41	9.5	50.5	33	17.4	50.4
Lithuania	*2002*	*41.2*	*16.4*	*57.6*	*26.6*	*15.8*	*42.4*
Luxembourg	N.A.	45.6	15.3	60.9	30.7	13.9	44.6
Malta	*2003*	*46.5*	*22.9*	*69.4*	*34.3*	*16.9*	*51.2*
Netherlands	1998–2002	43.5	10.4	53.9	28.5	10.1	38.6
Poland	2000	41	15.4	56.4	28.7	18.9	47.6
Portugal	2003/2004	44.1	14.5	58.6	31.9	14.6	46.5
Slovakia	*1992–1999*	*49.7*	*19.3*	*69*	*32.1*	*18.9*	*51*
Slovenia	*2001*	*50*	*16.5*	*66.5*	*30.9*	*13.8*	*44.7*
Spain	1990–2000	45	13.4	58.4	32.2	15.8	48
Sweden (Göteborg)	2002	43.5	14.8	58.3	26.6	11	37.6

Age range and year of data in surveys may differ. With the limited data available, prevalences are not age-standardized. Self reported surveys (italicized) may underestimate true prevalence. © International Association for the Study of Obesity/International Obesity TaskForce London – May 2007. See www.iotf.org/database/.

by two studies, both conducted by the US Centers for Disease Control and Prevention (CDC). The annual Behavioral Risk Factor Surveillance System (BRFSS), which uses self-reported data from telephone interviews, estimated the prevalence of obesity among adult Americans in 2006 to be 25% (Yun *et al.*, 2006). By contrast, the more rigorous National Health and Nutrition Examination Survey (NHANES) reported that 33% of American men and 35% of women were obese in 2003–2004 (National Health and Nutrition Examination Survey, 2003). (NHANES examines a stratified probability sample of the population, who are interviewed and examined in a standardized fashion by trained staff.) It is clearly important for decision-makers to use accurate data when setting priorities and allocating resources in healthcare (Connor Gorber *et al.*, 2007).

Another problem is the time taken to collect and process data. Some reports are based on information that may be years out of date – a potentially important consideration when the incidence of obesity is rising so rapidly.

Across European countries, surveys of adult overweight and obesity are inconsistent in their timing, sample size and methodology, with several countries relying heavily on self-reported data (see Table 2.2). The International Obesity Task Force (IOTF) has highlighted the need for rigorous and systematic surveillance of obesity throughout Europe, including robust measurements of height, weight and waist circumference (International Obesity Task Force, 2005). As a result, the European Commission has established the European Health Interview Survey (EHIS) to standardize the collection of self-reported data on height, weight, physical activity and consumption of fruit and vegetables. This will be followed in 2010 by the European Health Examination Survey (EHES), introducing objective measures of height, weight, blood pressure and cholesterol in a randomly-sampled population (European Commission, 2007).

Current and recent prevalences of obesity

Worldwide, obesity is common and rapidly increasing. Prevalences among adults in developed Western countries are up to 30%, while the highest prevalence worldwide is currently 80%,

among some Pacific Islanders (WHO, 2007). The rising prevalence of obesity among children and adolescents is discussed separately below.

The global distribution of obesity (BMI >30 kg/m^2) among men and women in 2005 is shown in Figures 2.3 and 2.4. Figure 2.5 shows the increasing prevalence of overweight (BMI ≥25 kg/m^2) among adults in the US over the last 10 years.

Europe

Data (based on BMI criteria) from member states within Europe are regularly updated on the IOTF web site. Recent findings are presented in Table 2.2. As already noted, some countries rely primarily on self-reported data, which are likely to underestimate the prevalences of overweight and obesity. The reported prevalence of obesity varies widely, from <10% in men (Latvia and Italy) and women (Italy), to >20% in men (Austria, Cyprus, Czech Republic, England, Germany and Malta) and women (Austria, Cyprus, Czech Republic, England, Germany and Hungary).

In most European countries, the prevalence of obesity in adults has been increasing. This trend is well illustrated by the annual Health Survey for England, which provides comprehensive data on height, weight, BMI and WHR, as well as blood pressure, smoking and alcohol use, fruit and vegetable consumption and physical activity levels. Between 1993 and 2006, the prevalence of obesity rose in men from 13% to 24.9% and in women from 16% to 25.2%, with morbid obesity (BMI >40 kg/m^2) in women increasing from 1.4% to 2.7% (Department of Health, 2006a). Concurrently, the proportion of normal-weight adults fell to 32% of men and 42% in women. Obesity is predicted to continue rising, affecting 33% of men and 28% of women by 2010, and the UK Government's Foresight Report, *Tackling Obesities: Future Choices*, published in October 2007, suggests that 60% of men and 50% of women in England will be obese by 2050 (Department of Health, 2006b).

North America

Data from NHANES show that obesity, including morbid levels, is very common in adult Americans, and that the prevalence in men

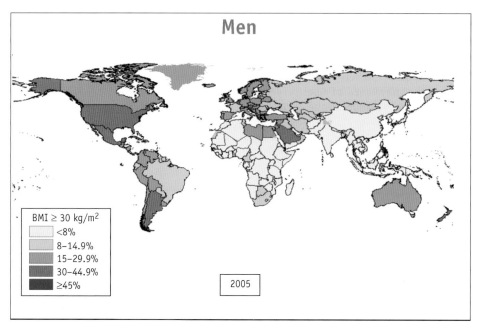

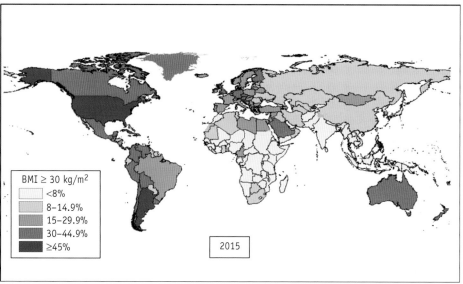

Figure 2.3 Global prevalence of obesity in men in 2005 showing the percentage of adults with BMI $\geq$30 kg/m^2 in each country (upper panel). Data are age-standardized to WHO world population. Predicted prevalences in 2015 are shown in the lower panel. Maps available at www.who.int/globalatlas. Reproduced with kind permission of the WHO.

continues to rise (Ogden *et al.*, 2006). Between 1999 and 2000 and 2003–2004, the prevalence among men rose from 28% to 31%, but appeared stable at 33% among women. The frequency of morbid obesity (BMI >40 kg/m^2) has risen steadily in both genders, reaching 2.8% in men and 6.9% in women in 2003–2004. The relentless and accelerating spread of obesity across America in recent years is shown graphically in Figure 2.5.

The NHANES data also provide vivid comparisons between genders and ethnic and

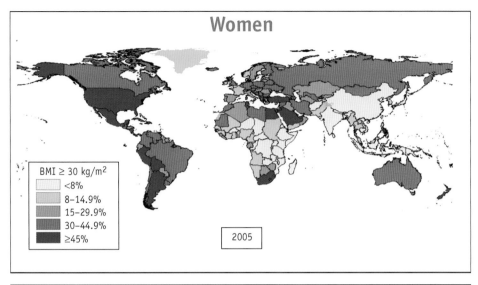

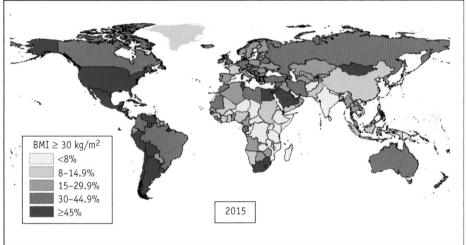

Figure 2.4 Global prevalence of obesity in women in 2005, showing the percentage of adults with BMI ≥30kg/m² in each country (upper panel). Data are age-standardized to WHO world population. Predicted prevalences in 2015 are shown in the lower panel. Maps available at www.who.int/globalatlas. Reproduced with kind permission of the WHO.

age groups in the USA. In 2003–2004, about 30% of non-Hispanic white adults, 37% of Mexican Americans and 45% of non-Hispanic black adults were obese. Across all groups, the middle-aged showed the highest prevalences, with obesity affecting 29% of subjects aged 20–39 years, 37% of those aged 40–59 years and 31% among those aged ≥60 years (Ogden *et al.*, 2006). Closer analysis reveals further influences of age and gender. The highest prevalence was among Black American women

aged 40–59 years, with 30% overweight, 58% obese and 17% with BMI ≥40kg/m². Mexican American women aged 40–59 years were also severely affected: prevalences of overweight, obesity and BMI ≥40kg/m² were 31, 48 and 8%, respectively. As discussed below and in Chapters 9 and 12, the high prevalences of obesity have variable relationships with susceptibility to the metabolic and cardiovascular complications of obesity in these different populations.

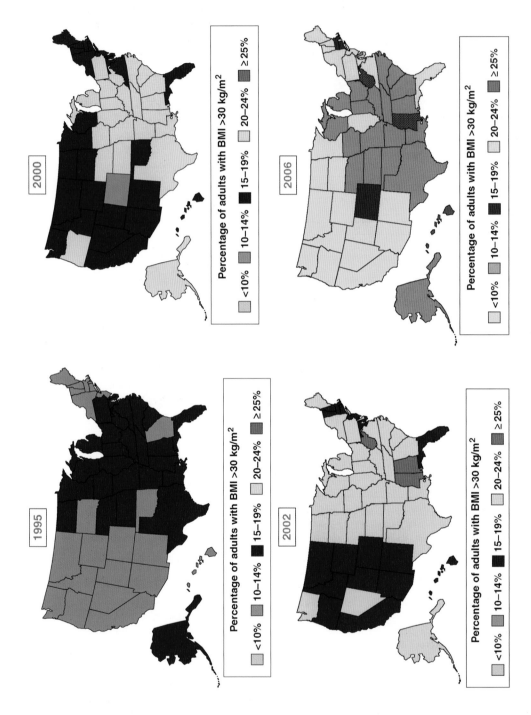

Figure 2.5 Spread of overweight/obesity across the USA between 1995 and 2006. Each panel shows the percentage of adults with BMI $>25\,kg/m^2$ in each state. A more extensive series of images is available at (www.cdc.gov). Reproduced with kind permission of the US Centers for Disease Control and Prevention.

Percentage of adults with BMI $>30\,kg/m^2$

<10%   10–14%   15–19%   20–24%   ≥25%

Middle East

These countries show generally increasing levels of obesity, but with marked variations, especially between rural and urban populations. In Iran, adults in Teheran City aged ≥20 years show high prevalences of overweight (43% in men, 38% in women) and obesity (14% in men, 30% in women) that are comparable with many Western countries (Azizi, 2001). By contrast, prevalences are much lower in rural areas of Iran, where only 17% of men aged <40 years are overweight or obese (Ghaseemi *et al.*, 2002). In adults from Bahrain aged 30–79 years, prevalences of overweight and obesity are 35% and 21%, respectively, for men and 31% and 40% for women (Musaiger and Al-Mannai, 2001). In Egypt, urban dwellers showed prevalences of 40% overweight and 45% obesity among women, and of 45% overweight and 20% obesity among men; in rural areas, prevalences were 30% overweight and 21% obese for women, and 28% and 6%, respectively, among men (Galal, 2002). Data from the WHO Global InfoBase show that the prevalence of obesity has reached 26% in men and 40% in women in the United Arab Emirates, 28% in men and 30% in women in Kuwait, and 26% in men and 74% in women from Saudi Arabia (WHO Global Infobase, 2007).

Africa

Obesity is an emerging problem in this continent, alongside its long-established burdens of malnutrition and wasting conditions, HIV/AIDS and other chronic infections. Urbanization, with its associated obesogenic lifestyle factors, is spreading in many African countries; it is predicted that by 2025, half of Africa's total population will live in urban areas, where the number of people aged ≥60 years will double to 80 million.

The recent South Africa Demographic Health Survey reported that obesity affected almost 30% of women and 10% of men (Steyn *et al.*, 2006). A much more limited study in Gambia found a remarkably high prevalence of overweight among women aged 35–50 years, with 34% pre-obese and 50% obese – levels on a par with those in Black American women. Obesity rates were lower among younger women (aged 14–25 years), with only 10% overweight and 6% obese; 12% of men aged 35–80 were obese, but strikingly, no younger men examined were

obese (Siervo *et al.*, 2006). In Cameroon, urban women aged ≥15 years showed prevalences of overweight 29% and obesity 20%; corresponding values for men were 21% and 7%. Among females, obesity rates ranged from 12% for those aged <35 years to 41% in those aged 45–54 years, while men in these age categories showed prevalences of 13% and 16% (Kamadjeu *et al.*, 2006).

Asia and the Pacific

The prevalence of obesity, defined by conventional BMI thresholds, is relatively low in Asian countries, where typically <10% of adults have BMI >30 kg/m². However, this disguises a higher prevalence of visceral (central) obesity and the significantly higher total body fat content of Asian subjects, which confer higher risks of type 2 diabetes and cardiovascular disease at relatively low BMI thresholds.

China has adopted its own modified criteria defining overweight at BMI ≥24 and obesity at BMI ≥28 kg/m². The 2002 China National Nutrition and Health Survey showed that 200 million Chinese adults (23% of the total) were overweight, while 60 million (7%) were obese (Wu, 2006). Although overweight and obesity are also rising in rural areas, the main cause of China's rapidly increasing obesity epidemic is urbanization and particularly increased consumption of dietary fat.

The high frequency of central adiposity, even against a background of relatively low BMI, and its predisposition to type 2 diabetes and cardiovascular disease, is already having an adverse impact on health (Reddy *et al.*, 2002; Li *et al.*, 2002), and this will inevitably worsen. The prevalences of diabetes and other obesity-related comorbidities already match or even exceed those found in the West, and the prevalence of type 2 diabetes is forecast to double by 2030 (Lee *et al.*, in press; Wild *et al.*, 2004).

Causes of the rise in obesity

Various obesogenic factors contribute to the rising prevalence of obesity, operating to varying degrees with time and among populations (see Chapter 8). These range from declining levels of physical labour as populations move from rural to urban settings and abandon walking in favour of driving, to labour-saving devices in the home and the replacement of active sport and play by television and computer games. Also relevant in some populations is an increase in energy intake, or in energy density (particularly fat content) of food, although this can be difficult to ascertain from self-reported data (see Chapter 3). An example is in China, where nutritional surveys have shown that energy intake from animal sources increased threefold between 1982 and 2002, from 8 to 25% (Wu *et al.*, 2005). In rapidly expanding urban Chinese populations, dietary fat now accounts for 35% of total energy intake – above the recommended limit for Western populations.

Socio-economic and educational factors

Socio-economic status and educational status are inversely related to the prevalence of obesity in many populations, suggesting that they may also play a role. However, the relationship is complex, often differs between men and women, and depends on the general level of economic and nutritional development in the population (see Chapter 14).

One of the most comprehensive analyses of the association between obesity and educational status comes from the MONICA study. The WHO initiated this large cross-sectional survey in the late 1970s to measure 10-year trends in the major cardiovascular disease risk factors and the incidence of coronary heart disease and stroke (Molarius *et al.*, 2000). The results indicated a statistically significant, inverse correlation between educational attainment and BMI in males and almost all female populations, especially in Western countries. Interestingly, this pattern of a shifting burden of obesity towards the poor is emerging in several developing countries such as Brazil, where a 10% decrease in the prevalence of obesity has been reported among more affluent women, in contrast to a 26% increase among the least affluent women (Monteiro *et al.*, 2007).

A recent analysis of data from the Framingham Heart Study poses broader questions about the biological, ecological and social factors contributing to obesity (Christakis and Fowler, 2007). This study of the changing distribution of obesity within neighbourhoods suggests that obesity may spread through social networks in a striking pattern that is underpinned by social ties involving kinship and friendship (Figure 2.6). The

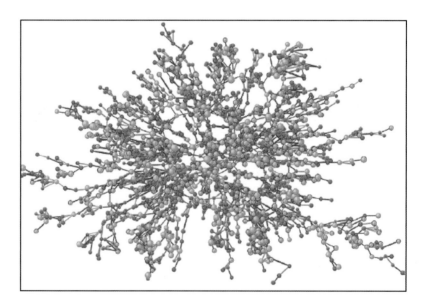

Figure 2.6 Distribution of obesity within a social network of over 2000 people in the Framingham Heart Study population. Each circle represents an individual. Blue and red borders respectively denote females and males, while a yellow fill indicates obesity (BMI >30 kg/m²; size proportional to BMI) and green a non-obese subject. Purple lines indicate non-genetic ties (friendship or marital) between individuals, and orange lines a familial tie. From Finkelstein, Fiebelkorn and Wang (2003), with kind permission of the editor of the *New England Journal of Medicine*. An animation showing the spread of obesity through the social networks with time can be downloaded at www.nejm.org.

associations identified were strong and, although not fully explained, indicate that shared social factors influence behaviours that presumably include food consumption and physical activity. This is an interesting new area for further exploration of both gene-environment interactions and the impact of social factors on obesogenic behaviours.

Childhood obesity

Defining obesity in children is not straightforward, mainly because of the need to account for their growth trajectories, but also because the early development of childhood overweight and obesity in some populations makes it difficult to identify a 'reference' population (see Chapter 21). As yet, there are only limited data on long-term outcomes for people who became obese in childhood, although becoming obese earlier in life clearly amplifies certain health risks, particularly for type 2 diabetes. Reliable data on outcomes are needed to improve the precision of anthropometric thresholds to predict the risk of comorbidities. Moreover, the differences in regional fat distribution, total fat body content, and ethnic variation need to be more fully explored in children.

Various measures and definitions of childhood obesity have been proposed, but none has been universally accepted – which greatly complicates the comparison and interpretation of national epidemiological data. They have included:

- BMI $\geq$95th centile for age, or BMI $>30\,kg/m^2$ (whichever is smaller), in individuals aged 2–18 years. Overweight is defined by a BMI lying between the 85th and 95th centiles. These criteria are used in the UK, adopting centiles derived from a reference population of children in 1990, established by Cole, Freeman and Preece (1995) (see Figure 21.1). They have also been recommended for use in the USA, to replace the previous terminology of 'at risk of overweight' and 'overweight' (American Medical Association, 2007).
- BMI >98th centile representing obesity, and BMI >91st centile for overweight (Scottish InterCollegiate Guidelines Network, 2003). Many practising clinicians appear to base judgements on these more stringent levels.
- BMI cut-off levels throughout childhood that, at age 18 years, match the WHO adult cut-offs that define overweight (BMI $\geq$25 kg/m²) and obesity (BMI $\geq$30 kg/m²) (see Figure 21.2).

These have been developed from several national data sets by an International Obesity Task Force group (Cole et al., 2000) and provide continuity with the adult population; they facilitate comparisons between different international surveys, but may underestimate the prevalence of obesity, especially in Asian populations.

- In 2006, WHO (2006b) published new anthropometric standards for pre-school children. These are based on a carefully selected reference population of 8440 children from 6 countries, with trained field staff to ensure consistent data collection. Because of concerns that formula feeds may over-nourish infants and alter their growth, the survey included only children who had been exclusively breast-fed for six months, and whose parents had received education about feeding and weaning. The results showed that healthy children receiving optimal nourishment grow remarkably similarly across different countries and environments. The published growth charts include indicators such as weight-for-age, length and height-for-age, weight-for-length ÷ height and BMI, all for children up to 18 years of age. Adoption of these criteria would probably increase substantially the detection rates of both under-nutrition and overweight in children.
- WHO Reference 2007 is a new standard for children from 6 to 19 years, proposed by a WHO expert group, and is complementary to the recommendations for children under 6 years of age (De Onis et al., 2007a; De Onis et al., 2007b). This defines growth curves throughout the age range, with overweight approximating to BMI $>25\,kg/m^2$ and obesity approximating to BMI $>30\,kg/m^2$ at the age of 19.

Current and recent prevalences of childhood obesity

Childhood obesity is already common, especially in westernized countries. In 2004, according to IOTF criteria, it was estimated that ~10% of children worldwide aged 5–17 years were overweight and that 2–3% were obese (Lobstein et al., 2004). Prevalence rates vary considerably between different regions and countries, from <5% in Africa and Asia to >20% in Europe and 30% in the Americas.

The prevalence of obesity continues to increase at an alarming rate in many parts of the world, including developing countries. Repeated surveys in most countries show a clear rise in the prevalence of obesity and overweight, in some instances increasing faster than in adults. Some examples are shown in Table 2.3 and Figure 2.7.

Table 2.3 Reported prevalence of overweight (including obesity) among children in selected countries, showing rises with time.

	Date of survey	Prevalence of overweight (%)[a]
Canada	1978–1999	14
	2004	29
USA	1971–1994	14
	1988–1994	25
	2003–2004	36
Brazil	1974	4
	1997	14
Chile	1987	13
	2000	27
England	1984	7
	1994	12
	2004	29
Iceland	1978	12
	1998	24
Netherlands	1980	5
	1996–1997	11
Spain	1980	13
	1995	19
	2000–2002	34
Russia	1992	15
	1998	9
China	1991	6 (urban 8)
	1997	8 (urban 12)
Japan	1976–1980	10
	1992–2000	19
Australia	1985	11
	1995	21
New Zealand	1989	13
	2000	30

[a]Overweight (includes obesity) defined by Cole-IOTF criteria.

Europe

Within Europe, the Southern region shows the highest prevalences of childhood overweight and obesity. Using IOTF criteria, 26% of boys and 19% of girls aged 6–17 years in northern Greece in 2000 were overweight or obese, as were 44% of 15-year old boys from Crete in 2004. A survey conducted in Spain in 2000 found that 35% of boys and 32% aged 13–14 years were overweight or obese, while in 2001, 36% of 9-year olds from central Italy were overweight, including 12% who were obese.

By contrast, Northern European countries – except for the UK – report generally lower prevalences. Overweight affected 18% of 10-year old Swedish children in 2000–2001, and only 10% of Dutch children aged 5–17 (of whom only 2% were obese) in 1997. England has strikingly higher rates: among children aged 2–15 years in 2006, 13.6% were overweight and 15.9% were obese. Russia reported a reduction in overweight between 1992 and 1995, reflecting severe economic difficulties. Otherwise, other North European countries are showing increases in prevalence, and many are predicted to reach the UK's current levels by 2010.

The North-South gradient through Europe is unexplained. Similar gradients have been reported within some countries, perhaps reflecting social inequalities.

The Americas

The USA has shown particularly rapid increases in childhood obesity (defined as BMI >95th centile of a reference population from the early 1970s). The prevalence has risen from 4% to 6% across various age groups in 1971–1994, to 14–19% in 2003–2004 (Figure 2.8). A further 17% had a BMI >85th centile in 2003–4, so that over 34% of all children were overweight or obese (USA CDC, 2003). In Latin America, obesity is spreading rapidly among children in Brazil and Chile. In Chile, the rise has outpaced even that in the USA: between 1979 and 1997, overweight among 6–18 year olds increased threefold, from 4 to 14%, while 6-year old children showed a doubling in prevalence of overweight between 1987 and 2000, from 12 to 26% in boys and 14 to 27% in girls (see Figure 2.7).

Africa and the Middle East

North Africa and the Middle East show increasing evidence of overweight, in some instances approaching levels found in the USA and UK. In

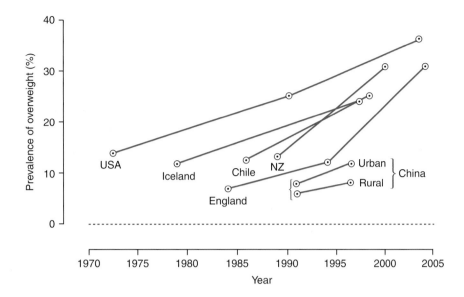

Figure 2.7 Increasing prevalence of overweight among children in selected countries. Overweight includes obesity and is defined by the IOTF criteria (Scottish InterCollegiate Guidelines Network, 2003). Data from Table 2.3.

Egypt, overweight (defined as a BMI >1 standard deviation above a reference population mean) was >25% in pre-school children and 14% in adolescents. Twenty per cent of adolescents aged 15–16 years in Saudi Arabia were defined as overweight (based on a BMI >120% of a reference median value). In Bahrain on 2002, and using IOTF criteria, 15% of boys and 27% of girls aged 12–17 years were overweight, while over 15% of both sexes were obese.

In Sub-Saharan Africa, obesity is eclipsed by undernutrition and there are few data on children. In South Africa, the Youth Behavioural Study of high-school students, using IOTF criteria, reported overweight in 25% of girls (with 5% obese) and 7% of boys (2% obese). Within ethnic groups, Indian females had the highest prevalence of overweight (13%) and obesity (14%), with 18% overweight and 6% obese among males (National Health Promotion

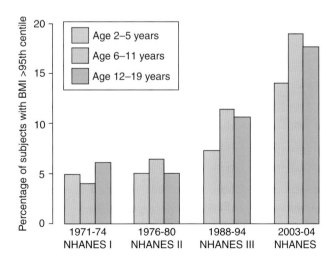

Figure 2.8 Prevalence of obesity (defined as BMI ≥95th centile of a reference population in the early 1970s) among children in the USA, stratified by age, in NHANES surveys between 1971 and 2004. Reproduced with kind permission of the US Center for Disease Control and Prevention.

Research and Development Group of the Medical Research Council, 2002).

Asia and the Pacific

In Asia, the gap in overweight and obesity prevalence between rich and poor is very apparent. In India, 20% of children in the upper social class are overweight, while those in the lower social class are more likely to suffer malnutrition and have an overweight prevalence of <5%. In Sri Lanka, only 2% of children are estimated to be overweight. In the Western Pacific region, overweight prevalences among children range from 15% to 20%. At present, the rate is lower in China; using China-specific cut-off points, overweight affects approximately 6% of those aged up to 17 years – but this still represents over 20 million children. Although adult obesity is overwhelmingly common in the Pacific Islands, adequate data for children are not yet available.

Predicted increases in obesity in adults

Extrapolating from the progressive rise in the prevalences of obesity and overweight between 1995 and 2005, the WHO estimates that 700 million people (age 15 and above) worldwide will be obese by 2015 – a 3.5-fold increase over the number in 1995. During the same period, the number of overweight people is expected to reach 2.3 billion overall (Figure 2.1).

These predictions derive from the WHO Global InfoBase (www.who.int/infobase/), which collates data from national surveys and provides judicious estimates from countries where information is insufficient. The global prevalences of obesity by country in 2005, and the predicted prevalence in 2015, are shown in Figure 2.3 (for men) and Figure 2.4 (for women). The most obvious increases are expected to be in North and South America, Europe, Central Asia and the Pacific Rim. In the USA, 75% of all adults are predicted to have a BMI $\geq 25\,\mathrm{kg/m^2}$ by 2015, and the prevalence of obesity in some ethnic groups will approach the highest levels that were seen worldwide during the late twentieth century: among non-Hispanic black women, 87% will be overweight and 63% obese (Wang and Beydounet, 2004). In China, obesity is a recent phenomenon but the rate of increase is likely to be high. The future prevalence in central and sub-Saharan Africa and India remains difficult to predict but there are indications of rising levels of overweight and obesity in some populations.

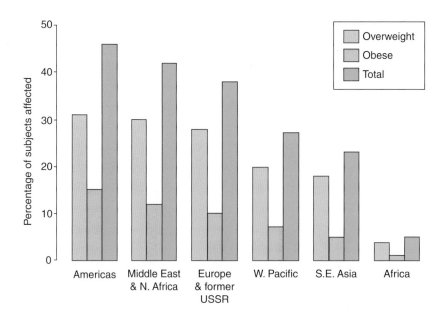

Figure 2.9 Predicted prevalences of overweight (BMI 25–29.9 kg/m²) and obesity (BMI $\geq 30\,\mathrm{kg/m^2}$) in school-age children by 2010, according to WHO regions. Data from Wang Y, Lobstein T (2006) Worldwide trends in childhood overweight and obesity. *International Journal of Pediatric Obesity*, 1: 11–25.

As the WHO surveys and predictions define obesity as BMI ≥30 kg/m², the prevalence of clinically significant obesity (and of obesity-related comorbidities) may be substantially underestimated in many large Asian populations.

Future trends in children

Without intervention, obesity is expected to continue rising among children in most regions of the world, notably North and South America, Europe and the former USSR, North Africa and the Middle East. Prevalences in South-East Asia and China have started to increase relatively late but are now gaining momentum. As in adults, obesity is likely to remain rare in much of Sub-Saharan Africa. Predictions for the various WHO regions are shown in Figure 2.9.

Comorbidities of obesity

Obesity increases the risk for a wide range of chronic diseases, including type 2 diabetes, cardiovascular disease (leading to myocardial infarction, heart failure and stroke) and several types of cancer. Other comorbidities include gall-bladder disease, fatty liver, sleep apnoea and osteoarthritis of weight-bearing joints (see Chapters 9–13).

The estimated proportions of the burden of disease attributed to obesity vary according to the population surveyed and the definition of obesity,

as illustrated in Figure 2.10. Overall, increased BMI is thought to account for about 60% of the risk of developing type 2 diabetes, 30–40% of the risk for hypertension and endometrial carcinoma, 20–25% of risk for coronary-heart disease and stroke, and about 10% of carcinoma of the breast and colon.

The disability attributable to obesity and its consequences in 2000 was calculated at over 30 million disability-adjusted life years (DALYs), due primarily to ischaemic heart disease and type 2 diabetes (WHO, 2004). Ultimately, obesity shortens life expectancy. In 2000, increased BMI alone was estimated to account for 2.5 million deaths in 2000, while the combined total with physical inactivity (itself a major contributor to obesity) was 4.5 million (WHO, 2004) – comparable with the excess mortality associated with raised cholesterol, and approaching that due to tobacco (Figure 2.11).

Predicted rises in obesity-related morbidity and mortality

It is expected that the near-global spread of obesity will be accompanied by widespread and marked increases in the comorbidities to which it predisposes, and ultimately in obesity-related deaths.

Diabetes will become one of the world's largest health challenges, with the vast majority

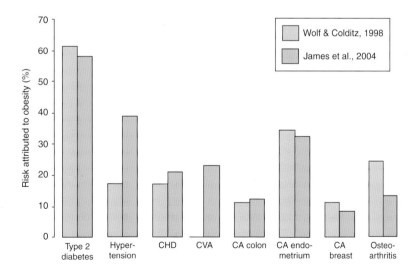

Figure 2.10 Percentage of risk attributed to obesity in developing certain diseases. Estimates by Wolf and Colditz (1998) and James *et al.* (2004) are shown, for North American and global populations respectively, and BMI risk thresholds of 29 kg/m² and 30 kg/m², respectively.

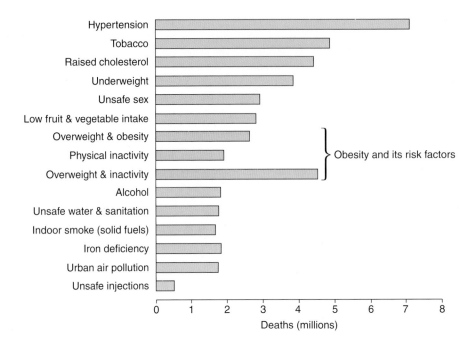

Figure 2.11 Leading causes of death worldwide in 2000. Data from World Health Report (De Onis *et al.*, 2007).

(>95%) of new cases having type 2 diabetes in which obesity plays an important aetiological role (see Figure 2.10). The incidence of diabetes is increasing ever faster in many countries, and estimates and predictions of prevalence are continually having to be revised upwards (Venkat Narayan *et al.*, 2006). Worldwide, predictions of a doubling in cases over a 10–15 year period are apparently being fulfilled (Figure 2.12). Current estimates are that the 150 million cases

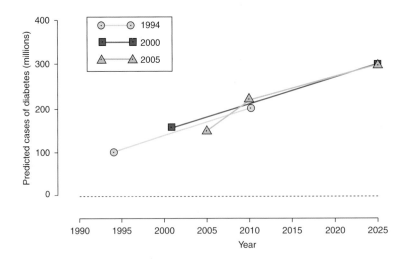

Figure 2.12 Worldwide estimates of current numbers of cases of diabetes and of future numbers of cases, reported in (1) 1994, (2) 2000, and (3) 2005. Data from: (1) WHO Study Group. *Prevention of Diabetes Mellitus*. Technical Report, WHO, Geneva 1994; (2) International Diabetes Federation. Diabetes and cardiovascular disease: time to act. Brussels: IDF, 2001; (3) Roglic *et al.*, (2005). The burden of mortality attributable to diabetes: realistic estimates for the year 2005. *Diabetes Care* 28: 2130–5.

of diabetes in 2005 will increase to 366 million by 2030. The number of deaths due to diabetes is forecast to double from 1.1 million in 2005 to 2.2 million by 2030. Most of those affected will live in developing countries, notably the Asian-Pacific region, where it will be very difficult to meet the large financial and social costs inflicted by the disease.

Cardiovascular disease. Obesity is now recognized as an independent risk factor for coronary-heart disease (CHD) and hypertension (see Chapter 12). CHD stands out as the leading single cause of death in the world (30% of all deaths) and is forecast by the WHO to remain so, with the estimated number of deaths rising from 17.5 million in 2005 to 23.3 million by 2030.

Cancers. There is convincing evidence that excess body fat increases the risk for numerous malignancies, notably cancers of the colon, kidney, pancreas, endometrium, oesophagus, and breast cancer in post-menopausal women (see Chapter 13). Obesity has been held responsible for up to 72 000 additional cases of cancer within 15 European Union countries, and will undoubtedly contribute to increases in the prevalences of malignancies in many populations (Bergstrom *et al.*, 2001).

Impact of childhood obesity

The spread of childhood obesity has also led to gloomy predictions concerning the risks for comorbidities and life expectancy for today's children. In the USA alone, recently revised estimates from the Centres for Disease Control forecast a threefold increase in type 2 diabetes between 2005 and 2050, from 16.2 million to 48.3 million – 9.3 million more cases than previously estimated (Venkat Narayan *et al.*, 2006). It is inevitable that major health burdens associated with childhood obesity will fall on countries that will find it difficult to bear the associated healthcare and social costs.

Controversy has surrounded predictions of premature mortality. For example, one study in the USA suggested that nearly 112 000 of current deaths could be attributed to obesity, but that none were associated with being overweight; this study did not attempt to estimate the prevailing level of morbidity (Flegal *et al.*, 2005). Nonetheless, these uncertainties have not deterred forecasters from warning of the potential for obesity to curtail life expectancy. A group of eminent US researchers has stated

that children born in the early twenty first century may have their life expectancy shortened as a result of the escalating epidemic of obesity. Among obese children, the overall lifetime risk for developing type 2 diabetes may now be as high as 33%, rising to 50% among certain ethnic minorities in the USA, while life expectancy may be reduced by up to 13 years because of diabetes (Olshansky *et al.*, 2005).

Costs of obesity to society

Overweight and obesity, and the burden of associated chronic diseases, have significant economic and social impact because of disability and death. Obesity incurs considerable direct and indirect costs. Direct medical costs include preventative, diagnostic and treatment services related to overweight and obesity; the costs associated with comorbidities are overlooked in some analyses, thus underestimating the total economic burden. Indirect costs relate to income lost from decreased productivity, reduced opportunities and restricted activity, illness, absenteeism and premature death, as well as the numerous changes that societies have to make for obese people.

Indirect costs

The indirect costs incurred by death, lost productivity and related loss of income may be substantially greater than direct costs, but are often neglected – as are the societal costs associated with obesity. These 'invisible costs' are now beginning to be documented and are attracting attention in the media.

Wide-ranging adjustments to the infrastructure of many countries have been required to cope with the reality of most of the population being overweight. Within the health system, additional costs may result from the need for stronger beds, operating tables and wheel chairs, and even for double crews in reinforced ambulances to cope with lifting heavier patients. The impact of obesity is ultimately reflected in the growing requirements for bigger coffins and larger-capacity crematorium equipment to accommodate obese cadavers.

Elsewhere, the progressive increase in mean population weights has necessitated ergonomic alterations for larger people, such as enlargement of turnstiles and seats in sports-grounds. Obesity is also having important consequences for transport safety standards. The US car industry has had to adopt new benchmarks for safety: the weight of standard adult dummies used in crash tests is now 101 kg (223 pounds), compared with 77 kg (170 pounds) before 2001. Following a tourboat accident in which 20 passengers drowned, and which was partly blamed on the passengers' excessive weight, the US Coast Guard has raised the assumed weight for a standard passenger on light vessels to 90 kg (185 pounds).

Air travel also provides a graphic illustration of how safety standards must keep up with the spread of obesity. A warning to check passengers' true weights was issued following an air crash in Canada in 1988, and this is now mandatory for light aircraft. Investigation of an aircraft accident in the USA in 1991 revealed identical structural failures in seats that carried people weighing over 90 kg, but none in seats bearing lighter passengers. Finally, the crash of a scheduled-service passenger aircraft in North Carolina in 2003 (killing all 21 on board) was attributed to problems with weight and balance because official guidance had underestimated the average passenger's weight by 9 kg. Accordingly, the Federal Aviation Authority (FAA) issued new advice on calculating passenger loading in 2005.

Total costs of obesity and overweight

Overall, the cost to society is substantial, accounting for up to 6% of total direct health expenditure in Europe, and 1% or more of the gross domestic product (GDP) in some countries. In the USA, using 1998 data, overweight and obesity were initially thought to account for at least $52 billion (9% of total medical expenditure), rising to $79 billion if nursing-home costs are included. Obesity alone accounted for $27–48 billion, half of which was borne by federally-funded Medicare and Medicaid programmes (Finkelstein, Fiebelkorn and Wang, 2004). These estimates were subsequently revised to $75 billion for obesity alone, of which $18 billion was borne by Medicare and £21 billion by Medicaid. None of these calculations includes indirect and societal costs (Finkelstein, Fiebelkorn and Wang, 2004).

In other countries, the costs of obesity may be harder to calculate, and vary widely. In England, the National Audit Office (NAO) estimates that obesity accounted for 18 million sick days and 31 000 deaths each year, resulting in 40 000 lost years of working life; deaths associated with obesity shorten life by an average of 9 years. The NAO's conservative estimates of costs in 1998 were £2.6 billion (US $5.2 billion), predicted to rise to £3.6 billion (US $7.2 billion) by 2010. In Spain, the costs attributable to obesity are calculated at €2.5 billion (US $3.4 billion) per year. In 2002, and applying the methodology used by the UK's NAO, estimated costs across 15 EU countries were €33 billion (US $44 billion) (Fry and Finley, 2005). This has been extrapolated in 2005 to the expanded European Union (25 countries), where obesity was estimated to cost €41 billion per year and the combined cost with overweight reached €81 billion annually (Impact Assessment Report, 2007).

The estimated costs of obesity per capita in selected Western countries are shown in Figure 2.13.

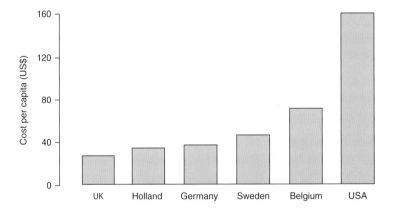

Figure 2.13 Estimated costs of obesity (per capita, in US dollars) in selected Western countries. Data from WHO Europe web site, November 2006.

Costs to the individual: psychological and employment disadvantage

As discussed in Chapter 14, the psychological problems of obesity are common, wide-ranging and potentially serious – and often neglected. Some issues are controversial: some observers suggest that discussion about body-weight and the control of eating might tip vulnerable individuals towards anorexia, while others consider that the growing world-wide awareness of obesity has reinforced prejudice against the obese, who are often stigmatized.

The relentless increase in the prevalence of obesity suggests that most people are undeterred by such concerns; some people may have become less sensitive about the issue, or less aware of their weight and appearance. Evidence from the South Africa Demographic and Health Survey points to important shortfalls in awareness, with only 10% of men and 22% of women considering themselves overweight, while actual prevalences were 29 and 57%, respectively. Awareness of obesity differed between population groups: white women were the most aware, while the greatest discrepancies between perceived and actual body weight were seen in the least-educated groups of men and women (Puoane et al., 2002).

Cultural and ethnic factors undoubtedly modulate the social impact of obesity, as well as its perception. The NHANES data indicate that obesity is much more common among US ethnic minorities (Black Americans, Hispanic Americans, Asian and Pacific Islander Americans, American Indians and Alaska Natives, and Native Hawaiians) than in whites, especially in women, and is forecast to increase substantially particularly among Black American females. In the latter group, low socio-economic status, poverty and poor educational achievement have long been associated with the higher prevalence of obesity (Kumanyika, 1993). In some parts of the world – notably the Pacific Islands and some African countries – obesity may still carry historic and cultural connotations of power, beauty and affluence; however, this does not necessarily equate with an individual's satisfaction with body size.

The psychological impact of obesity, and the many ways in which it can affect an individual's quality of life, mental health, educational achievement and employment prospects, are discussed in detail in Chapter 14.

Conclusions

Obesity is now reaching pandemic proportions across much of the world, and the rapid rise of overweight and obesity among children is of particular concern. Obesity and its consequences are set to impose unprecedented health, financial and social burdens on global society, unless effective actions are taken to reverse the trend. The scale of the problem and the pervasive influence of the westernized cultural changes that underlie it, pose major challenges for the preventative strategies described in Chapter 22.

References

American Medical Association, DHHS Health Resources and Services Administration, and the Centers for Disease Control and Prevention (2007) Expert Commission Recommendations on the Assessment, Prevention and Treatment of Child and Adolescent Overweight and Obesity.

Azizi, F. (2001) Tehran Lipid and Glucose Study, Endocrine Research Center, Tehran.

Bergstrom, A., Pisani, P., Tenet, V. et al. (2001) Overweight as an avoidable cause of cancer in Europe. International Journal of Cancer, **91** (3), 421–30.

Christakis, N.A. and Fowler, J.H. (2007) The spread of obesity in a large social network over 32 years. New England Journal of Medicine, **357**, 370–79.

Cole, T., Freeman, J. and Preece, M. (1995) Body mass index reference curves for the UK 1990. Archives of Disease in Childhood, **73**, 25–9.

Cole, T.J., Bellizzi, M.C., Flegal, K.M. and Dietz, W.H. (2000) Establishing a standard definition for child overweight and obesity worldwide: international survey. BMJ (Clinical Research Ed), **320**, 1240–3.

Connor Gorber, S., Tremblay, M., Moher, D. and Gorber, B. (2007) A comparison of direct vs. self-report measures for assessing height, weight and body mass index: a systematic review. Obesity Reviews, **8** (4), 307.

De Onis, M. et al. (2007) Development of WHO growth reference for school-aged children and adolescents. Bulletin of the World Health Organization, **85** (9), 660–7. http://www.who.int/growthref/.

Department of Health. (2006a) The Health Survey for England, Department of Health, England.

Department of Health (2006b) Forecasting obesity to 2010. Department of Health.

European Commission (2007) White Paper: A Strategy for Europe on Nutrition, Overweight and Obesity Related Health Issues.

Finkelstein, E.A., Fiebelkorn, I.C. and Wang, G. (2003) National medical spending attributable to overweight and obesity: How much, and who's paying? *Health Affairs*, (W3), 219–26.

Finkelstein, E.A., Fiebelkorn, I.C. and Wang, G. (2004) State-level estimates of annual medical expenditures attributable to obesity. *Obesity Research*, **12** (1), 18–24.

Flegal, K.M., Graubard, B.I., Williamson, D.F. and Gail, M.H. (2005) Excess deaths associated with underweight, overweight, and obesity. *The Journal of the American Medical Association*, **293**, 1861–7.

Fry, J. and Finley, W. (2005) The prevalence and costs of obesity in the EU. *Proceedings of the Nutrition Society*, **64**, 359–62.

Galal, O. (2002) The nutrition transition in Egypt: obesity, undernutrition and the food consumption context food consumption. *Public Health Nutrition*, **5** (1A), 141–8.

Ghaseemi, H. *et al.* (2002) *An Accelerated Nutrition Transition in Iran*, Public Health Nutrition.

Gillum, R.F. and Sempos, C.T. (2005) Ethnic variation in validity of classification of overweight and obesity using self-reported weight and height in American women and men: the Third National Health and Nutrition Examination Survey. *Nutrition Journal*, **4**, 27.

Huxley, R. *et al.* (2008) The Obesity in Asia Collaboration. Ethnic comparisons of the cross-sectional relationships between measures of body size with diabetes and hypertension. *Obesity Reviews*, **9** (Suppl. 1), 53–61.

Impact Assessment Report accompanying the White Paper from the European Commission. (2007) A Strategy For Europe On Nutrition, Overweight and Obesity Related Health Issues (Com(2007) 279 FinalSec(2007)707).www.ec.europa.eu/health/ph_determinants/life_style/nutrition/documents/nutrition_impact_en.pdf (accessed 28 June 2008).

International Obesity Task Force (2005) EU Platform Briefing Paper March. Available as download from www.iotf.org/media/euobesity3.pdf (accessed 28 June 2008).

James, W.P., Chunming, C. and Inoue, S. (2002) Appropriate Asian body mass indices? *Obesity Reviews*, **3** (3), 139.

James, W.P.T., Jackson-Leach, R., Ni Mhurchu, C. *et al.* (2004) Comparative quantification of health risks: Global and regional burden of disease attributable to selected major risk factors, Vol. 1. Ezzati, M., Lopez, A., Roger, A. and Murray, C. (eds). WHO: Geneva, pp. 495–596.

Kamadjeu, R.M., Edwards, R., Atanga, J.S. *et al.* (2006) Anthropometry measures and prevalence of obesity in the urban adult population of Cameroon: an update from the Cameroon Burden of Diabetes Baseline Survey. *BMC Public Health*, **6**, 228.

Kumanyika, S.K. (1993) Special issues regarding obesity in minority populations. *Annals of Internal Medicine*, **119** (7 Pt 2), 650–4.

Lee, C.M.Y., Martiniuk, A.L.C., Woodward, M. *et al.* on behalf of the Asia Pacific Cohort Studies Collaboration

(APCSC) The burden of overweight and obesity in the Asia-Pacific region. *Obesity Reviews*, 8(3), 191–6.

Li, G., Chen, Y., Jang, Y. *et al.*(2002) Obesity, coronary heart disease risk factors and diabetes in China: an approach to the criteria of obesity in the Chinese population. *Obesity Reviews*, **3**, 167–72.

Lobstein, T., Baur, L. and Uauy, R. IOTF Childhood Obesity Working Groups (2004) Obesity in children and young people: a crisis in public health. *Obesity Reviews*, **5** (Suppl 1), 4–85.

Molarius, A., Seidell, J.C., Sans, S. *et al.* (2000) Educational level, relative body weight, and changes in their association over 10 years: an international perspective from the WHO MONICA Project. *American Journal of Public Health*, **90**, 1260–8.

Monteiro, C. *et al.* (2007) Income-specific trends in obesity in Brazil 1975–2003. *AJPH*, **97**, 1808–12.

Musaiger, A.O. and Al-Mannai, M.A. (2001) Weight, height, body mass index and prevalence of obesity among the adult population in Bahrain. *Annals of Human Biology*, **28** (3).

National Health and Nutrition Examination Survey 2003–4. US Centers for Disease Control, Atlanta.

National Health Promotion Research and Development Group of the Medical Research Council (2002) The 1st South African National Youth Risk Behaviour Survey 2002 prepared for the South African National Department of Health, South Africa.

Ogden, C.L., Carroll, M.D., Curtin, L.R. *et al.* (2006) Prevalence of overweight and obesity in the United States, 1999–2004. *The Journal of the American Medical Association*, **295**, 1549–55.

Olshansky, S.J., Passaro, D.J., Hershow, R.C. *et al.* (2005) A potential decline in life expectancy in the United States in the 21st century. *The New England Journal of Medicine*, **352**, 1138–45.

Puoane, T., Steyn, K., Bradshaw, D. *et al.* (2002) Obesity in South Africa: the South African demographic and health survey. *Obesity Research*, **10**, 1038–48.

Reddy, K.S., Prabhakaran, D., Shah, P. and Shah, B. (2002) Differences in body mass index and waist: hip ratios in North Indian rural and urban populations. *Obesity Reviews*, **3**, 197–202.

Scottish InterCollegiate Guidelines Network. (2003) SIGN Guideline 69, http://www.sign.ac.uk/guidelines/fulltext/69/index.html (accessed 28 June 2008).

Siervo, M., Grey, P., Nyan, O.A. and Prentice, A.M. (2006) Urbanization and obesity in The Gambia: a country in the early stages of the demographic transition. *European Journal of Clinical Nutrition*, **60** (4), 455–63.

Steyn, N.P., Bradshaw, D., Norman, R. *et al.* (2006) Dietary Changes and the Health Transition in South Africa: Implications for Health Policy, Cape Town, South African Medical Research Council.

USA CDC, National Health and Nutritional Examination Survey NHANES 2003–4.

Venkat Narayan, K.M., Boyle, J.P., Geiss, L.S. *et al.* (2006) Impact of recent increase in incidence on future diabetes burden: U.S., 2005–2050. *Diabetes Care*, **29**, 2114–6

Wang, Y. and Beydounet, M. (2007) The Obesity Epidemic in the United States – Gender, Age, Socioeconomic, Racial/Ethnic, and Geographic Characteristics: A Systematic Review and Meta-Regression Analysis. *Epidemiologic Reviews*, **29**, 6–28. Advance Access published May 17.

WHO (2004) Overweight and obesity (high body mass index). Chapter 8. WPT James *et al.* in *Comparative Quantification of Health Risks Global and Regional Burden of Diseases Attributable to Selected Major Risk Factors*. WHO, Geneva.

WHO (2006a) Factsheet 311 September. http://www.who.int/mediacentre/factsheets/fs311/en/index.html (accessed 17 June 2008).

WHO (2006b) Child Growth Standards: Length/Height-for-age, Weight-for-age, Weight-for-length, Weight-for-height and Body Mass Index-for age WHO, ISBN 9789241546935.

WHO (2007) WHO statement: Controlling the global obesity epidemic. http://www.who.int/nutrition/topics/obesity/en/ (accessed 8 July 2007).

WHO Expert Committee (1997) Physical status: the use and interpretation of anthropometry. Report of a WHO Expert Committee. Technical Report Series No. 854.

WHO Expert Consultation (2004) Appropriate body-mass index for Asian populations and its implications for policy and intervention strategies. *Lancet*, **363**, 157–63.

WHO Global Infobase http://www.who.int/infobase/ (accessed 8 July 2007).

WHO/IASO/IOTF (2000) *The Asia-Pacific Perspective: Redefining Obesity and its Treatment*, Health Communications Australia, Melbourne.

WHO/NUT/NCD (2000) Obesity: Preventing and Managing the Global Epidemic. Report of a WHO Consultation in Obesity. WHO TRS 894: Geneva.

Wild, S., Roglic, G., Green, A. *et al.* (2004) Global prevalence of diabetes: estimates for the year 2000 and projections for 2030. *Diabetes Care*, **27** (5), 1047–53.

Wolf A.M. and Colditz G.A. (1998) *Obes Res*, **6**, 97–106.

Wu, Y. (2006) Overweight and obesity in China. *BMJ (Clinical Research ed)*, **333**, 362–3.

Wu, Y. *et al.* (2005) The current prevalence status of body overweight and obesity in China: data from the China nutrition and health survey. *Chinese Journal of Preventive Medicine*, **39**, 316–20.

Yun, S., Zhu, B.P., Black, W. *et al.* (2006) A comparison of national estimates of obesity prevalence from the behavioral risk factor surveillance system and the National Health and Nutrition Examination Survey. *International Journal of Obesity (London)*, **30**, 164–70.

Key Methodologies in Obesity Research and Practice

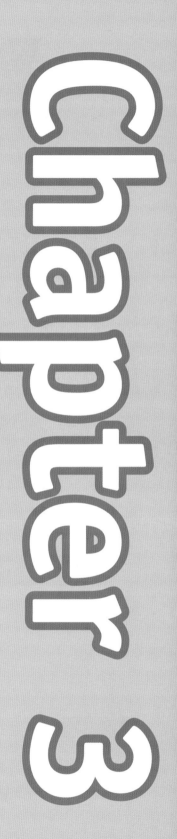

Key points

- Body mass index (BMI), calculated as (weight in kg)/(height in m)^2, is a convenient measure of obesity that predicts overall health risk. Overweight and obesity are defined as BMI $\geq$25 and $\geq$30 kg/m^2, respectively; lower thresholds are appropriate in Asian populations.

- Waist circumference is correlated with visceral fat mass and predicts diabetes and cardio-vascular risk more powerfully than BMI; values of $\geq$88 cm in women and $\geq$102 cm in men indicate substantially increased risk. A waist:hip ratio (WHR) of $\geq$0.95 (men) or $\geq$0.8 (women) also indicates increased cardiovascular risk.

- Body composition components comprise total body water (TBW), fat mass (FM), fat-free (lean) mass (FFM) and bone mineral content (BMC). TBW can be measured by isotope dilution, while FFM can be estimated from body density, calculated from underwater weighing or air-displacement plethysmography. Whole-body DEXA (dual-energy X-ray absorptiometry) scanning can be used to estimate FM, FFM and BMC. Bioimpedance, a non-invasive method that measures the body's electrical resistance, can yield estimates of TBW and hence FFM and FM.

- Regional fat distribution is best measured by magnetic resonance imaging (MRI) or computerized tomographic (CT) scanning. Both are expensive and the latter incurs.

- Food intake can be assessed from various questionnaires and food diaries. Under-reporting of food intake, a consistent finding among obese people, can compromise these methods.

- Total energy expenditure (TEE) comprises basal metabolic rate (BMR), thermogenesis (e.g. heat generated by food, fever or drugs) and physical activity. BMR typically accounts for two-thirds of TEE and is proportional to FFM. TEE rises with increasing body weight because FFM also rises, and is therefore higher in obese than in lean subjects.

- Energy expenditure can be calculated from indirect calorimetry (using a portable 'ventilated hood' apparatus, or a whole-body chamber suitable for studies lasting several days), or the isotopic doubly-labelled water method, which yields the carbon dioxide production rate over several days. Physical activity can be measured by movement-sensitive accelerometers or from heart rate.

- Insulin sensitivity and β-cell function can both be estimated from fasting blood levels of insulin and glucose using homeostatic model assessment (HOMA). The intravenous glucose tolerance test (IVGTT) derives insulin sensitivity from the rate of disappearance of glucose following an intravenous bolus injection. The euglycaemic hyperinsulinaemic clamp (EHC) determines insulin sensitivity from the amount of glucose that has to be administered intravenously to maintain a normal blood glucose level during intravenous infusion of insulin to stimulate glucose uptake into skeletal muscle.

Chapter 3   Key Methodologies in Obesity Research and Practice

Susan A. Jebb, Alexandra M. Johnstone, Janet Warren, Gail R. Goldberg, and Les Bluck

Extreme overweight is easily identified, and indeed has been recognized since antiquity. An obese person can also be readily distinguished from a muscular athlete, but mild or moderate obesity – which may still have adverse health consequences – may be difficult to judge. As in all scientific disciplines, the systematic study of obesity requires well-established definitions of adiposity that are based on rigorous and relevant measurements. This is particularly important for clarifying the relationships between obesity and its health consequences, and for determining the indications for treatment and monitoring its outcome.

This chapter reviews the key measures and methodologies used to quantify obesity and its principal metabolic sequelae, notably insulin resistance. Their applications to obesity research and clinical practice, and their advantages and disadvantages, are highlighted throughout.

Anthropometric indices

Tall, lean people may weigh more than short, obese subjects – demonstrating that measuring weight alone is inadequate to define obesity. Individual differences in stature, age, gender and ethnicity demand more sophisticated analyses in order to identify a 'healthy' weight range that reflects the lowest risk of ill-health (Seidell and Flegal, 1997).

Various methods have been devised to allow for differences in height and shape when interpreting weight, including weight/height, weight/surface area and weight/(height^2). The Belgian statistician, Quételet, originally suggested that weight/(height^2) was an appropriate way to correct weight for height, and this is the basis for the body mass index (BMI), which is widely used to define obesity.

BMI, also known as the Quételet index, is calculated as the weight in kilograms divided by the square of the height in metres (kg/m^2). Within populations, BMI is closely correlated to percentage body fat content, and it also predicts the health risks of obesity. The World Health Organization (1999) classifies a healthy BMI in adults as between 18.5 and 24.9 kg/m^2 (see Table 3.1), with overweight and obesity represented by BMI 24.9–29.9 and ≥30 kg/m^2, respectively. The thresholds for overweight and obesity are derived from the relationship between BMI and premature mortality, and also agree well with increasing risk of various comorbidities of obesity such as type 2 diabetes, hypertension and coronary-heart disease (Chapter 9). At a BMI below the cut-off point for underweight (18.5 kg/m^2), there is an increase in other health risks, notably in females for low bone density, amenorrhoea and infertility.

For children, the use of constant cut-off BMI levels is not appropriate since body weight and height vary naturally during growth and development and especially around puberty (see Chapter 21). Instead, BMI percentile charts are used to describe the typical pattern of growth in boys and girls aged 0–18 years (Figure 3.1). The BMI of an individual child is plotted on the distribution for the appropriate age and sex, and values lying above the 85th or 95th percentiles are clinically defined as overweight or obese, respectively. However, this classification creates a difficult transition to the BMI-based criteria for defining overweight and obesity in adults, which apply from the age of 18 years. The International Obesity Task Force have therefore proposed an alternative method, in which overweight and obesity are defined by the BMI percentiles that extrapolate to match a BMI of 25 or 30 kg/m^2, respectively, at age 18 years (Cole et al., 2005). Figure 3.2 shows these charts

Obesity: Science to Practice   Edited by Gareth Williams and Gema Frühbeck
© 2009 John Wiley & Sons, Ltd

Table 3.1   Classification of weight status and comorbid risk in adults, based on BMI.

Weight category	Risk of BMI (kg/m²) comorbidities
Underweight	<18.5 Low
Healthy/normal weight	18.5–24.9 Average
Overweight (pre-obese)	25–29.9 Increased
Obesity: moderate (class 1)	30–34.9 Moderate-severe
Obesity: severe (class 2)	35–39.9 Moderate-severe
Obesity: morbid (class 3)	≥40 Severe

From World Health Organization (1999).

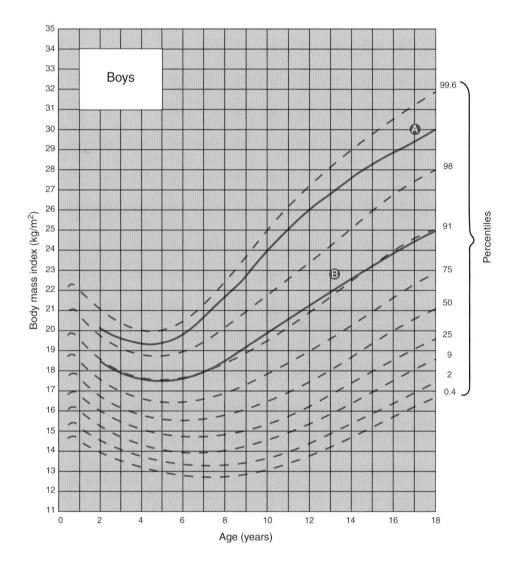

Figure 3.1 BMI percentile charts for boys (above) and girls (next page), aged up to 18 years. Overweight and obesity are defined as a BMI that exceeds the 85th and 95th percentiles, respectively, for the appropriate age and gender. These charts are in use in the UK, based on data collected in 1990. Some BMI percentile charts in clinical use also show the recently-defined thresholds for overweight (B) and obesity (A) that are illustrated in Figure 3.2.

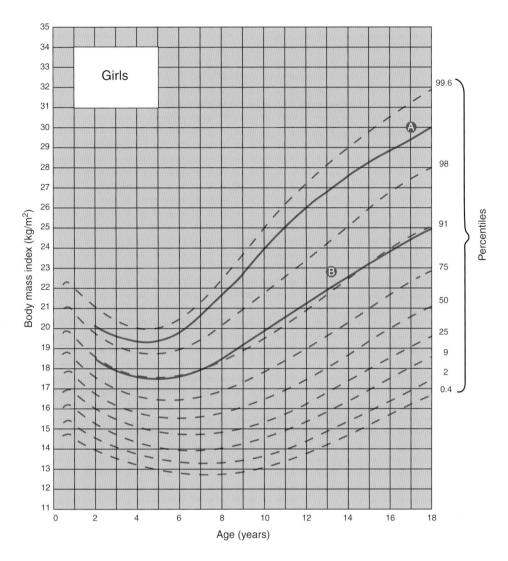

Figure 3.1 *(Continued)*

for boys and girls, from which age- and gender-specific cut-off levels of BMI for overweight and obesity can be read.

The measurement of BMI is simple, accurate and well-suited to population surveillance and to monitoring trends in the prevalence of obesity. However, BMI assumes that excess weight has a fixed fat:lean ratio and therefore cannot distinguish between individuals who have similar build but who may have marked differences in body composition and fat content (Prentice and Jebb, 2001). Differences in the amount and distribution of body fat between individuals of comparable BMI are strikingly illustrated in Figure 3.7 (on page 55). Body fat content also

shows considerable variation with gender, age and ethnic origin. At a given BMI, men have a lower proportion of fat than women, while even individuals who maintain constant weight throughout adult life will have a progressive increase in fat and a reduction in lean tissue mass (Elia, 2001).

The original WHO classification is based on data derived from mainly Caucasian subjects. It is now clear that there are important ethnic differences in body composition that can affect the interpretation of BMI and its associated risks (Deurenberg and Deurenberg-Yap, 2003). In particular, Asian people have a relatively high body fat content at a given

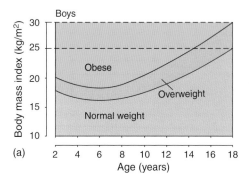

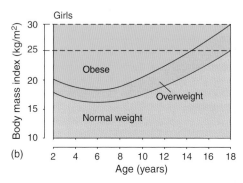

Figure 3.2 BMI cut-off curves defining overweight and obesity for (a) boys and (b) girls. The cut-off curves are constructed so as to coincide with the BMI values of 30 kg/m² (obesity) and 25 kg/m² (overweight) at age 18 years, the age from which the adult BMI thresholds apply. Adapted from T.J. Cole, M.S. Faith, A. Pietrobelli, M. Heo (2005). 'What is the best measure of adiposity change in growing children: BMI, BMI %, BMI z-score or BMI centile?' *European Journal of Clinical Nutrition*, **59**(3): 419–25.

BMI; accordingly, the risks of obesity-related diseases such as type 2 diabetes begin to appear at a lower BMI than in Caucasians (see Chapter 9).

Further limitations of BMI are apparent when measuring the response to obesity treatments. Weight loss induced by exercise is associated with smaller losses of lean tissue (which is denser than fat), compared with dietary restriction alone. Thus, weight and BMI may change little during an exercise programme, even though significant loss of fat may occur. BMI alone may also fail to detect important differences in the change in body composition between dietary treatments. These subtle effects can be identified using sophisticated research techniques, such as imaging or multi-compartment modelling (see below).

Body circumferences

Body fat distribution is also an important risk factor for obesity-related diseases, and in some cases (e.g. type 2 diabetes and cardiovascular risk) may be a more powerful predictor than BMI (see Chapter 9). Central fat mass – the major correlate of risk – can be crudely assessed using body circumferences. Typically, women (at least pre-menopausal) carry excess weight over the hips and thighs in the gluteo-femoral distribution, whereas men tend to deposit excess fat in and around the abdomen.

Measures of the relative size of the waist and hips (the waist:hip ratio, WHR) have been used as a proxy for central fat distribution. Waist circumference can be measured using various anatomical landmarks, including the midpoint between the lowest rib and the iliac crest, at the umbilicus, and the narrowest girth (Klein *et al.*, 2007). It should be measured at the end of expiration, using a non-stretching metal tape measure. Hip circumference is measured as the maximal circumference at the level of the greater trochanters, measured with the subject standing with his/her feet together (WHO, 1995). Consistent definition of these sites and careful training are essential to obtain reproducible and reliable measures. A WHR above 0.95 for men and 0.8 in women is considered to indicate increased cardiovascular risk (WHO, 1999).

It is now more common to use the waist circumference alone as an index of abdominal fat; indeed, waist circumference correlates well with both abdominal and intra-abdominal visceral fat (Janssen *et al.*, 2002), and can be used to stratify cardio-metabolic risk (see Chapter 9). Table 3.2 shows the waist circumference thresholds identified as conferring increased (Level 1) and substantially increased risk (Level 2) of cardiovascular disease (Lean, Han and Morrison, 1995). Because risk is consistently higher in Asian subjects, lower cut-off values have been proposed in these populations (see Chapter 9).

Skinfold thickness

The thickness of the subcutaneous fat depot at various key sites has been shown to be related to total fat content, and was widely used before the advent of more sophisticated methods, especially in epidemiological studies.

Table 3.2 Comorbid risks of obesity according to waist circumference, in men and women.

	Waist circumference (cm)
Men	
Level 1: Increased risk	94–102
Level 2: Substantially increased risk	>102
Women	
Level 1: Increased risk	80–88
Level 2: Substantially increased risk	>88

From M.E. Lean, T.S. Han and C.E. Morrison (1995) 'Waist circumference as a measure for indicating need for weight management'. *British Medical Journal*, **311**(6998): 158–61.

A skinfold thickness (SFT) is the double thickness of the epidermis, underlying fascia and subcutaneous fat, when the tissues are pinched between measuring callipers (Lohman, 1981). Measurements made at one or more sites can be combined to give an estimate of total body fat, using predictive equations derived from body density measurements (see below). This assumes, first, that there is a constant relationship between total body fat and subcutaneous fat at the sites measured, and second, that the density of FFM is constant.

Measurements are usually made at four sites: biceps, triceps, subscapular and suprailiac. Using sex- and age-dependent, population-based linear regression equations, the sum of these values (in mm) can be used to estimate total body fat (Durnin and Womersely, 1974). For trained observers, the total error (biological and technical) in estimating body fat is 3.3% (Lohman, 1981), which compares favourably with more sophisticated body composition techniques (Johnstone *et al.*, 2006; Jebb *et al.*, 1993). However, the practical difficulties of consistently locating the correct site and applying the callipers, particularly in obese subjects, can introduce considerable observer error. This limits the usefulness of this technique outside research environments; it is unreliable in routine clinical practice when used to estimate body fat changes over time.

Single skinfolds have been used to monitor regional fat loss or gain, but as the metabolic consequences of obesity are more strongly related to visceral rather than subcutaneous fat, the value of this approach is questionable.

Measurements of body composition

Fat and fat-free mass (FFM)

The specific measurement of body composition requires more sophisticated understanding and techniques. In the simplest model, the body is considered to comprise two compartments: fat mass (FM) and fat-free mass (FFM). Fat mass is relatively homogeneous, but the FFM component includes bone mineral, protein, water and glycogen and other minor constituents. Analysis of a limited number of cadavers has shown that the main constituents exist in relatively predictable proportions; thus, the measurement of one or more components can allow the composition of the whole body to be inferred (reviewed by Ellis, 2000) (Table 3.3).

Although these proportions are assumed to be constant in the 2-compartment model, a change in one of these compartments will affect the estimate of FFM and therefore of FM (which is calculated as the difference from body weight). The greater the number of compartments modelled, the more accurate is the estimate of body composition. Multi-compartment models are commonly used for research purposes (Heymsfield, Wang and Withers, 1996). A 3-compartment model usually combines measures of total body water with densitometry to estimate the contents

Table 3.3 The body composition of 'reference man' (a normal adult male weighing 75 kg), showing individual components, their density and percentage contribution to body weight.

Component	Density (g/ml)	Percentage of whole body weight
Water	0.994	62.4
Protein	1.34	16.4
Mineral: Osseous	3.038	5.9
Non-osseous	3.317	4.8
Fat	0.901	15.3
Fat-free mass	1.100	84.7
Whole body	1.064	100.0

of water, fat and (dry) fat-free tissue (Coward, Parkinson and Murgatroyd, 1988), whereas a 4-compartment model also includes bone mineral (usually measured by dual energy X-ray absorptiometry) and yields the contents of bone, water, fat and (dry) fat-free tissue (Fuller et al., 1992; Ellis, 2000).

Three main methods of measuring body composition measurement have been employed, namely total body potassium, total body water (TBW) and body densitometry. Nowadays, total body potassium is infrequently used and will not be considered further (see Lukaski, 1987). Densitometry and TBW measurements are important techniques in their own right and, in combination, are the cornerstones of more sophisticated measurements of body composition. The newer technique of dual energy X-ray absorptiometry (DEXA), widely used to measure bone mineral, can also be used to measure fat and fat-free components.

Densitometry

Density is calculated as body mass/volume. Traditionally, density has been measured by directly measuring mass on weighing scales, and body volume by underwater weighing, using the basic principle of water displacement that accounts for the difference between the weight in air and weight in water. Underwater weighing requires total submergence, and can therefore be both difficult and frightening, particularly for children and the elderly. Instead, air-displacement plethysmography can be used to measure body density, using the commercial system Bod Pod® (Figure 3.3), or its paediatric equivalent, the PeaPod. This apparatus uses the inverse relationship between pressure and volume (Boyle's law) to derive the body volume of a subject sealed inside a chamber, with appropriate corrections for the air in the lungs and gut. Density measurements derived from the Bod Pod® show excellent agreement with underwater weighing, and are more reproducible as well as being much more acceptable to the subject (McCrory et al., 1995). The precision of measuring fat mass using the Bod Pod® is ±0.3 kg fat (Dewit et al., 2000), with a coefficient of variation of 1.7% (McCrory et al., 1995).

When the body's density is known, and assuming the density of fat to be 0.9 kg/l and that of fat-free

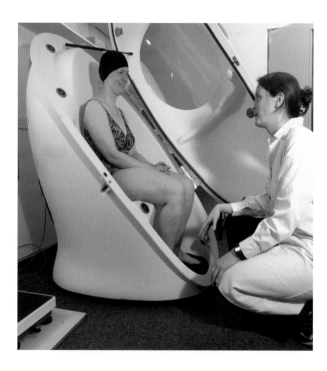

Figure 3.3 Subject seated in an air displacement plethysmograph (Bod Pod®) for measuring body density. By applying standard equations, body fat mass and composition can be estimated from the density.

mass 1.1 kg/l, the percentage of body fat can be estimated using a standard equation (Siri, 1961).

Total body water (TBW)

Fat is essentially anhydrous and the FFM contains a known proportion of water; it is therefore possible to estimate FFM if the total body water content is known, when fat mass can be calculated as the difference from body weight (Heymsfield, Wang and Withers, 1996). Total body water is conveniently measured by the isotope dilution method. The chosen tracer must mix rapidly with water in all body compartments and be metabolized and lost from the body in a constant proportion to unlabelled water (Schoeller and Jones, 1987); these assumptions are not universally applicable, but the technique is valid under most experimental conditions.

Deuterium is usually the label of choice, being the cheapest and most easily obtained. The subject drinks a precisely weighed dose of deuterium oxide (D_2O), usually diluted in water, and samples of body water (usually saliva or urine) are collected at intervals for 3–6 hours to measure the relative abundance of D_2O and H_2O. D_2O concentration at steady state is then divided into the weight of the dose administered, to yield the TBW content. The method is amenable to use in various settings outside the laboratory, although sophisticated methods – mass spectrometry or Fourier-Transform Infrared Spectroscopy (FITR) – are required to measure the abundance of the isotope within the samples. With careful attention to detail, TBW can be measured with a precision and accuracy of 1–2% for both adults and children (Van Marken Lichtenbelt, Westerterp and Wouters, 1994; Sopher et al., 2004)

Dual energy X-ray absorptiometry

Dual energy X-ray absorptiometry (DEXA) is most commonly used to assess bone mineral density (BMD) in the vertebral column and femoral neck to determine osteoporosis risk. Many machines can also measure whole-body bone mineral content (BMC), and because X-rays are attenuated differently by bone and soft tissues, DEXA can also be used to estimate regional and whole-body composition.

The scanner detects X-rays that are generated at two discrete energies, typically 140 keV and 70 keV. This allows two components to be distinguished in each pixel, initially bone and soft tissue, or in those pixels that do not contain bone, fat and fat-free tissue (Jebb, 1997). Sequential scanning along the length of the body allows an image of bone, fat and fat-free tissue to be built up (Figure 3.4).

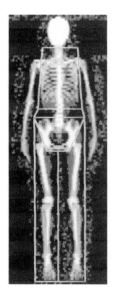

	BMD (g/cm^2)	BMC (g)	Lean mass (g)	Fat mass (g)
Head	2.65	616	2,766	6,668
Trunk	0.97	897	15,651	9,533
Abdomen	1.10	380	7,554	4,181
Arms	0.86	351	4,249	3,888
Legs	1.01	882	12,446	7,272
Total	1.13	2,746	35,113	21,361

Figure 3.4 Whole-body DEXA scan, of a woman with a BMI of 22 kg/m². Regional body composition, measured in the sectors indicated on the scan, is shown in the panel on the right. BMD: bone mineral density; BMC: bone mineral content.

Regional BMC, FM and FFM data can be determined for the trunk, head, limbs and abdomen.

The dose of radiation received during each whole-body scan depends on the type of scanner, but is typically 1–3 µSv, less than the total daily background radiation dose to the whole body (Njeh *et al.*, 1999). Nonetheless, this method must conform to local Radiation Protection guidelines. Scanning extremely obese subjects can be problematic, in that the bed may not hold their weight and/or the scanning surfaces may not be wide enough; newer machines are addressing these practical issues. Even for moderately overweight subjects, regional analysis becomes very difficult because the limbs cannot be separated easily from the trunk. As DEXA measurements are influenced by the thickness of body tissues, results may be affected by substantial changes of weight and/or extremes of body size.

A typical coefficient of variation for whole-body BMC is around 1.4% (Tothill, Avenell and Reid, 1994a), and for fat mass around 2.6% (Tothill, Avenell and Reid, 1994b). With the widespread availability of DEXA scanners, this is an increasingly popular technique to measure body composition.

Bioelectrical impedance (Bioimpedance)

Numerous devices are now available to measure bioelectrical impedance, that is, the resistance to a weak (100 µA) current generated by a small battery. The underlying principle is that lean tissue is a more efficient conductor than fat, because of its water and electrolyte content. Using height as a proxy for conductor length, bioimpedance can provide a measure of total body water (TBW) and, assuming a known and constant hydration fraction for fat-free tissue, FFM can be estimated and body fat then calculated as the difference from total body weight.

The current is applied to the body using electrodes attached to the skin, sensors on a footplate, or metal handles that are gripped (Figure 3.5). Measurements are usually made from hand to foot, or foot to foot. Measurements across each of these sites can allow impedance in different segments of the body to be determined, and thus regional body composition to be estimated; however, the accuracy of segmental and regional measurements remains uncertain. Some models apply the current at multiple frequencies to distinguish between different body water compartments. At the standard frequency (50KHz), the

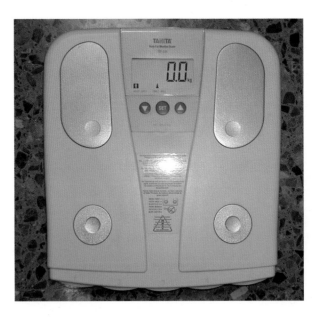

Figure 3.5 Measurement of bioelectrical impedance (bioimpedance) using a commercially available unit. The electrical resistance of the body, measured using a weak current delivered through the foot plate, is used to derive total body water and fat-free mass.

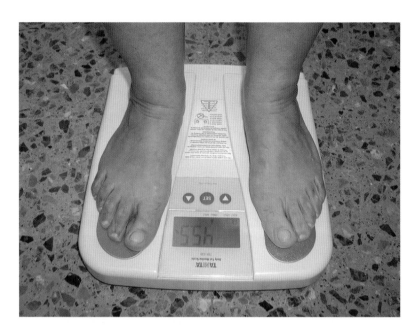

Figure 3.5 (*Continued*)

current overcomes the capacitance of the cell membrane and thus measures total body water, whereas lower frequencies detect only extra-cellular water; the intracellular water content may therefore be calculated. This modified technique may allow body composition to be measured in oedematous subjects.

In groups of subjects, whole-body measurements of TBW, FFM and fat mass using bioimpedance show good agreement with deuterium dilution, densitometry and DEXA (Jebb *et al.*, 2000). At an individual level, bioimpedance is generally superior to skinfold thickness measurements, with within- and between-subject coefficients of variation of around 1–2% in determining body fat mass. Moreover, bioimpedance provides a good estimate of the composition of weight change in individuals, presumably because geometrical assumptions of the method are consistent within the same subject (Jebb *et al.*, 2006). The apparatus is quick and convenient to use, and units are now relatively inexpensive.

Measurements of fat distribution

The importance of abdominal fat as a risk factor for insulin resistance and the metabolic syndrome has focused attention on the measurement of body fat in specific depots. In the idealized 'reference man' (Ellis, 2000) most adipose tissue (~85%) is subcutaneous, with much of the remainder within the abdomen and a small amount in the mediastinum and around the heart (see Chapters 4 and 12). The amount of intra-abdominal fat is influenced by gender, age, race and ethnicity, habitual physical activity and overall adiposity (Rodriguez *et al.*, 2007). The term 'visceral' fat is commonly used to describe intra-abdominal adipose tissue, which includes both intraperitoneal fat (i.e. mesenteric and omental fat), which drains directly into the portal system, and retroperitoneal fat, which drains into the systemic venous circulation. The portal venous drainage of intraperitoneal fat means that its products have particular impact on the liver, which is relevant to the metabolic consequences of visceral obesity (see Chapter 10).

Magnetic resonance (MR) and computed tomography (CT) imaging are considered 'gold-standard' methods for determining the quantity of subcutaneous abdominal adipose tissue (SAT) and visceral-abdominal adipose tissue (VAT). There is growing interest in novel, non-invasive approaches to measuring body shape and composition, such as 3-D imaging (Wells, Treleaven and Cole, 2007) and ultrasound technologies (Gong *et al.*, 2007), respectively.

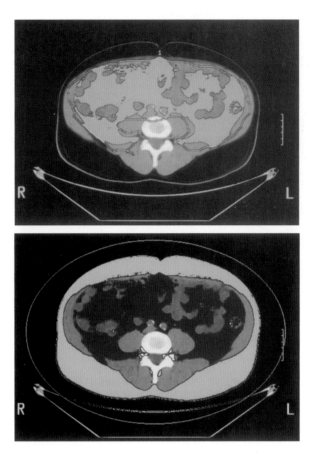

Figure 3.6 CT images of the abdomen (at L4/L5 level) of a man with central obesity, with visceral (upper panel) and subcutaneous fat (lower panel) highlighted in yellow. Reproduced by kind permission of Professor Luc van Gaal.

Computed tomography (CT) imaging

CT scans provide high-resolution cross-sectional areas of adipose tissue, muscle and bone at any body site (Ross, 2003), with a within-subject coefficient of variation for measuring adipose tissue volumes of <1% (see Figure 3.6). Stacks of single-plane CT images can be assembled to reconstruct a 3-D image; this can also be produced by the newer technique of spiral CT. The high cost of CT scanning and the significant exposure to ionizing radiation limit its use for body composition measurements.

Magnetic resonance (MR) imaging

MR spectroscopy and imaging are based on the principle that applying a powerful magnetic field (typically 1.5 Tesla, about 10 000 times the strength of the Earth's magnetic field) to the body causes its protons to align with the field; when a radiofrequency pulse is then applied, the protons return to their original state, releasing the energy absorbed. The resulting signal intensity is determined by the local concentration of protons and other properties, notably the 'relaxation time' of the various tissues.

A whole-body scan is rapid (~30 seconds) and involves no radiation exposure; MRI is therefore well suited to obtaining multiple slice images from which the whole body can be reconstructed. Fat and lean tissue can be highlighted by adjusting the scan conditions, and the volume of various adipose tissue depots can be determined (Figure 3.7). MRI is also useful in determining abdominal body composition at a single transverse level, conventionally at L4–L5.

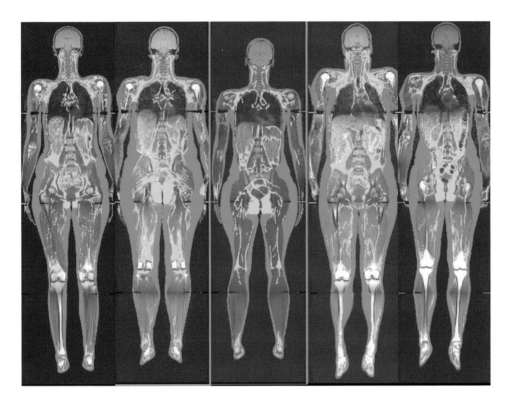

Figure 3.7 MRI whole-body scans and fat maps of young adult women (24–30 y), each of whom has a BMI around 25 kg/m². Total body fat is subdivided into subcutaneous fat (green) and visceral fat (yellow). Abdominal fat can be further subdivided for anatomical and metabolic studies, according to horizontal reference planes at the top of the liver and the top of the femoral heads. Note the marked differences in subcutaneous and internal fat masses, even at comparable BMI. Images courtesy of Prof. Jimmy D. Bell, MRI Unit, Imaging Sciences Department, MRC Clinical Sciences Centre, Hammersmith Hospital, Imperial College London, UK.

The precision of MRI is poorer than CT; the coefficient variation for repeated measures of subcutaneous adipose tissue in an individual ranges from 1 to 10%, and for visceral adipose tissue from 5 to 11% (Després, Ross and Lemieux, 1996). MRI has been used to demonstrate the preferential loss of visceral fat during exercise regimens (Ross *et al.*, 2000).

Measuring energy balance

Excess fat accumulates when energy intake consistently exceeds energy expenditure. The relative importance of intake and expenditure in the aetiology of obesity has been much debated (see Chapter 8), and various methodological errors and uncertainties have helped to cloud this issue. Accurate measurements of dietary intake and energy expenditure are important in understanding the aetiology of obesity, and can

also help to establish an individualized approach to weight management.

Dietary assessment

The assessment of dietary intake presents challenges to both clinicians and researchers. Both prospective and retrospective methods have been used (see Table 3.4). The method must be chosen on a case-by-case basis, and guided by the objectives of the study or clinical situation, the aims of the dietary assessment and the types of dietary data required. The costs, including the personnel and other resources needed to manage and analyse the data must also be considered, together with the characteristics of the study population, including cognitive ability, literacy and cultural factors.

For detailed individual estimates of habitual intake, dietary recall records over several days are

Table 3.4 Common dietary assessment methods.

	Dietary assessment method	Description	Analysis	Advantages	Disadvantages
Prospective Collects information about current intake	Weighed or estimated food records	Usually a written log of food consumption and preparation during a specific time period	Food records require coding by trained personnel with access to nutritional expertise	Assesses actual or usual diet of individuals	Costly and time-consuming to analyse
	The 7-day dietary record was considered the 'gold standard' in dietary assessment	Maintaining the food record either by digital recording or electronically is possible	Nutritional database required for analysis	If of sufficient length may capture diet variability	High burden on respondent, especially if longer-term
		Quantified by weighing foods, or estimated by household measures, food photographs, food models or by duplicate portions Several days required to evaluate habitual intake	Provides mean daily intake for energy and nutrients	Does not rely on subject's memory	Requires participants be motivated and literate Habitual eating patterns may be influenced or changed by the recording process
Retrospective Collects information about food intake from previous months or years	Diet history	A trained interviewer asks about habitual dietary intake and patterns over a relatively long period (e.g. a month); structured interview lasting up to 2 hours	As above for nutritional analysis	Detailed information on food intake and habits is obtained	Expensive, labour- intensive and time- consuming
	Method developed by Burke (1947)	Usually includes a 24-hour recall	Additional analyses depend on specific research question		Requires trained and skilled interviewer Method relies on subject's memory
	Food recalls	A trained interviewer asks about food and drink consumed during a specified time for example previous 24 hours	Analysis as for food records	Respondent burden is relatively low	Single 24-hour recall may not be representative of habitual intake; may be useful for group studies

Method	Description	Advantages	Disadvantages
	Can be conducted in person or by phone Food portions estimated by household measures, food photographs or food models Provides mean daily intake for energy and nutrients Repeated 24 hours required to assess individual intake Number of repeat days will depend on nutrients of interest for example 3–10 days for total energy and macronutrient intakes	Procedure does not alter food intake patterns Literacy not required Short interview (e.g. 20 minutes), compared with a diet history	Method dependent on respondent's recall ability Participant recall may be intentionally selective Expensive to administer; phone interviews can reduce cost Multiple recall days increases time and cost of analysis
Food Frequency Questionnaire (FFQ) The best known FFQs are by Willet (Willett et al., 1985) and Block (Block et al., 1986)	Respondents report how often they have consumed foods from a set list over a specified time- period for example 6–12 months The number of questions asked can vary widely (e.g. 20–200) Can be semi-quantitative Often self- administered Computer based questionnaires available Some FFQs can be scanned electronically for analysis Semi-quantitative questionnaires are used to provide nutritional intake data	Relatively cheap to administer and analyse Rapid method of assessment Suitable for large-scale studies investigating disease risk or prevalence Low respondent burden Ranks individuals into broad consumption categories Can provide nutrient intake data	Cognitively demanding; unsuitable for children and elderly Memory of food patterns in the past is required Quantification may be inaccurate, due to reliance on standard portions Accuracy of this method for providing nutritional data is unclear

appropriate and flexible. For some epidemiological purposes, it may be adequate to rank individuals as high, medium or low consumers of specific foods or nutrients, when a food-frequency questionnaire may be used.

Some limitations apply. A single recall or record is only suitable for group analysis (Gibson, 2005). A food-frequency questionnaire developed in one population may not be suitable for use in another, due to differences in food habits. Grouping of particular foods may not be appropriate for the analysis of all diet-health relationships: for example, a questionnaire developed to segregate high-fibre from low-fibre foods will not adequately distinguish between high and low glycaemic index foods. Finally, seasonal effects on food intake should also be considered.

Advances in technology have improved assessment techniques and reduced the burden on both respondent and interviewer. Ongoing research into the cognitive processes involved in the recall of food intake has led to the development of the 'multiple pass recall', which is a staged process building on an initial quick list of foods reported eaten the previous day. Each successive stage is known as a 'pass'. An automated version of this technique was recently used in the US Department of Agriculture national food survey (Raper et al., 2004). Dietary assessment in children and the elderly can pose particular problems due to immaturity or cognitive impairment, and surrogate reporters (e.g. parents or carers) may be required.

Errors, either systematic or random, can affect dietary assessment at all stages of collecting and analysing data (Gibson, 2005). Increasing the number of observations can reduce random errors due to diet variability, and using standard protocols throughout dietary assessment and data processing can decrease mistakes.

Errors associated with the assessment tool and biases introduced by the respondents can be problematic. Under-reporting of dietary intake is widespread, particularly in the obese who consistently fail to account for up to one-third of their total daily energy intake. This was originally described by Prentice et al. (1986) and has been confirmed in a review of the validity of reported energy intake (Livingstone and Black, 2003). Over-reporting is unusual, but can occur in children. Influences such as social desirability may distort dietary assessments: respondents may provide the response expected by the questioner rather than the true one. The estimation

of portion size is particularly troublesome, and can be subject to systematic error. The development of statistical models to overcome bias is an active area of research (Kipnis et al., 2002).

Validity refers to the accuracy (i.e. the 'truth') of the measure, while reliability describes the precision or repeatability. It is possible for a tool to be precise but not accurate. Many dietary assessments have been 'validated' – or more correctly, their relative validity has been assessed against other reference techniques. As far as possible, the reference tool should not be subject to the same systematic errors as the comparison tool. Independent validation is therefore preferable. This can be done by using nutritional biomarkers that are related in a dose-dependent way to a particular nutrient, for example urinary nitrogen as a marker of protein intake (Bingham, 2002).

Biomarkers can also be used to assess the validity of dietary data obtained (Livingstone and Black, 2003), as can the measurement or estimation of energy expenditure. Energy expenditure can be measured by doubly labelled water, or estimated from basal metabolic rate (BMR) and physical activity level (see below). Plausible and implausible reported energy intakes can be identified using the Goldberg cut-off (Goldberg et al., 1991; Black, 2000), which compares the subject's reported energy intake (expressed as a multiple of BMR) with total energy expenditure calculated from BMR and physical activity; in steady state, energy intake equals expenditure. The method is applicable to those in energy balance and takes into account the number of subjects studied and the numbers of days of measurement; it is not appropriate in those trying to lose weight or in growing children. More recently individualised estimates of energy expenditure have been used to examine the accuracy of dietary records in national surveys (Rennie et al., 2005; Rennie, Coward and Jebb, 2007).

Some situations may not require a quantitative assessment. These methods also allow the structured collection of qualitative data that allow the practitioner to match dietary advice to the subject's habitual eating behaviour, or as a platform to explore areas where change is needed. For research studies focusing on a particular aspect of dietary change, tailored questionnaires may be developed to probe specific behaviours such as consumption of fruit and vegetables and low-fat or high-fibre foods.

Energy expenditure

Total energy expenditure comprises three main elements: basal metabolism, thermogenesis and physical activity (Figure 3.8). Various methods are available to measure or estimate these components and total energy expenditure, and are described below.

Individual energy requirements and expenditure vary widely, mainly according to body size and composition, gender, age and physical activity levels. Special circumstances such as active growth, pregnancy and the catabolic response to trauma can also influence energy expenditure.

Body weight and composition are key determinants of total energy expenditure (TEE). Lean (fat-free) mass is broadly proportional to basal metabolic rate (BMR), which usually accounts for about two-thirds of TEE (Figure 3.8). As fat mass increases with obesity, lean mass also rises (although not as rapidly). Energy expenditure is therefore higher in obese subjects than in the lean, and as energy intake must equal output at steady rate, it follows that an obese person's intake must be higher than for a lean subject, in order to maintain the greater weight (Figure 3.9). Apart from profound hypothyroidism, there are no known exceptions to this rule – an important practical point when explaining and managing the causes of obesity in a clinical setting. Average adult values for daily energy expenditure are generally 2000–2500 kcal; the lowest levels recorded (in terminally malnourished subjects) were ~900 kcal/day.

Energy is generated mainly by the oxidation of carbohydrate (which yields 4 kcal/g) and fat

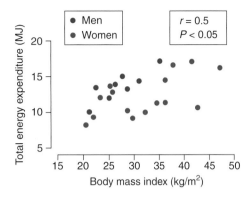

Figure 3.9 Relationship between BMI and total energy expenditure (TEE). TEE rises with increasing BMI and is higher in obese than in lean subjects. From Ravussin *et al.* (1982). *American Journal of Clinical Nutrition*, 35: 566–73.

(9 kcal/g), each of which contribute 40–45% of total basal requirements. Most of the remainder is provided by oxidation of amino acids derived from protein breakdown, yielding 4 kcal/g (see Chapter 7).

Tissue synthesis and maintenance demand additional energy cost in growing infants, children, pregnant and lactating women, as do tissue breakdown or repair due to disease or trauma. These extra energy costs may be reflected in some or all of the measurements discussed below, but are difficult to quantify; estimates are usually derived from stoichiometric equations based on rates and composition of weight gain or loss, milk production, tissue synthesis and the effects of infection or trauma (FAO/WHO/UNU, 2004; Elia, 1992a, 1992b).

Basal metabolic rate (BMR)

BMR is the minimum energy expenditure required to maintain essential functions (breathing, circulation, body temperature, autonomic activities) that sustain life. Compared with adults, infants and growing children have a higher BMR relative to body size. After adolescence, the main determinants of BMR are weight and particularly FFM (Figure 3.9). Generally, BMR is higher in men than in women of equivalent surface area, and it declines gradually with age in both genders (Schofield, 1985; FAO/WHO/UNU, 2004). As already mentioned and contrary to popular belief, BMR is always higher in obese than in lean subjects because of the greater energy costs of

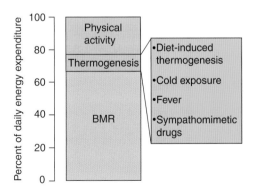

Figure 3.8 Energy expenditure and its components in humans.

maintaining lean and fat tissue (Prentice *et al.*, 1986; see Figure 3.11). Skeletal muscle – the main component of fat-free mass – accounts for about 30% of BMR, other quantitatively important tissues being the viscera (25%), brain (20%) and heart (10%) (see Chapter 7).

BMR can be measured accurately and reproducibly (coefficient of variation <2%) using the indirect calorimetric techniques described below. Standard conditions must be observed, with the subject fasted for 13 hours, and immediately upon waking, lying at complete rest but awake, at a thermoneutral ambient temperature of 24 °C (Schofield *et al.*, 1985; FAO/WHO/UNU, 2003). Measurements can be made over a few minutes or up to an hour, and results expressed as kJ/min or MJ/day as appropriate. Many investigators measure resting metabolic rate (RMR) for which the conditions are less stringent, typically 2 hours post-absorptive, and/or at unspecified time of day and/or sitting and/or having had a period of rest after arriving at the laboratory. Sleeping metabolic rate (which represents 90–100% of BMR) is also less demanding and can be used as a proxy for BMR.

BMR can also be estimated by predictive equations using weight, age, gender and physical activity level (Table 3.5). These formulae are reasonably accurate, provided that appropriate population-specific equations are used.

Thermogenesis

Thermogenesis is the energy expended above BMR through factors other than exercise. These include physiological responses to the ingestion of food (diet-induced thermogenesis: the energy costs of digesting, absorbing, utilizing and storing ingested nutrients), exposure to cold (shivering) or heat (sweating), and compounds such as alcohol, nicotine, caffeine and some thermogenic drugs (see Chapter 7).

The effect of food depends on the size and macronutrient composition of the meal ingested, but generally is equivalent to about 10% of the total energy content of a mixed meal or diet (Goran and Astrup, 2002). In rodents, an important heat-producing tissue is brown adipose tissue (BAT); this is present in human neonates but atrophies and eventually disappears through infancy (See Chapter 4).

Thermogenesis can be measured using indirect calorimetry, as the energy expended above BMR under the test conditions.

Physical activity

Physical activity comprises all bodily movements produced by the contraction of skeletal muscle and, in healthy adults under normal circumstances, is the part of TEE not accounted for by BMR and thermogenesis. Physical activity is the most variable component of energy expenditure, and may account for 15–30% of an individual's TEE, depending on occupation, lifestyle and exercise habits; strenuous and weight-bearing activities expend more energy than light or sedentary ones. Physical activity can be measured and expressed in absolute terms (kJ/min, MJ/day) or expressed as the physical activity level (PAL) that is the ratio of TEE:BMR.

Various methods can measure the energy cost, types and patterns of movement and the physiological responses to activity, but no single technique can cover all these aspects (Wareham and Rennie, 1998). In free-living people, this is the most difficult component of energy expenditure to measure, and because it is the most variable, is the most difficult to predict.

Table 3.5 Formulae to calculate BMR and total energy expenditure (TEE) in men and women. From FAO/WHO/UNU, Technical Report Series Vol 724. Geneva: WHO 1985

BMR (MJ/24h): Age	Men	Women
18–30	(0.063 × weight) + 2.896	(0.062 × weight) + 2.036
31–60	(0.048 × weight) + 3.653	(0.034 × weight) + 3.538
>60	(0.049 × weight) + 2.459	(0.038 × weight) + 2.755
Total energy expenditure: BMR ×	• 1.55 (light activity) • 1.79 (moderate activity) • 2.10 (very heavy activity)	• 1.56 (light activity) • 1.64 (moderate activity) • 1.82 (very heavy activity)

Weight in kg. Conversion factor: 0.43 MJ = 100 kcal.

Habitual physical activity is usually estimated from self-recall (through questionnaires, diaries or logs), or by monitoring body movement (using accelerometers or pedometers) or physiological responses such as heart rate; direct recording by an observer is occasionally used in children (Table 3.6).

Numerous questionnaires are available, and the commonly used tools, together with their validation, have been comprehensively reviewed (Kriska *et al.*, 1997). The use of accelerometers combined with a log book has been cited as the best method for assessing the validity of self-recall questionnaires (Ainsworth *et al.*, 2000). As

Table 3.6 Methods to assess physical activity, with their main advantages and disadvantages.

Measure	Advantages	Disadvantages
Self-report	Captures quantitative and qualitative information	Reliability and validity may be reduced by poor recall of activities
	Inexpensive, allowing large sample size	Potential problems with content validity due to misinterpretation of physical activity in different populations
	Usually low participant burden	
	Can be administered quickly	
	Information available to estimate energy expenditure from daily living	
Activity monitors	Objective indicator of body movement (acceleration)	High cost may prohibit assessment of large numbers of participants
	Useful in both field and laboratory settings	Inaccurate assessment of a large range of activities (e.g. upper body movement, incline walking, swimming)
	Provides an indicator of intensity, frequency and duration	Lack of field-based equations to accurately estimate energy expenditure in specific populations
	Non-invasive	Cannot guarantee accurate monitor placement on participants during long, unobserved periods of data collection
	Ease of data collection and analyses	
	Provides minute-by-minute information	
	Allows extended periods of recording (weeks)	
Heart rate monitoring	Physiological parameter	Cost may prohibit assessment of large numbers of participants
	Good association with energy expenditure	Some discomfort for participants especially over extended recording periods
	Valid in laboratory and field settings	Useful only for aerobic activities
	Low participant burden for limited recording periods (30 minutes to 6 hours)	Heart rate characteristics and the subject's training state can affect interpretation
	Describes intensity, frequency and duration well (adults)	Accurate prediction of energy expenditure from heart rate remains uncertain
	Easy and quick for data collection and analyses	
	Potential to provide participants with educational information	

(Continued)

Table 3.6   (*Continued*)

Measure	Advantages	Disadvantages
Pedometers	Inexpensive, non-invasive	Loss of accuracy when jogging or running is assessed
	Potential for use in a wide variety of settings, including workplace and school	Possibility of participant tampering
	Easy to administer to large groups	Specifically designed to assess walking only
	Potential to promote behaviour change	
	Objective measure of common activity behaviour (i.e. walking)	
Direct observation	Provides excellent quantitative and qualitative information	Time-intensive training needed to establish between-observer and within-observer agreement
	Physical activity categories established *a priori*, allowing specific targeting of physical activity behaviours	Labour-intensive and time-intensive data collection, which limits the number of participants
	Software programs now available to enhance data collection and recording	Observer's presence may change the subject's normal physical activity patterns
		Limited research reporting on validation of direct observation coding systems against physiological criteria

Adapted from: D. Dale, G.J. Wells and C.E. Matthews; Chapter 1: Methods for assessing physical activity and challenges for research. In Welk (2002) *Physical Activity Assessments for Health Related Research*, Champaign, IL, Human Kinetics.

well as being validated in a representative population, questionnaires should be unambiguous and cover the relevant dimensions of physical activity, such as leisure time, gardening, household chores, active transport (walking, cycling) and occupational. The International Physical Activity Questionnaire (IPAQ) has recently been developed as a valid measure suitable for between-country comparisons. A short-format questionnaire is useful for surveillance, whereas a longer version is suitable for more detailed assessment; both versions are available in many languages (http://www.ipaq.ki.se/).

Activity monitors typically use an electronic component within the device to register the acceleration of the body in a single dimension (uniaxial) or in multiple dimensions (Dale *et al.*, 2002). It is important to note that movement of the hip (or wherever the monitor is worn) is assessed, not the absolute acceleration of the person, and that accelerometers do not detect a complete range of body movement: bicycling or upper-body work and its intensity are not captured. A practical point is that most monitors cannot be worn in water and cannot be used to evaluate swimming. Activity monitors have been extensively validated in both children and adults (Dale *et al.*, 2002). The cut-off values of movement counts that relate to intensity levels of exercise are somewhat arbitrary, and accurate energy expenditure prediction equations for free-living individuals have not yet been developed for certain populations.

Heart rate monitoring can be used to measure physical activity, and above a threshold known as the 'flex heart rate', there is a linear relationship between heart rate and energy expenditure by large muscle groups; moderate and vigorous activity can be defined from heart rate once this threshold is exceeded. This is important because heart rate can change considerably under these conditions, but energy expenditure much less so.

Heart rate is also affected by many other factors, such as environmental conditions and psychological state. The estimation of energy expenditure from heart rate can be improved by individual calibration equations, which include the measurement of resting energy expenditure, and/or by using statistical models that account for influences on heart rate such as sex, age and fitness level. It has also been shown that the type of muscular contraction affects the linear relationship between heart rate and energy expenditure (Janz, 2002). Recently, a movement sensor has been combined with measurements of heart rate to predict energy expenditure related to physical activity, and one such device has been validated (Brage *et al.*, 2005).

Choice of methods

Each approach yields different information. Questionnaires and diaries provide details of specific activities and their duration, and can be used to estimate energy expenditure by making assumptions about the relative energy expended (the 'metabolic equivalents' or 'METS') with each activity category. A compendium of METS for a wide range of activities has been compiled (Ainsworth *et al.*, 2000).

Accelerometers provide a summary of overall activity 'counts' and may be combined with a diary to provide more detail. Intensity of activity is best measured by heart rate. The energy expended through specifically physical activity is best measured by a combination of doubly-labelled water and indirect calorimetry (see below).

The method to measure physical activity should be selected according to the purpose of the evaluation, the nature of the study population, the resources available and the limitations of the various techniques. Measuring physical activity in children demands particular considerations (Sirard and Pate, 2001). Where self-reported assessments are used, questionnaires should have been suitably validated. The measurement of physical activity will continue to advance as technology develops, for example with the application of Global Positioning System (GPS) methods.

Indirect calorimetry

Indirect calorimetry (respirometry) uses gas exchange (O_2 consumption, CO_2 generation) to measure the rate at which heat is produced by the body and thus energy expenditure. Each litre of O_2 consumed and each litre of CO_2 produced is associated with a known amount of heat, the 'energy equivalent'. Indirect calorimetry can be based on O_2 consumption, CO_2 production or both. Energy expenditure can be inferred mainly from consumption of O_2, which reflects the oxidation of endogenous or dietary macronutrients to release heat; the total contribution of CO_2 to energy expenditure is relatively trivial. If energy expenditure alone is to be measured, only O_2 consumption needs to be quantified (see Chapter 7).

To evaluate the contributions of different nutrients to energy expenditure, CO_2 generation has to be measured as well, when knowledge of the respiratory quotient (RQ) can be exploited. RQ is the (volume of CO_2 generated)/(volume of O_2 consumed) when nutrients are oxidized. Oxidation of fat has an RQ of 0.7 and of carbohydrate, 1.0. At rest and during moderate exercise, and with a normal diet the whole-body RQ is about 0.8–0.85, indicating that roughly equal proportions of fat and carbohydrate are being oxidized; with increasingly heavy exercise, the RQ rises progressively towards 1.0, reflecting the preponderance of carbohydrate utilization. Unlike carbohydrate and fat, which are ultimately broken down to water and CO_2, protein is not metabolized completely and nitrogenous compounds are excreted in urine. Protein oxidation can therefore be inferred by measuring urinary nitrogen and applying an appropriate constant that relates nitrogen excretion to protein oxidation. Macronutrient oxidation rates are calculated from the net oxidation of fat and carbohydrate, expressed in terms of O_2 consumption, CO_2 production and nitrogen excretion (Murgatroyd, Shetty and Prentice, 1993).

Indirect calorimetry techniques include the classic Douglas bag (which collects expired air for analysis of O_2 and CO_2 after breathing for a known time) and various automated bedside or portable equipment using masks or hoods with continuous gas analysis (Figure 3.10). These methods are useful for measuring energy expenditure over short periods of time, for example for BMR, resting or sleeping energy expenditure, after eating, or during exercise.

Minute-by-minute changes in energy expenditure over hours or longer can be measured accurately using whole-body calorimeters, or respiration chambers. The chamber is a well-sealed room, ventilated with a constant and

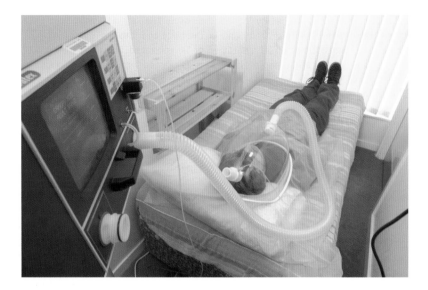

Figure 3.10 Measuring energy expenditure with a portable indirect calorimetry system ('ventilated hood').

measured supply of fresh air. Samples of well-mixed air are drawn off for analysis and the differences in O_2 and CO_2 concentrations in the ingoing and outgoing air are calculated. Depending on the protocol and equipment used, the data can be manipulated to yield BMR, thermogenesis, exercise and physical activity and macronutrient oxidation.

Whole-body chambers are comfortably furnished, and subjects are not impeded by close-fitting apparatus; most include a bed, chair, desk, television and exercise equipment (cycle ergometer, step block, treadmill), and some also have an inbuilt toilet and showers. Food and drink and other necessary items, and urine and faecal samples, are passed in and out of the chamber through separate air-lock hatches. Some chambers also including a hermetically-sealed hatch for collecting blood samples from the subject's arm. Measurement periods are typically 24 or 36 hours, but can be up to 14 days. The technique is most valuable for assessing within-subject responses, or the effects of manipulations of diet or activity, or changes in physiological state such as pregnancy, weight loss or gain. Whole-body calorimetry is not appropriate for those who need close care (e.g. infants, young children, or frail, ill or other vulnerable people).

Whole-body calorimetry enables very accurate and precise measurement to be made of 24-hr energy expenditure and its components, with a within-subject coefficient of variation of TEE measurement of ~1%. It cannot mimic the complexity of all daily activities, but the use of strictly standardized protocols under highly controlled artificial conditions removes behavioural influences on energy balance and allows the underlying physiological mechanisms to be explored (Prentice *et al.*, 1991).

Whole-body calorimetry has provided graphic confirmation of the principle that energy expenditure is greater in obese than in lean subjects (Figure 3.11).

Doubly-labelled water

The doubly-labelled water (DLW) method is an ingenious isotopic tracer technique that allows the CO_2 production rate, integrated over several days, to be calculated (IDECG, 1990; Speakman, 1997). DLW is water labelled with two stable (non-radioactive) isotopes, deuterium ^2H and ^{18}O. ^2H labels the body's water pool and its rate of disappearance from the body (as vapour from the lungs and skin, and in urine, stool, sweat and breast milk) provides a measure of water turnover. ^{18}O labels both the water and bicarbonate (HCO_3^-) pools, which are in equilibrium through the carbonic anhydrase reaction,

$$H_2O + CO_2 \rightleftharpoons H_2CO_3 \rightleftharpoons H^+ HCO_3^-.$$

The disappearance rate of ^{18}O thus reflects the combined turnover of water and HCO_3^-, and HCO_3^- turnover (i.e. the CO_2 production rate) can be calculated as the difference between these two

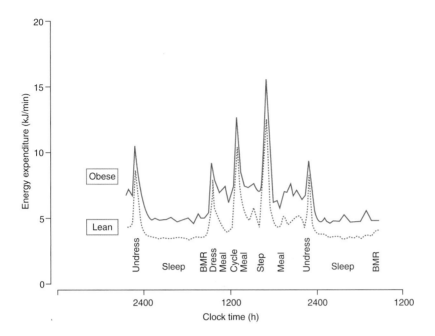

Figure 3.11 Minute-by-minute measurements of energy expenditure, recorded in a whole-body calorimeter chamber, in individual representative obese and lean subjects. Programmed activities at set times during the 37-hour study period are shown. Note that energy expenditure is consistently higher in the obese subject.

rates (Figure 3.12). CO_2 production can then be converted to energy expenditure using classical

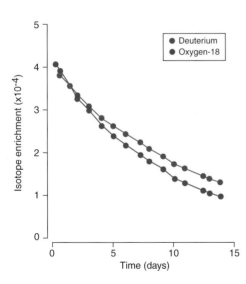

Figure 3.12 The doubly-labelled water technique for measuring average energy expenditure over a period of days. CO_2 production is estimated from the differences between the disappearance curves of ^2H and ^{18}O, following oral administration of $^2H_2$ ^{18}O.

indirect calorimetry equations. After collection of a baseline sample (urine or saliva), the subject drinks an accurately weighed oral loading dose of $^2H_2$ ^{18}O. Over about 14 days, depending on age and physical activity levels, concentrations of the two isotopes return to background levels. Isotope enrichments are measured by mass spectrometry.

DLW can provide a non-invasive measure of total energy expenditure under genuinely free-living conditions, and can be used in any situation where biological samples can be collected (Black *et al.*, 1996; Prentice *et al.*, 1996). Total energy expenditure estimated by DLW, used with predicted or measured BMR, allows the energy expended on physical activity and thermogenesis to be quantified. As the latter is small and reasonably constant, the difference between TEE and BMR essentially represents the energy expended on physical activity. Physical activity levels (PAL = TEE/BMR) can also be calculated (Prentice *et al.*, 1991).

DLW data can also be used to assess body composition, as total body water is measured; and as an independent biomarker of energy intake. However, because DLW gives a measure of total energy expenditure integrated over many days the data cannot be partitioned into the different components of energy expenditure, and different activity patterns within the measurement period cannot be distinguished. Also, the method is not appropriate for short-term measurements over less than several days (see Figure 3.12).

Assessing insulin sensitivity

Important consequences of obesity are type 2 diabetes and its associated metabolic and cardiovascular abnormalities, collectively termed the 'metabolic syndrome' (Chapter 10). The associations are partly explained by excess adiposity interfering with the ability of insulin to exert its normal metabolic and other actions – so-called 'insulin resistance'. The mechanisms through which obesity induces insulin resistance (or decreases insulin sensitivity) are described in detail in Chapter 10; suggested factors include raised levels of free fatty acid (FFA) and the 'ectopic' deposition of triglyceride in key tissues such as liver and skeletal muscle.

Insulin sensitivity is generally measured as insulin's impact on glucose metabolism, and particularly its ability to lower blood glucose concentrations, and this is the basis of the methods described below. However, insulin has many other actions – including the suppression of very low density lipoprotein (VLDL) production by the liver, vasodilation and the stimulation of sympathetic tone – and some of these effects may be impaired to different degrees (or even relatively spared) in individuals found to be 'insulin resistant' by methods that assess glucose metabolism.

Insulin lowers blood glucose both by inhibiting its endogenous production by the liver, and by decreasing its removal from the bloodstream, especially by skeletal muscle. The effect on the liver is quantitatively more important. Insulin inhibits both the processes that contribute to the glucose secreted into the bloodstream, that is, gluconeogenesis (the generation of glucose from other metabolites such as alanine, lactate and pyruvate) and glycogen breakdown (glycogenolysis). Hepatic glucose production maintains the normal fasting and basal blood glucose concentrations and is extremely insulin-sensitive: glucose output is constantly restrained by even low fasting levels of insulin, and is rapidly shut off when insulin concentrations increase after eating. The ability of insulin to suppress endogenous glucose production is referred to as 'hepatic insulin sensitivity', as the main source (usually 90%) is the liver; however, the kidney can also generate glucose through gluconeogenesis.

In skeletal muscle, insulin enhances glucose uptake from the bloodstream (by causing the translocation of GLUT4 glucose transporters from deep within the cytosol to the cell membrane), and then its utilization and storage as glycogen. These processes operate at relatively high insulin concentrations (particularly after eating) and are referred to as 'peripheral' insulin sensitivity. Interestingly, impairment of insulin action in skeletal muscle appears to be less important in causing hyperglycaemia than the failure to restrain hepatic glucose production: individuals with type 2 diabetes often have peripheral insulin resistance that is comparable with (or even less than) that in subjects with IGT or even normoglycaemia.

Insulin sensitivity can be measured in various ways, and with different degrees of complexity and precision. The methods range from simple tests that require a single blood-sample, which are useful in epidemiological studies, to sophisticated laboratory-based research techniques. No single test is suitable for all circumstances (Wallace and Matthews, 2002). Many of the methods described below cannot distinguish between the hepatic and peripheral components, and therefore provide a composite measure of whole-body insulin sensitivity.

Indices from fasting samples

Various methods infer whole-body insulin sensitivity from the relationship between fasting concentrations of insulin and glucose. These methods have the advantages of being simple, inexpensive and non-invasive, and are widely used; however, the information provided is limited because they cannot capture the dynamic changes occurring in response to a glucose challenge.

The underlying rationale for these tests is that an impairment in insulin sensitivity is compensated by increased insulin secretion and therefore higher circulating insulin concentrations; if this compensation is inadequate then circulating glucose levels will also increase (Table 3.7). Indices derived from measurements of fasting glucose and insulin are more indicative of the hepatic rather than the peripheral component of insulin sensitivity.

Table 3.7 Fasting indices of insulin sensitivity, showing representative values in lean and obese subjects.

Index	Formula	Representative values	
		Lean	Obese
Fasting plasma glucose	G_b	4.97	5.15
Fasting plasma insulin	I_b	48.3	71.1
HOMA	Original formula	1.10	0.75
	$\dfrac{156.3}{I_b G_b}$	0.65	0.43
FIRI	$\dfrac{173.6}{I_b G_b}$	0.72	0.47
QUICKI	$\dfrac{1}{Log(2.592 I_b G_b)}$	0.358	0.336
Fasting Belfiori Index	$\dfrac{2 \bar{I_b} \bar{G_b}}{I_b G_b + I_b G_b}$	1.16	0.95
FPG/FPI	$\dfrac{G_b}{I_b}$	0.103	0.072

Notation: G_b fasting plasma glucose (mmol/l), I_b fasting plasma insulin (pmol/l). $\bar{G_b}$ and $\bar{I_b}$ represent population values. All indices are based on the glucose and insulin data reported by Matthews *et al.* (1985). Note that the values yielded by the downloadable HOMA calculator (see text) differ from those derived using the original HOMA formula.

The homeostasis model assessment (HOMA)

This computer-based model, devised by Matthews *et al.* (1985), assumes that a constant basal glucose turnover rate is maintained through the feedback of glucose on the β cells to stimulate insulin secretion, and that for a given fasting blood glucose level, the prevailing insulin concentration reflects both insulin resistance and any degree of β-cell dysfunction. The relationship is complex (Figure 3.13) but can be used to estimate both insulin resistance (IR) and β-cell function (β). By this model, insulin resistance (HOMA-R) is calculated as the product of fasting plasma glucose (in mmol/l) and insulin (mU/l) concentrations, divided by a constant (22.5) that is introduced to produce a 'reference' value of 1.0 for healthy young adults. HOMA-R increases as insulin resistance worsens (see Figure 3.13).

A downloadable calculator, based on HOMA, which produces R and β from fasting plasma glucose and insulin measurements, is available at www.dtu.ox.ac.uk. This version is recalibrated to take into account recent refinements in insulin assays, so that HOMA values obtained from the calculator do not correspond exactly to those derived using the original formula.

HOMA-R values correlate well with values of whole-body insulin resistance obtained by the euglycaemic hyperinsulinaemic clamp (EHC), which is regarded as the gold standard technique (see below).

Other fasting indices

Several other methods based on the [insulin]× [glucose] product have been described (Table 3.7). The FIRI index differs from HOMA only in the normalizing constant, whereas the Quantitative Insulin Sensitivity Check Index (QUICKI) uses the product of log [insulin]×log [glucose], in recognition of the skewed distributions of insulin and glucose concentrations, especially in the context of obesity (Radziuk, 2000). QUICKI is a reliable index for epidemiological work, which correlates with the EHC technique better than HOMA (Katz *et al.*, 2000).

Data from all these methods are difficult to compare between centres because of differences between local insulin assays and thus in the absolute values of insulin concentration obtained. The fasting Belfiori Index was developed to circumvent this problem: plasma insulin and glucose concentrations are related to reference values derived from each laboratory's own reference population.

Legro, Finegood and Dunaif (1998) have suggested that the ratio of fasting glucose to insulin, rather than the product, can be used as an index

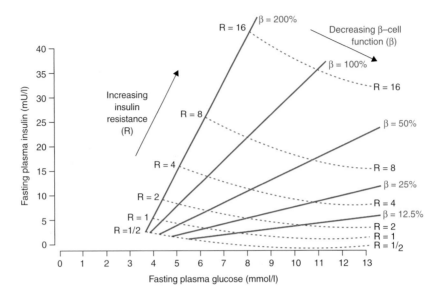

Figure 3.13 Homeostatic model assessment (HOMA) uses fasting plasma glucose and insulin concentrations to estimate both insulin resistance (R) and β-cell function (β), both of which are expressed relative to values in normal lean subjects (R = 1, β = 100%). An individual's levels of insulin resistance and β-cell function can be estimated by plotting the fasting glucose and insulin values on to this grid. Adapted from Matthews *et al.* (1985), with kind permission of the editor of *Diabetologia*.

of insulin sensitivity; reference to Figure 3.13 will confirm that this approach is flawed.

Indices from an oral glucose challenge

The 75-g oral glucose tolerance test (OGTT) is the time-honoured method for diagnosing diabetes and IGT (Alberti and Zimmet, 1999). The conventional test employs two blood samples, one fasted and the second two hours after the glucose challenge, and allows the subject to be categorized as normal glucose-tolerant, impaired fasting glucose, impaired glucose tolerance or diabetes (Table 3.8).

Table 3.8 Definition of states of glucose tolerance. From WHO consultation. *Definition*, Diagnosis and Classification of diabetes *mellitus* Part 1, Geneva: WHO 1999.

		2-h plasma glucose, mmol/l(mg/dl)		
		< 7.8 (140)	7.8–11.0 (140–199)	≥ 11.1(200)
Fasting plasma glucose, mmol/l (mg/dl)	< 6.1 (110)	Normal	IGT	Diabetes on an isolated 2-h hyperglycaemia IPH (isolated postchallenge hyperglycaemia)
	6.1–6.9 (110–125)	IFG	IFG and IGT	
	≥ 7.0 (126)	Diabetes on an isolated fasting hyperglycaemia		Diabetes on both fasting and 2-h hyperglycaemia

IFG, impaired fasting glucose; IGT, impaired glucose tolerance; IPH, isolated postchallenge hyperglycaemia.

Various methods have been proposed to devise measures of insulin sensitivity from the changes in insulin and glucose levels during the OGTT. For these, it is assumed that post-absorptive glucose uptake occurs only by non-insulin dependent routes (Matsuda and DeFronzo, 1999), and that hepatic and peripheral insulin sensitivity are closely related (Matthews et al., 1985).

The complex dynamic changes in plasma insulin after ingesting glucose make it difficult to evaluate insulin sensitivity, and several approaches have been explored. First, and most simply, single insulin and glucose measurements can be made at a defined time-point after the glucose ingestion, as in the Insulin Sensitivity Index (ISI) (Hanson et al., 2000). Second, insulin and glucose values can be averaged over a time-period, such as in the index proposed by Cederholm (Cederholm and Wibell, 1990) and Gutt (Gutt et al., 2000). Here, insulin sensitivity is expressed by estimating glucose disposed of during 2 hours after dosing, and dividing this by the product of [mean blood glucose]×log [mean insulin]. Third, the relationship between the areas under the glucose and insulin curves can be used; one method, analogous to the Belfiori fasting index, estimates insulin sensitivity from the product of the areas under the plasma insulin and glucose concentration-time curves, both related to reference population values (Belfiore, Iannello and Volpicelli, 1998).

Finally, in a refinement of the ISI, the Matsuda or Composite Index (Matsuda and DeFronzo, 1999) uses average plasma concentrations over the 2 hours following a glucose load rather than at a single time-point, and expresses insulin resistance as the geometric mean of this product and HOMA-R (calculated from the fasting sample); this measure is said to take account of both peripheral and hepatic components of insulin sensitivity.

All these approaches are subject to error because of the variability in intestinal glucose absorption.

The minimal model

Unlike most other procedures, the minimal model of glucose kinetics is based on a physiological definition of insulin sensitivity from which quantitative estimates can be obtained. The model was first developed to interpret the results of intravenous glucose tolerance tests (Bergman et al., 1979), but more recently has been adapted

for use with an oral glucose challenge and even a test meal (Bluck, Clapperton and Coward, 2006).

The model assumes that endogenous glucose production (by the liver) is suppressed because insulin levels rise rapidly after glucose administration, and that there are two routes for glucose uptake, one insulin-assisted and the other insulin-independent. As the increase in plasma insulin following intravenous glucose is transient, and yet insulin-dependent disposal lasts much longer, it is assumed that plasma insulin is transported to a 'remote', non-accessible region from where it exerts its action. These assumptions can be embodied in a pair of time-dependent differential equations, which describe the simplest model that explains data originally obtained from intravenous glucose tolerance tests performed in dogs (Bergman et al., 1979). This minimal model yields two parameters. *Glucose effectiveness* (S_G) is defined as the incremental change in the rate of glucose disappearance due to an increment in the circulating glucose, while *insulin sensitivity* (S_I) is defined as the incremental change in glucose effectiveness due to an increment in plasma insulin. Both parameters apply in the basal (fasted) state.

Intravenous glucose tolerance test

Numerous variants exist, but the core protocol involves the intravenous injection of a bolus of about 20 g of glucose (300 mg/kg), followed by frequent blood sampling at defined intervals for the determination of plasma glucose and insulin (Bergman et al., 1979) (Figure 3.14). The acute insulin response following the glucose injection is short-lived and, in subjects whose insulin secretion is impaired, may be insufficient for the precise determination of insulin sensitivity (Yang, Youn and Bergman, 1987); to overcome this problem, circulating insulin levels are augmented by either tolbutamide (Welch and Gebhart, 1987) or insulin itself (Finegood, Hramiak and Dupre, 1990) given intravenously 20 minutes after the glucose bolus. Insulin administration, either as a bolus (Vessby et al., 2001) or short infusion (Toffolo, Cefalu and Cobelli, 1999), is now widely accepted as a standard protocol. The number of samples (~30) required in the original test can be reduced to approximately 12 with only a slight loss of precision (Steil et al., 1993).

Estimation of the S_G and S_I requires nonlinear fitting mathematics, and specific software packages

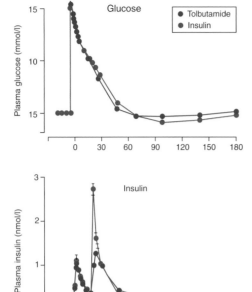

Figure 3.14 The intravenous glucose tolerance test (IVGTT) is used to estimate both insulin sensitivity and 'glucose effectiveness', that is the degree to which a rise in blood glucose per se enhances glucose disposal. Profiles of insulin and glucose are shown during two modified versions of the test, with intravenous injection of tolbutamide or insulin to enhance the endogenous insulin response. Adapted from Saad et al. (1997) *Diabetes* 46: 1167–71.

are commercially available (Boston *et al.*, 2003; Boston *et al.*, 2005). There is good agreement between S_I and insulin sensitivity measures obtained by clamp techniques. The combination of the IVGTT with the minimal model is currently widely used, with around 50 major studies being reported annually.

The addition of a glucose tracer (radioactive or stable label) to the glucose dose allows glucose disposal to be estimated separately from endogenous glucose production (Avogaro *et al.*, 1989; Bluck, Clapperton and Coward, 2005). When data from these studies are analysed in conjunction with those using unlabelled glucose, some anomalies are found, which are probably due to oversimplification of the minimal model. Accordingly, a more sophisticated model of glucose distribution has been proposed (Toffolo and Cobelli, 2003), which provides estimates of S_G and S_I (Vicini, Caumo and Cobelli,

1997), as well as a realistic profile of endogenous glucose production during the course of the test (Vicini *et al.*, 1999).

Minimal model with glucose ingestion

Using the minimal model to investigate the kinetics of glucose disposal after oral glucose is complicated by the unpredictability of glucose absorption from the gut, and is subject to wide inter- and intra-individual variation. Various approaches have been proposed. The meal glucose tolerance test (MGTT) (Steil *et al.*, 2004) describes the absorption of glucose from either a glucose drink or a meal by the simplest possible equation that is predictive of the observed plasma profile, and allows insulin sensitivity to be calculated from simple area under the curve measurements of plasma insulin and glucose. An alternative method uses a parametric model for glucose absorption and has been refined by incorporating isotopically-labelled glucose to allow meal-based glucose to be investigated separately from endogenous release (Dalla Man *et al.*, 2005). In addition, a hybrid method uses oral glucose to provoke the insulin response and an intravenous bolus of tracer to estimate glucose disposal kinetics (Bluck, Clapperton and Coward, 2006). Unlike the other oral tests (which use the original minimal model with a single pool for glucose disposal), this Oral dose intravenous label experiment (ODILE) requires the more sophisticated modelling of the IVGTT.

Euglycaemic hyperinsulinaemic clamp (EHC)

As the name implies, this technique aims to 'clamp' blood glucose concentration at a fixed level within the normal range in the presence of a raised insulin concentration; blood glucose is maintained at the reference value by infusing exogenous glucose at the necessary rate (DeFronzo, Tobin and Andres, 1979). Under hyperinsulinaemic conditions, hepatic glucose production is assumed to be completely suppressed, and glucose disposal to occur solely by uptake into skeletal muscle. Thus, the amount of glucose administered to maintain euglycaemia is a measure of insulin sensitivity: the more glucose required, the greater is the individual's sensitivity.

The procedure is lengthy, complicated and requires near-instantaneous measurements of

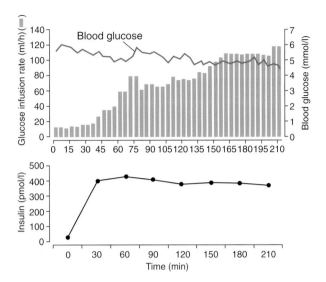

Figure 3.15 The euglycaemic, hyperinsulinaemic clamp (EHC). Insulin is infused intravenously at a constant rate to achieve stable hyperinsulinaemia that maximally stimulates peripheral glucose uptake. Glucose is infused simultaneously and the rate adjusted to maintain blood glucose at ~5 mmol/l. At steady state (the last 30 min of the infusions), the glucose delivery rate equals the glucose disposal rate.

blood glucose so that the glucose infusion rate can be accurately titrated. Soluble insulin is infused intravenously at a fixed rate of 50 mU/kg/h into one arm, together with an infusion of 20% glucose at a variable rate, adjusted on the basis of blood glucose levels (sampled from the other arm) every 5 minutes, to keep blood glucose within the range 4–7 mmol/l. The infusions are continued for 3 hours and steady-state is assumed during the last 30 minutes, when the glucose infusion rate and final blood glucose concentration are measured (Figure 3.15).

Insulin sensitivity can be expressed simply as the average glucose infusion rate during the last 30 minutes of the clamp – which, at a steady rate, equals the glucose disposal rate. Alternatively, the glucose metabolic clearance rate (G_{mcr}) can be derived as (glucose disposal rate)/(steady-state blood glucose level), and the insulin sensitivity index (S_i) as (glucose disposal rate)/(steady-state plasma insulin concentration).

The EHC is generally regarded as the most reliable method for determining insulin sensitivity, and is the 'gold-standard' used to validate other techniques. However, the steady-state insulin concentrations achieved are supraphysiological, and assumptions about glucose disposal break down if individuals lose substantial amounts of glucose in the urine, or (as may happen in cases

with severe hepatic insulin resistance) the output of glucose from the liver is not completely suppressed.

Continuous infusion of glucose with model assessment

This method uses sophisticated computer modelling analogous to that of HOMA to evaluate the relationship between plasma insulin and glucose concentrations when glucose is infused intravenously at a constant rate to raise blood glucose and stimulate insulin secretion (Turner *et al.*, 1979). Measures of both insulin resistance (CIGMA-R) and β-cell function (expressed as a percentage of the 'normal' value found in healthy young adults) can be derived.

The protocol involves infusing glucose (5 mg/kg ideal body weight) for 60 minutes and sampling blood for insulin and glucose levels at near steady-state, during the last 10 minutes. CIGMA-R is calculated as the ratio of final [insulin] to that in 'normal' subjects; the estimation of β-cell efficiency is complicated.

CIGMA measurements of both insulin resistance and β-cell efficiency are relatively reproducible and correlate well with those obtained by the EHC; it is cheap and simple to perform and also avoids the supraphysiological insulin levels of the EHC.

Insulin suppression test (IST)

This method assesses insulin sensitivity from the steady-state plasma glucose concentration when exogenous glucose and insulin are infused together, and in the presence of somatostatin or its analogue, sandostatin, to switch off endogenous insulin secretion (Greenfield *et al.*, 1981). Under steady-state conditions, the final plasma glucose level can be used as an index of insulin resistance.

The insulin tolerance test (ITT)

The ITT measures insulin sensitivity as the rate or fall of plasma glucose, or the total fall during the 15 minutes after an intravenous bolus of insulin. The dose used is small (0.05–0.01 U/kg) to lower blood glucose but without causing clinical hypoglycaemia, which provokes the release of counter-regulatory hormones (glucagon, catecholamines, growth hormone) that antagonize insulin action and aggravate insulin resistance. The simplified version, which measures the fall in glucose over 15 minutes (Akinmokun *et al.*, 1992), requires sampling of 'arterialized' blood (with the hand or arm heated to induce vasodilation) to produce reproducible and valid findings. The fall in glucose correlates closely with measures of insulin sensitivity obtained by the EHC, ISIVGTT and HOMA.

References

Ainsworth, B.E., Haskell, W.L. *et al.* (2000) Compendium of physical activities: an update of activity codes and MET intensities. *Medicine and Science in Sports and Exercise*, **32** (9), S498–S516.

Akinmokun, A. *et al.* (1992) The Short Insulin Tolerance Test for determination of insulin sensitivity – a comparison with the Euglycaemic Clamp. *Diabetic Medicine*, **9** (5), 432–37.

Alberti, K.G.M.M. and Zimmet, P.Z. (1999) *Definition, Diagnosis and Classification of Diabetes Mellitus and its Complications*, World Health Organization, Geneva, pp. 1–59.

Avogaro, A. *et al.* (1989) Stable-Label Intravenous Glucose-Tolerance Test Minimal Model. *Diabetes*, **38** (8), 1048–55.

Belfiore, F. and Iannello, S. (1998) Insulin resistance in obesity: Metabolic mechanisms and measurement methods. *Molecular Genetics and Metabolism*, **65** (2), 121–8.

Belfiore, F., Iannello, S. and Volpicelli, G. (1998) Insulin sensitivity indices calculated from basal and OGTT-induced insulin, glucose, and FFA levels. *Molecular Genetics and Metabolism*, **63** (2), 134–41.

Bergman, R. *et al.* (1979) Quantitative estimation of insulin sensitivity. *American Journal of Physiology*, **236** (6), E667–77.

Bingham, S.A. (2002) Biomarkers in nutritional epidemiology. *Public Health Nutrition*, **5**, 821–7.

Black, A. (2000) Critical evaluation of energy intake using the Goldberg cut-off for energy intake: basal metabolic rate. A practical guide to its calculation, use and limitations. *International Journal of Obesity*, **24**, 1119–30.

Black, A.E., Coward, W.A., Cole, T.J. and Prentice, A.M. (1996) Human energy expenditure in affluent societies: an analysis of 574 doubly-labelled water measurements. *European Journal of Clinical Nutrition*, **50**, 72–92.

Block, G., Hartman, A.M., Dresser, C.M. *et al.* (1986) A data-based approach to diet questionnaire design and testing. *American Journal of Epidemiology*, **124**, 453–69.

Bluck, L.J.C., Clapperton, A.T. and Coward, W.A. (2005) 13C and 2H-labelled glucose compared for minimal model estimates of glucose metabolism in man. *Clinical Science*, **109**, 513–21.

Bluck, L.J.C., Clapperton, A.T. and Coward, W.A. (2006) A stable isotope minimal model protocol with oral glucose administration. *Rapid Communications in Mass Spectrometry*, **20** (3), 493–98.

Boston, R.C. *et al.* (2003) MINMOD Millennium: A computer program to calculate glucose effectiveness and insulin sensitivity from the frequently sampled intravenous glucose tolerance test. *Diabetes Technology and Therapeutics*, **5** (6), 1003–15.

Boston, R.C. *et al.* (2005) AKA-Glucose: A program for kinetic and epidemiological analysis of frequently sampled intravenous glucose tolerance test data using database technology. *Diabetes Technology and Therapeutics*, **7** (2), 298–306.

Brage, S., Brage, N. *et al.* (2005) Reliability and validity of the combined heart rate and movement sensor Actiheart. *European Journal of Clinical Nutrition*, **59** (4), 561–70.

Burke, B. (1947) The dietary history as a tool in research. *Journal of the American Dietetic Association*, **23**, 1041–46.

Cederholm, J. and Wibell, L. (1990) Insulin release and peripheral sensitivity at the oral glucose tolerance test. *Diabetes Research and Clinical Practice*, **10** (2), 167–75.

Cole, T.J., Faith, M.S., Pietrobelli, A. and Heo, M. (2005) What is the best measure of adiposity change in growing children: BMI, BMI %, BMI z-score or BMI centile? *European Journal of Clinical Nutrition*, **59** (3), 419–25.

Coward, W.A., Parkinson, S.A. and Murgatroyd, P.R. (1988) Body composition measurements for nutrition research. *Nutrition Research Reviews*, **1**, 115–24.

Dale, D., Welk, G.J. *et al.* (2002) *Physical Activity Assessments for Health-Related Research* (ed. G.J. Welk), Human Kinetics, Champaign IL.

Dalla Man, C. *et al.* (2005) Measurement of selective effect of insulin on glucose disposal from labelled glucose oral test minimal model. *American Journal of Physiology-Endocrinology and Metabolism*, **289** (5), E909–14.

DeFronzo, R.A., Tobin, J.D. and Andres, R. (1979) Glucose Clamp Technique: a method for quantifying insulin secretion and resistance. *The American Journal of Physiology*, **237** (3), E214–23.

Despres, J.P., Ross, R. and Lemieux, S. (1996) Imaging techniques applied to the measurement of human body composition, in *Human Body Composition* (eds A.F. Roche, S.B. Heymsfield and T.G. Lohman), Human Kinetics, Chicago, IL, pp. 149–66.

Deurenberg, P. and Deurenberg-Yap, M. (2003) Validity of body composition methods across ethnic population groups. *Forum of Nutrition*, **56**, 299–301.

Dewit, O., Fuller, N.J., Fewtrell, M.S. *et al.* (2000) Whole body air displacement plethysmography compared with hydrodensity for body composition analysis. *Archives of Disease in Childhood*, **82** (2), 159–64.

Durnin, J.V.G.A. and Womersely, J. (1974) Body fat assessed from body density and its estimation from skinfold thickness: measurement on 481 mean and women from 16–72 years. *The British Journal of Nutrition*, **32**, 77–97.

Elia, M. (1992a) *Energy Metabolism: Tissue Determinants and Cellular Corollaries* (eds J. Kinney and H.N. Tucker), Raven Press Ltd, New York, pp. 19–47.

Elia, M. (1992b) Organ and tissue contribution to metabolic rate, in *Energy Metabolism: Tissue Determinants and Cellular Corollaries* (eds J. Kinney and H.N. Tucker), Raven Press Ltd, New York, pp. 61–79.

Elia, M. (2001) Obesity in the elderly. *Obesity Research*, **9** (Suppl 4), 244S–248S.

Ellis, K.J. (2000) Human body composition: in vivo methods. *Physiological Reviews*, **80**, 649–80.

Finegood, D.T., Hramiak, I.M. and Dupre, J. (1990) A modified protocol for estimation of insulin sensitivity with the minimal model of glucose kinetics in patients with insulin-dependent diabetes. *Journal of Clinical Endocrinology and Metabolism*, **70** (6), 1538–49.

Fuller, N.J., Jebb, S.A., Laskey, M.A. *et al.* (1992) Four-compartment model for the assessment of body composition in humans: comparison with alternative methods and evaluation of the density and hydration of fat-free mass. *Clinical Science*, **82**, 687–93.

Gibson, R. (2005) *Principles of Nutritional Assessment*, Oxford University Press, Oxford.

Goldberg, G.R., Black, A.E., Jebb, S.A. *et al.* (1991) Critical evaluation of energy intake data using fundamental principles of energy physiology. 1. Derivation of cut-off limits to identify under-recording. *European Journal of Clinical Nutrition*, **45**, 569–81.

Gong, W., Ren, H., Tong, H. *et al.* (2007) A comparison of ultrasound and magnetic resonance imaging to assess visceral fat in the metabolic syndrome. *Asia Pacific Journal of Clinical Nutrition*, **16** (Suppl1), 339–45.

Goran, M.I. Astrup, A., and on behalf of the Nutrition Society (2002) *Introduction to Human Nutrition* (eds M. Gibney, H.H. Vorster and F.J. Kok), Blackwell Science, Oxford.

Greenfield, M.S. *et al.* (1981) Assessment of insulin resistance with the insulin suppression test and the euglycemic clamp. *Diabetes*, **30** (5), 387–92.

Gutt, M. *et al.* (2000) Validation of the insulin sensitivity index (ISI0,120): comparison with other measures. *Diabetes Research and Clinical Practice*, **47** (3), 177–84.

Hanson, R.L. *et al.* (2000) Evaluation of simple indices of insulin sensitivity and insulin secretion for use in epidemiologic studies. *American Journal of Epidemiology*, **151** (2), 190–8.

Heymsfield, S.B., Wang, Z. and Withers, R.T. (1996) *Human Body Composition* (eds A.F. Roche, S.B. Heymsfield and T.G. Lohman), Human Kinetics, UK, pp. 129–47.

IDECG, International Dietary Energy Consultancy Group (1990) *The Doubly-Labelled Water Method for Measuring Energy Expenditure: Technical recommendations for use in humans [AM Prentice ed]*, NAHRES-4, IAEA, Vienna, http://www.unu.edu/unupress/food2/UID05E/uid05e00.htm.

International Physical activity Questionnaire (2007) http://www.ipaq.ki.se/, (accessed 1 August 2007).

Janssen, I., Heymsfield, S.B., Allison, D.B. *et al.* (2002) Body mass index and waist circumference independently contribute to the prediction of nonabdominal, abdominal subcutaneous, and visceral fat. *The American Journal of Clinical Nutrition*, **75** (4), 683–88.

Janz, K.F. (2002) *Physical Activity Assessments for Health Related Research* (ed. G.J. Welk), Human Kinetics, Champaign IL.

Jebb, S.A. (1997) Measurement of soft tissue composition by dual energy X-ray absorptiometry. *The British Journal of Nutrition*, **77** (2), 151–63.

Jebb, S.A., Cole, T.J., Doman, D. *et al.* (2000) Evaluation of the novel Tanita body-fat analyser to measure body composition by comparison with a four-compartment model. *The British Journal of Nutrition*, **83** (2), 115–22.

Jebb, S.A., Murgatroyd, P.R., Goldberg, G.R. *et al.* (1993) *In vivo* measurement of changes in body composition: description of methods and their validation against 12-d continuous whole-body calorimetry. *The American Journal of Clinical Nutrition*, **58** (4), 455–62.

Jebb, S.A., Siervo, M., Murgatroyd, P.R. *et al.* (2006) Validity of the leg-to-leg bioimpedance to estimate changes in body fat during weight loss and regain in overweight women: a comparison of multi-compartment models. *International Journal of Obesity*, **31**, 756–62.

Johnstone, A.M., Rance, K.A., Murison, S.D. et al. (2006) Additional anthropometric measures may improve the predictability of basal metabolic rate in adult subjects. *European Journal of Clinical Nutrition*, **60** (12), 1437–444.

Katz, A. et al. (2000) Quantitative insulin sensitivity check index: A simple, accurate method for assessing insulin sensitivity in humans. *Journal of Clinical Endocrinology and Metabolism*, **85** (7), 2402–10.

Kipnis, V., Midthune, D., Freedman, L. et al. (2002) Bias in dietary-report instruments and its implications for nutritional epidemiology. *Public Health Nutrition*, **5**, 915–23.

Klein, S., Allison, D.B., Heymsfield, S.B. et al. (2007) Association for Weight Management and Obesity Prevention; NAASO, The Obesity Society; American Society for Nutrition; American Diabetes Association. Waist circumference and cardiometabolic risk; a consensus statement from Shaping America's Health: Association for Weight Management and Obesity Prevention; NAASO, The Obesity Society; the American Society for Nutrition; and the American Diabetes Association. *The American Journal of Clinical Nutrition*, **85** (5), 1197–202.

Kriska, A. and Caspersen, C., (ed.) (1997) A collection of physical activity questionnaires. *Medicine and Science in Sports and Exercise*, **29** (Supplement), 1–205.

Lean, M.E., Han, T.S. and Morrison, C.E. (1995) Waist circumference as a measure for indicating need for weight management. *British Medical Journal (Clinical research edition)*, **311** (6998), 158–61.

Legro, R.S., Finegood, D. and Dunaif, A. (1998) A fasting glucose to insulin ratio is a useful measure of insulin sensitivity in women with polycystic ovary syndrome. *Journal of Clinical Endocrinology and Metabolism*, **83** (8), 2694–8.

Livingstone, M. and Black, A. (2003) Markers of the validity of reported energy intake. *Journal of Nutrition*, **133**, 895S–920S.

Lohman, T.G. (1981) Skinfolds and body density and their relation to body fatness: a review. *Human Biology*, **53**, 181–225.

Lukaski, H.C. (1987) Methods for the assessment of human body composition: traditional and new. *The American Journal of Clinical Nutrition*, **46** (4), 537–56.

Matsuda, M. and DeFronzo, R.A. (1999) Insulin sensitivity indices obtained from oral glucose tolerance testing – Comparison with the euglycaemic insulin clamp. *Diabetes Care*, **22** (9), 1462–70.

Matthews, D.R. et al. (1985) Homeostasis Model Assessment – Insulin resistance and beta-cell function from fasting plasma-glucose and insulin concentrations in man. *Diabetologia*, **28** (7), 412–19.

McCrory, M.A., Gomez, T.D., Bernauer, E.M. and Mole, P.A. (1995) Evaluation of a new air displacement plethysmograph for measuring human body composition. *Medicine and Science in Sports and Exercise*, **27** (12), 1686–91.

Murgatroyd, P.R., Shetty, P.S. and Prentice, A.M. (1993) Techniques for the measurement of human energy expenditure: a practical guide. *International Journal of Obesity*, **17**, 549–68.

Njeh, C.F., Fuerst, T., Hans, D. et al. (1999) Radiation exposure in bone mineral density assessment. *Applied Radiation and Isotopes*, **50** (1), 215–36.

Prentice, A.M., Black, A.E., Coward, W.A. et al. (1986) High levels of energy expenditure in obese women. *British Medical Journal*, **292**, 983–7.

Prentice, A.M., Diaz, E.O., Murgatroyd, P.R. et al. (1991) *New Techniques in Nutritional research*. Bristol-Myers Squibb/Mead Johnson Nutrition Symposia (eds R.G. Whitehead and A. Prentice), Academic Press Inc., Cambridge, pp. 177–206.

Prentice, A.M. and Jebb, S.A. (2001) Beyond body mass index. *Obesity Reviews*, **2** (3), 141–7.

Prentice, A.M., Black, A.E., Coward, W.A. and Cole, T.J. (1996) Energy expenditure in overweight and obese adults in affluent societies: an analysis of 319 doubly-labelled water measurements. *European Journal of Clinical Nutrition*, **50**, 93–7.

Radziuk, J. (2000) Insulin sensitivity and its measurement: Structural commonalities among the methods. *Journal of Clinical Endocrinology and Metabolism*, **85** (12), 4426–33.

Raper, N., Perloff, B., Ingwersen, L. et al. (2004) An overview of USDA's dietary intake data system. *Journal of Food Composition and Analysis*, **17**, 545–55.

Rennie, K.L., Jebb, S.A., Wright, A. and Coward, W.A. (2005) Secular trends in under-reporting in young people. *British Journal of Nutrition*, **93** (2), 241–7.

Rennie, K.L., Coward, A. and Jebb, S.A. (2007) Estimating under-reporting of energy intake in dietary surveys using an individualised method. *British Journal of Nutrition*, **97** (6), 1169–76.

Report of a Joint FAO/WHO/UNU Expert Consultation (2004) Human energy requirements. FAO Food and Nutrition Technical Report Series No 1. Rome: Food and Agriculture Organization of the United Nations.

Rodriguez, A., Catalan, V., Gomez-Ambrosi, J. and Fruhbeck, G. (2007) Visceral and subcutaneous adiposity: Are both potential therapeutic targets for tackling the metabolic syndrome? *Current Pharmaceutical Design*, **13** (21), 2169–75.

Ross, R. (2003) Advances in the application of imaging methods in applied and clinical physiology. *Acta Diabetologica*, **40** (Suppl 1), S45–S50.

Ross, R., Goodpaster, B., Kelley, D. and Boada, F. (2000) Magnetic resonance imaging in human body composition research. From quantitative to qualitative tissue measurement. *Annals of the New York Academy of Sciences*, **904**, 12–17.

Saad, M.F., Steil G.M., Kades W.W. et al. (1997) Differences between the tolbutamide-boosted and insulin-modified minimal model protocols. *Diabetes* **46**, 1167–71.

Schoeller, D.A. and Jones, P.J.H. (1987) Measurement of total body water by isotope dilution: A unified approach to calculations, in *In vivo Body Composition Studies* (eds K.J. Ellis, S. Yasumara and W.D. Morgan), The Institute of Physical Sciences in Medicine, London, pp. 13–7.

Schofield, W.N., Schofield, C. and James, W.P.T. (1985). Basal metabolic rate–review and prediction together with an annotated bibliography of source material. *Human Nutrition Clinical Nutrition*, 36CPB, Suppl.

Seidell, J.C. and Flegal, K.M. (1997) Assessing obesity: classification and epidemiology. *British Medical Bulletin*, **53** (2), 238–52.

Sirard, J.R. and Pate, R.R. (2001) Physical activity assessment in children and adolescents. *Sports Medicine*, **31** (6), 439–54.

Siri, W.S. (1961) Body composition from fluid spaces and density: analysis of methods, in *Techniques for measuring body composition* (eds J. Brozek and A. Henschel), Washington D.C. National Academy of Sciences - National Research Council, pp. 223–44.

Speakman, J.R. (1997) *Doubly Labelled Water: Theory and Practice*, Chapman & Hall, London.

Sopher, A.B., Thornton, J.C., Wang, J. *et al.* (2004) Measurement of percentage of body fat in 411 children and adolescents: a comparison of dual-energy X-ray absorptiometry with a four-compartment model. *Pediatrics*, **113** (5), 1285–90.

Steil, G.M. *et al.* (1993) Reduced sample number for calculation of insulin sensitivity and glucose effectiveness from the minimal model – suitability for use in population studies. *Diabetes*, **42** (2), 250–6.

Steil, G.M. *et al.* (2004) Evaluation of insulin sensitivity and beta-cell function indexes obtained from minimal model analysis of a meal tolerance test. *Diabetes*, **53**, 1201–7.

Toffolo, G., Cefalu, W.T. and Cobelli, C. (1999) Beta-cell function during insulin-modified intravenous glucose tolerance test successfully assessed by the C-peptide minimal model. *Metabolism-Clinical and Experimental*, **48** (9), 1162–6.

Toffolo, G. and Cobelli, C. (2003) The hot IVGTT two-compartment minimal model: an improved version. *American Journal of Physiology-Endocrinology and Metabolism*, **284** (2), E317–21.

Tothill, P., Avenell, A. and Reid, D.M. (1994a) Comparisons between Hologic, Lunar and Norland dual-energy X-ray absorptiometers and other techniques used for whole-body soft tissue measurements. *European Journal of Clinical Nutrition*, **48**, 781–94.

Tothill, P., Avenell, A. and Reid, D.M. (1994b) Precision and accuracy measurements of whole-body bone mineral: comparisons between Hologic, Lunar and Norland dual-energy X-ray absorptiometers. *British Journal of Radiology*, **67**, 1210–7.

Turner, R. *et al.* (1979) Insulin deficiency and insulin resistance interaction in diabetes: Estimation of their relative contribution by feedback analysis from basal plasma insulin and glucose concentrations. *Metabolism: Clinical and Experimental*, **28** (11), 1086–96.

Van Marken Lichtenbelt, W.D., Westerterp, K.R. and Wouters, L. (1994) Deuterium dilution as a method for determining total body water: effect of test protocol and sampling time. *The British Journal of Nutrition*, **72** (4), 491–7.

Vessby, B. *et al.* (2001) Substituting dietary saturated for monounsaturated fat impairs insulin sensitivity in healthy men and women: The KANWU study. *Diabetologia*, **44** (3), 312–9.

Vicini, P., Caumo, A. and Cobelli, C. (1997) The hot IVGTT two-compartment minimal model: indexes of glucose effectiveness and insulin sensitivity. *American Journal of Physiology-Endocrinology and Metabolism*, **36** (5), E1024–32.

Vicini, P. *et al.* (1999) Glucose production during an IVGTT by deconvolution: validation with the tracer-to-tracee clamp technique. *American Journal of Physiology-Endocrinology and Metabolism*, **276** (2), E285–94.

Wallace, T.M. and Matthews, D.R. (2002) The assessment of insulin resistance in man. *Diabetic Medicine*, **19** (7), 527–34.

Wareham, N.J. and Rennie, K.L. (1998) The assessment of physical activity in individuals and populations: Why try to be more precise about how physical activity is assessed? *International Journal of Obesity*, **22**, S30–8.

Welch, N.S. and Gebhart, S.S.P. (1987) Evaluation of a simple method for determining insulin sensitivity in non-insulin-dependent diabetics. *Clinical Research*, **35** (1), A26–126.

Welk, G.J. (2002) *Physical Activity Assessments for Health-Related Research*, Human Kinetics, Champaign IL.

Wells, J.C., Treleaven, P. and Cole, T.J. (2007) BMI compared with 3-dimensional body shape: the UK National Sizing Survey. *The American Journal of Clinical Nutrition*, **85** (2), 419–25.

WHO (1995). Physical status: The use and interpretation of anthropometry. Technical Report Series no. 845 Geneva: WHO.

World Health Organization (1998) Obesity: Preventing and managing the global epidemic. Report of a WHO consultation on obesity, Geneva, 3–5 June 1997. Geneva, (WHO/NUT/NCD/98.1).

Willett, W.C., Sampson, L., Stampfer, M.J. *et al.* (1985) Reproducibility and validity of a semiquantitative food frequency questionnaire. *American Journal of Epidemiology*, **122**, 51–65.

Yang, Y.J., Youn, J.H. and Bergman, R.N. (1987) Modified protocols improve insulin sensitivity estimation using the minimal model. *American Journal of Physiology*, **253** (6), E595–602.

Adipose Tissue: Development, Anatomy and Functions

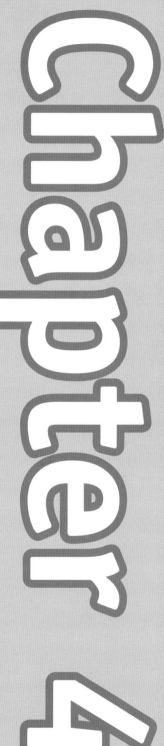

Key points

- Fat tissue comprises two types: white adipose tissue (WAT), the body's main energy store, and brown adipose tissue (BAT), specialised for heat production (thermogenesis). WAT comprises 15–20% of body weight in normal-weight adults, and its stored triglyceride contains about 7,000 kcal of energy per kg.

- White adipocytes are derived from mesenchymal stem cells via lipoblasts and preadipocytes. Specific transcription factors guide differentiation and the expression of key receptors, enzymes and adipokines during maturation. Mature adipocytes cannot proliferate; numbers increase (hyperplasia) by differentiation of local or immigrant preadipocytes.

- Adipocytes comprise 60–70% of cells in WAT, the remaining stroma-vascular fraction (SVF) including fat precursors, immune cells and blood vessels. Mature adipocytes range from 20–200 μm in diameter, and have a single (unilocular) large lipid droplet, sparse mitochondria and a compressed peripheral nucleus.

- WAT occurs in specific depots in subcutaneous (80% of total fat) and internal sites. Fat distribution varies among ethnic groups, and with various diseases (lipodystrophies, Cushing syndrome) and drugs (glucocorticoids, protease inhibitors). In obesity, ectopic lipid deposition occurs in liver, muscle and heart.

- Visceral fat, typically prominent in males, is more strongly associated with cardiovascular and metabolic disease than the gluteo-femoral deposition characteristic of women. Possible reasons include regional differences in production of adipokines (e.g. leptin and adiponectin, which both enhance insulin sensitivity) and the adverse metabolic effects (impaired glucose metabolism, increased hepatic triglyceride secretion) of FFA released from visceral fat into the portal circulation.

- Lipogenesis (triglyceride synthesis and storage) in the adipocyte is almost all derived from FFA (taken up from the circulation or cleaved from circulating triglyceride by lipoprotein lipase) and glycerol-3-phoosphate (derived from glucose). Lipogenesis is strongly stimulated at several levels by insulin.

- Lipolysis (hydrolysis of triglyceride) releases FFA and glycerol. Rate-limiting steps involve hormone-sensitive lipase (HSL) and other lipases, which are powerfully stimulated by catecholamines (via β-adrenoceptors), natriuretic peptides and growth hormone, and strongly inhibited by insulin. TNF-α, a potent lipolytic agent, interferes with insulin signalling. Perilipin, a protein coating lipid storage droplets, also regulates lipolysis by inhibiting HSL.

- Adipokines are specific cytokines secreted by adipose tissue (by adipocytes and/or SVF cells). Leptin inhibits feeding, mobilises intracellular triglyceride and improves insulin sensitivity; mutations that disable leptin production or signalling cause hyperphagia, obesity and insulin resistance, while obese subjects may develop 'leptin resistance'. Adiponectin, whose levels fall paradoxically in obesity, enhances insulin sensitivity (possibly, like leptin, by stimulating AMP-activated kinase) and protects against atheroma formation. Other adipokines include resistin, apelin and interleukins (produced by SVF immune cells).

- BAT adipocytes are derived from specific myogenic precursors and can also transdifferentiate from white adipocytes under catecholamine stimulation. They contain numerous (multilocular) small lipid droplets and mitochondria (whose cytochromes produce the brown colour), and a rounded nucleus.

- BAT is present at birth in mammals and in rodents, persists throughout life in large inter-scapular, mediastinal and perirenal depots; it rapidly involutes in humans, although small but metabolically active foci of BAT may survive.

- Thermogenesis in BAT comes from oxidation of FFA, with production of heat rather than ATP by a specific uncoupling protein (UCP-1) which short-circuits the mitochondrial proton gradient. BAT thermogenesis is stimulated by the sympathetic nervous system and catechol-amines, acting via the β_3 adrenoceptor.

Chapter 4   Adipose Tissue: Development, Anatomy and Functions

Dominique Langin, Gema Frühbeck, Keith N. Frayn, and Max Lafontan

Introduction

Adipose tissue serves an obvious role in regulating energy homeostasis, because it is the body's main depot for energy storage and mobilization. Adipose tissue is also a complex tissue with important regulatory functions. It secretes key signalling molecules that impact on multiple target organs, and expresses a wide range of receptors that make it responsive to numerous metabolic and endocrine cues. It is also richly innervated and vascularized, and contains specialized immune cells; the latter have recently attracted increasing attention, with the recognition that obesity is associated with chronic, systemic low-grade inflammation that may mediate some aspects of obesity-related morbidity. Finally, the mass of adipose tissue and its distribution within the body are important determinants of the metabolic, cardiac and other comorbidities of obesity.

This chapter reviews the development, structure and distribution of white adipose tissue (WAT), together with its metabolic, endocrine and immune functions. The specialized brown adipose tissue (BAT, or brown fat), which is specifically adapted for heat production, is described at the end of the chapter.

Development of white adipose tissue

There are two main phases of fat formation in the fetus (Pond, 1999). Primary fat formation occurs relatively early in humans (14th–16th week of gestation) and around the 15th day in the rat, with gland-like aggregates of lipoblasts laid down in specific sites such as the upper thoracic region, dorso-lateral to the vertebral column. Secondary fat formation extends from the 23rd week of gestation into the early neonatal period. With differentiation, the precursor cells accumulate triglyceride, initially in numerous cytoplasmic lipid droplets; this 'multilocular' morphology predominates in the sites of early fat development. Coalescence of the multiple lipid droplets ultimately yields the single, large droplet and the 'unilocular' form characteristic of the mature adipocyte. The second trimester represents a critical period for the development of obesity in later life, because it determines the number of fat cells. At the start of the third trimester, small fat cells are already present in the main fat depots. As it grows, adipose tissue is partitioned by connective tissue septa into lobules, which expand continuously during subsequent growth.

In a newborn human, white fat accounts for about 700 g (16% of total body weight). During the first year, fat mass increases rapidly to about 2.8 kg, this being accompanied by marked proliferation of fat cell precursors. A second peak of accelerated fat expansion occurs before puberty; thereafter, adipocyte proliferation increases during adolescence and then remains fairly constant throughout adult life in individuals whose weight is stable. During old age, adipose tissue depots tend to increase again.

Differentiation of white adipocytes

Adipocytes are derived from mesenchymal stem cells that populate the primordial fat pad. These precursor cells can enter several other cell lineages, which culminate in the formation of bone, cartilage, muscle, nerve or blood cells (Rosen and MacDougald, 2006; Liu et al., 2007); those destined to become mature white adipocytes

Obesity: Science to Practice   Edited by Gareth Williams and Gema Frühbeck
© 2009 John Wiley & Sons, Ltd

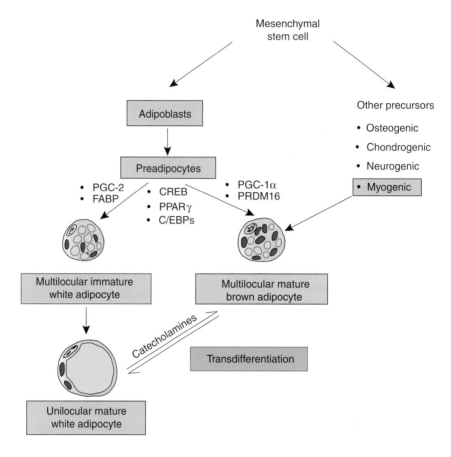

Figure 4.1 Differentiation pathways of white and brown adipocytes. CREB: (cAMP-response-element)-binding protein; PPARγ: peroxisome proliferator-activated receptor-gamma; C/EBPs: CCAAT/enhancer-binding proteins; PGC-2: peroxisome proliferator-activated receptor-gamma co-activator-2; FABP: fatty-acid binding protein; PGC-1α: peroxisome proliferator-activated receptor-gamma co-activator-1alpha; PRDM16: PR domain containing 16.

first differentiate into epithelioid-like lipoblasts and then preadipocytes (Figure 4.1). It has proved difficult to characterize distinct cellular intermediates between stem cells and mature adipocytes, and for practical purposes two main phases of adipogenesis are described. The first or 'determination' phase results in the conversion of the stem cell to a preadipocyte, which cannot be distinguished morphologically from its precursor cell but has lost the potential to differentiate into other cell types. In the second phase of 'terminal differentiation', the preadipocyte takes on the characteristics of the mature adipocyte by acquiring all the machinery needed for lipid transport synthesis and mobilization, hormonal responsiveness and the secretion of adipocyte-specific proteins (Figure 4.2).

The sequence of differentiation of precursor cells into mature adipocytes has been extensively studied *in vitro*. Pluripotent stem cells (e.g. C3H10T1/2) can be forced to commit to the adipocyte lineage through carefully-timed exposure to key regulators such as PPARγ (peroxisome proliferator-activated receptor-gamma) agonists and C/EBPs (CCAAT/enhancer-binding proteins), and rodent preadipocyte cell-lines (e.g. 3T3-L1) have also provided much information (Rosen and MacDougald, 2006). When implanted subcutaneously into immune-tolerant (athymic) mice, these cell lines produce fat pads that are histologically and biochemically normal. Some aspects of differentiation remain uncertain, including how stem cells become committed to the adipocyte lineage, early markers of adipoblasts, and the epigenetic regulatory factors that control gene transcription and therefore differentiation *in vivo* (Chun *et al.*, 2006).

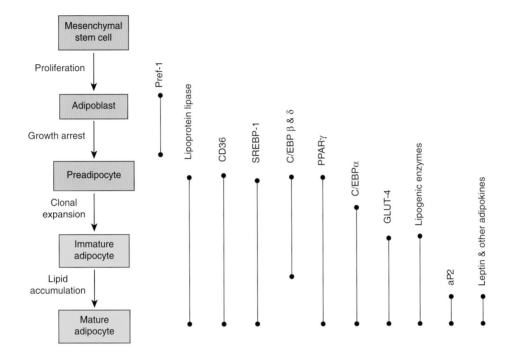

Figure 4.2 Key events and regulators of adipogenesis, showing the sequence of expression of markers of the mature, fully competent adipocyte. Pref-1: preadipocyte factor-1; CD36: cluster-designated 36; SREBP-1: sterol regulatory element-binding protein-1; C/EBPβ and δ: CCAAT/enhancer-binding protein beta and delta; PPARγ: peroxisome proliferator-activated receptor-gamma; C/EBPα: CCAAT/enhancer-binding protein alpha; GLUT-4: glucose transporter 4; aP2: adipocyte fatty acid-binding protein.

The later stages of differentiation into mature adipocytes have been relatively well characterized (Figure 4.1). The differentiation programme is complex and orchestrated by multiple transcription factors some of which are common for both white and brown fat cells (CREB, (cAMP-response-element-binding protein), PPARγ and C/EBPs), whereas a few preferentially favour the differentiation into white adipocytes (PGC-2, peroxisome proliferator-activated receptor-gamma co-activator-2; FABP, fatty-acid binding protein) or brown adipocytes (PGC-1α, PRDM16). Some of these, and the key markers of the mature adipocyte's wide repertoire of enzymes, adipokines and transcription factors, are shown in Figure 4.2.

Cells carrying specific marker antigens can be identified and harvested in various ways, e.g. using antibodies coupled to magnetic microbeads or in fluorescence-activated cell sorting (FACS). These techniques have been used to identify various types of precursor cell in fat depots, and to investigate their source and fate. For example, undifferentiated stromal cells from fat share specific markers (presence of CD105, absence of CD34; i.e. CD105$^+$/CD34$^-$) with both stromal cells in bone marrow and mesenchymal stem cells that can be induced to differentiate into adipocytes (Liu *et al.*, 2007). However, the only fat stromal cell-type able to differentiate into adipocytes was CD34$^+$/CD31$^-$, which also did not express the mesenchymal marker CD105; this subset includes preadipocytes, and also endothelial progenitor cells (Sengenes *et al.*, 2005; Miranville *et al.*, 2004). Thus, differentiation from stem cell to preadipocyte involves the loss of CD105 and the expression of CD34.

The source of the CD34$^+$/CD31$^-$ progenitor cells remains controversial: they may be derived from 'resident' precursor cells *in situ*, or originate in the bone marrow and travel in the bloodstream to home in on fat depots. Such trafficking of bone marrow-derived adipocyte precursors has recently been demonstrated in mice fed a high-fat diet and given a thiazolidinedione (TZD) (Crossno *et al.*, 2006). Moreover, experimental disruption of vascularization in the adipose tissue of mice significantly reduces fat accumulation in genetic and diet-induced obesity (Rupnick *et al.*, 2002; Kolonin *et al.*, 2004; Brakenhielm *et al.*, 2004). The endothelium of blood vessels in adipose tissue presumably carries specific markers that permit 'docking' of marrow-derived adipocyte precursors, but these have not yet been identified. It is not known whether this mechanism explains fat expansion in humans treated with TZDs.

Hyperplasia (increased number) of adipocytes occurs when the maximal storage capacity of the adipocyte is reached. This effect has been demonstrated in both rodents and humans (Gregoire, Smas and Sul, 1998). As mature adipocytes cannot proliferate, 'new' adipocytes have been assumed to originate from the proliferation and differentiation of resident preadipocytes pre-existing in the fat depots. In rodents made obese by feeding a high-fat diet, adipocyte size first increases, followed by a rise in adipocyte numbers, which is partly explicable by the proliferation of resident preadipocytes (Faust *et al.*, 1978; Ellis, McDonald and Stern, 1990). As mentioned above, other precursor cells may also originate in the marrow and enter the fat depot from the circulation.

Structure of white adipose tissue

White adipose tissue is a specialized loose connective tissue, in which clusters of individual adipocytes are held together by delicate reticulin fibres to form lobules, bounded by fibrous septa and surrounded by a rich network of capillaries and nerves. Adipocytes comprise only 60–70% of the total cell population. The remaining cell types, comprising the 'stroma-vascular fraction' (SVF), include fat precursor cells, fibroblasts, immune cells and the endothelial cells and pericytes of the blood vessels (Figure 4.3). The striking multi-cellularity of WAT is reflected in its ability to produce and respond to a wide range of endocrine, metabolic and immune signals, and in the numerous functions that it serves. Some of the secretory products of the adipocyte – 'adipokines' – are discussed in detail below.

Stroma-vascular fraction

The importance of the SVF cells in fat has been neglected until recently. These include immune cells (macrophages and lymphocytes) embedded in the extracellular matrix of collagen

and elastin fibres, and the vascular bed. Like adipocytes, SVF cells in the primordial fat pad are derived from mesenchymal stem cells and various other cells with phenotypes also found in bone marrow; some marrow-derived precursors may also arrive via the circulation.

SVF cells make important contributions to the development and function of adipose tissue. The CD34$^+$/CD31$^-$ fraction that contains preadipocytes also includes endothelial cells; we have already mentioned the crucial importance of normal vascularization of fat, and the possible role of the endothelium in attracting marrow-derived adipocyte precursors to home into fat pads.

The SVF also contains numerous immune cells, which can be isolated using antibody-coated microbeads, FACS and other techniques. In human adipose tissue, the number of resident macrophages was found to correlate with BMI (Weisberg *et al.*, 2003; Curat *et al.*, 2004; Clément *et al.*, 2004; Cancello *et al.*, 2005, 2006), and a similar correlation has been observed in various mouse obesity models (Weisberg *et al.*, 2003; Xu *et al.*, 2003). Significant numbers of T lymphocytes occur in the SVF of rodents (Caspar-Bauguil *et al.*, 2005), and T lymphocytes accumulate in the fat pads of obese subjects (Wu *et al.*, 2007). Preferential infiltration into intra-abdominal versus subcutaneous fat has been observed, with approximately twice as many lymphocytes being present in omental as compared with subcutaneous depots. The immune activities of the increased number of both macrophages and T lymphocytes may influence preadipocyte and adipocyte functions, as well as contributing to the generalized chronic inflammatory state that characterizes obesity.

Structure of white adipocytes

Young white adipocytes are transiently multilocular, containing multiple lipid droplets, with a round or oval nucleus. In the mature unilocular adipocyte, 90% of the cell volume is occupied by the lipid droplet, stretching the cytoplasm into a thin peripheral rim and flattening the nucleus into a semilunar shape that occupies only 2–3% of the cell's volume (Figure 4.4). A thin interface membrane separates the lipid droplet from the cytoplasm, which contains sparse mitochondria with loose, membranous cristae, a small Golgi zone, plentiful free ribosomes (but relatively little granular endoplasmic

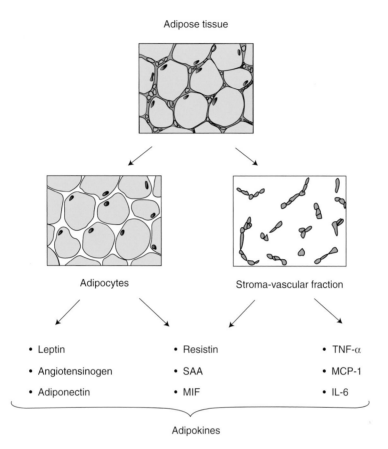

Adipose tissue

Adipocytes

Stroma-vascular fraction

- Leptin
- Angiotensinogen
- Adiponectin

- Resistin
- SAA
- MIF

- TNF-α
- MCP-1
- IL-6

Adipokines

Figure 4.3 Cell types present in white adipose tissue and some of their secreted products. Adipocytes comprise about two-thirds of total cell numbers, the remainder being the stroma-vascular function (SVF). Some products are secreted mainly by adipocytes or SVF cells, and some (e.g. resistin) are produced by both. SAA: serum amyloid A; MIF: macrophage migration inhibitory factor; TNF-α: tumour necrosis factor-alpha; MCP-1: monocyte chemoattractant protein-1; IL-6: interleukin 6.

reticulum) and occasional lysosomes. Externally, a thin basal lamina surrounds the adipocyte (Figure 4.5). The central lipid droplet is mostly (95%) triglyceride, which is rich in oleic and palmitic acids, with small amounts of diacylglycerols, free fatty acids, phospholipids and cholesterol.

Individual adipocytes vary enormously in diameter (from 20 to 200 μm) depending on species, sex, cell populations and location. To accommodate a large lipid load, adipocytes can increase their volume by a thousand-fold, from a few picolitres to about 1–3 nanolitres (in omental adipocytes from morbidly obese subjects). Adipocytes cannot expand indefinitely; when they reach their maximum capacity, new adipocytes are recruited from the precursor pool.

Distribution of WAT

In mammals, WAT occurs throughout the body in discrete depots, which are homologous among all species but show considerable variation in size and functional importance (Pond, 1992; Pond, 1999). This dispersed distribution has frustrated many attempts to classify fat depots according to anatomical location or physiological function (Shen et al., 2003), and improved understanding of the molecular biology of WAT has now rendered some previous classifications obsolete.

Total body fat, comprising the sum of all depots, is usually subdivided into subcutaneous and internal adipose tissue (Shen et al., 2003) (Table 4.1). Subcutaneous fat constitutes the layer between the dermis and the outer surface

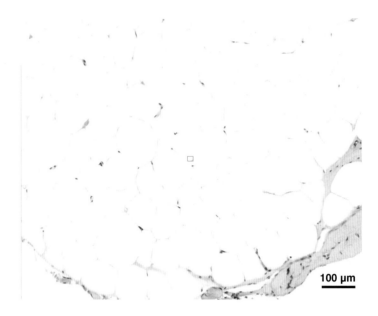

Figure 4.4 White adipocytes shown by light microscopy (human omental white adipose tissue with haematoxylin and eosin stain; original magnification 10×; bar=100 μm). Image courtesy of Dr María Angela Burrell, Department of Histology and Pathology, University of Navarra, Pamplona, Spain.

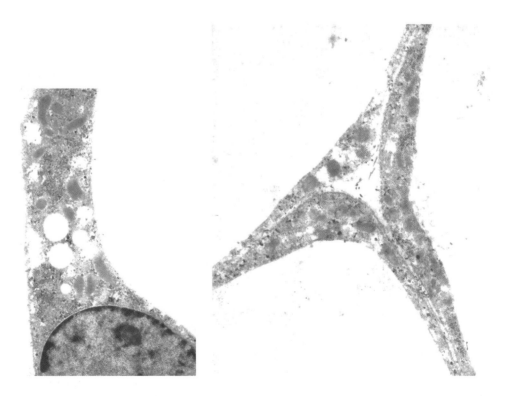

Figure 4.5 White adipocytes: electron micrograph of the perinuclear area (left; magnification 15,000×) and the junction between three adipocytes (right; magnification 7,725×). Note the basal lamina separating the adipocyte membrane from the extracellular matrix. Images courtesy of Dr María Angela Burrell, Department of Histology and Pathology, University of Navarra, Pamplona, Spain.

Table 4.1 Main adipose tissue depots.

White adipose tissue (WAT)

Subcutaneous – ~80% of total body fat
(superficial and deep adipose tissue layers)
   Truncal
      Cervical
      Dorsal
      Lumbar
   Abdominal
   Gluteo-femoral
   Mammary

Internal – ~20% of total body fat
   Visceral
      Intrathoracic (pericardial, epicardial)
      Intraabdominopelvic
         Intraperitoneal
            Omental (greater and lesser omentum)
            Mesenteric
            Umbilical
         Extraperitoneal
         Intraabdominal
            Preperitoneal
            Retroperitoneal (peripancreatic,
               periaortic, pararenal, perirenal –
               infiltrated with brown adipocytes)
         Intrapelvic
            Gonadal (parametrial, retrouterine,
               retropubic)
            Urogenital (paravesical, pararectal)
      Ectopic (e.g., hepatic steatosis,
         intramyocardial fat)

   Non-visceral
      Periarticular
         Paraosseal
      Muscular
         Perimuscular
         Intermuscular
         Intramuscular
      Other depots (bone marrow; cranial, facial,
         retro-orbital adipose tissue)

Brown adipose tissue (BAT)
   Cervical
   Paravertebral
   Supraclavicular
   Interscapular
   Mediastinal
   Para-aortic
   Suprarenal

(aponeuroses and fasciae) of the musculature. In the lower trunk, gluteal region and thighs, a fascial plane within the subcutaneous fat subdivides it into deep and superficial layers. Internal fat includes all the remaining visceral depots (lying within the thorax, abdomen and pelvis as well as triglyceride deposited in 'ectopic' sites such as muscle, heart and liver) and non-visceral sites such as the orbits and marrow cavities.

Overall, fat can be one of the body's largest compartments and is quantitatively the most variable. The normal range is 10–20% of body weight in males and 20–30% in females, but can range from only a few percent in elite athletes to over half the body's weight in the morbidly obese. As in most species, pregnant women lay down additional fat to support the growth of the fetus and prepare for lactation.

Variations in fat distribution

In humans, the various fat depots vary considerably with sex, age and ethnic origin (Wajchenberg, 2000; Lafontan and Berlan, 2003). Sexual dimorphism is marked, and mainly accounts for differences in body build between males and females. The 'gynoid' distribution typical of women shows abundant subcutaneous fat in the gluteo-femoral region and breasts, whereas the main subcutaneous depots in men include the nape of the neck, the upper arm, overlying deltoid and triceps muscles, and the lumbosacral area (Figure 4.6). These patterns become more obvious with advancing age in well-nourished, sedentary individuals, and men in particular tend to accumulate visceral fat in the abdomen, especially in the mesentery and omentum and in the retroperitoneal area.

There are significant ethnic variations in body fat content and distribution that may account for racial differences in the metabolic and cardiac risks of obesity. Asian subjects have a higher total body fat mass than Caucasians matched for BMI, which may explain their greater susceptibility to obesity-related type 2 diabetes (Chapter 9).

With increasing obesity, all the fat depots expand, including the visceral components in the abdomen. As discussed below, visceral fat is one of the contributors to central (abdominal) obesity, which can be measured by waist circumference, and which is particularly associated

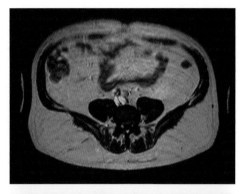

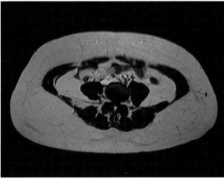

Figure 4.6 Sexual dimorphism in human fat distribution, illustrated by magnetic resonance (MR) images at the level of L4/L5. Men (upper) tend to accumulate fat around and within the abdominal cavity and subcutaneously over the upper body, while women (lower) deposit subcutaneous fat preferentially in the gluteo-femoral region. Images by courtesy of Dr. Julian Kabala, University Hospitals Bristol, Bristol, U.K.

with type 2 diabetes, dyslipidaemia and cardio-vascular disease (Chapter 10). Worsening obesity is also accompanied by increasing ectopic triglyceride deposition in the liver and in skeletal and cardiac muscle, and appears to contribute to cardiometabolic risk (Chapters 11 and 12).

Conversely, weight loss is accompanied by shrinkage of the expanded fat depots. Certain factors preferentially decrease visceral depots, including exercise, caloric restriction, the anti-obesity drug rimonabant (apparently a specific effect of cannabinoid CB1 receptor blockade) and bariatric surgery. This may explain why these treatments improve insulin sensitivity and cardiovascular risk more than might be expected for the degree of weight loss.

Various diseases can modify the distribution of body fat. Inherited and acquired lipodystro-phies are characterized by the failure to develop, or the loss, of fat in specific distributions. The anatomical predilection of these conditions is unexplained. For example, all adipose tissue is absent from birth in congenital generalized

lipodystrophy (Berardinelli-Seip syndrome), an autosomal recessive genetic disorder (Figure 4.7). Generalized body fat loss, possibly through auto-immune attack, occurs in the Lawrence syndrome of acquired generalized lipodystrophy. By con-trast, familial partial lipodystrophy (Dunnigan-Köbberling syndrome), inherited as an autosomal dominant trait, affects the limbs and buttocks but spares the face and neck. Severe insulin resistance accompanies all these conditions, pos-sibly because triglyceride is taken up into muscle and liver instead of fat (see Chapter 10).

Hormones and drugs can also alter fat mass and distribution. Cushing syndrome and gluco-corticoid therapy induce marked central obe-sity, with a rounded face and a 'buffalo hump', while the protease inhibitors used to treat HIV infection cause loss of fat from the face and the development of a 'buffalo hump'.

Site-specific differences in fat accumulation or mobilization relate not only to the adipo-cytes' metabolic activity, but also to the depot's capacity to produce new adipocytes; regional

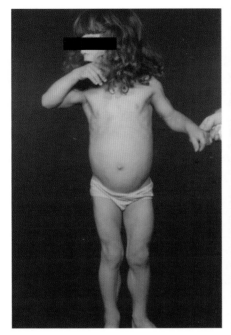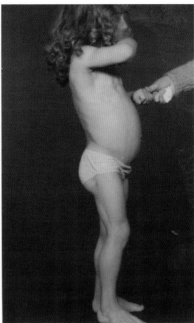

Figure 4.7 Congenital generalised lipodystrophy (Berardinelli-Seip syndrome). Body fat comprised only 3% of total body weight in this 3-year old girl, who also had severe insulin resistance and acanthosis nigricans. Image reproduced by courtesy of Dr. David Savage, University of Cambridge.

variations in adipokine expression, hormone receptor density, vascularization and innervation are also important (Wajchenberg, 2000; Linder *et al.*, 2004; Fontana *et al.*, 2007).

Disease correlates of fat distribution

The regional distribution of body fat is an important determinant of metabolic and cardiovascular risk (Chapters 9 and 10). A dominant effect of 'android' (central) obesity was noted by Jean Vague in the 1950s and has been amply confirmed by numerous prospective studies showing a strong association with type 2 diabetes, hypertension, atherosclerosis and premature death. By contrast, 'gynoid' or gluteo-femoral adiposity appears relatively benign and may even protect against insulin resistance, dyslipidaemia and ischaemic heart disease (Yusuf *et al.*, 2005).

Possible explanations for the diabetogenic and other adverse effects of central obesity are discussed in Chapters 9 and 10. Abdominal visceral fat mass provides an important link with the many facets of the metabolic syndrome, notably insulin resistance, glucose intolerance, dyslipidaemia and hypertension (Wajchenberg, 2000; Lafontan and Berlan, 2003; Després and Lemieux, 2006). However, the cause and nature of the association are poorly understood; it is still uncertain whether insulin resistance predisposes to central fat deposition or *vice versa*.

Suggested factors include the delivery to the liver of high levels of free fatty acids (FFA), generated by active lipolysis in intra-abdominal fat that drains directly into the portal veins. High FFA levels are thought to interfere with glucose utilization, thus inducing insulin resistance, increased hepatic glucose output and hyperglycaemia (see Chapter 10). The notion that FFA derived from visceral fat can induce hepatic insulin resistance is supported by studies in dogs fed a high-fat diet that produced visceral obesity (Kabir *et al.*, 2005). Excess FFA supplied to the liver also increases production of atherogenic lipids such as VLDL. Compared with adipocytes from lower-body fat depots, those from central or upper-body depots show more active lipolysis when stimulated with catecholamines and are less readily suppressed by insulin (Zierath *et al.*, 1998). Moreover, visceral adipose tissue is more active lipolytically that subcutaneous abdominal fat. These depot-specific differences appear to arise from variations in the expression of adrenoreceptors and other receptors (Wajchenberg, 2000), and to differences in lipoprotein lipase (LPL) activity that may affect their ability to absorb and store extra FFA under various physiological and pathological conditions. The relative sluggishness of lower-body adipocytes may suggest a role as long-term fuel reserves to cover pregnancy and lactation, and these depots are relatively spared during periods of fat loss in women (Jones and Edwards, 1999).

Regional differences in the expression and secretion of key products may also contribute, such as leptin (Van Harmelen *et al.*, 1998) and adiponectin (Motoshima *et al.*, 2002) and pro-inflammatory and pro-atherogenic factors such as interleukins and plasminogen activator inhibitor 1 (PAI-1). These regional variations in adipose tissue secretion may also contribute to the differing cardio-metabolic risk associated with specific fat depots, and especially the pathogenic effects of visceral fat (Bastelica *et al.*, 2002). Leptin is preferentially secreted by subcutaneous adipose tissue, while expression levels of adiponectin, IL-1β, IL-8 and PAI-1 are greater in visceral fat (Lafontan and Berlan, 2003; Bouloumie *et al.*, 2005; Maury *et al.*, 2007). Moreover, compared with subcutaneous adipose tissue, visceral and omental fat express higher levels of immunoglobulins and complement proteins (Yang *et al.*, 2003; Gabrielsson *et al.*, 2003) and of several cytokines such as IL-6, interferon regulator factor-1, visfatin, chemokine (C-C-motif) ligands 2, 3, 4, 8 and 21 (Vohl *et al.*, 2004). With central obesity, changes in the overall profile of products secreted by adipose tissue could play a role in the development of insulin resistance and type 2 diabetes, such as decreased concentrations of insulin-sensitizing factors such as adiponectin and increased levels of pro-inflammatory cytokines.

The accumulation of macrophages in human visceral WAT has been associated with hepatic inflammation and fibrosis in morbidly obese subjects (Curat *et al.*, 2004; Cancello *et al.*, 2006; Clément *et al.*, 2004; see Chapter 11); these observations strengthen the notion that the pro-inflammatory mediators secreted by visceral fat may be mainly produced by macrophages. As discussed in Chapters 10 and 12, increased levels of pro-inflammatory and pro-atherogenic mediators are associated with other features of the metabolic syndrome and are likely to contribute to the increased cardiovascular risk.

Fat storage and mobilization

Adipose tissue serves several functions, including insulation and mechanical cushioning, but its major physiological role is to store energy in the form of triglyceride, and to supply energy in the form of FFA as needed by other tissues.

Many other tissues contain reserves of glycogen, lipid or protein, but these contain only limited energy stores. Total glycogen stores (about 500 g, in liver and skeletal muscle) equate to about one day's worth of normal energy expenditure, and liver glycogen is completely depleted after fasting for 24 hours. Proteins tend to be conserved and are only catabolized in large amounts during prolonged starvation.

The triglyceride stored in WAT is therefore the body's main long-term repository for storing energy that is excess to requirements, and the most important fuel store for survival during starvation. Due to the high energy content of triglyceride (9 kcal/g) and its hydrophobicity, the storage of energy as triglyceride is highly efficient: 1 kg of adipose tissue contains only 100 g of water, but 800 g of triglyceride, and thus about 7,000 kcal of energy. In theory, a typical body fat mass of 15 kg would provide enough energy for 50–60 days of total starvation, and this is in agreement with the survival limit of initially normal-weight adults under famine conditions. Obese subjects, by virtue of their increased fat mass, can survive starvation for much longer – over 120 days in some cases (Forbes, 1970). This highlights the crucial importance of fat storage as a survival advantage during most of human evolution, during which famine has been a powerful selection force (Prentice, 2005). Until relatively recently, the ability to store excess energy safely as triglyceride in adipocytes must have conferred enormous survival benefits; however, in an energy-replete environment, the continuing effect of the same 'thrifty' genes that have been selected to promote triglyceride storage will encourage the spread of obesity. However, the 'thrifty' gene hypothesis has been recently challenged by Speakman (2007), who presents a 'predation release' hypothesis as a nonadaptive scenario explaining the genetic predisposition to obesity (Chapter 8).

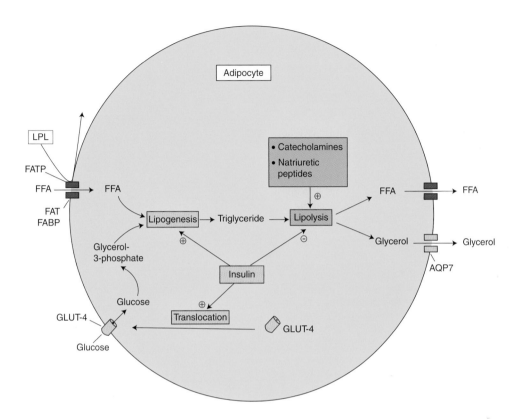

Figure 4.8 Overview of lipogenesis and lipolysis in the white adipocyte. FFA: free fatty acids; LPL: lipoprotein lipase; GLUT4: glucose transporter 4; FAT: fatty acid translocase (also known as CD36); FATP: fatty acid transport protein; FABP: fatty-acid binding protein; AQP7: aquaporin 7.

The processes of fat deposition (lipogenesis) and mobilization (lipolysis) are key functions of the adipocyte (Figure 4.8). Both are carefully regulated by integrated endocrine and neural mechanisms, which cooperate to keep fat mass relatively constant under habitual conditions. This is achieved in part by the adipocyte's ability to signal the size of the body's triglyceride stores to the brain, through leptin and other mechanisms (see below).

Lipogenesis

In humans, almost all the triglyceride stored in adipocytes is derived from the uptake of FFA from the blood stream, either from FFA bound to albumin or released by the hydrolysis of circulating triglyceride under the action of the adipocyte-produced enzyme, lipoprotein lipase (LPL) (Figure 4.8). In turn, circulating triglyceride comes either from VLDL secreted by the liver or, after eating, from chylomicrons that transport triglyceride reconstituted from the digestion products of dietary fat.

LPL is a complex enzyme, expressed by adipocytes and various other tissues, and its regulation is tissue-specific (Fielding and Frayn, 1998). In WAT, LPL is powerfully up-regulated by insulin, and this gives WAT a special role in clearing circulating triglyceride after eating, and in reconstituting it for storage in adipocytes. LPL is synthesized in adipocytes and then exported to the capillaries, where it binds to the luminal surface of the endothelial cells by inte-racting with cell-surface glycosaminoglycans, especially heparan sulphate. The LDL and chylomicrons are too large to penetrate the endothelium; the endothelial-bound LPL acts upon these lipoprotein particles in the vascular space to liberate FFA, which then cross the endothelium to be taken up by adipocytes.

FFA appear to enter the adipocyte by facilitated diffusion, with fatty acid translocase (FAT; also known as CD36) playing an important role (Hajri and Abumrad, 2002); adipocytes from CD36 knockout mice lack the normal high-affinity uptake of long-chain FFA (Febbraio et al., 1999), resulting in impaired triglyceride synthesis in WAT (Coburn *et al.*, 2000). Also involved in FFA uptake in adipocytes are fatty-acid binding proteins (FABP) (Chmurzyńska, 2006) and fatty acid transport proteins (FATP) (Gimeno, 2007). There is also evidence that the transport of FFA across the adipocyte membrane is intimately associated with their 'activation', i.e. esterification with co-enzyme A to form fatty acyl-CoA (Gargiulo, Stuhlsatz-Krouper and Schaffer, 1999).

An alternative pathway for generating FFA from glucose – '*de novo* lipogenesis' – is physiologically significant in lower mammals and in the human breast during lactation, but only minor in human WAT. This is because the activity of the rate-limiting enzyme, ATP:citrate lyase, is normally very low in human adipose tissue (Swierczynski *et al.*, 2000). This enzyme is, however, up-regulated by insulin (O'Brien and Granner, 1996), and this pathway could theoretically become significant in subjects eating a high-carbohydrate, high-energy diet (Aarsland, Chinkes and Wolfe, 1997). *De novo* lipogenesis also operates in subjects with complete deficiency of LPL, which results in the inability to clear chylomicrons and VLDL from the circulation (type 1 hyperlipoproteinaemia); these subjects still have normal fat depots and replete adipocytes (Peeva *et al.*, 1992), indicating that an alternative pathway is functioning.

The process for esterifying fatty acids to form triglyceride in adipocytes is shown in Figure 4.9. This involves the sequential addition of fatty acyl Co-A residues to a glycerol 'backbone', mainly via the glycerol 3-phosphate (or phosphatidic acid) pathway. This starts with glycerol 3-phosphate, produced in the fed state from glucose by glycolysis in the adipocyte; the glycerol generated by hydrolysis of circulating triglyceride cannot be used to any significant extent by adipocytes, because the critical enzyme, glycerokinase, shows little activity (Coleman and Lee, 2004). Importantly, the esterification pathway is also stimulated by insulin. Data from transgenic animals suggest that the conversion of diacylglycerol to triglycerides, mediated by diacylglycerol acyltransferase (DGAT), is a critical step *in vivo* (Smith *et al.*, 2000).

During fasting, a significant proportion of the FFA is re-esterified into triglycerides. The amount of released FFA is therefore a balance between triglyceride breakdown and resynthesis (Figure 4.9). Re-esterification requires glyceroneogenesis, i.e. the *de novo* synthesis of glycerol-3-phosphate from pyruvate, lactate or certain amino acids (Beale *et al.*, 2002). The key enzyme in this process is the cytosolic isoform of phosphoenolpyruvate carboxykinase (PEPCK-C). The enzyme is also induced by TZD treatment in rodent and human adipocytes (Tordjman *et al.*, 2003; Leroyer *et al.*, 2006). Recent advance has stressed the role of glyceroneogenesis and of PEPCK-C in fatty acid release from adipose tissue (Cadoudal *et al.*, 2005). Stimulating the pathway that promotes an increased re-esterification of fatty acids is probably an attractive strategy to restrain fatty acid release during fasting and even exercise (Frayn, 2002).

Thus, triglyceride synthesis in adipose tissue is stimulated by insulin at multiple stages, notably the activation of LPL and the stimulation of fatty acid esterification; *de novo* fatty acid synthesis and perhaps enhanced FFA uptake into adipocytes may also contribute. In parallel, as explained below, insulin also inhibits fat mobilization, and so the net effect on adipocyte triglyceride stores is strongly anabolic.

Lipolysis

The release of stored lipid energy by adipose tissue as needed by other tissues is achieved by a highly active and tightly-regulated pathway that hydrolyses triglyceride and delivers FFA into the circulation (Figure 4.9). Lipolysis is controlled by multiple mechanisms that, in general, ensure reciprocal regulation with fat deposition, so that fatty acids flow in and out of the adipocyte according to the animal's nutritional and physiological state.

The rate-limiting steps in lipolysis are the hydrolysis of triglyceride by lipases. Triglycerides are broken down first into diacylglycerols and then monoacylglycerols, releasing one molecule of fatty acid at each step; the final step generates a fatty acid and glycerol (Figure 4.9).

Fat mobilization is stimulated most strongly (at least acutely) by catecholamines and natriuretic peptides such as atrial natriuretic peptide (ANP). Circulating catecholamines (adrenaline and noradrenaline) act on β-adrenoceptors to stimulate adenylyl cyclase to produce cAMP from adenosine triphosphate (ATP) (Figure 4.10). Noradrenaline released from sympathetic nerve endings in fat acts similarly. Atrial and brain natriuretic peptides,

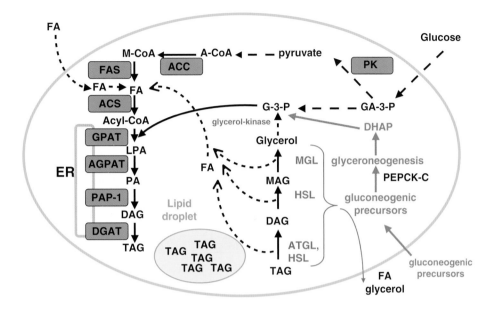

Figure 4.9 Triglyceride synthesis, fatty acid esterification and release. Adipocyte triglyceride lipase (ATGL) predominantly mediate the initial step in triacylglycerol (TAG) hydrolysis, resulting in the formation of diacylglycerol (DAG; diglyceride) and fatty acid (FA). Hormone-sensitive lipase (HSL) catalyzes hydrolysis of TAG, DAG, and monoacylglycerol (MAG; monoglyceride). Monoacylglycerol lipase (MGL) catalyzes hydrolysis of MAG to form glycerol and FA. ER: endoplasmic reticulum; DGAT: diacylglycerol acyltransferase; PA: phosphatidic acid; LPA: lysophosphatidic acid; PAP-1: phosphatidate phosphatase; AGPAT: 1-acylglycerol-3-phosphate O-acyltransferase; GPAT: glycerol-3-phosphate acyltransferase; ACS: acyl-CoA synthetase; FAS: fatty acid synthase; ACC: acetyl-CoA carboxylase; M-CoA: malonyl-CoA; A-CoA; acetyl-CoA; G-3-P: glycerol 3-phosphate; PK: pyruvate kinase; GA-3-P; glyceraldehyde-3-phosphate; DHAP; dihydroxyacetone phosphate; PEPCK: phosphoenolpyruvate carboxykinase.

acting through the natriuretic peptide receptor A, which possesses guanylyl cyclase activity, generate cGMP. The two second messengers, cAMP and cGMP, stimulate lipolysis by activating the enzyme hormone-sensitive lipase (HSL). Another enzyme, adipose triglyceride lipase (ATGL) is also involved together with HSL in the first stage of lipolysis. Other hormones that stimulate lipolysis include growth hormone, glucocorticoids and thyroxine, all of which increase β-adrenoceptor expression.

Another powerful lipolytic agent is tumour necrosis factor-α (TNF-α), originally termed 'cachectin' because of its association with fat loss in malignancy and heart failure (Langin and Arner, 2006). TNF-α requires prolonged exposure to stimulate lipolysis, which it does through at least three separate mechanisms: inhibiting insulin signalling by interfering with insulin receptor substrate (IRS) proteins; inhibiting signalling through the adenosine receptor that normally suppresses lipolysis; and direct stimulation of basal (hormone-independent)

lipolysis by interacting with perilipin, the cytoplasmic lipid-binding protein that normally restrains lipolysis (see below).

There is also powerful inhibitory control of fat mobilization, notably by insulin acting through its usual metabolic signalling pathway, i.e. phospatidylinositol-3 kinase (PI3 kinase) and protein kinase B (PKB); the latter in turn phosphorylates and activates phosphodiesterase 3B, which hydrolyses cAMP and reduces cAMP concentrations. Other anti-lipolytic pathways involve α_2-adrenoceptors, A_1-adenosine receptors, EP_3-prostaglandin E_2 receptors and neuropeptide Y/PYY (NPY1) receptors. The existence of inhibitory nicotinic acid receptors has also been postulated to explain the powerful anti-lipolytic action of nicotinic acid (Karpe and Frayn, 2004). Apart from insulin receptors, these are all 7-transmembrane domain receptors that are coupled through inhibitory GTP-binding (Gi) proteins to the enzyme adenylyl cyclase, and thus reduce cAMP levels. These multiple controls presumably reflect the importance of

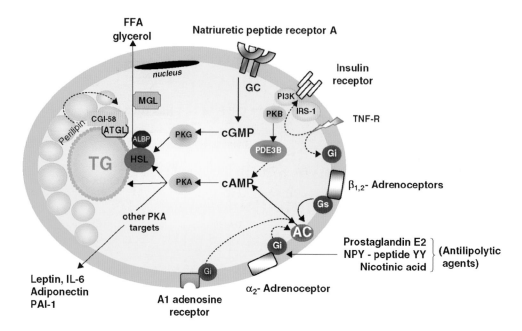

Figure 4.10 Regulation of lipolysis: hormone-sensitive lipase (HSL) is powerfully stimulated by catecholamines (acting through β₁ and β₂ adrenoceptors) and natriuretic peptides (acting through NPR-A receptors), and inhibited by insulin and adenosine. Tumour necrosis factor-alpha (TNF-α) is a potent lipolytic agent that inhibits insulin signalling. FFA: free fatty acids; TG: triglycerides; ATGL: adipocyte triglyceride lipase; CGI-58: ATGL coactivator comparative gene identification-58; ALBP: adipocyte lipid-binding protein; PKG: protein kinase G; PKA: protein kinase A; GC: guanylyl cyclase; PI3K: phospatidylinositol-3 kinase; IRS-1: insulin receptor substrate-1; PKB: protein kinase B; PDE3B: phosphodiesterase 3B; AC: adenylate cyclase; Gi: inhibitory GTP-binding proteins; Gs: stimulatory GTP-binding proteins; NPY: neuropeptide Y; IL-6: interleukin-6; PAI-1: plasminogen activator inhibitor-1. MGL: monoacylglycerol; TNF-R: TNF-α receptors.

precisely regulating fatty acid delivery into the circulation.

Intracellular cAMP concentration is therefore a major integrator for regulating fat mobilization (Figure 4.10). Raised cAMP levels were long assumed to activate protein kinase A (PKA), which in turn phosphorylated and activated HSL. However, other lipases, as well as lipid droplet-associated proteins such as perilipins, are now known to participate.

HSL is a multi-functional enzyme that can hydrolyse triglyceride and diacylglycerol, as well as cholesterol and other esters (Langin, Lucas and Lafontan, 2000). In unstimulated adipocytes, HSL is distributed diffusely throughout the cytosol, some being associated with lipid droplets. When phosphorylated by PKA, HSL is translocated to the surface of small lipid storage droplets, which lie peripherally and are coated with perilipin – a protein that blocks access of lipases to the lipid and thus suppresses lipolysis (Moore *et al.*, 2005) (Figure 4.11). Consistent with this, basal lipolysis is greatly elevated in perilipin knockout mice

(Martinez-Botas *et al.*, 2000: Tansey *et al.*, 2001). Perilipin phosphorylation appears essential for the dispersal of the lipid droplets, which is essential for full lipolytic stimulation by catecholamines and other hormones (Miyoshi *et al.*, 2006; Marcinkiewicz *et al.*, 2006; Miyoshi *et al.*, 2007). HSL is also regulated by adipocyte lipid-binding protein (ALBP), which interacts with it to form a complex (ALBP-HSL) with enhanced lipolytic activity that translocates to the surface of the lipid droplets following lipolytic stimulation (Smith *et al.*, 2004). The importance of ALBP in HSL activation is underlined by the observation that ALBP-knockout mice exhibit decreased lipolytic activity (Baar *et al.*, 2005).

HSL is not the only lipase involved, as HSL-knockout mice show normal basal lipolysis and some residual response to catecholamines (Zechner *et al.*, 2005). An important player is a novel lipase, ATGL, which confers most of the residual lipolytic activity in HSL-knockout mice (Zimmermann *et al.*, 2004; Villena *et al.*, 2004; Jenkins *et al.*, 2004). In mouse adipocytes, HSL and

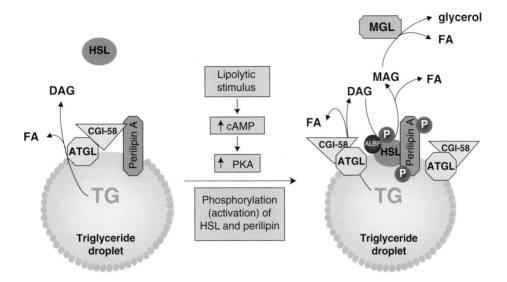

Figure 4.11 Regulation of hormone-sensitive lipase (HSL). HSL is activated by increased intracellular cAMP and cGMP (e.g. generated by binding of catecholamines and natriuretic peptides with their receptors) and inhibited by insulin (which decreases cAMP). Perilipin, a protein that coats lipid droplets, blocks access of HSL to the droplets' triglyceride content. FA: free fatty acids; ATGL: adipocyte triglyceride lipase; CGI-58: ATGL coactivator comparative gene identification-58; ALBP: adipocyte lipid-binding protein; DAG: diacylglycerol; MAG: monoacylglycerol; MGL, monoacylglycerol lipase; TG: triglyceride.

ATGL together account for >95% of total triacyl-hydrolase activity (Schweiger *et al.*, 2006). At present, the respective roles of HSL and ATGL in human fat cell lipolysis have not been well established. ATGL is activated by a cofactor, comparative gene identification (CGI)-58 (Lass *et al.*, 2006). Because CGI-58 interacts with perilipins on the surface of the lipid droplets, a complex interplay has been proposed between ATGL, perilipins and CGI-58 (Granneman *et al.*, 2007). Both PKA and PKG phosphorylate and activate human HSL. Thus, the catecholamine and natriuretic peptide pathways converge on HSL to induce lipolysis in human fat cells, while ATGL participates in basal lipolysis (Langin *et al.*, 2005). In mice, ATGL seems to participate in stimulated lipolysis because ATGL deficiency causes a drastic reduction in stimulated lipolysis and ATGL is required for PKA-stimulated lipolysis (Zechner *et al.*, 2005). HSL, but not ATGL, shows significant diacylglycerol lipase activity.

The final step in the hydrolysis of triglycerides is catalysed by monoacylglycerol lipase, an abundant and non-hormonally regulated lipase (Fredrikson, Tornqvist and Belfrage, 1986) (Figure 4.9).

Thus, each triglyceride molecule generates three FFA molecules that are released from the cell into the plasma, where they bind to albumin and circulate for distribution to other tissues. The pathway by which FFA leave the adipocyte is not clear; no specific fatty acid transporter, analogous to FAT, has yet been identified.

Lipolysis also yields glycerol, which leaves the cell membrane by facilitated diffusion involving AQP7, a member of the aquaporin channel family (Kuriyama *et al.*, 1997). Glycerol release from adipocytes or fat tissue is often taken as a measure of lipolysis, because fat expresses little if any glycerol kinase activity, which is necessary to reutilize glycerol (Coleman and Lee, 2004). It has recently been suggested that, in rodents, TZDs can up-regulate glycerol kinase in WAT, thus increasing local re-esterification of FFA and reducing FFA delivery into the circulation (Guan *et al.*, 2002). However, this is not supported by the human data available (Tan *et al.*, 2003; Mazzucotelli *et al.*, 2007).

Adipokines

Adipose tissue produces and releases a wide range of specific factors in addition to its major metabolic products, FFA and glycerol (see Figure 4.3). Some of these factors have only a local paracrine action on adjacent cells (adipocytes or SVF cells), whereas others exert hormonal effects on distant tissues. Collectively, these products may influence insulin sensitivity, glucose homeostasis and cardiovascular function.

Strictly, adipokines are cytokines that are secreted by adipocytes into the extravascular space and/or the circulation, such as leptin and adiponectin. Other adipose tissue products include LPL (exported to the vascular endothelium), various binding proteins, prostaglandins and sterol hormones. The latter include oestrogens produced from circulating androgens under the influence of the aromatase enzyme, which is located in mesenchymal cells and preadipocytes cells rather than in mature adipocytes (Simpson et al., 2002).

In addition, numerous bioactive factors and cytokines are now known to be expressed and released by the SVF cells, not adipocytes (Fain, 2006) – a distinction that has not always been made clear (Rajala and Scherer, 2003; Trayhurn and Wood, 2004). Some examples are shown in Figure 4.3. Mainly SVF-specific products include various cytokines and other factors important in inflammation, such as the interleukins (IL-1β, IL-6, IL-8, IL-10 and IL-18), the interleukin receptor antagonist, IL1-Ra, and TNF-α (Fain et al., 2004; Bruun et al., 2004; Curat et al., 2006). Some other products are released by both adipocytes and SVF cells, such as cathepsins, resistin, serum amyloid (SAA-1 and -2), haptoglobin, pentraxin-3 and macrophage migration inhibitory factor (MIF) (Fain, 2006).

This account focuses on leptin and adiponectin. Other adipokines include resistin (Steppan et al., 2001); apelin, a peptide also secreted by hypothalamic neurones (Boucher et al., 2005); visfatin, which apparently has insulin-mimetic effects (Fukuhara et al., 2005, 2007); and retinol-binding protein-4 (RBP-4), which may induce insulin resistance in rodents (Yang et al., 2005), but remains of uncertain significance in humans (Graham et al., 2006; Vitkova et al., 2007).

Leptin

Leptin is a protein expressed by white adipocytes and, to a limited extent, by other tissues such as placenta and stomach. It is encoded by the LEP gene in humans and in mice by ob – which was identified by positional cloning in the genetically obese ob/ob mouse (Chapter 6). Leptin is secreted, and circulates in the bloodstream, as a 146-amino acid (12-kDa) protein. Despite its size, it readily enters the hypothalamus and other brain regions involved in energy regulation, by active transport across the blood-brain barrier mediated by a short form of the leptin receptor (ObRa).

The leptin receptor, encoded by the LEP-R in humans and db (ObR) in the mouse, is a member of the class I cytokine receptor family that has a single transmembrane-spanning domain. Six isoforms, resulting from alternative splicing of a single mRNA and differing in the length of the intracellular tail, share the same extracellular-binding domain. The long isoform (ObRb) mediates most of the known effects of leptin via its intracellular tail. Leptin signalling operates through various pathways involving Janus kinase and signal transducer and activator of transcription (JAK-STAT), mitogen-activated protein kinase (MAPK), phosphatidyl-inositol 3-kinase (PI3 kinase) and AMPK – the pattern of signalling depending on the cell type (Ceddia, 2005).

Leptin was originally named for its experimental effects in reducing feeding and body weight, and it appears to operate as an important regulator of feeding in rodents, especially in the face of starvation and other states that reduce body fat (see Chapter 6). It also helps to regulate lipid turnover and thus metabolism in adipose tissue, skeletal muscle, liver and the β cell (Ceddia, 2005). In particular, it acts to prevent ectopic triglyceride deposition in these tissues, by up-regulating FFA oxidation and down-regulating lipogenesis (Chapter 10); these effects lead to enhanced insulin sensitivity (Figure 4.12). In rodent skeletal muscle, leptin inhibits the expression of FAT and thus decreases FFA uptake (Steinberg, Bonen and Dyck, 2002; Unger, 2005). In humans, leptin also increases fatty acid oxidation in skeletal muscles from lean, but not obese subjects (Steinberg, Bonen and Dyck, 2002).

Plasma leptin levels increase in parallel with BMI and body fat mass, and are therefore higher in obese subjects than in lean (Figure 4.13). This is in contrast to the ob/ob mouse, in which leptin is absent from the circulation and explains the increased appetite and excessive weight gain (Chapter 6). The fact that obese humans do not display the predicted features of high leptin levels – hypophagia and insulin sensitivity – implies that leptin's actions are attenuated to some degree in obesity. This possible 'leptin resistance' is discussed below.

Humans and rodents that lack adipose tissue (e.g. through lipodystrophies, or experimental ablation of WAT) have low circulating leptin levels and show marked ectopic triglyceride

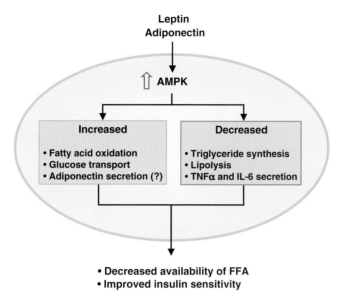

Figure 4.12 Metabolic actions of leptin and adiponectin. Both activate AMPK, leading to decreased free fatty acids (FFA) utilization and enhanced insulin sensitivity.

deposition in muscle, liver and the β cell. Manifestations of this 'lipotoxicity' include insulin resistance and impaired insulin secretion (Garg and Misra, 2004; Unger, 2003). Treatment of lipodystrophic subjects or animals with exogenous leptin reduces appetite, and clears triglycerides from liver and skeletal muscle (Oral *et al.*, 2002; Petersen *et al.* 2002). As discussed below, the insulin-sensitizing effects of both leptin and adiponectin may be partly explained by their direct stimulation of AMPK, a key enzyme in cellular energy homeostasis (Figure 4.12).

As discussed in Chapters 6 and 21, mutations affecting either leptin (*LEP* or *ob*) or its receptors (*LEP-R* or ObR) in humans and rodents lead to overeating, early-onset obesity and insulin resistance that may be accompanied by type 2 diabetes. The severe obesity found in congenitally leptin-deficient subjects provided the first evidence that leptin is an important regulator of energy balance in humans (Montague *et al.*, 1997). Moreover, treating these patients with exogenous leptin reduces obesity and resolves the associated diabetes and hypogonadism (Licinio *et al.*, 2004). By contrast, most obese patients – who have raised leptin levels in relation to their body fat mass – do not respond to leptin treatment. This apparent 'leptin resistance' (Munzberg and Myers, 2005) may be due to over-activity of the protein suppressor of

cytokine signalling (SOCS-3), which is induced by leptin but acts to inhibit leptin signalling and thus decrease the central anorexic effect of leptin (Howard and Flier, 2006). Of note, silencing of the ob-receptor gene related protein in the hypothalamus prevents 'leptin resistance' in dietary-obese mice (Couturier *et al.*, 2007).

A homozygous mutation in the human leptin receptor (*LEP-R*) gene results in a truncated leptin receptor that lacks both the transmembrane and intracellular domains. In addition to early-onset morbid obesity, affected subjects have no pubertal development and impaired secretion of growth hormone and thyrotrophin, indicating that leptin is an important physiological regulator of several endocrine functions in humans (Clément *et al.*, 1998). Leptin receptor mutations were recently demonstrated in 3% of a cohort of subjects with severe, early-onset obesity (Farooqi *et al.*, 2007).

Adiponectin

This adipocyte-specific plasma protein, discovered by four groups using different approaches, is also called AdipoQ, Acrp30 or GBP28. Adiponectin is a product of the apM1 gene, highly expressed in adipocytes (Kadowaki and Yamauchi, 2005; Kadowaki *et al.*, 2006). Various factors

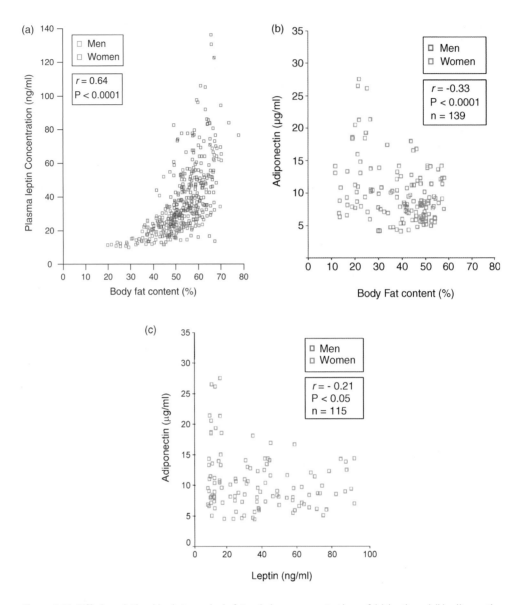

Figure 4.13 Differing relationships between body fat and plasma concentrations of (a) leptin and (b) adiponectin. Leptin is positively correlated with body fat, whereas adiponectin shows a negative correlation. These divergent relationships are emphasized in the negative correlation between plasma leptin and adiponectin concentrations (c).

inhibit adiponectin expression and production in adipocytes, notably TNF-α, insulin, glucocorticoids, β-adrenergic agonists and reactive oxygen species. Sex, ageing, lifestyle and diet are likely to play roles in the regulation of adiponectin levels.

Adiponectin is structurally similar to the complement protein 1q, and possesses a C-terminal globular domain and an N-terminal collagen-like domain. It circulates in a wide range of complexes, which complicates its plasma measurement. It is secreted from the adipocyte as oligomeric complexes of various sizes, namely a trimeric low molecular weight (LMW) form, a middle molecular weight (MMW) hexamer comprising two trimers, and high molecular weight (HMW) forms consisting of up to 18 molecules (Pajvani *et al.*, 2003; Lara-Castro *et al.*, 2006). All three isoforms are present in plasma, probably circulating in humans complexed with other high molecular weight glycoproteins such as α_2-macroglobulin and thrombospondin-1; the latter are involved in regulating inflammation and tissue remodelling (Wang *et al.*, 2006), and may interfere with adiponectin's bioavailability. The HMW form is the most closely related to insulin resistance and the metabolic syndrome (Hara *et al.*, 2006). Serum HMW complexes correlate better with glucose tolerance than total adiponectin levels (Fisher *et al.*, 2005; Lara-Castro *et al.*, 2006; Aso *et al.*, 2006), and HMW levels increase selectively when insulin sensitivity improves in type 2 diabetic patients treated with TZDs (Pajvani *et al.*, 2004). Moreover, relative increases in HMW and MMW isoforms, and a reduction in LMW adiponectin, occur after weight reduction (Bobbert *et al.*, 2005).

Two types of adiponectin receptor, encoded on different chromosomes, have been described (Yamauchi *et al.*, 2003). Both AdipoR1 and AdipoR2 are 7-transmembrane receptors, with the atypical feature of the N-terminus lying on the inside and the C-terminus outside the membrane; both can form homo- or hetero-multimers. In humans, AdipoR1 is ubiquitously expressed, with highest levels in skeletal muscle, whereas AdipoR2 is predominantly expressed in liver. Little is known about their regulation in humans (Kadowaki *et al.*, 2006; Staiger *et al.*, 2004). Exercise training up-regulates AdipoR1 and AdipoR2 expression in human skeletal muscle (Blüher *et al.*, 2006), while no significant change is reported in subcutaneous adipose tissue during energy restriction (Viguerie *et al.*, 2005). An adiponectin receptor interacting protein, APPL1, has recently been identified (Mao *et al.*, 2006). This 70-amino acid protein occurs in insulin-sensitive tissues that also express adiponectin receptors; APPL1 binds to adiponectin receptors and enhances downstream responses such as fatty acid oxidation, GLUT4 translocation and glucose uptake, AMPK protein levels and phosphorylation.

Unlike leptin and other adipokines, circulating levels of adiponectin are inversely related to BMI and body fat mass (Matsubara, Maruoka and Katayose, 2002) (Figure 4.13). This relationship is interesting, in light of the evidence that adiponectin enhances insulin sensitivity and protects against atherogenesis, and suggests a potential link between obesity and its cardio-metabolic risks. Adiponectin may confer beneficial metabolic and cardiovascular

effects, notably improved insulin sensitivity and protection against atheroma formation, at least in rodents. Adiponectin-deficient mice show insulin resistance, hyperlipidaemia and hypertension, characteristic of the metabolic syndrome, while adiponectin administration improves insulin sensitivity in these and other rodent models of insulin resistance (Kadowaki *et al.*, 2006). Adiponectin ameliorates insulin resistance by activating muscle glucose utilization and by promoting fatty acid oxidation in muscle and liver, thus clearing triglyceride from these tissues and reducing 'lipotoxicity' (see Chapter 10). By inhibiting gluconeogenic enzymes, it also decreases hepatic glucose production.

The effects of adiponectin in humans are less clear. *In vitro*, it enhances insulin-stimulated glucose uptake and fatty acid oxidation in human skeletal muscle, although these effects are impaired in tissue from obese and type 2 diabetic subjects (Bruce *et al.*, 2005). In humans, plasma adiponectin levels are inversely correlated with the degree of insulin resistance (Figure 4.14). In addition, low adiponectin levels are associated with dyslipidaemia, hypertension and oxidative stress; with hepatic steatosis and insulin resistance (Bajaj *et al.*, 2004); and, in Pima Indians, with increased risk of developing type 2 diabetes (Krakoff *et al.*, 2003). Paradoxically elevated adiponectin levels are observed in humans with mutations of the insulin receptor and severe insulin resistance; the increase in adiponectin could represent an attempt to compensate for insulin resistance in these cases (Semple *et al.*, 2006).

In addition to its beneficial metabolic effects, adiponectin may also protect against atheroma formation (Hug and Lodish, 2005; Han *et al.*, 2007). It exerts several anti-atherogenic actions on both the arterial wall and macrophage functions. It stimulates the production of nitric oxide (NO) and thus improves endothelium-dependent vasodilatation (see Chapter 12); it also reduces the expression of adhesion molecules and of growth factors by endothelial cells, and suppresses the proliferation and migration of vascular smooth muscle cells (Arita *et al.*, 2002). Its multiple inhibitory effects on macrophages include down-regulation of scavenger receptor class A-1 expression, inhibition of the transformation of macrophages to foam cells, and a switch from the production of pro-inflammatory cytokines such as IL-1β in favour of anti-inflammatory factors such as

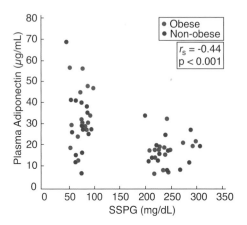

Figure 4.14 The inverse relationship between plasma adiponectin and insulin sensitivity as inferred from steady-state plasma glucose (SSPG) concentration during infusion of fixed amounts of glucose and insulin. Higher values of SSPG indicate greater insulin resistance. From Abbasi *et al.* (2004) with permission of the editor of *Diabetes*.

IL-10 and the IL-1R antagonist (Ouchi *et al.*, 2001; Yokota *et al.*, 2000).

The metabolic and insulin-sensitizing effects of both leptin and adiponectin can be explained, at least partially, by their direct activation of AMP-activated protein kinase (AMPK), a key enzyme in cellular energy homeostasis (Figure 4.12). Although operating through different receptors and distinct signalling pathways, the actions of leptin and adiponectin converge on the control of AMPK activity in skeletal muscle, liver and adipose tissue. Important effects are to enhance fatty acid oxidation, preventing triglyceride accumulation and lipotoxicity in these tissues (Lafontan and Viguerie, 2006).

AMPK functions as an integrated energy sensor that controls energy balance by activating catabolic processes that generate ATP (fatty acid oxidation, glucose uptake), while inhibiting anabolic processes that consume energy, such as lipogenesis, protein synthesis and gluconeogenesis (Carling, 2004; Kahn *et al.*, 2005; Long and Zierath, 2006). This role is discussed further in Chapter 6.

Receptors expressed by adipose tissue

It is clear from the previous sections of this chapter that white adipose tissue is tightly regulated in its metabolic and secretory functions.

Consistent with its various roles, adipose tissue expresses a wide variety of receptors for hormones, neurotransmitters, cytokines and growth factors.

Brown adipose tissue

BAT is a specialized tissue that differs markedly from WAT in its structure and function. It is distinguished macroscopically by its brown appearance (Figure 4.15), which is due to the cytochrome pigments in its abundant mitochondria (Cinti, 2001). Brown adipocytes differ structurally from the unilocular white adipocytes in several respects. They are generally smaller (15–60 µm in diameter), with a larger oval nucleus, small multilocular lipid droplets and abundant cytoplasm that contains plentiful, densely-packed mitochondria with numerous, complex cristae (see Figures 4.16(a) and 4.16(b)).

Brown adipocytes are thought to be derived from adipoblasts and preadipocytes that exhibit a particular molecular signature, with specific transcriptional factors such as PRDM16 being induced in precursor cells during brown fat adipogenesis (see Figure 4.1). Recent evidence suggests that specific myogenic precursors differentiate into brown adipocytes (Seale *et al.*, 2008; see Note added in proof, page 102). PRDM16 activates a broad programme of brown fat determination, including expression of the transcriptional co-activator PGC-1α, which controls the expression of uncoupling protein-1 (UCP-1, see below) and other thermogenic genes (Seale *et al.*, 2007).

BAT is present throughout life in rodents. In the human neonate, BAT is found in conspicuous depots in the mediastinum, surrounding the great vessels, around the kidneys and between the scapulae. At birth, its total weight is about 150–250 g (2–5% of body weight). Until recently, it was generally accepted that BAT involutes steadily during the first few months, with clearly recognizable depots having essentially disappeared within the first 1–2 years of age. In normal adults, it was thought that only occasional brown adipocytes were scattered through white fat masses, although brown adipocytes can be induced under certain conditions (see below). However, recent findings using positron emission tomography (PET) have suggested that active BAT occurs in adults (Nedergaard, Bengtsson and Cannon, 2007). This is discussed further below.

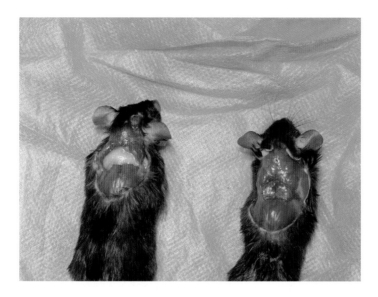

Figure 4.15 Interscapular brown adipose tissue (BAT) in an obese *ob/ob* mouse (left) and a lean control (right). In the obese mouse, white adipose tissue (WAT) is prominent in this site, whereas the lean mouse shows typically well developed BAT; the dark colour is due to the high content of mitochondrial cytochromes.

Functions of BAT

BAT is specialized for heat production (Himms-Hagen, 1990). Its lipid stores turn over rapidly, and the liberated fatty acids are oxidized by the brown adipocyte's mitochondria in a process that generates heat directly (Figure 4.17). The tissue shows intense metabolic activity, explained by

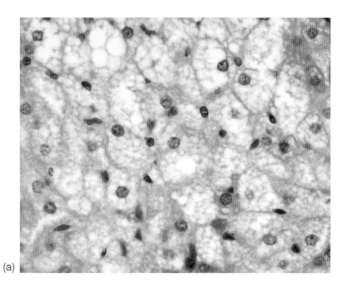

(a)

Figure 4.16 (a) Brown adipocytes, shown by light microscopy (haematoxylin and eosin stain; original magnification, 40×; bar ▬▬▬ 100 μm. Note the numerous multilocular lipid droplets and rounded nuclei. Image courtesy of Dr. María Angela Burrell, Department of Histology and Pathology, University of Navarra, Pamplona, Spain. And (b) Electron micrograph of a brown adipocyte (original magnification, 15,000×). Note the numerous complex mitochondria. Image courtesy of Dr. María Pilar Sesma, Department of Histology and Pathology, University of Navarra, Pamplona, Spain.

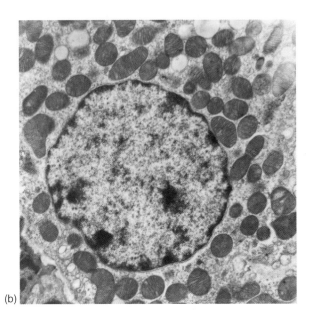

(b)

Figure 4.16 *(Continued)*

its plentiful mitochondria. Heat is produced by fatty acid oxidation, which is 'uncoupled' – i.e. does not result in ATP synthesis. This is due to uncoupling protein-1 (UCP-1), a 32-kDa protein expressed only in brown adipocytes, and which spans the inner mitochondrial membrane (Ricquier and Bouillaud, 2000) (Figure 4.17). Oxidative phosphorylation normally drives protons into the intermembrane space, generating an electrochemical gradient that pushes protons back into the mitochondrial matrix, activating ATP synthetase. In the presence of UCP-1, the proton electrochemical gradient is short-circuited by protons re-entering the matrix through this channel; the energy generated is therefore in the form of heat, rather than ATP.

UCP-1 expression and protein levels increase rapidly in response to cold, the experimental administration of β_3 agonist drugs, and activation of the sympathetic nervous system. BAT is densely innervated with sympathetic nerve terminals, and its thermogenic activity is regulated by the sympathetic system. Noradrenaline released from sympathetic nerve endings acts through β_3-adrenoceptors to activate adenylyl cyclase, thus increasing cAMP production. This in turn activates HSL, to generate the fatty acids that are the substrate for heat production, and also increases the expression and activity of UCP-1 (Figure 4.17). BAT is a highly vascular tissue, and sympathetic activity greatly increases its blood flow, thus delivering the heat generated to the rest of the body.

In neonatal mammals, hibernators and rodents, a crucial function of BAT is the maintenance of body temperature through cold-induced thermogenesis. In addition, BAT thermogenesis is activated in rats that overeat – an important aspect of diet-induced thermogenesis. Rothwell and Stock (1979) suggested that this response could help to restrain body fat mass under conditions of over-nutrition, thus highlighting the importance of BAT in the normal control of energy balance in lower mammals. Subsequently, the role of BAT in counteracting excess adiposity in rodents has been confirmed by other studies. The thermogenic activity of BAT is reduced, as is whole-body energy expenditure, in *ob/ob* mice and *fa/fa* rats (see Chapter 6). UCP-1 levels are low in retroperitoneal brown fat pads in genetically obese rodents (Himms-Hagen, 1990). Targeted ablation of BAT in mice leads to obesity and increased body weight (Lowell *et al.*, 1993), whereas transgenic mice whose white adipocytes express UCP-1 are protected against genetic and dietary-induced obesity, even though their normal BAT atrophies under these conditions (Valet *et al.*, 2002).

BAT in humans

As mentioned above, macroscopically visible BAT disappears soon after birth in normal humans.

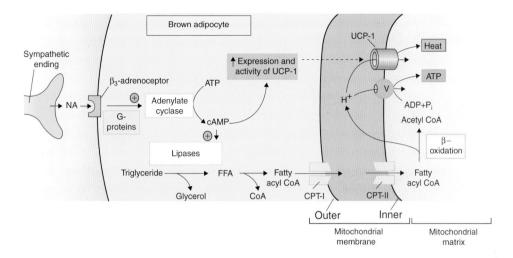

Figure 4.17 The process of thermogenesis in the brown adipocyte. FFA, produced by lipolysis of stored triglyceride, are oxidized in mitochondria. Oxidative phosphorylation generates a proton gradient across the inner mitochondrial membrane; instead of driving ATP production, this is dissipated as heat because the protons re-enter the matrix through the uncoupling protein, UCP-1, in the inner mitochondrial membrane.

UCP-1 mRNA can only be detected at very low levels in WAT of adults (Lean and James, 1986; Oberkofler *et al.*, 1997), and BAT does not contribute significantly to thermogenesis in humans (Astrup *et al.*, 1985). However, UCP-1 expression and a 'brown' phenotype can be induced under certain rare conditions, including 'hibernomas' (tumours consisting of brown fat) and in the perirenal WAT of patients with phaeochromocytoma (Gonzalez-Barroso, Ricquier and Cassard-Doulcier, 2000). The connection with phaeochromocytoma can be explained by high levels of catecholamines activating β_3-adrenoceptors on brown adipocytes persisting from the neonatal period.

Recent PET studies using fluorodeoxyglucose (a marker of metabolic activity, used in clinical practice to map tumour tissue) have provided evidence that active BAT exists in adults (Nedergaard, Bengtsson and Cannon, 2007). These have shown symmetrical areas of increased tracer uptake in the upper parts of the body, broadly corresponding to the distribution of BAT in lower mammals and in human neonates (Figure 4.18). The main depots are found in the supraclavicular region and neck, with additional activity in the paravertebral, mediastinal, paraaortic and suprarenal areas; however, there was no interscapular localization. This presumed BAT activity is acutely enhanced by cold exposure and stimulated by the sympathetic nervous system.

The prevalence of active BAT in normal adults can be only estimated indirectly, but is thought to be present in around 10% of the general population (Nedergaard, Bengtsson and Cannon, 2007). BAT therefore has the potential to play a role in normal energy balance and could become a pharmacological target for new drugs to treat obesity.

Interestingly, human white adipocytes can be manipulated *in vitro* to develop 'brown' characteristics. The phenotype of human subcutaneous fat cells, which are prototypical white adipocytes, can be modified by forced expression of PGC-1α (Tiraby *et al.*, 2003; Mazzucotelli *et al.*, 2007). This transcriptional coactivator switches on genes involved in fatty acid oxidation and the mitochondrial respiratory chain and induces the expression of UCP-1. The coordinated upregulation of gene expression results in an increased capacity to oxidize fatty acids. Moreover, induction of glycerol kinase, which catalyses the phosphorylation of glycerol into glycerol-3-phosphate, is also observed. If the cells are stimulated by catecholamines, increased glycerol kinase activity generates a futile cycle through the direct reincorporation into triglycerides of glycerol and fatty acids generated by triglyceride hydrolysis. Therefore, turning on the expression of PGC-1α may favour the utilization of FFA within the fat cell instead of their release into the bloodstream.

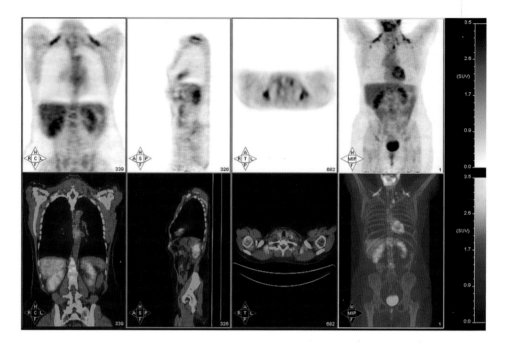

Figure 4.18 PET scan of an adult, showing discrete areas of increased metabolic activity in the fat of the upper thorax and neck, which are thought to correspond to functionally active brown adipose tissue (BAT). Other organs with high metabolic activity are the heart, kidneys and liver; residual isotope (fluorodeoxyglucose) is also seen in the bladder. Images courtesy of Dr María José García Velloso, Department of Nuclear Medicine, Clínica Universitaria de Navarra, Pamplona, Spain.

Note added in proof

Adipose tissue development and dynamics

Recent studies, published just before this book went to press, have cast new light on some important aspects of the origins and turnover of white and brown fat.

First, Spalding *et al.* (2008) have succeeded in clarifying the turnover of white adipocytes in adults, and in calculating rates of adipocyte death and renewal. They did this by measuring the relative abundance of ^{14}C in genomic DNA from adipocytes; this isotope was derived from atmospheric nuclear bomb testing during a defined period in the 1950s and effectively pulse-labelled the DNA. Spalding *et al.* (2008) found that an individual's total number of adipocytes remained roughly constant at all stages of adult life, but that ~10% of adipocytes died, while a comparable proportion were renewed, each year. Thus, white adipose tissue turns out to be a more dynamic tissue than was previously assumed. These findings were consistent across a wide

range of BMI, including subjects with early-onset obesity, and following weight loss. Adipocyte number has been shown to be a major determinant of fat mass in the adult, and the number of adipocytes in both lean and obese subjects appears to be set during childhood. However, it remains possible that the common scenario of gradual but significant weight gain throughout adult life may be underpinned by an initial increase in triglyceride loading until an adipocyte size threshold is reached, when additional new adipocytes are recruited from committed precursor cells or mesenchymal stem cells (see pages 79–82)

New information about the identity of the precursor cells that give rise to white adipocytes has come from the studies of Tang *et al.* (2008). These now appear to be pericytes, the cells that surround the endothelium tubes of the microvasculature. These progenitor cells become committed to the white adipocyte lineage either prenatally or in the early postnatal period (Tang *et al.*, 2008). Adipose tissue has long been recognised to expand in conjunction with its vasculature, but these new findings suggest that the blood vessels may actively direct the process; as well as serving as a progenitor niche, they may also produce signals for adipocyte development.

Finally, the origin and development of brown adipocytes have been further elucidated by Seale *et al.* (2008) and Tseng *et al.* (2008). Seale *et al.* (2008) have shown that the white and brown adipocyte precursors diverge earlier than previously believed, with the latter originating in the early embryo from distinct precursors that express Myf5, a gene thought to be expressed exclusively by the myogenic lineage. Thus, brown fat appears to share a common origin with skeletal muscle. Tseng *et al.* (2008), in seeking specific cues that direct the differentiation of white and brown adipocytes, found that bone morphogenetic protein 7 plays a key role in the development of brown adipocytes.

References

Aarsland, A., Chinkes, D. and Wolfe, R.R. (1997) Hepatic and whole-body fat synthesis in humans during carbohydrate overfeeding. *The American Journal of Clinical Nutrition*, **65**, 1774–82.

Abbasi, F., Chu, J.W., Lamendola, C. *et al.* (2004) Discrimination between obesity and insulin resistance in the relationship with adiponectin. *Diabetes*, **53**, 585–90.

Arita, Y., Kihara, S., Ouchi, N. *et al.* (2002) Adipocyte-derived plasma protein adiponectin acts as a platelet-derived growth factor-BB-binding protein and regulates growth factor-induced common postreceptor signal in vascular smooth muscle cell. *Circulation*, **105**, 2893–8.

Aso, Y., Yamamoto, R., Wakabayashi, S. *et al.* (2006) Comparison of serum high-molecular weight (HMW) adiponectin with total adiponectin concentrations in type 2 diabetic patients with coronary artery disease using a novel enzyme-linked immunosorbent assay to detect HMW adiponectin. *Diabetes*, **55**, 1954–60.

Astrup, A., Bulow, J., Madsen, J. and Christensen, N.J. (1985) Contribution of BAT and skeletal muscle to thermogenesis induced by ephedrine in man. *American Journal of Physiology. Endocrinology and Metabolism*, **248**, E507–15.

Baar, R.A., Dingfelder, C.S., Smith *et al.* (2005) Investigation of in vivo fatty acid metabolism in AFABP/aP2(−/−) mice. *American Journal of Physiology. Endocrinology and Metabolism*, **288**, E187–93.

Bajaj, M., Suraamornkul, S., Piper, P. *et al.* (2004) Decreased plasma adiponectin concentrations are closely related to hepatic fat content and hepatic insulin resistance in pioglitazone-treated type 2 diabetic patients. *The Journal of Clinical Endocrinology and Metabolism*, **89**, 200–6.

Bastelica, D., Morange, P., Berthet, B. *et al.* (2002) Stromal cells are the main plasminogen activator inhibitor-1-producing cells in human fat: evidence of differences between visceral and subcutaneous deposits. *Arteriosclerosis, Thrombosis, and Vascular Biology*, **22**, 173–8.

Beale, E.G., Hammer, R.E., Antoine, B. and Forest, C. (2002) Glyceroneogenesis comes of age. *The FASEB Journal*, **16**, 1695–6.

Blüher, M., Bullen, J.W., Jr., Lee, J.H. *et al.* (2006) Circulating adiponectin and expression of adiponectin receptors in human skeletal muscle: associations with metabolic parameters and insulin resistance and regulation by physical training. *The Journal of Clinical Endocrinology and Metabolism*, **91**, 2310–6.

Bobbert, T., Rochlitz, H., Wegewitz, U. *et al.* (2005) Changes of adiponectin oligomer composition by moderate weight reduction. *Diabetes*, **54**, 2712–9.

Boucher, J., Masri, B., Daviaud, D. *et al.* (2005) Apelin, a newly identified adipokine up-regulated by insulin and obesity. *Endocrinology*, **146**, 1764–1.

Bouloumie, A., Curat, C.A., Sengenes, C. *et al.* (2005) Role of macrophage tissue infiltration in metabolic diseases. *Current Opinion in Clinical Nutrition and Metabolic Care*, **8**, 347–54.

Brakenhielm, E., Cao, R., Gao, B. *et al.* (2004) Angiogenesis inhibitor, TNP-470, prevents diet-induced and genetic obesity in mice. *Circulation Research*, **94**, 1579–88.

Bruce, C.R., Mertz, V.A., Heigenhauser, G.J. and Dyck, D.J. (2005) The stimulatory effect of globular adiponectin on insulin-stimulated glucose uptake and fatty acid oxidation is impaired in skeletal muscle from obese subjects. *Diabetes*, **54**, 3154–60.

Bruun, J.M., Lihn, A.S., Madan, A.K. *et al.* (2004) Higher production of IL-8 in visceral vs. subcutaneous adipose tissue. Implication of nonadipose cells in adipose tissue. *American Journal of Physiology. Endocrinology and Metabolism*, **286**, E8–13.

Cadoudal, T., Leroyer, S., Reis, A.F. *et al.* (2005) Proposed involvement of adipocyte glyceroneogenesis and phosphoenolpyruvate carboxykinase in the metabolic syndrome. *Biochimie*, **87**, 27–32.

Cancello, R., Henegar, C., Viguerie, N. *et al.* (2005) Reduction of macrophage infiltration and chemoattractant gene expression changes in white adipose tissue of morbidly obese subjects after surgery-induced weight loss. *Diabetes*, **54**, 2277–86.

Cancello, R., Tordjman, J., Poitou, C. *et al.* (2006) Increased infiltration of macrophages in omental adipose tissue is associated with marked hepatic lesions in morbid human obesity. *Diabetes*, **55**, 1554–61.

Carling, D. (2004) The AMP-activated protein kinase cascade – a unifying system for energy control. *Trends in Biochemical Sciences*, **29**, 18–24.

Caspar-Bauguil, S., Cousin, B., Galinier, A. *et al.* (2005) Adipose tissues as an ancestral immune organ: site-specific change in obesity. *FEBS Letters*, **579**, 3487–92.

Ceddia, R.B. (2005) Direct metabolic regulation in skeletal muscle and fat tissue by leptin: implications for glucose and fatty acids homeostasis. *International Journal of Obesity*, **29**, 1175–83.

Chmurzyńska, A. (2006) The multigene family of fatty acid-binding proteins (FABPs): function, structure and polymorphism. *Journal of Applied Genetics*, **47**, 39–48.

Chun, T.H., Hotary, K.B., Sabeh, F., *et al.* (2006) A pericellular collagenase directs the 3-dimensional development of white adipose tissue. *Cell*, **125**, 577–91.

Cinti, S. (2001) The adipose organ: morphological perspectives of adipose tissues. *Proceedings of the Nutrition Society*, **60**, 319–28.

Clément, K., Vaisse, C., Lahlou, N. *et al.* (1998) A mutation in the human leptin receptor gene causes obesity and pituitary dysfunction. *Nature*, **392**, 398–401.

Clément, K., Viguerie, N., Poitou, C. *et al.* (2004) Weight loss regulates inflammation-related genes in white adipose tissue of obese subjects. *The FASEB Journal*, **18**, 1657–69.

Coburn, C.T., Knapp, F.F., Jr., Febbraio, M. *et al.* (2000) Defective uptake and utilization of long chain fatty acids in muscle and adipose tissues of CD36 knockout mice. *The Journal of Biological Chemistry*, **275**, 32523–9.

Coleman, R.A. and Lee, D.P. (2004) Enzymes of triacylglycerol synthesis and their regulation. *Progress in Lipid Research*, **43**, 134–76.

Couturier, C., Sarkis, C., Séron, K. *et al.* (2007) Silencing of OB-RGRP in mouse hypothalamic arcuate nucleus increases leptin receptor signaling and prevents diet-induced obesity. *Proceedings of the National Academy of Sciences of the United States of America*, **104**, 19476–81.

Crossno, J.T. , Jr., Majka, S.M., Grazia, T. *et al.* (2006) Rosiglitazone promotes development of a novel adipocyte population from bone marrow-derived circulating progenitor cells. *The Journal of Clinical Investigation*, **116**, 3220–8.

Curat, C.A., Miranville, A., Sengenes, C. *et al.* (2004) From blood monocytes to adipose tissue-resident macrophages: induction of diapedesis by human mature adipocytes. *Diabetes*, **53**, 1285–92.

Curat, C.A., Wegner, V., Sengenes, C. *et al.* (2006) Macrophages in human visceral adipose tissue: increased accumulation in obesity and a source of resistin and visfatin. *Diabetologia*, **49**, 744–7.

Després, J.P. and Lemieux, I. (2006) Abdominal obesity and metabolic syndrome. *Nature*, **444**, 881–7.

Ellis, J.R., McDonald, R.B. and Stern, J.S. (1990) A diet high in fat stimulates adipocyte proliferation in older (22 month) rats. *Experimental Gerontology*, **25**, 141–8.

Fain, J.N. (2006) Release of interleukins and other inflammatory cytokines by human adipose tissue is enhanced in obesity and primarily due to the nonfat cells. *Vitamins and Hormones*, **74**, 443–77.

Fain, J.N., Madan, A.K., Hiler, M.L. *et al.* (2004) Comparison of the release of adipokines by adipose tissue, adipose tissue matrix, and adipocytes from visceral and subcutaneous abdominal adipose tissues of obese humans. *Endocrinology*, **145**, 2273–82.

Farooqi, I.S., Wangensteen, T., Collins, S. *et al.* (2007) Clinical and molecular genetic spectrum of congenital deficiency of the leptin receptor. *The New England Journal of Medicine*, **356**, 237–47.

Faust, I.M., Johnson, P.R., Stern, J.S. and Hirsch, J. (1978) Diet-induced adipocyte number increase in adult rats: a new model of obesity. *American Journal of Physiology. Endocrinology and Metabolism*, **235**, E279–86.

Febbraio, M., Abumrad, N.A., Hajjar, D.P. *et al.* (1999) A null mutation in murine CD36 reveals an important role in fatty acid and lipoprotein metabolism. *The Journal of Biological Chemistry*, **274**, 19055–62.

Fielding, B.A. and Frayn, K.N. (1998) Lipoprotein lipase and the disposition of dietary fatty acids. *The British Journal of Nutrition*, **80**, 495–502.

Fisher, F.F., Trujillo, M.E., Hanif, W. *et al.* (2005) Serum high molecular weight complex of adiponectin correlates better with glucose tolerance than total serum adiponectin in Indo-Asian males. *Diabetologia*, **48**, 1084–7.

Fontana, L., Eagon, J.C., Trujillo, M. *et al.* (2007) Visceral fat adipokine secretion is associated with systemic inflammation in obese humans. *Diabetes*, **56**, 1010–3.

Forbes, G.B. (1970) Weight loss during fasting: implications for the obese. *The American Journal of Clinical Nutrition*, **23**, 1212–9.

Frayn, K.N. (2002) Adipose tissue as a buffer for daily lipid flux. *Diabetologia*, **45**, 1201–10.

Fredrikson, G., Tornqvist, H. and Belfrage, P. (1986) Hormone-sensitive lipase and monoacylglycerol lipase are both required for complete degradation of adipocyte triacylglycerol. *Biochimica et Biophysica Acta*, **876**, 288–93.

Fukuhara, A., Matsuda, M., Nishizawa, M. *et al.* (2005) Visfatin: a protein secreted by visceral fat that mimics the effects of insulin. *Science*, **307**, 426–30. Retraction: Fukuhara *et al.* (2007). *Science*, **318**, 565.

Gabrielsson, B.G., Johansson, J.M., Lonn, M. *et al.* (2003) High expression of complement components in omental adipose tissue in obese men. *Obesity Research*, **11**, 699–708.

Garg, A. and Misra, A. (2004) Lipodystrophies: rare disorders causing metabolic syndrome. *Endocrinology and Metabolism Clinics of North America*, **33**, 305–31.

Gargiulo, C.E., Stuhlsatz-Krouper, S.M. and Schaffer, J.E. (1999) Localization of adipocyte long-chain fatty acyl-CoA synthetase at the plasma membrane. *Journal of Lipid Research*, **40**, 881–92.

Gimeno, R.E. (2007) Fatty acid transport proteins. *Current Opinion in Lipidology*, **18**, 271–6.

Gonzalez-Barroso, M., Ricquier, D. and Cassard-Doulcier, A.M. (2000) The human uncoupling protein-1 gene (UCP1): present status and perspectives in obesity research. *Obesity Reviews*, **1**, 61–72.

Graham, T.E., Yang, Q., Blüher, M. *et al.* (2006) Retinol-binding protein 4 and insulin resistance in lean, obese, and diabetic subjects. *The New England Journal of Medicine*, **354**, 2552–63.

Granneman, J.G., Moore, H.P., Granneman, R.L. *et al.* (2007) Analysis of lipolytic protein trafficking and interactions in adipocytes. *The Journal of Biological Chemistry*, **282**, 5726–35.

Gregoire, F.M., Smas, C.M. and Sul, H.S. (1998) Understanding adipocyte differentiation. *Physiological Reviews*, **78**, 783–809.

Guan, H.P., Li, Y., Jensen, M.V. *et al.* (2002) A futile metabolic cycle activated in adipocytes by antidiabetic agents. *Nature Medicine*, **8**, 1122–8.

Hajri, T. and Abumrad, N.A. (2002) Fatty acid transport across membranes: relevance to nutrition and metabolic pathology. *Annual Review of Nutrition*, **22**, 383–415.

Han, S.H., Quon, M.J., Kim, J.A. and Koh, K.K. (2007) Adiponectin and cardiovascular disease: response to therapeutic interventions. *Journal of the American College of Cardiology*, **49**, 531–8.

Hara, K., Horikoshi, M., Yamauchi, T. *et al.* (2006) Measurement of the high-molecular weight form of adiponectin in plasma is useful for the prediction of insulin resistance and metabolic syndrome. *Diabetes Care*, **29**, 1357–62.

Himms-Hagen, J. (1990) Brown adipose tissue thermogenesis: interdisciplinary studies. *The FASEB Journal*, **4**, 2890–8.

Howard, J.K. and Flier, J.S. (2006) Attenuation of leptin and insulin signaling by SOCS proteins. *Trends in Endocrinology and Metabolism*, **17**, 365–71.

Hug, C. and Lodish, H.F. (2005) The role of the adipocyte hormone adiponectin in cardiovascular disease. *Current Opinion in Pharmacology*, **5**, 129–34.

Jenkins, C.M., Mancuso, D.J., Yan, W. *et al.* (2004) Identification, cloning, expression, and purification of three novel human calcium-independent phospholipase A2 family members possessing triacylglycerol lipase and acylglycerol transacylase activities. *The Journal of Biological Chemistry*, **279**, 48968–75.

Jones, P.R. and Edwards, D.A. (1999) Areas of fat loss in overweight young females following an 8-week period of energy intake reduction. *Annals of Human Biology*, **26**, 151–62.

Kabir, M., Catalano, K.J., Ananthnarayan, S. *et al.* (2005) Molecular evidence supporting the portal theory: a causative link between visceral adiposity and hepatic insulin resistance. *American Journal of Physiology. Endocrinology and Metabolism*, **288**, E454–61.

Kadowaki, T. and Yamauchi, T. (2005) Adiponectin and adiponectin receptors. *Endocrine Reviews*, **26**, 439–51.

Kadowaki, T., Yamauchi, T., Kubota, N. *et al.* (2006) Adiponectin and adiponectin receptors in insulin resistance, diabetes and the metabolic syndrome. *The Journal of Clinical Investigation*, **116**, 1784–92.

Kahn, B.B., Alquier, T., Carling, D. and Hardie, D.G. (2005) AMP-activated protein kinase: ancient energy gauge provides clues to modern understanding of metabolism. *Cell Metabolism*, **1**, 15–25.

Karpe, F. and Frayn, K.N. (2004) The nicotinic acid receptor – a new mechanism for an old drug. *Lancet*, **363**, 1892–4.

Kolonin, M.G., Saha, P.K., Chan, L. *et al.* (2004) Reversal of obesity by targeted ablation of adipose tissue. *Nature Medicine*, **10**, 625–32.

Krakoff, J., Funahashi, T., Stehouwer, C.D. *et al.* (2003) Inflammatory markers, adiponectin, and risk of type 2 diabetes in the Pima Indian. *Diabetes Care*, **26**, 1745–51.

Kuriyama, H., Kawamoto, S., Ishida, N. *et al.* (1997) Molecular cloning and expression of a novel human aquaporin from adipose tissue with glycerol permeability. *Biochemical and Biophysical Research Communications*, **241**, 53–8.

Lafontan, M. and Berlan, M. (2003) Do regional differences in adipocyte biology provide new pathophysiological insights? *Trends in Pharmacological Sciences*, **24**, 276–83.

Lafontan, M. and Viguerie, N. (2006) Role of adipokines in the control of energy metabolism: focus on adiponectin. *Current Opinion in Pharmacology*, **6**, 580–5.

Langin, D. and Arner, P. (2006) Importance of TNF-alpha and neutral lipases in human adipose tissue lipolysis. *Trends in Endocrinology and Metabolism*, **17**, 314–20.

Langin, D., Dicker, A., Tavernier, G. *et al.* (2005) Adipocyte lipases and defect of lipolysis in human obesity. *Diabetes*, **54**, 3190–7.

Langin, D., Lucas, S. and Lafontan, M. (2000) Millenium fat-cell lipolysis reveals unsuspected novel tracks. *Hormone and Metabolic Research*, **32**, 443–52.

Lara-Castro, C., Luo, N., Wallace, P. *et al.* (2006) Adiponectin multimeric complexes and the metabolic syndrome trait cluster. *Diabetes*, **55**, 249–59.

Lass, A., Zimmermann, R., Haemmerle, G. *et al.* (2006) Adipose triglyceride lipase-mediated lipolysis of cellular fat stores is activated by CGI-58 and defective in Chanarin-Dorfman Syndrome. *Cell Metabolism*, **3**, 309–19.

Lean, M.E.J. and James, W.P.T. (1986) Brown adipose tissue in man, in *Brown Adipose Tissue* (eds P. Trayhurn and D.G. Nicholls), Edward Arnold, London, pp. 339–65.

Leroyer, S.N., Tordjman, J., Chauvet, G. *et al.* (2006) Rosiglitazone controls fatty acid cycling in human adipose tissue by means of glyceroneogenesis and glycerol phosphorylation. *The Journal of Biological Chemistry*, **281**, 13141–9.

Licinio, J., Caglayan, S., Ozata, M. *et al.* (2004) Phenotypic effects of leptin replacement on morbid obesity, diabetes mellitus, hypogonadism and behavior in leptin-deficient adults. *Proceedings of the National Academy of Sciences of the United States of America*, **101**, 4531–6.

Linder, K., Arner, P., Flores-Morales, A. *et al.* (2004) Differentially expressed genes in visceral and subcutaneous adipose tissue of obese men and women. *Progress in Lipid Research*, **45**, 148–54.

Liu, T.M., Martina, M., Hutmacher, D.W. *et al.* (2007) Identification of common pathways mediating differentiation of bone marrow- and adipose tissue-derived human mesenchymal stem cells into three mesenchymal lineages. *Stem Cells (Dayton, Ohio)*, **25**, 750–60.

Long, Y.C. and Zierath, J.R. (2006) AMP-activated protein kinase signaling in metabolic regulation. *The Journal of Clinical Investigation*, **116**, 1776–83.

Lowell, B.B., S-Susulic, V., Hamann, A. *et al.* (1993) Development of obesity in transgenic mice after genetic ablation of brown adipose tissue. *Nature*, **366**, 740–2.

Mao, X., Kikani, C.K., Riojas, R.A. *et al.* (2006) APPL1 binds to adiponectin receptors and mediates adiponectin signalling and function. *Nature Cell Biology*, **8**, 516–23.

Marcinkiewicz, A., Gauthier, D., Garcia, A. and Brasaemle, D.L. (2006) The phosphorylation of serine 492 of perilipin A directs lipid droplet fragmentation and dispersion. *The Journal of Biological Chemistry*, **281**, 11901–9.

Martinez-Botas, J., Anderson, J.B., Tessier, D. *et al.* (2000) Absence of perilipin results in leanness and reverses obesity in Leprdb/db mice. *Nature Genetics*, **26**, 474–9.

Matsubara, M., Maruoka, S. and Katayose, S. (2002) Inverse relationship between plasma adiponectin and leptin concentrations in normal-weight and obese women. *European Journal of Endocrinology/ European Federation of Endocrine Societies*, **147**, 173–80.

Maury, E., Ehala-Aleksejev, K., Guiot, Y. *et al.* (2007) Adipokines oversecreted by omental adipose tissue in human obesity. *American Journal of Physiology. Endocrinology and Metabolism*, **293**, E656–65.

Mazzucotelli, A., Viguerie, N., Tiraby, C. *et al.* (2007) The transcriptional coactivator peroxisome proliferator activated receptor (PPAR) gamma coactivator-1 alpha and the nuclear receptor PPAR alpha control the expression of glycerol kinase and metabolism genes independently of PPAR gamma activation in human white adipocytes. *Diabetes*, **56**, 2467–75.

Miranville, A., Heeschen, C., Sengenes, C. *et al.* (2004) Improvement of postnatal neovascularization by human adipose tissue-derived stem cells. *Circulation*, **110**, 349–55.

Miyoshi, H., Souza, S.C., Zhang, H.H. *et al.* (2006) Perilipin promotes hormone-sensitive lipase-mediated adipocyte lipolysis via phosphorylation-dependent and -independent mechanisms. *The Journal of Biological Chemistry*, **281**, 15837–44.

Miyoshi, H., Perfield, J.W., Souza, S.C. *et al.* (2007) Control of adipose triglyceride lipase action by serine 517 of perilipin A globally regulates protein kinase A-stimulated lipolysis in adipocytes. *The Journal of Biological Chemistry*, **282**, 996–1002.

Montague, C.T., Farooqi, I.S., Whitehead, J.P. *et al.* (1997) Congenital leptin deficiency is associated with severe early-onset obesity in humans. *Nature*, **387**, 903–8.

Moore, H.P., Silver, R.B., Mottillo, E.P. *et al.* (2005) Perilipin targets a novel pool of lipid droplets for lipolytic attack by hormone-sensitive lipase. *The Journal of Biological Chemistry*, **280**, 43109–20.

Motoshima, H., Wu, X., Sinha, M.K. *et al.* (2002) Differential regulation of adiponectin secretion from cultured human omental and subcutaneous adipocytes: effects of insulin and rosiglitazone. *The Journal of Clinical Endocrinology and Metabolism*, **87**, 5662–7.

Munzberg, H. and Myers, M.G., Jr. (2005) Molecular and anatomical determinants of central leptin resistance. *Nature Neuroscience*, **8**, 566–70.

Nedergaard, J., Bengtsson, T. and Cannon, B. (2007) Unexpected evidence for active brown adipose tissue in adult humans. *American Journal of Physiology. Endocrinology and Metabolism*, **293**, E444–52.

O'Brien, R.M. and Granner, D.K. (1996) Regulation of gene expression by insulin. *Physiological Reviews*, **76**, 1109–61.

Oberkofler, H., Dallinger, G., Liu, Y.M. *et al.* (1997) Uncoupling protein gene: quantification of expression levels in adipose tissues of obese and non-obese humans. *Journal of Lipid Research*, **38**, 2125–33.

Oral, E.A., Simha, V., Ruiz, E. *et al.* (2002) Leptin-replacement therapy for lipodystrophy. *The New England Journal of Medicine*, **346**, 570–8.

Ouchi, N., Kihara, S., Arita, Y. *et al.* (2001) Adipocyte-derived plasma protein, adiponectin, suppresses lipid accumulation and class A scavenger receptor expression in human monocyte-derived macrophages. *Circulation*, **103**, 1057–63.

Pajvani, U.B., Du, X., Combs, T.P. *et al.* (2003) Structure-function studies of the adipocyte-secreted hormone Acrp30/adiponectin. Implications for metabolic regulation and bioactivity. *The Journal of Biological Chemistry*, **278**, 9073–85.

Pajvani, U.B., Hawkins, M., Combs, T.P. *et al.* (2004) Complex distribution, not absolute amount of adiponectin, correlates with thiazolidinedione-mediated improvement in insulin sensitivity. *The Journal of Biological Chemistry*, **279**, 12152–62.

Peeva, E., Brun, L.D., Ven Murthy, M.R. *et al.* (1992) Adipose cell size and distribution in familial lipoprotein lipase deficiency. *International Journal of Obesity and Related Metabolic Disorders*, **16**, 737–44.

Petersen, K.F., Oral, E.A., Dufour, S. *et al.* (2002) Leptin reverses insulin resistance and hepatic steatosis in patients with severe lipodystrophy. *The Journal of Clinical Investigation*, **109**, 1345–50.

Pond, C.M. (1992) An evolutionary and functional view of mammalian adipose tissue. *Proceedings of the Nutrition Society*, **51**, 367–77.

Pond, C.M. (1999) Physiological specialisation of adipose tissue. *Progress in Lipid Research*, **38**, 225–48.

Prentice, A.M. (2005) Early influences on human energy regulation: thrifty genotypes and thrifty phenotypes. *Physiology & Behavior*, **86**, 640–5.

Rajala, M.W. and Scherer, P.E. (2003) Minireview: The adipocyte – at the crossroads of energy homeostasis, inflammation, and atherosclerosis. *Endocrinology*, **144**, 3765–73.

Ricquier, D. and Bouillaud, F. (2000) Mitochondrial uncoupling proteins: from mitochondria to the regulation of energy balance. *The Journal of Physiology*, **529**, 3–10.

Rosen, E.D. and MacDougald, O.A. (2006) Adipocyte differentiation from the inside out. *Nature Reviews. Molecular Cell Biology*, **7**, 885–96.

Rothwell, N.J. and Stock, M.J. (1979) A role for brown adipose tissue in diet-induced thermogenesis. *Nature*, **281**, 31–5.

Rupnick, M.A., Panigrahy, D., Zhang, C.Y. et al. (2002) Adipose tissue mass can be regulated through the vasculature. *Proceedings of the National Academy of Sciences of the United States of America*, **99**, 10730–5.

Schweiger, M., Schreiber, R., Haemmerle, G. et al. (2006) Adipose triglyceride lipase and hormone-sensitive lipase are the major enzymes in adipose tissue triacylglycerol catabolism. *The Journal of Biological Chemistry*, **281**, 40236–41.

Seale, P., Kajimura, S., Yang, W. et al. (2007) Transcriptional control of brown fat determination by PRDM16. *Cell Metabolism*, **6**, 38–54.

Seale, P., Bjork, B., Yang, W. et al. (2008) PRDM16 controls a brown fat/skeletal muscle switch. *Nature*, **454**, 961–7.

Semple, R.K., Soos, M.A., Luan, J. et al. (2006) Elevated plasma adiponectin in humans with genetically defective insulin receptors. *The Journal of Clinical Endocrinology and Metabolism*, **91**, 3219–23.

Sengenes, C., Lolmede, K., Zakaroff-Girard, A. et al. (2005) Preadipocytes in the human subcutaneous adipose tissue display distinct features from the adult mesenchymal and hematopoietic stem cells. *Journal of Cellular Physiology*, **205**, 114–22.

Shen, W., Wangm, Z., Punyanita, M. et al. (2003) Adipose quantification by imaging methods: a proposed classification. *Obesity Research*, **11**, 5–16.

Simpson, E.R., Clyne, C., Rubin, G. et al. (2002) Aromatase – a brief overview. *Annual Review of Physiology*, **64**, 93–127.

Smith, A.J., Sanders, M.A., Thompson, B.R. et al. (2004) Physical association between the adipocyte fatty acid-binding protein and hormone-sensitive lipase: a fluorescence resonance energy transfer analysis. *The Journal of Biological Chemistry*, **279**, 52399–405.

Smith, S.J., Cases, S., Jensen, D.R. et al. (2000) Obesity resistance and multiple mechanisms of triglyceride synthesis in mice lacking Dgat. *Nature Genetics*, **25**, 87–90.

Spalding, K.L., Arner, E., Westermark, P.O. et al. (2008) Dynamics of fat cell turnover in humans. *Nature*, **453**, 783–7.

Speakman, J.R. (2007) A nonadaptive scenario explaining the genetic predisposition to obesity: the 'predation release' hypothesis. *Cell Metabolism*, **6**, 5–12.

Staiger, H., Kaltenbach, S., Staiger, K. et al. (2004) Expression of adiponectin receptor mRNA in human skeletal muscle cells is related to in vivo parameters of glucose and lipid metabolism. *Diabetes*, **53**, 2195–201.

Steinberg, G.R., Bonen, A. and Dyck, D.J. (2002) Fatty acid oxidation and triacylglycerol hydrolysis are enhanced after chronic leptin treatment in rats. *American Journal of Physiology. Endocrinology and Metabolism*, **282**, E593–600.

Steppan, C.M., Bailey, S.T., Bhat, S. et al. (2001) The hormone resistin links obesity to diabetes. *Nature*, **409**, 307–312.

Swierczynski, J., Goyke, E., Wach, L. et al. (2000) Comparative study of the lipogenic potential of human and rat adipose tissue. *Metabolism: Clinical and Experimental*, **49**, 594–9.

Tan, G., Debard, C., Tiraby, C. et al. (2003) A 'futile cycle' induced by thiazolidinediones in adipose tissue? *Nature Med*, **9**, 811–2.

Tang, W., Zeve, D., Suh, J.M. et al. (2008) White fat progenitor cells reside in the adipose vasculature. *Science*, **322**, 583–6.

Tansey, J.T., Sztalryd, C., Gruia-Gray, J. et al. (2001) Perilipin ablation results in a lean mouse with aberrant adipocyte lipolysis, enhanced leptin production, and resistance to diet-induced obesity. *Proceedings of the National Academy of Sciences of the United States of America*, **98**, 6494–9.

Tiraby, C., Tavernier, G., Lefort, C. et al. (2003) Acquirement of brown fat cell features by human white adipocytes. *The Journal of Biological Chemistry*, **278**, 33370–6.

Tordjman, J., Chauvet, G., Quette, J. et al. (2003) Thiazolidinediones block fatty acid release by inducing glyceroneogenesis in fat cells. *The Journal of Biological Chemistry*, **278**, 18785–90.

Trayhurn, P. and Wood, I.S. (2004) Adipokines: inflammation and the pleiotropic role of white adipose tissue. *The British Journal of Nutrition*, **92**, 347–55.

Tseng, Y.H., Kokkotou, E., Schulz, T.J. et al. (2008) New role of bone morphogenetic protein 7 in brown adipogenesis and energy expenditure. *Nature*, **454**, 1000–4.

Unger, R. (2003) Lipid overload and overflow: metabolic trauma and the metabolic syndrome. *Trends in Endocrinology and Metabolism*, **14**, 398–403.

Unger, R.H. (2005) Hyperleptinemia: protecting the heart from lipid overload. *Hypertension*, **45**, 1031–4.

Valet, P., Tavernier, G., Castan-Laurell, I. *et al.* (2002) Understanding adipose tissue development from transgenic animal models. *Journal of Lipid Research*, **43**, 835–60.

Van Harmelen, V., Reynisdottir, S., Eriksson, P. *et al.* (1998) Leptin secretion from subcutaneous and visceral adipose tissue in women. *Diabetes*, **47**, 913–7.

Viguerie, N., Vidal, H., Arner, P. *et al.* (2005) Adipose tissue gene expression in obese subjects during low-fat and high-fat hypocaloric diets. *Diabetologia*, **48**, 123–31.

Villena, J.A., Roy, S., Sarkadi-Nagy, E. *et al.* (2004) Desnutrin, an adipocyte gene encoding a novel patatin domain-containing protein, is induced by fasting and glucocorticoids: ectopic expression of desnutrin increases triglyceride hydrolysis. *The Journal of Biological Chemistry*, **279**, 47066–75.

Vitkova, M., Klimcakova, E., Kovacikova, M. *et al.* (2007) Plasma levels and adipose tissue mRNA expression of retinol-binding protein 4 are reduced during calorie restriction in obese subjects but are not related to diet-induced changes in insulin sensitivity. *The Journal of Clinical Endocrinology and Metabolism*, **92**, 2330–5.

Vohl, M.C., Sladek, R., Robitaille, J. *et al.* (2004) A survey of genes differentially expressed in subcutaneous and visceral adipose tissue in men. *Obesity Research*, **12**, 1217–22.

Wajchenberg, B.L. (2000) Subcutaneous and visceral adipose tissue: their relation to the metabolic syndrome. *Endocrine Reviews*, **21**, 697–738.

Wang, Y., Xu, L.Y., Lam, K.S. *et al.* (2006) Proteomic characterization of human serum proteins associated with the fat-derived hormone adiponectin. *Proteomics*, **6**, 3862–70.

Weisberg, S.P., McCann, D., Desai, M. *et al.* (2003) Obesity is associated with macrophage accumulation in adipose tissue. *The Journal of Clinical Investigation*, **112**, 1796–1808.

Xu, H., Barnes, G.T., Yang, Q. *et al.* (2003) Chronic inflammation in fat plays a crucial role in the development of obesity-related insulin resistance. *The Journal of Clinical Investigation*, **112**, 1821–30.

Wu, H., Ghosh, S., Perrard, X.D. *et al.* (2007) T-cell accumulation and regulated on activation, normal T cell expressed and secreted upregulation in adipose tissue in obesity. *Circulation*, **115**, 1029–38.

Yamauchi, T., Kamon, J., Ito, Y. *et al.* (2003) Cloning of adiponectin receptors that mediate antidiabetic metabolic effects. *Nature*, **423**, 762–9.

Yang, Q., Graham, T.E., Mody, N. *et al.* (2005) Serum retinol binding protein 4 contributes to insulin resistance in obesity and type 2 diabetes. *Nature*, **436**, 356–62.

Yang, Y.S., Song, H.D., Li, R.Y. *et al.* (2003) The gene expression profiling of human visceral adipose tissue and its secretory functions. *Biochemical and Biophysical Research Communications*, **300**, 839–46.

Yokota, T., Oritani, K., Takahashi, I. *et al.* (2000) Adiponectin, a new member of the family of soluble defense collagens, negatively regulates the growth of myelomonocytic progenitors and the functions of macrophages. *Blood*, **96**, 1723–32.

Yusuf, S., Hawken, S., Ounpuu, S. *et al.* (2005) Obesity and the risk of myocardial infarction in 27,000 participants from 52 countries: a case-control study. *Lancet*, **366**, 1640–9.

Zechner, R., Strauss, J.G., Haemmerle, G. *et al.* (2005) Lipolysis: pathway under construction. *Current Opinion in Lipidology*, **16**, 333–40.

Zierath, J., Livingston, J., Thorne, A. *et al.* (1998) Regional difference in insulin inhibition of non-esterified fatty acid release from human adipocytes: relation to insulin receptor phosphorylation and intracellular signalling through the insulin receptor substrate-1 pathway. *Diabetologia*, **41**, 1343–54.

Zimmermann, R., Strauss, J.G., Haemmerle, G. *et al.* (2004) Fat mobilization in adipose tissue is promoted by adipose triglyceride lipase. *Science*, **306**, 1383–6.

The Regulation of Energy Balance: An Overview

Key points

- The maintenance of adequate nutrition and energy stores is essential for survival and reproductive success. Numerous interdependent control pathways, involving both the central nervous system (CNS) and peripheral mechanisms, have evolved to maintain energy balance and body fat (the main energy store in mammals) at optimal levels.

- Body fat and weight are regulated around a predetermined trajectory through life, which probably represents the net result of numerous genetic and environmental factors rather than a genetic 'set-point'.

- Homeostatic circuits that regulate body fat mass include those based on insulin and leptin. Concentrations of both hormones are proportional to fat mass, and both act on the CNS to reduce feeding and increase energy expenditure; this induces an energy deficit that mobilizes triglyceride and thus acts to restrain fat mass from increasing. Mutations that disable leptin (*ob/ob* mouse) or its receptor (*db/db* mouse, *fa/fa* rat), or transgenic knockout of insulin receptors selectively in the CNS, lead to overeating and obesity.

- Food-seeking and eating behaviour are affected by numerous central and peripheral mechanisms. Effectors include neurotransmitters that stimulate feeding (e.g. neuropeptide Y) or inhibit feeding (e.g. α-melanocyte stimulating hormone); gut peptides that increase or decrease feeding (ghrelin and cholecystokinin, respectively); gastric distension, sensed by vagal endings, which induces satiety; and altered metabolite availability (e.g. hypoglycaemia, detected by specific glucose-sensitive neurones, which powerfully induces hunger).

- The CNS also regulates energy expenditure, notably through the sympathetic nervous system outflow that stimulates heat production in thermogenic tissues, including brown adipose tissue, which is prominent in lower mammals. Central pathways controlling energy expenditure overlap with those that regulate feeding.

- Many aspects of energy homeostasis in lower mammals also operate in humans. Very rare cases of human obesity arise through mutations affecting leptin, its receptor and the melanocortin pathway. However, humans also show specific eating behaviours, including eating more in sociable company ('social facilitation').

- Human obesity is mostly (>95%) due to variable lifestyle factors (relative overconsumption of food and/or decreased physical activity), superimposed on an individually determined polygenic genetic susceptibility to fat gain through life. Genetic susceptibility may determine many aspects of human energy homeostasis, ranging from the capacity to oxidize triglyceride to a preference for palatable foods and social facilitation.

Chapter 5 The Regulation of Energy Balance: An Overview

Gareth Williams

Although the worldwide increase in the prevalence of obesity might suggest otherwise, the regulation of energy balance in mammals is usually remarkably accurate. Elucidating how genetic and environmental factors can overcome normal energy homeostatic controls and cause obesity is of great scientific interest, and could potentially lead to effective treatments for the condition. The efficacy of normal energy homeostatic mechanisms may also hinder therapeutic attempts to manage obesity, by stimulating hunger and other compensatory responses when weight is lost. Thus, knowledge of how energy balance is regulated in animals and humans is essential for understanding, diagnosing and treating obesity.

This chapter aims to provide a brief overview of the mechanisms that control energy intake and expenditure, and the ways in which they are coordinated so as to maintain body energy stores at optimal levels. It also serves as an introduction to the following three chapters, which provide detailed accounts of normal energy homeostasis and the causes of obesity in humans and other mammals.

Chapter 6 focuses on the various regulatory signals that enable mammals to adapt their behaviours (food-seeking and eating) and metabolic processes (anabolism versus catabolism) in response to short- and long-term energetic demands, and on the pathways in the central and peripheral nervous systems that transmit, integrate and prioritize the resulting mass of information. This account is based largely on experimental work in lower mammals, including various syndromes of genetic obesity in rodents that have helped to identify key regulatory signals and their target neurones in the central nervous system (CNS). Throughout, evidence of physiological relevance is critically reviewed, highlighting both the links to human energy balance and obesity and the areas where animal data cannot be validly extrapolated to humans.

Chapters 7 and 8 concentrate on humans, and respectively the physiological control of normal energy balance, and the various genetic and environmental factors that lead to obesity by subverting these regulatory mechanisms.

Regulation of body fat and composition

Adequate energy stores are crucially important to the survival and reproductive capacity of individual animals and thus the future of the species. Given this, it is perhaps not surprising that many regulatory systems appear to be involved in controlling feeding and energy expenditure. Even primitive organisms have elaborate defences to conserve energy balance – for example, the nematode *Caenorhabditis elegans* has over 400 genes involved in regulating its triglyceride energy stores (Ashrafi *et al.*, 2003). In mammals, energy homeostasis is necessarily more complex, with a plethora of central and peripheral mechanisms that affect food-seeking and ingestive behaviours, the fate of ingested nutrients, and energy expenditure through heat production in thermogenic tissues.

Body weight is maintained surprisingly constant in most adult mammals whose habitual environmental conditions (notably food availability and physical activity) are generally steady. In mammals, the vast majority of the body's energy stores are in the form of triglyceride, largely deposited in adipose tissue, with most of the remainder being represented by relatively limited amounts of glycogen in liver and muscle. Body fat mass is therefore a better surrogate for long-term energy balance and, in adult humans under steady conditions, varies by only a small percentage over periods of days to months.

As discussed in Chapters 6 and 7, the weight of evidence favours the existence of concerted control mechanisms for regulating energy

Obesity: Science to Practice Edited by Gareth Williams and Gema Frühbeck
© 2009 John Wiley & Sons, Ltd

homeostasis and fat mass. Many studies in animals and humans have convincingly demonstrated that body fat is a regulated variable; that is, that body fat content (and hence body weight) is actively defended by compensatory responses in energy intake and expenditure in response to imposed changes in energy status that alter body fat mass (e.g. Langhans and Geary (2006); Sandoval, Cota and Seeley (2008); see Figure 5.1). However, it is unclear whether this remarkable precision reflects active regulation around a genetically determined 'set-point', or whether body weight 'settles' at a level that results from the sum of various physiological controls and environmental influences. The wide variety of social and hedonic (i.e. pleasure-related) factors that can markedly alter human eating behaviour, such as the social setting of eating and the hedonic properties of food itself (see Chapter 8), would suggest that an individual's weight is more malleable than might be expected with a genetic 'set-point'. Moreover, the rapid spread of obesity – whether globally or through local social networks (see Figure 8.8) – also indicates that environmental influences can dominate energy homeostasis in humans, even though individual susceptibility to obesity may have an important genetic component (see Chapter 8).

The ability of energy homeostasis to react rapidly and appropriately to a wide range of environmental and nutritional challenges is essential to survival. This demands great versatility in the mechanisms that sense and respond to such challenges, and in the higher centres that integrate this information and coordinate responses such as prioritizing the seeking and eating of food, or altering the activity of the sympathetic nervous system outflow that drives heat production in thermogenic tissues. Table 5.1 illustrates the diversity of nutritional and environmental factors to which energy homeostatic mechanisms in mammals have to respond, together with some of the signals and effector pathways that underpin these responses.

At first sight, many different pathways within the CNS appear to serve similar functions and to converge on the same outcome. For example, the hypothalamus – a brain region that is crucial to both feeding and energy expenditure – contains dozens of neurotransmitters and peptides that increase or decrease food intake when injected into specific hypothalamic sites or the adjacent cerebroventricular system (see Figure 5.2). This apparent reduplication has been described as 'redundancy',

although it may be more appropriate in physiological terms to regard the multiplicity of control systems as providing a 'backup' or 'failsafe' function that will continue to maintain energy balance if one particular pathway is disabled by genetic or environmental causes. Thus, a degree of overlap between the various regulatory systems could assist survival and confer the ability to respond to a wide range of nutritional challenges.

In addition, individual control systems respond to specific signals and may assume particular importance under specific circumstances. For example, hunger can be induced by numerous conditions as diverse as food deprivation, insulin-deficient diabetes, hypoglycaemia and the absence of food in the stomach. In each of these conditions, quite different central and/or peripheral signals and pathways drive the common response (hunger) (see Table 5.1). Hunger in food deprivation and insulin-deficient diabetes (e.g. induced by experimental destruction of the islet β cells) may be partly explained by falls in circulating insulin and leptin concentrations, resulting both in disinhibition of hypothalamic neurones that release neuropeptide Y (a powerful stimulant of feeding) and inhibition of the appetite-suppressing melanocortin neurones (Figure 5.3; see Chapter 6). By contrast, the intense hunger triggered by acute hypoglycaemia is apparently related to the fall in glucose availability to specific glucose-sensing neurones in various sites in the CNS and periphery.

All the above conditions represent immediate or longer-term threats to survival. By contrast, overconsumption of palatable food – which is due to its hedonic properties – apparently cuts across these regulatory controls and may have deleterious metabolic and survival consequences. This occurs in the diet-induced obesity that can develop in animals presented with palatable and varied foods, and which may be an experimental surrogate for 'common' lifestyle-related obesity in humans (see below).

How is fat mass regulated?

Many attempts have been made to explain how fat mass could be maintained at an essentially constant level that presumably reflects optimal survival value for the individual animal. Various models have been based around classical endocrine concepts of homeostasis, in which signals generated by (or closely related to) body fat mass would act on target sites, presumed to lie with

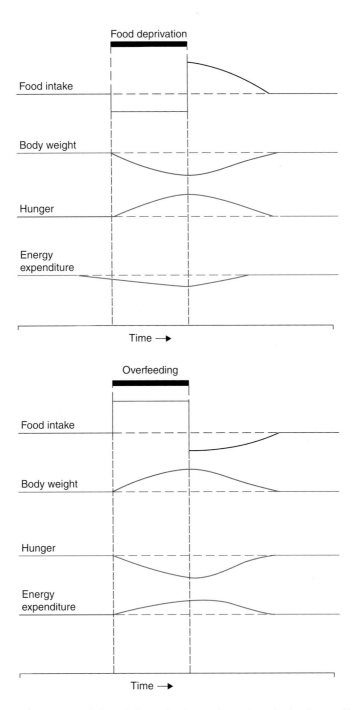

Figure 5.1 Body weight in mammals is actively regulated around a predetermined trajectory. Upper panel: food deprivation leads to weight and fat loss, with compensatory changes including increased hunger and a reduction in energy expenditure. When food again becomes available, animals overeat and hyperphagia persists (although diminishing with time) until body weight has been restored. Concurrently, energy expenditure remains subnormal but increases towards normal levels as weight is regained. Lower panel: forced overfeeding results in weight and fat gain, accompanied by a reduction in hunger and an increase in energy expenditure. When overfeeding ceases, spontaneous food intake is low initially and returns gradually to normal as the excess weight is lost. Conversely, energy expenditure falls steadily towards normal as weight returns to the predetermined level.

Table 5.1 Some examples of nutritional and environmental challenges to energy homeostasis, and the physiological responses which they elicit. NTS: nucleus of the solitary tract (see Chapter 6); POMC: proopiomelanocortin (precursor peptide in melanocortin neurones)

Condition →	Trigger →	Signal →	Effector pathway →	Outcomes
• Starvation • Diabetes	↓ Fat mass	• ↓ Leptin • ↓ Insulin	• ↑ NPY neurones • ↓ POMC neurones	• Food seeking • Hunger • Thermogenesis
• Starvation • Insulin excess	↓ Blood glucose	↓ Glucose Availability	• ↑ Glucose-inhibited neurones • ↓ Glucose-stimulated neurones	• Food seeking • Hunger • Counter-regulatory hormone release
Empty stomach	↓ Nutrients in Stomach lumen	↑ Ghrelin release	• NPY neurones • Orexin neurones	↑ Hunger
Full stomach	↑ Gastric distension	Firing of gastric stretch receptors	Vagal afferents (Via NTS)	↑ Satiety
Food in small intestine	↑ Nutrients in gut lumen	• ↑ CCK release • ↑ GLP-1 release	• Vagal afferents • Hypothalamic and NTS neurones	↑ Satiety

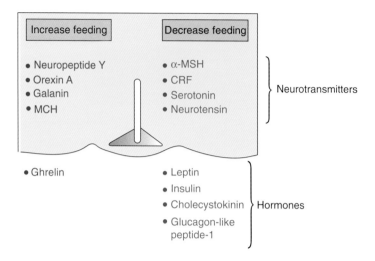

Figure 5.2 Examples of neurotransmitters and circulating hormones that act on the hypothalamus to affect feeding in rodents.

the CNS, so as to decrease feeding and/or increase energy expenditure. These latter changes would induce an overall energy deficit and thus introduce the negative feedback link that is needed to complete the homeostatic circuit; under conditions of energy deficit, triglyceride is mobilized, leading to a fall in fat mass that would counteract any tendency for body fat content to increase above a predetermined level.

Classical cross-circulation experiments conducted during the 1970s on genetic obesity syndromes in mice (*ob/ob* and *db/db*) supported this view, with the *ob* mutation suggested to disable an anti-obesity signal, while the *db* mutation was thought to inactivate the receptor that normally recognized this signal (see Chapter 1). At the time, some 20 years before the discovery of leptin, both the anti-obesity signal and its receptor were speculative entities.

A strong contender for the anti-obesity signal was insulin, whose circulating levels increase broadly in parallel with fat mass and the associated insulin resistance (see Chapter 6). Insulin injected experimentally into the third ventricle of the rat hypothalamus was shown to reduce food intake and body weight, while increasing energy expenditure by activating the sympathetic nervous system outflow that stimulates thermogenesis in rodents. It was also found that insulin is transported actively across the blood-brain barrier into the hypothalamus; that it inhibits hypothalamic neurones that release the orexigenic (feeding-stimulating) neuropeptide Y (NPY); and more recently, that selective knockout of insulin receptors on neurones leads to increased food intake and body weight (Schwartz and Porte, 2005). In addition, certain genetically obese rodents such as

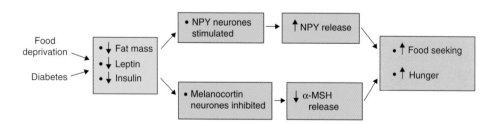

Figure 5.3 Mechanisms of hunger in rodents subjected to food deprivation and insulin-deficient diabetes.

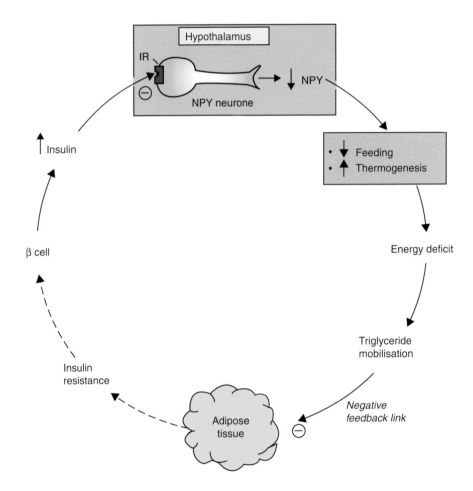

Figure 5.4 Insulin as a potential regulator of body fat mass. Should fat mass increase, circulating insulin levels would increase in parallel with insulin resistance. Insulin acts on the hypothalamus (e.g. by inhibiting NPY neurones) and other CNS sites to decrease feeding and increase energy expenditure through sympathetic stimulation of thermogenic tissues. These effects would induce an energy deficit, leading to triglyceride mobilization that would tend to reduce fat mass back to normal. IR: insulin receptor.

the *fa/fa* Zucker rat were found to be relatively insensitive to the central appetite-suppressing and anti-obesity actions of insulin (Schwartz and Porte, 2005). Thus, insulin is a plausible candidate for a fat-related signal that gains access to physiologically relevant CNS neurones, and whose central actions produce the energy deficit that is necessary to complete a negative-feedback homeostatic circuit that could regulate fat mass (Figure 5.4).

With the discovery of leptin in 1994, the maintenance of fat mass appeared initially to be completely explained (Chapter 6). Leptin, secreted by adipose tissue and circulating at concentrations proportional to fat mass, was shown – like insulin – to enter the hypothalamus

and inhibit NPY neurones; it also stimulates the melanocortin neurones of the hypothalamus, which powerfully inhibit eating and decrease body weight, and which provide a critical counterbalance to the NPY system. Leptin's actions on these and other target neurones underpin its central actions of decreasing food intake while stimulating sympathetically-mediated thermogenesis and energy expenditure, again leading to an overall energy deficit and weight loss (Figure 5.5). Consistent with the cross-circulation experiments, the *ob* mutation was found to affect the leptin gene, while *db* (and *fa* in the rat) disables the leptin receptor. Moreover, very rare cases of human obesity have been discovered that are due to mutations of either leptin or its receptor, proving

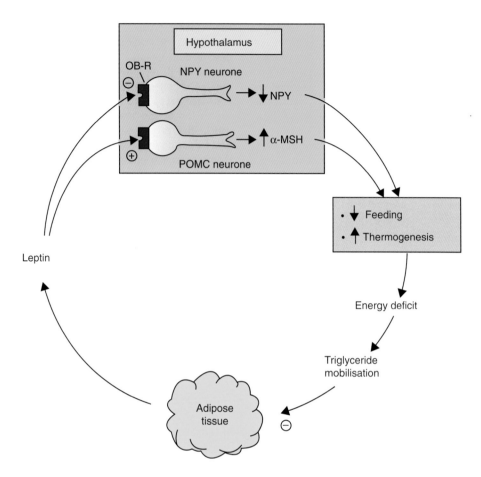

Figure 5.5 Leptin as a regulator of body fat mass. See legend for Figure 5.4. OB-R: leptin receptor; POMC: proopiomelanocortin (melanocortin precursor).

the concept that at least minimal levels of leptin signalling are required for normal energy homeostasis in humans (see Chapters 8 and 21).

Although intellectually satisfying, clarification of the role of leptin has not provided all the answers to the mysteries of energy homeostasis. Evidence that supports roles of other candidates such as insulin cannot be discounted simply because leptin was discovered. It seems reasonable to conclude that leptin is just one of many signals contributing to the regulation of body fat mass, and that different signals may play more or less significant roles in different species and under different circumstances. The significance of physiological leptin concentrations in humans is uncertain: in humans with 'common', lifestyle-related obesity, leptin levels are increased in proportion to fat mass, but evidently fail to limit body weight. This may indicate that leptin is less potent or relevant

as a regulator of feeding and energy balance in humans than in rodents, although it is possible that obese humans might become insensitive to leptin in the same way that they develop resistance to the actions of insulin (see Chapter 8).

A further complexity is that body weight and composition in mammals, including humans, show physiological, age-related variations. Body fat and weight are regulated around a trajectory that is defined throughout the individual's lifespan. After rapid growth during childhood and adolescence, body weight usually increases more slowly during adulthood and decreases again in older age – this being accompanied by a progressive rise in the proportion of body fat at the expense of lean tissue (Morley, 2007; Zafon, 2007). Thus, there may be active regulation of both body fat and of other components of body composition, although the mechanisms controlling the latter are yet to be identified.

Overall, both body fat and lean tissue may be regulated within genetically determined boundaries by a variety of external and internal factors (Speakman, 2004). External factors range from the availability and energy density of food and (in humans) opportunities for physical exercise, to day length and other cues that drive feeding behaviour in animals preparing for hibernation. Internal modulatory factors include operation of the reproductive axis – an activity that is essential for survival of the species, and which in turn depends critically on the individual animal having adequate nutrition and energy stores (Asarian and Geary, 2006).

Regulation of energy intake and expenditure

Much previous research on the regulation of energy homeostasis has concentrated on a single candidate (e.g. a neurotransmitter or peptide) and its impact on either food intake or energy expenditure. Accordingly, the scientific literature on energy homeostasis has tended to portray energy intake and expenditure as separate processes that are regulated by factors described as short-term or long-term, peripheral or central, humoral or neural, and gastrointestinal or metabolic.

It is now clear that there is no single overriding factor controlling energy intake or expenditure; instead, energy balance is controlled by a regulatory system that is built around bidirectional interactions between peripheral organs and the brain. Moreover, any implied dichotomy between food intake and energy expenditure is in part artificial, in that the mechanisms controlling energy intake and expenditure are extensively intertwined. Many key neurotransmitters affect both energy intake and expenditure in a concerted fashion: NPY, for example, promotes net energy gain in rodents by both stimulating feeding and inhibiting energy expenditure, whereas the melanocortin α-MSH has the opposite effects and induces an overall energy deficit (Chapter 6). These neurotransmitters, as well as circulating signals such as leptin and insulin, act on pathways that descend from the hypothalamus to the sympathetic motoneurones in the spinal cord and thus modulate the activity of the sympathetic nerves that supply the

thermogenic tissues, notably brown adipose tissue (BAT) in lower mammals (Figure 5.6). As described in Chapter 3, sympathetic stimulation of the β_3 receptors in BAT results in coordinated changes in fat metabolism, including enhanced fatty acid oxidation and increased expression of the 'uncoupling protein' UCP-1, which diverts the energy liberated by fatty acid oxidation into the production of heat rather than adenosine triphosphate (ATP). Thus, the CNS pathways that regulate food intake overlap with those that control peripheral metabolism and energy expenditure through the autonomic outflow (Schwartz and Porte, 2005).

An important distinction between energy intake and energy expenditure in mammals is that expenditure may be increased or decreased more or less continuously for prolonged periods, whereas feeding occurs discontinuously in discrete meals. Accordingly, any physiological mechanism that alters body weight or body fat through changes in food intake must modulate the size and/or frequency of single meals. Prototypic adiposity signals that reflect the size of the body's fat stores, such as leptin and insulin, regulate energy intake primarily by affecting meal size (see Langhans and Geary, 2006), and they do so by modulating the effectiveness of the physiological controls of meal termination (or satiation), such as cholecystokinin (CCK) (Emond et al., 1999; Morton et al., 2005; Riedy et al., 1995). This effect needs to be considered when analysing the impact of 'long-term' adiposity signals and 'short-term' meal controls, in particular at the neurochemical level where most of this modulation takes place.

Integrative role of the CNS

The brain does not act in isolation to control energy intake and expenditure. Rather, it receives and integrates peripheral signals from the gastrointestinal tract and from currently available and stored metabolic fuels. These peripheral signals are both humoral and neural. Neural inputs are largely relayed via afferent (sensory) fibres of the vagus nerve; an example is gastric distension, sensed and transmitted to the CNS by vagal afferents in the stomach wall. Humoral factors include hormones (e.g. insulin and leptin), gut peptides such as the orexigenic peptide, ghrelin, released from the stomach under fasting conditions, and

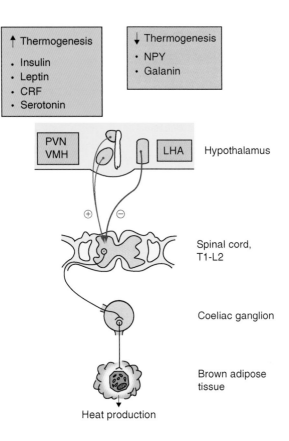

Figure 5.6 CNS control of energy expenditure through the sympathetic nervous system (SNS) outflow that activates heat production in thermogenic tissues, notably brown adipose tissue (BAT) in lower mammals and human neonates, and skeletal muscle. Various hormonal and neurochemical regulators of the SNS and thermogenesis are shown. Both the ventromedial (VMH) and paraventricular (PVN) nuclei give rise to descending pathways that stimulate SNS motoneurones in the intermedio-lateral column of the thoracic spinal cord, while outflow from the lateral hypothalamic area (LHA) is inhibitory.

circulating metabolites. Certain metabolites (e.g. glucose, fatty acids and amino acids) and hormones can act in a concerted fashion at different levels, for example by triggering a vagally mediated signal in the periphery to influence food intake, while also affecting eating and energy expenditure by direct actions in the brain. Thus, any distinction between 'gastrointestinal' and 'metabolic' controls of energy intake is tenuous.

The extent to which these diverse signals converge is illustrated by the recent realization that various metabolic and endocrine factors activate overlapping intracellular signalling cascades in the brain areas that control energy intake and expenditure (Cota *et al.*, 2006; Minokoshi *et al.*, 2004). This has reawakened interest in an earlier 'ischymetric' hypothesis that there may be a mechanism that can sense the body's overall energy status and needs. Such a mechanism could be based around the interactions in key CNS regulatory neurones between two fuel-sensitive kinases, AMP kinase (AMPK) and the 'mammalian target of rapamycin' (mTOR). Activity of AMPK, the enzyme that converts AMP to adenosine diphosphate (ADP) and ATP, is increased under conditions of energy deficit, whereas mTOR is inhibited by fuel deficits. Energy status is signalled to AMPK and mTOR by numerous factors, including leptin, ghrelin, the fat-derived hormone adiponectin, and metabolites such as glucose and free fatty acids (see Chapter 6 and Figure 6.8).

Lessons from other species: informative or misleading?

Much of our understanding of the basic mechanisms of energy homeostasis is derived from work in experimental animals, using techniques that range from stereotactically targeted microinjection of peptides into selected brain areas, to transgenic overexpression or deletion of a chosen gene. The outcome of many experiments must be interpreted with caution, and by employing stringent criteria for physiological relevance. Microinjection, despite its seeming precision, delivers test substances at vastly supraphysiological dosages that may diffuse far beyond the target area (and can even enter the circulation). Non-specific effects of the test substance leading, for example, to malaise, anxiety or drowsiness can produce hypophagia, especially in short-term experiments. Conversely, the absence of a phenotype such as alterations in food intake or body weight in a transgenic knockout model does not necessarily mean that the target gene is irrelevant to energy homeostasis; instead, the absence of its product (or of its downstream effects) may have triggered compensatory changes in other 'redundant' or 'failsafe' mechanisms. It is evident that permanent knockouts are more likely to provide misleading findings than are conditional knockouts, in which the target gene can be effectively switched off at a chosen time-point in adult life.

All this begs the question as to how far findings in other species can be assumed to apply to humans. There are undoubtedly differences between species in the cognitive control of eating. For example, humans show robust increases in the amount of food consumed during a meal when eating with company, and especially in the company of friends (Figure 5.7); this so-called 'social facilitation' is not seen with laboratory rodents. On the other hand, lower mammals – like humans – are susceptible to a variety of non-regulatory influences, such as the pleasurable aspects of eating, and to certain learned associations that have little or no regulatory value. Moreover, several peripheral signals and neurochemically-defined pathways in the CNS that regulate aspects of energy homeostasis in rodents and primates have been shown to operate, at least to some degree, in humans. These include eating-inhibiting factors such as CCK, serotonin (the

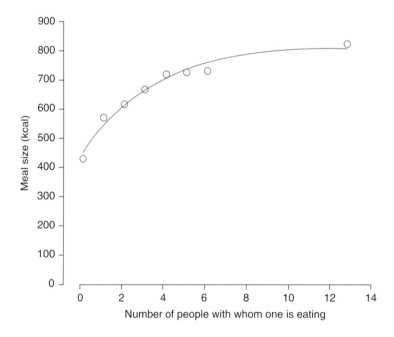

Figure 5.7 Social facilitation of eating behaviour. An individual's food intake increases with the number of people present at the meal, by up to 400 kcal at a single meal. From de Castro *et al.* (1990), with permission of the editor of *Physiology & Behavior*.

neurotransmitter whose action is exploited by various centrally-acting anti-obesity drugs), the melanocortin-4 receptor (MC4-R) and leptin; and the endocannabinoids and the gastric peptide, ghrelin, both of which stimulate eating in humans and lower mammals (see Chapters 6 and 21).

These perspectives underscore the general validity of animal research in the field of energy homeostasis. However, they also highlight the importance of corroborating initial findings that have been derived from other species, ideally using a variety of different experimental approaches, before concluding that these can safely be extrapolated to humans.

Causes of obesity

Obesity results from the failure of energy homeostasis and represents the breakdown of one or more of the mechanisms that normally maintain body fat mass. It is now clear that obesity can be due to many different causes, including certain drugs, endocrine disorders and inherited syndromes (Table 5.2). Extreme obesity is a striking condition that has caught the attention of humans since the Stone Age (see Chapter 1). However, with few exceptions – such as when it is accompanied by characteristic features of endocrinopathies or genetic syndromes – obesity is an uninformative clinical phenotype that reveals little or nothing about its underlying causes.

It is important to be aware of the possibility of 'secondary' obesity, because these conditions may require special diagnostic and therapeutic approaches. The list of potential causes of obesity

Table 5.2 Causes of obesity.

'Common', 'idiopathic' or 'lifestyle-related' (>95% of cases)
Secondary causes (<5% of cases)
• Drugs (e.g. corticosteroids, antipsychotics, antiepileptics)
• Endocrine disorders (e.g. Cushing syndrome, hypothalamic damage)
• Specific genetic syndromes (e.g. Prader-Willi syndrome)
• Mutations affecting energy control mechanisms (e.g. leptin mutations)

is long, although they account in total for less than 5% of cases among adults in westernized and developing countries. In the remaining 95% of cases with no identifiable underlying cause (at least using current diagnostic methods), obesity has been variously described as 'common', 'idiopathic' or 'lifestyle-related'.

Overall, 'common' obesity can be attributed to the impact of obesogenic lifestyle factors on individuals who have a variable genetic susceptibility to fat gain. Across populations, lifestyle changes such as decreased levels of everyday physical activity and increased consumption of energy-dense foods can be related to the spread of obesity, and in general terms, common obesity can be attributed to a cumulative excess of energy intake over expenditure. However, there is no doubt that common obesity is a heterogeneous condition, and that the term 'idiopathic' simply reflects the inability of available investigative methods to make a more precise diagnosis. Existing evidence already points to differing genetic susceptibilities for obesogenic factors as diverse as social facilitation, preference for energy-dense foods and the capacity to store triglyceride rather than oxidize fatty acids (see Chapters 7 and 8). Other obesity susceptibility genes will undoubtedly be identified, and ultimately it may prove possible to subdivide common obesity into categories defined by an individual's genetic susceptibility profile. However, the vast majority of common obesity appears to be a polygenic trait, and the contribution of any individual susceptibility gene is likely to be small.

In the same way that genetic predisposition varies widely between individuals, there are considerable individual and population differences in environmental exposure to factors such as the availability of energy-dense food and opportunities for active exercise or sedentary pursuits. The roles of genetic and environmental factors in human obesity are examined in detail in Chapter 8, which also discusses the relative importance of overconsumption of food versus reduced energy expenditure, notably through decreased levels of physical activity.

Some of these issues remain controversial, partly because of the difficulties of making accurate measurements of energy intake and expenditure in freely-living humans; some of the methodological pitfalls are described in Chapter 3. Relatively subtle aspects of energy homeostasis may also be involved, including 'non-exercise activity thermogenesis' (NEAT), which is the energy expended through minor involuntary muscle activity such as fidgeting or maintaining posture (Chapter 7). In addition, the ability to use particular metabolites could, in the long term, affect body fat mass. The hypothesis of 'nutrient balance' suggests that for energy balance to be stable, the relative intake of a particular nutrient must match the proportion of that nutrient used in fuelling metabolism. Although this view of energy homeostasis may be over-simplistic, there is increasing evidence that a decrease in the ability to oxidize fatty acids may predispose some individuals towards weight gain (Chapter 7).

Animal models of obesity

Striking obesity can also develop in animals, and several genetic obesity syndromes in rodents have been heavily investigated; some well-known examples related to mutations of leptin or its CNS targets are shown in Figure 5.8. These have sometimes been regarded as experimental models of human obesity and its associated metabolic disorders, notably insulin resistance and type 2 diabetes. Now that their underlying mechanisms have been elucidated, it is apparent that human counterparts of these syndromes do exist, but that they are extremely rare causes of obesity in humans and have no aetiological relationship to common human obesity (see Chapter 6). Nonetheless, unravelling the mysteries of genetic obesity syndromes such as the *ob/ob* and *db/db* mice has helped to broaden understanding of how energy balance is regulated at both central and peripheral levels in rodents, and has also provided some new insights into human energy homeostasis.

Animal models have been developed that attempt to mimic common, lifestyle-related obesity in humans. When unselected rodents are presented with a varied and palatable diet, a variable proportion (usually about half) overeat and become obese (Figure 5.9). In some cases, this diet-induced obesity may be accompanied by features characteristic of the human metabolic syndrome, notably insulin resistance, dyslipidaemia and endothelial dysfunction (Elliott *et al.*, 2004; see Chapter 10). It is not known why some

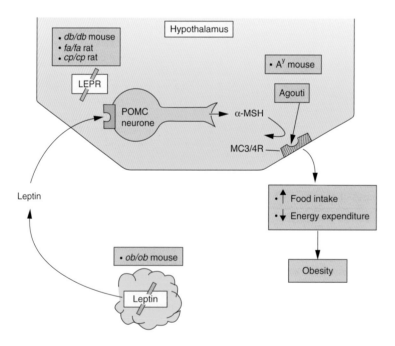

Figure 5.8 Genetic syndromes of obesity in rodents that are related to mutations in the genes encoding leptin (*ob/ob* mouse) or the leptin receptor (*db/db* mouse, *fa/fa* rat). The A^y (yellow obese) mouse has overexpression of agouti protein, an endogenous antagonist of MC4 receptors (causing hyperphagia and obesity) and MC1 receptors (preventing melanin production by α-MSH in hair follicles, thus producing yellow fur).

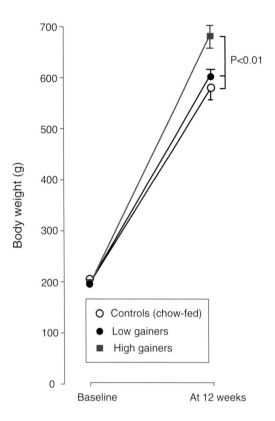

Figure 5.9 Diet-induced obesity. About one-half of unselected rats presented with palatable, varied food overeat significantly and become obese, and have significantly higher body weight and fat mass than chow-fed controls (designated 'high gainers' in this 12-week study). The remainder ('low gainers') appear relatively restrained, with weight gain that is slightly but not significantly higher than in controls. Muscle mass did not differ significantly between the groups. Data from Elliott *et al.* (2004) *Molecular Brain Research*, 128: 150–9.

animals develop diet-induced obesity, whereas others are seemingly resistant to the pleasurable properties of the food. Rodents with diet-induced obesity typically have raised insulin and leptin levels, suggesting that some property of the palatable food or the consequences of its ingestion can override the normal tendency of these signals to decrease feeding. One suggested explanation is intrinsic overactivity of the endocannabinoid system (which is involved in hedonic eating) in rats that over-eat palatable food, although the molecular basis is unknown (Harrold *et al.*, 2002).

Behavioural and neurochemical basis of human obesity

For humans in affluent societies, where palatable and varied foods are freely available, eating behaviour is driven primarily by social and hedonic cues; these show considerable variability in their impact on individuals and probably contribute a significant role to susceptibility to obesity (see Chapter 8). Elucidating the neural and neurochemical basis of these effects seems most likely to advance the understanding and treatment of human obesity. Current evidence points to the involvement of dopaminergic pathways in the 'reward' circuit of the brain, as well as endocannabinoids acting in the hypothalamus and elsewhere. Consistent with the latter suggestion, rimonabant (an antagonist of cannabinoid CB1 receptors) has been shown to reduce food intake and body weight in obese subjects (see Chapter 17). Susceptibility to obesity could be partly determined by polymorphisms in specific dopamine, cannabinoid or other receptors that influence the activity of the reward or related pathways.

References

This brief list of references is intended only as a supplement to the comprehensive references provided in Chapters 6, 7 and 8.

Asarian, L. and Geary, N. (2006) Modulation of appetite by gonadal steroid hormones. *Philosophical Transactions of the Royal Society of London. Series B, Biological Sciences*, **361**, 1251–63.

Ashrafi, K., Chang, F.Y., Watts, J.L. *et al.* (2003) Genome-wide RNAi analysis of Caenorhabditis elegans fat regulatory genes. *Nature*, **421**, 268–72.

Cota, D., Proulx, K., Smith, K.A. *et al.* (2006) Hypothalamic mTOR signaling regulates food intake. *Science*, **312**, 927–30.

de Castro, J.M. (1990) Social facilitation of duration and size but not rate of the spontaneous meal intake of humans. *Physiology & Behavior*, **47**, 1129–35.

Elliott, J.C., Harrold, J.A., Brodin, P. *et al.* (2004) Increases in melanin-concentrating hormone and MCH receptor levels in the hypothalamus of dietary-obese rats. *Molecular Brain Research*, **128**, 150–9.

Emond, M., Schwartz, G.J., Ladenheim, E.E. and Moran, T.H. (1999) Central leptin modulates behavioral and neural responsivity to CCK. *The American Journal of Physiology*, **276**, R1545–9.

Harrold, J.A., Elliott, J.C., King, P.J. *et al.* (2002) Down-regulation of cannabinoid-1 (CB-1) receptors in specific extrahypothalamic regions of rats with dietary obesity: a role for endogenous cannabinoids

in driving appetite for palatable food? *Brain Research*, **952**, 232–8.

Langhans, W. and Geary, N. (2006) Regulation of body weight, in *Obesity and Binge Eating Disorder* (eds S. Munsch and C. Beglinger), Karger, Basel, pp. 21–40.

Minokoshi, Y., Alquier, T., Furukawa, N., Kim, Y.B. *et al.* (2004) AMP-kinase regulates food intake by responding to hormonal and nutrient signals in the hypothalamus. *Nature*, **428**, 569–74.

Morley, J.E. (2007) Weight loss in older persons: new therapeutic approaches. *Current Pharmaceutical Design*, **13**, 3637–47.

Morton, G.J., Blevins, J.E., Williams, D.L. *et al.* (2005) Leptin action in the forebrain regulates the hindbrain response to satiety signals. *The Journal of Clinical Investigation*, **115**, 703–10.

Riedy, C.A., Chavez, M., Figlewicz, D.P. and Woods, S.C. (1995) Central insulin enhances sensitivity to cholecystokinin. *Physiology & Behavior*, **58**, 755–60.

Sandoval, D., Cota, D. and Seeley, R.J. (2008) The integrative role of CNS fuel-sensing mechanisms in energy balance and glucose regulation. *Annual Review of Physiology*, **70**, 513–35.

Schwartz, M.W. and Porte, D., Jr. (2005) Diabetes, obesity, and the brain. *Science*, **307**, 375–9.

Speakman, J.R. (2004) Obesity: the integrated roles of environment and genetics. *The Journal of Nutrition*, **134** (8 Suppl), 2090S–105S.

Zafon, C. (2007) Oscillations in total body fat content through life: an evolutionary perspective. *Obesity Reviews*, **8**, 525–30.

Control of
Eating

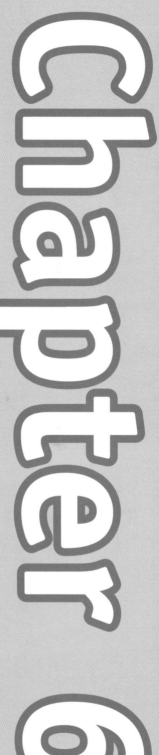

- Eating behaviour is complex and regulated by metabolic, endocrine and neural signals, as well as by learning and cognitive and social factors. Meals are initiated by increasing hunger and waning postprandial satiety from the previous meal, and terminated by satiation signals. Hedonic (pleasurable) and reward aspects of food and eating greatly influence the amount eaten.

- Flavour is sensed by specific receptors and relayed by cranial nerves to the nucleus tractus solitarii (NTS) in the brainstem (for taste) and the olfactory bulb (smell) and thence to the hypothalamus. Flavour and flavour variety determine hedonic and reward properties of foods, which can lead to long-term changes in food intake and body weight.

- Satiation signals generated by food in the gut help to terminate eating. These include gastric stretch receptors and cholecystokinin (CCK), released from the proximal small intestine; both signals are carried to the NTS via vagal afferents. Glucagon-like peptide-1 (GLP-1), released from the more distal gut on eating, also inhibits eating in rodents and humans.

- Ghrelin is secreted by endocrine cells in the stomach during fasting and stimulates hunger and eating in rodents and humans; levels fall on eating. It may act as a physiological hunger signal.

- Metabolic signals that stimulate hunger and eating include reduced availability and use of fuels, notably glucose and perhaps free fatty acids. Glucose is sensed by specific neurones in the brain (NTS and hypothalamus) and by vagal afferents in the hepatic portal vein. Small dips in blood glucose may trigger feeding in rodents and perhaps humans. The balance between two metabolic fuel sensors – AMP kinase (AMPK) and mammalian target of rapamycin (mTOR) – in the hypothalamus may determine eating.

- Leptin, a 14-kDa protein secreted by adipose tissue, acts on hypothalamic regions and the NTS and decreases food intake and body weight. Leptin levels are proportional to fat mass and could therefore signal body energy stores to the brain. Mutations in leptin and its receptor (LepR) lead to overeating and obesity in the *ob/ob* and *db/db* mice, respectively.

- Insulin may also act as an adiposity signal: circulating levels parallel fat mass, and it enters the hypothalamus and NTS and decreases eating and weight through central effects. Amylin, a β-cell peptide co-secreted with insulin, may function similarly, inhibiting eating via specific receptors in the area postrema (AP).

- Important target neurones for leptin and insulin lie in the hypothalamic arcuate nucleus. Both hormones stimulate POMC neurones that release α-MSH, an eating-inhibitory peptide that acts via MC4 and MC3 receptors. Conversely, leptin and insulin inhibit orexigenic (eating-stimulatiing) neurones that release both neuropeptide Y (NPY) (a powerful appetite stimulant, acting via Y1, Y4 and Y5 receptors) and AgRP, which increases eating by blocking MC4 receptors.

- Other key hypothalamic regions include the paraventricular nucleus (PVN), an important integrating centre (including inputs from NPY and POMC neurones and the NTS) that overall restrains eating; the ventromedial hypothalamic nucleus (VMH), a major site for leptin action and glucose sensing; and the lateral hypothalamic area (LHA), containing neurones expressing the eating-stimulating peptides, orexin A and MCH.

- The NTS in the brainstem integrates taste and visceral inputs (including satiation signals carried by vagal afferents) and contains neurones sensitive to leptin, insulin, amylin, ghrelin and glucose. The NTS projects to the PVN and other forebrain sites.

- The reward circuit in the forebrain receives numerous neural inputs, notably dopaminergic projections, and also involves opioids and endocannabinoids. The reward pathways for eating overlap with those for other reward activities (e.g. sex). Rimonabant, a cannabinoid CB1 receptor antagonist, decreases food intake in humans and is used clinically to treat obesity.

- Infections and inflammation trigger an acute-phase response, with release of pro-inflammatory cytokines that act centrally to inhibit eating, contributing to the hypophagia and cachexia that can accompany chronic inflammatory diseases.

- The high heritability of human obesity arises from numerous genes. Extremely rare cases of morbid obesity have been discovered in humans with single-gene mutations affecting components of the eating-inhibitory pathways. These include leptin, the leptin receptor, and the CCK1 receptor. One to two percent of obese Europeans have complete or partial loss of function mutations in the MC4R gene, making this one of the most common human genetic diseases.

Chapter 6 **Control of Eating**

**Wolfgang Langhans, Joanne Harrold,
Gareth Williams, and Nori Geary**

Eating in mammals and especially humans is a highly complex and varied behaviour, co-determined by physiological reflexes and controls, the pleasures of sensation, and, especially in humans, habit. Despite steady progress in both basic and clinical research, the control of normal and disordered eating remains incompletely understood – as is evident from the limited effectiveness of current strategies to treat obesity.

In most mammals, including humans, eating is functionally organized into meals, whose onset, size and termination are controlled by stimulatory and inhibitory signals (Figure 6.1). 'Hunger' describes the processes that initiate a meal. The amount eaten may vary according to the hedonic (pleasurable or unpleasurable) evaluation of the food. Various inhibitory signals that follow food ingestion eventually terminate the meal ('satiation'), while 'postprandial satiety' denotes those processes that inhibit eating until the next meal.

This chapter reviews the internal and external factors that affect eating, the neural and humoral signals that convey this information to the central nervous system (CNS), and the CNS pathways that process and integrate it (Figure 6.2). Much of the material relates to laboratory animals, but aspects relevant to human eating and obesity are highlighted throughout.

Flavour and orosensory signals

Flavour is a complex perception arising from a combination of orosensory stimuli generated during eating, including gustatory (taste), olfactory (smell), tactile ('mouth-feel') and thermal stimuli.

Taste is sensed by epithelial sodium channels for salt and by G-protein coupled receptors (GPCR) with specificities for the other primary tastes – sweet, bitter, 'umami' (savoury, or protein), sour and, in rats, possibly starch. Taste receptors are

expressed in the taste buds of the tongue and oropharynx; these are innervated by the facial (VII), glossopharyngeal (IX) and vagus (X) cranial nerves, which convey gustatory signals to the nucleus of the solitary tract (NTS), an important integrating centre in the brainstem that projects via the thalamus and hypothalamus to the cortex. In addition, the trigeminal nerve (V) carries the flavour-related signals sensed by other GPCRs in the oropharynx, notably temperature, tactile and specific chemicals such as capsaicin, the hot ingredient of chillies that is detected by vanilloid (capsaicin) receptors. Trigeminal afferents synapse in the sensory trigeminal nucleus, which also projects to the NTS.

Smell is detected by olfactory receptors (also GPCR) in the olfactory epithelium of the nasopharynx, and relayed first to the olfactory bulb by the olfactory nerve (I) and from there to the olfactory cortex and various other brain sites including the limbic forebrain.

Flavour partly determines the pleasantness (or hedonic aspects) of eating and the reinforcing properties of food on learning. Orosensory pleasure is among the most powerful motivators of eating – so-called 'food reward' or 'orosensory reward' (see below). For example, sham-eating rats (whose stomachs are continually emptied through a gastric cannula) ingest food faster in proportion to the concentration of preferred flavours (sugar or oil), and slower in proportion to the concentration of non-preferred flavours (bitter or salt). Sham-eating humans, who spit out test foods without swallowing, show the same effects (Klein *et al.*, 2006). Flavour stimuli also contribute to discrimination (non-hedonic identification of food) and associative learning, which underlies certain behavioural responses (e.g. flavour-cued hunger and satiation) and physiological reflexes (e.g. cephalic-phase endocrine reflexes) (Kringelbach, 2007). Orosensory pleasure can also cause long-term

Obesity: Science to Practice   Edited by Gareth Williams and Gema Frühbeck
© 2009 John Wiley & Sons, Ltd

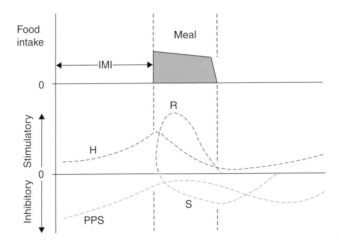

Figure 6.1 Processes controlling meal patterns. Food intake is a product of the size and number of meals, which in turn are thought to be controlled by four types of physiological processes, two stimulating eating and two inhibiting it. During fasting (i.e. intermeal meal intervals [IMI]), hunger (H) signals gradually increase, while postprandial satiety (PPS) signals gradually wane; when the sum of these reaches a certain threshold, the meal starts. During the meal, positive palatability or food reward (R) signals may further stimulate eating (and negative palatability may inhibit eating). Simultaneously, the postingestive consequences of food ingestion elicit satiation (S) signals that inhibit eating. When the sum of H, R and S falls to below a critical level, the meal ends. Note that during the IMI, S signals are thought to fall faster than PPS signals, whose strength probably increases for some time after meal end.

increases in food intake and obesity. Indeed, offering laboratory animals palatable, high-fat (and high energy density) diets is a common working model for human obesity (Rolls *et al.*, 1983).

Some basic flavour preferences (sweet, perhaps fat) and aversions (bitter, sour) appear to be innate, but most are learned. Such learning is sometimes reinforced by physiological consequences of eating (Gibson and Brunstrom, 2007).

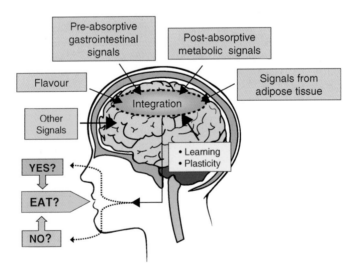

Figure 6.2 Integratory processes in the brain that control eating. The momentary decision to eat or not eat, made before each bite or sip, is the result of the brain's integration and evaluation of peripheral signals (blue boxes), information stored in the brain (e.g. learned effects of previous experiences, hedonic and other expectations) and other signals such as circadian effects, social context and energy demands.

Examples are conditioned aversions (e.g. for flavours associated with foods that caused nausea or vomiting) and 'specific hungers', that is preferences for flavours linked with foods containing certain vitamins or minerals, which can be learned during nutritional deficiencies. In these situations, the discriminative (non-hedonic) aspects of flavour are most important, although altered hedonic responses are part of the subsequent adaptation.

In humans, most flavour preferences seem to arise from the emotional, cognitive and cultural associations of foods, rather than their nutritional or physiological properties (Bowen, 1992; Gibson and Brunstrom, 2007; Zellner et al., 2004); indeed, mere exposure can be sufficient to condition flavour preferences. This probably explains much of the social and cultural variation in food choices, and perhaps the general fondness for dietary variety described below (Rozin, Hanko and Durlach, 2006).

Individual differences in flavour perception may contribute to human obesity. It has recently been shown that, compared with non-obese controls, obese subjects are less sensitive to the sensory intensity of sweet flavours, while also enjoying both sweet and fat flavours to a greater degree; both effects could favour overconsumption of sweet and fatty foods (Bartoshuk et al., 2006). Flavour variety can also increase food intake. Both rats and humans eat more if food contains multiple preferred flavours, compared with nutritionally-identical food that contains just one – even the individual's favourite. This is referred to as 'sensory-specific satiety' (Rolls, 1986). In rats, increased flavour variety also enhances long-term food intake and ultimately body weight (Rolls, Vanduijvenvoorde and Rowe, 1983).

Finally, an experiment of nature suggests a causal role of flavour perception in influencing food choices and body weight in humans. Otitis media often alters flavour perception, possibly because of the proximity of the trigeminal and glossopharyngeal nerves. Subjects who previously had severe otitis media have been shown to eat more sweets and have an increased risk of overweight and obesity (Bartoshuk et al., 2006).

Gut signals

Eating is affected by a wide variety of processes in the alimentary tract, which communicate with the brain through both hormonal and neural signals (Figure 6.3). This section focuses on gastric distension and some gut-related (gastrointestinal and pancreatic) peptide hormones that appear to act as feedback controls of eating; that is, their release is modulated by eating and, in turn, they affect eating. More details can be found in several recent reviews (Beglinger and Degen, 2006; Cummings and Overduin, 2007; Geary, 2004; Moran, 2006a; Ritter, 2004; Woods et al., 2006; Chaudri et al., 2008).

Gastric distension

The stomach is richly innervated with mechanoreceptors that respond to gastric filling and that signal to the brain via both vagal and spinal afferents. The effects of gastric mechanoreceptors on eating have been elegantly analysed in rats carrying both a gastric cannula (to drain the stomach), and a cuff around the pylorus that can be inflated to prevent gastric emptying. These studies found that meal size is significantly increased when the stomach is continually drained, and significantly decreased when the stomach is distended with fluid against a closed pylorus; the latter decreases were proportional to the volume of the fluid infused and occurred whether nutrient or non-nutrient fluids were used (Eisen et al., 2001; Kaplan and Moran, 2004; Phillips and Powley, 1996).

Thus, gastric distension can contribute to the control of eating, but this effect is normally rather small: the stomach has to be markedly distended for eating to be inhibited. As described below, however, it is possible that this mechanism may be enhanced by signals generated by food entering the gut beyond the stomach.

Cholecystokinin (CCK)

CCK is both a gut peptide hormone and CNS neurotransmitter. CCK expressed by neuroendocrine I cells in the duodenum and ileum is released into the circulation during and after meals, stimulated especially by high intraluminal concentrations of proteins and long-chain fatty acids derived from dietary triglyceride. Circulating CCK acts as a hormone, its actions including gall-bladder contraction. The classic demonstration by Gibbs, Young and Smith (1973) that intraperitoneal injections of CCK rapidly and selectively inhibited eating first implicated CCK in satiation, and CCK continues to be considered the prototypic endocrine satiation signal.

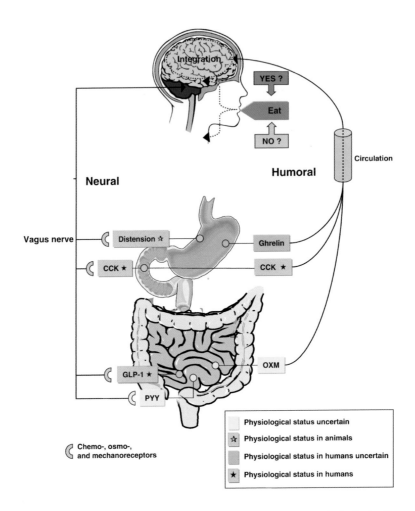

Figure 6.3 Some important gastrointestinal (GI) controls of eating. GI signals reach the brain via neural (left) and/or humoral (right) routes. CCK: cholecystokinin; GLP-1: glucagon-like peptide-1; OXM: oxyntomodulin; PYY: peptide YY.

The two most important empirical tests for normal physiological function of a hormone are related to the effects of 'physiological' doses of the hormone and the effects of antagonists (Beglinger and Degen, 2006; Geary, 2004). Reports that doses of CCK mimicking prandial levels are sufficient to inhibit eating in humans support the former criterion (Ballinger and Clark, 1994; Lieverse *et al.*, 1993), and in both humans and rats, the demonstration that selective CCK-1 receptor antagonists increase meal size and block the satiating effect of intraduodenal infusions of fat support the latter (Beglinger and Degen, 2004; Ritter, 2004; Asarian and Geary, 2007) (Figure 6.4). Comparably complete evidence is not yet available for other endocrine signals (Beglinger and Degen,

2004; Beglinger and Degen, 2006; Cummings and Overduin, 2007; Geary, 2004; Moran, 2006b; Woods *et al.*, 2006).

The satiating effect of CCK released from the intestines is mainly mediated by CCK-1 (originally named CCK-A) receptors on vagal sensory terminals in the upper gut, which project to the NTS; the satiating effect of CCK is abolished by selective destruction of abdominal vagal afferent fibres (Smith *et al.*, 1985). In both rodents and humans, mutations of the CCK-1 receptor gene produce hyperphagia and obesity (Geary, 2004; Moran and Kinzig, 2004), although lack of brain as well as gut CCK-1 receptors may contribute to this phenotype (see below). In humans, the common phenotype in all these cases is severe hyperphagia and morbid obesity,

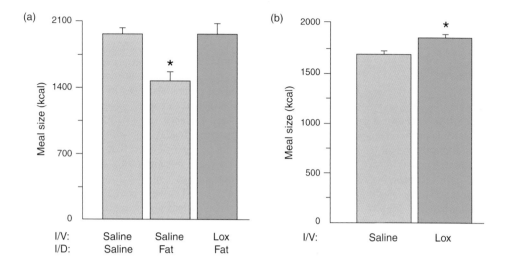

Figure 6.4 Evidence that CCK is a physiological satiation signal in humans. Both figures show the energy content of a buffet lunch eaten at midday by lean males, 4 h after a standard breakfast. (a) Intraduodenal (ID) infusion of a fat load (corn-oil), which releases CCK, significantly reduced meal size compared with a control ID saline infusion. This effect was blocked by intravenous infusion of the CCK1 receptor antagonist, loxiglumide, without producing physical or subjective side effects. From Matzinger *et al.* (1999) 'Inhibition of food intake in response to intestinal lipid is mediated by cholecystokinin in humans'. *American Journal of Physiology*, **277**: R1718, with permission of the editor. (b) Intravenous infusion of loxiglumide significantly increased meal size without affecting the subjects' enjoyment of their meals or their subjective sense of normal satiation. From Beglinger *et al.* (2001) 'Loxiglumide, a CCK-A receptor antagonist, stimulates calorie intake and hunger feelings in humans'. *American Journal of Physiology*, **280**: R1149, with permission of the editor.

which becomes apparent in early childhood or even infancy (see Chapters 8 and 21).

Proglucagon-derived peptides

Tissue-specific posttranslational processing of the proglucagon gene yields several peptide hormones that have been implicated in the control of eating. The first of these identified was glucagon itself (derived from proglucagon, amino acids 30–64), which is expressed by pancreatic α-cells and released during meals (Woods *et al.*, 2006; Holst, 2007). Intrameal infusion of glucagon during meals selectively reduces meal size, whereas infusion of glucagon antibodies has the opposite effect (Langhans *et al.*, 1982; Le Sauter, Noh and Geary, 1991). Glucagon acts in the periphery to generate a signal relayed to the brain by afferent fibres in the hepatic branch of the vagus nerve.

Glucagon-like peptide-1 (GLP-1; proglucagon residues 69–107/108) is expressed by intestinal L-cells and a specific group of neurones in the NTS in the brainstem. Intestinal GLP-1 is released during and after meals, and both central and peripheral GLP-1 administration dose-dependently inhibit eating (Chaudri *et al.*, 2008; Holst, 2007). The criteria for physiological endocrine function have not yet been tested extensively in rodents. In humans, however, physiological doses of GLP-1 appeared sufficient to inhibit eating, and the effect was markedly increased when GLP-1 was given together with protein-rich preloads (Degen *et al.*, 2006). Intestinal GLP-1 may reach CNS GLP-1 receptors, which are expressed in the PVN and other sites, to affect eating. Interestingly, mice lacking the GLP-1 receptor have unchanged body weight compared to controls, suggesting that GLP-1 is not normally a critical component in the control of energy homeostasis.

The two other proglucagon gene products implicated in the control of eating are glucagon-like peptide-2 (GLP-2; proglucagon residues 126–158) and oxyntomodulin (proglucagon 30–69), both of which are also expressed by intestinal L-cells. Peripheral administration of GLP-2 inhibits eating in rodents and humans (Cohen *et al.*, 2003). Central administration of GLP-2 selectively inhi-bited eating in rats (Tang-Christensen *et al.*, 2000), but intravenous

GLP-2 had no effect on appetite in humans (Schmidt *et al.*, 2003).

Ghrelin

Discovered in 1999, ghrelin is a 28-amino acid peptide that is the endogenous ligand at the growth hormone secretagogue receptor (GHS-R); it was originally named for its ability to stimulate growth hormone release. Ghrelin is expressed mainly in neuroendocrine cells of the stomach, and at much lower levels in the hypothalamus and elsewhere.

Gastric ghrelin has attracted great interest because it is the only gut peptide whose secretion and blood levels rise during fasting and fall on eating, and whose administration stimulates eating in the rat (Cummings, Foster-Schubert and Overduin, 2005; Cummings and Overduin, 2007). Moreover, chronic peripheral or central ghrelin administration causes sustained hyperphagia and decreased energy expenditure, thus increasing body fat and weight. Also, the GHS-R knockout mouse shows the expected lean phenotype, at least under some conditions (Wortley *et al.*, 2005; Zigman *et al.*, 2005). Importantly, ghrelin administration also increases hunger and food intake in humans (Cummings, Foster-Schubert and Overduin, 2005; Geary, 2004; Kojima *et al.*, 1999; Nakamura *et al.*, 2001; Tschop, Smiley and Heiman, 2000; Ueno *et al.*, 2005) (Figure 6.5). As yet, however, it is unknown whether physiological preprandial rises in circulating ghrelin are sufficient to trigger eating in humans.

Most evidence suggests that the orexigenic (appetite-stimulating) effect of ghrelin is mediated by neurones that express GHS-R in the arcuate nucleus (ARC) at the base of the hypothalamus and in the brain stem (Arnold *et al.*, 2006; Cowley *et al.*, 2003). Some neurones in these regions also express ghrelin itself, but their role is unknown.

Blocking GHS-R with antagonists or ghrelin 'RNA spiegelmers' (mirror-image oligonucleotides that bind and neutralize the endogenous peptide) is reported to decrease eating and weight gain in rodents (Helmling *et al.*, 2004; Monnikes *et al.*, 2005; Wang *et al.*, 2005). Overall, ghrelin may contribute to the control of energy homeostasis both by acting as a hunger signal and as an 'inverse adiposity signal', in that fasting ghrelin concentrations are negatively correlated with body weight in both rats and humans (Cummings, Foster-Schubert and Overduin, 2005; Cummings and Overduin, 2007).

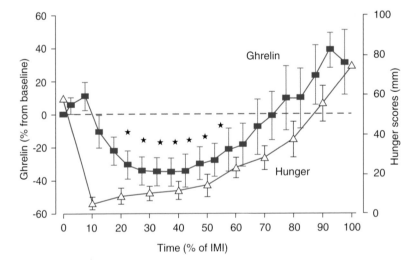

Figure 6.5 Hunger is closely related to plasma ghrelin concentrations in humans. Hunger scores (rated on a 100-mm visual analogue scale) and plasma ghrelin concentrations were measured between lunch (starting at time = 0) and a freely-requested dinner (starting at 100% of the intermeal interval in each case). Subjects were six healthy lean males. Mean lunch size was 800 kcal, mean lunch duration was 20 min, and mean intermeal interval was 359 min. Data are mean ± SEM of baseline values at the start of lunch. *$P < 0.05$ compared with baseline. From: Cummings *et al.* (2004). 'Plasma ghrelin levels and hunger scores in humans initiating meals voluntarily without time- and food-related cues'. *American Journal of Physiology*, **287**: E297, with permission of the editor.

Other gut peptides

Several further gut peptides are implicated in the control of eating. We mention here some of the more important candidates; the interested reader is referred to recent reviews for details (Lutz, 2006; Woods *et al.*, 2006; Chaudri *et al.*, 2008).

PYY$_{3-36}$, a cleavage product of peptide YY (PYY), is expressed by intestinal L cells and is released into the bloodstream during meals. PYY$_{3-36}$ may inhibit eating through an indirect action in the ARC: it activates the Y2 autoceptors on the neuropeptide Y (NPY)/agouti-related peptide (AgRP) neurones, which inhibit the release of their orexigenic (eating-stimulating) peptides, NPY and AgRP (Batterham *et al.*, 2002; Dumont *et al.*, 1995). Its physiological importance is unknown.

Apolipoprotein A-IV is a protein secreted during fat absorption that also seems to control eating, especially fat intake (Tso and Liu, 2004). Whether it acts peripherally or centrally remains in doubt.

Finally, in addition to glucagon, three further pancreatic hormones – insulin, amylin and pancreatic polypeptide – have been implicated in the control of eating (Woods *et al.*, 2006). Insulin and amylin are described further below.

Metabolic signals

Ultimately, eating is required to fuel metabolism, and it seems intuitive that some aspects of metabolism should control food intake. General evidence supports this notion: parenteral administration of energy-yielding substrates (e.g. glucose or fatty acids) can inhibit eating, while pharmacological agents that block utilization of these fuels can stimulate eating (Langhans, 1996). This suggests that fluctuations in the availability or utilization of metabolic fuels, or some common consequence of these, may control eating. There is now evidence that such changes can be sensed both centrally and peripherally (Figure 6.6) – although the physiological relevance

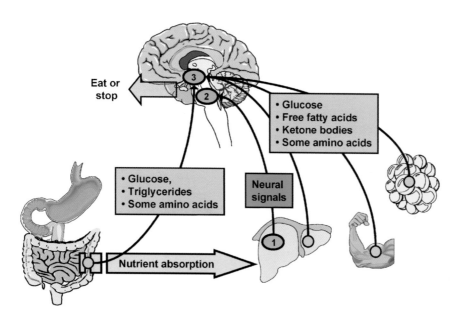

Figure 6.6 The availability or utilization of metabolic fuels can be sensed in the periphery and the brain to affect eating. Circulating metabolic substrates absorbed from the gut or mobilized from endogenous stores may act directly on the brain, or may signal via vagal afferent nerves from the liver. Metabolites may also be stored temporarily in peripheral tissues (liver, muscle, fat) and released later. Key sites include: (1) glucose sensors in the hepatic portal vein; (2) the nucleus tractus solitarii (NTS) in the caudal hindbrain, where vagal afferents first synapse and where neural inputs (visceral sensory, and descending from the hypothalamus) are integrated with locally- registered humoral and metabolic signals; and (3) the hypothalamus, a major focus for circulating metabolic signals that act on the brain to control eating.

of these effects is still debatable, especially in well-nourished people who eat regular ample meals.

Glucose

Glucose, with its marked increases in blood concentrations and utilization after carbohydrate ingestion, is an obvious candidate to control eating. As mentioned, peripheral intravenous infusions of glucose have been shown to inhibit eating (Langhans, 1996); in some studies, the satiating potency of glucose was enhanced by insulin (MacLagan, 1937), suggesting that the sensors responsible are partly insulin-sensitive. Conversely, eating is powerfully stimulated by profound reductions in glucose concentrations (e.g. insulin-induced hypoglycaemia) or in glucose utilization (e.g. blockade with the antimetabolite, 2-deoxyglucose) (Langhans, 1996).

Evidence for the role of glucose in normal eating comes from studies of transgenic mice with deletion (knockout) of the GLUT-2 glucose transporter in all tissues except for the pancreatic β cells (thus preserving insulin secretion). These GLUT-2 knockout mice eat significantly more than wild-type controls; their hypothalami show suppressed regulation of orexigenic (e.g. NPY) and appetite-suppressing peptides (e.g. melanocortins) during the transition from a 24-h fast to refeeding (Bady

et al., 2006). GLUT-2, which allows unrestricted glucose entry into cells, is expressed by glucose-sensing neurones in various CNS sites. Finally, and probably more relevant physiologically, is the intriguing observation that a small (~0.2 mmol/l) but consistent decline in blood glucose level precedes spontaneous meals in both rats (LouisSylvestre and LeMagnen, 1980) and humans (Melanson et al., 1999). This dip is suggested to contribute to the initiation of eating; its cause and the nature and site of the putative glucose sensors remain elusive.

Because of its unique location and function, the liver has long been considered to be involved in controlling food intake (Russek, 1963). In rats, infusion of physiological doses of glucose into the hepatic portal vein reduces food intake more than equivalent infusions into the jugular vein (Tordoff and Friedman, 1986; Tordoff and Friedman, 1988; Tordoff, Tluczek and Friedman, 1989), while intraportal infusions of small glucose doses (with or without insulin) during spontaneous meals selectively reduce the amount eaten (Langhans, Grossmann and Geary, 2001) (Figure 6.7). Thus, meal-related increases in hepatic portal glucose levels may contribute to satiation. Vagal afferents terminating in the wall of the portal vein apparently function as hepatic glucose sensors, as originally suggested by Niijima (Niijima, 1969). Fasting GLP-1 levels confer maximum sensitivity to the hepatoportal

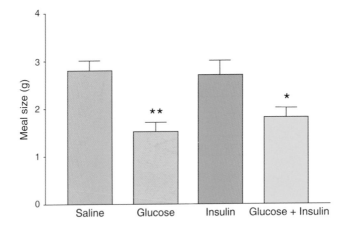

Figure 6.7 Infusion of low doses of glucose into the hepatic portal vein reduces spontaneous meal size in rats. Glucose (1 mmol), insulin (2 mU) or both were infused during the first nocturnal sponaneous meal via remotely controlled cannulas. Data are means ± SEM. *P < 0.05; **P < 0.01 versus control saline infusions. From W. Langhans, F. Grossmann and N. Geary (2001) 'Intrameal hepatic-portal infusion of glucose reduces spontaneous meal size in rats'. *Physiology & Behavior*, **73**: 499, with permission of the editor.

glucose sensor, suggesting that the GLP-1 receptor is a necessary part of the sensor (Burcelin et al., 2001). This recalls the synergy between glucose and GLP-1 in stimulating insulin secretion (Balkan and Li, 2000).

Carbohydrate metabolism within the liver may also influence eating. Hepatic over-expression of the enzyme 6-phosphofructo-2-kinase/fructose-2,6-bisphosphatase in transgenic mice reduces food intake and body weight (and also hypothalamic NPY expression), as compared with over-expression of glucokinase that has similar metabolic consequences (Wu et al., 2005). The underlying mechanism is not known.

CNS Glucose-sensing neurones

The CNS contains numerous populations of glucose-sensing neurones, which alter their membrane potentials and firing rates in responses to changes in ambient glucose levels They are found in the hypothalamus, NTS and other brain sites, and together with peripheral glucose sensors, they form a functional network that monitors glucose availability and participates in glucose homeostasis and eating control (Niijima, 1983).

Glucose-sensing neurones comprise two broad classes: glucose-excited and glucose-inhibited, whose firing rates are respectively increased and decreased by rising glucose concentrations. *Glucose-excited neurones* are abundant in the ventromedial hypothalamic area (VMH), where they comprise 30% of neurones, and in the NTS. They may sense glucose in the same way as the pancreatic β cell, because the same key components – GLUT-2, the adenosine triphosphate (ATP)-sensitive K^+ channel, the sulphonylurea receptor SUR-1, and glucokinase (GK) – are expressed in these areas; the GLP-1 receptor is also co-localized (Li et al., 2003; Marty et al., 2006; Navarro et al., 1996). Glucose phosphorylation by GK is the rate-limiting step in ATP production and is essential for the effects of glucose on the membrane potential and ion channel function of glucose-sensing neurones. *Glucose-inhibited neurones* are plentiful in the lateral hypothalamic area (LHA), comprising 40% of neurones, and include orexin-expressing neurones, which respond to very small increases in glucose due to the highly-sensitive glucose-regulated K^+ channels in their membranes (Burdakov, 2007).

Glucose-sensing neurones have functional connections with other neuronal populations, including the appetite-modulating pathways in the hypothalamus and other regions; glucose availability influences the expression and turnover of several appetite-regulating peptides (Levin, 2006), which presumably mediate some of the effects of glucose on eating. Some glucose-sensing neurones also respond to other metabolites and hormones such as insulin and leptin (Levin, 2006). Thus, these neurones appear to integrate a variety of signals, and their outputs control neuroendocrine and autonomic responses (e.g. those triggered by hypoglycaemia) as well as eating.

Free fatty acids

In animals and humans, acute pharmacological inhibition of fatty acid oxidation (FAO) is usually accompanied by transient hyperphagia (Leonhardt and Langhans, 2004). The importance of FAO as an energy source for the liver raises the possibility that hepatic sensors of FAO might mediate this response, but recent studies do not support this notion. Increases in FAO, induced in various ways (e.g. fasting, or administering a β_3 adrenergic agonist), could be blocked by the FAO inhibitor mercaptoacetate, but the expected increase in food intake did not occur (Brandt et al., 2006a; Brandt et al., 2006b; Jambor de Sousa et al., 2006). Moreover, increasing hepatic FAO through various transgenic manipulations in mice has failed to reduce food intake (An et al., 2004; Ishigaki et al., 2005; Savage et al., 2006). Overall, physiological changes in hepatic FAO appear to be of minor importance in initiating or terminating normal meals, but might affect eating under special circumstances, such as in diabetic rats fed a high-fat diet (Friedman et al., 1985; La Fleur et al., 2003).

Fatty acid availability does not seem to affect long-term food intake or body weight. Chronic administration of the FAO inhibitor etomoxir did not induce hyperphagia (Dobbins et al., 2001), while reduced peripheral FAO in transgenic mice (Wanders et al., 1999) or humans with genetic disorders of fatty acid metabolism (Wood, 2004) is not associated with hyperphagia or obesity.

Fatty acids and/or their use can apparently be sensed in the mediobasal hypothalamus and affect eating, because the fatty-acid synthase inhibitor, cerulenin, induces hypophagia and weight loss when infused intracerebroventricularly (ICV) (Lam, Schwartz and Rossetti, 2005). The physiological relevance of this effect is unclear.

An integrated metabolic signal?

Clarification of metabolic signalling pathways has revived an earlier hypothesis that eating is controlled by an 'energostatic' ('ischymetric') signal of overall metabolic status, rather than the use of a single metabolite (Langhans, 1996). One possible basis is the interaction in the brain between two fuel-sensitive kinases – AMP kinase (AMPK), a ubiquitous energy sensor and the enzyme that converts AMP to adenosine diphosphate (ADP) and ATP, and the 'mammalian target of rapamycin' (mTOR) (Cota *et al.*, 2006) (Figure 6.8). AMPK activity is increased by fuel deficits and by ghrelin, and decreased by glucose and free fatty acids and by leptin (Minokoshi *et al.*, 2004); also, activation of AMPK inhibits mTOR activity (Cota *et al.*, 2006). By contrast, mTOR is inhibited by fuel deficits and stimulated by leptin.

AMPK activation or deactivation in the rat hypothalamus respectively increases or decreases food intake (Andersson *et al.*, 2004; Minokoshi *et al.*, 2004), suggesting that changes in cellular energy status contribute to the control of eating. Conversely, increased mTOR signalling in the hypothalamus is associated with decreased food intake and body weight (Cota *et al.*, 2006). AMPK is widely distributed in the brain (Turnley *et al.*, 1999), whereas mTOR appears to be mainly confined to NPY/AgRP neurones in the ARC (Cota *et al.*, 2006).

The responsiveness of AMPK and mTOR to hormones as well as metabolites (Figure 6.8) suggests a broad role in integrating information about fuel availability and endocrine status. These two fuel-sensitive kinases therefore appear to have reciprocal functions, and the balance between them may reflect overall energy availability. An emerging concept is that changes in AMPK and mTOR sensing in the brain in response to fuel surplus inhibit eating, and vice versa.

Adiposity signals

Under steady conditions, body weight in mammals including humans is relatively constant, which implies close matching of energy intake and expenditure: in humans, an excess of intake over expenditure of only 1% would lead to a weight gain of over 1 kg per year. Moreover, experimental manipulations of body weight are readily compensated for by appropriate changes in energy intake and expenditure (Langhans and Geary, 2006). In adults, changes in body weight are largely attributable to fluctuations in body fat, suggesting that body fat mass is the regulated variable. This can be partly explained by specific circulating factors whose plasma levels reflect the size of the fat stores ('lipostatic' or adiposity signals) and which control food intake

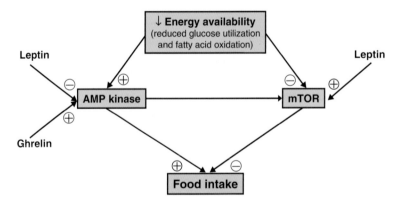

Figure 6.8 Suggested roles of hypothalamic AMP kinase (AMPK) and mTOR as metabolic fuel sensors controlling eating. AMPK in various neuronal systems is activated by falls in ATP relative to AMP, and leads to changes that stimulate eating. mTOR activation inhibits eating, and mTOR is inhibited by AMPK and stimulated by leptin, whereas AMPK is inhibited by leptin and stimulated by ghrelin.

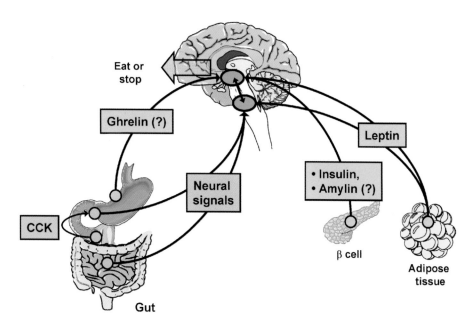

Figure 6.9 Suggested roles of adiposity signals in controlling eating. Adiposity signals (yellow boxes) act through receptors in the hypothalamus (leptin and insulin) and/or the NTS in the hindbrain (leptin); the roles of amylin and ghrelin as lipostatic signals remain uncertain. Hypothalamic actions of leptin and (presumably) insulin activate a descending pathway to the NTS. The adiposity signals modulate meal-related, vagally-mediated satiation signals such as cholecystokinin (CCK).

and energy expenditure so as to keep body fat mass constant (Figure 6.9).

Four hormones that circulate at levels proportional to fat mass have been proposed as adiposity signals; leptin, the only one secreted by the adipocytes themselves, and insulin, ghrelin (discussed earlier) and amylin.

Leptin

Elegant experiments in the 1970s suggested that the striking obesity and diabetes phenotypes of *ob/ob* and *db/db* mice were caused by single-gene mutations of an unknown hormone and its receptor, respectively. A significant new chapter in the physiology of eating opened in 1994 when Friedman's group (Zhang *et al.*, 1994) exploited molecular genetic methods to identify the *ob* gene product as an adipocyte-derived protein, which they termed leptin. This was quickly followed by identification of the *db* product as the leptin receptor, whose fully competent signalling form in humans is now known as LepRb (Chua *et al.*, 1996; Tartaglia *et al.*, 1995). The true role of leptin in the regulation

of energy balance remains controversial, but the scientific impact of this powerful demonstration of molecular genetics can hardly be underestimated (Kandel, Schwartz and Jessell, 2000).

Leptin is a 14-kDa protein, structurally related to the cytokines, and is highly conserved among mammals. It is expressed at high levels in adipose tissue, especially white adipose tissue; lower levels are found in stomach and placenta. Leptin fulfils many theoretical predictions for an adiposity signal. It is secreted by adipose tissue into the bloodstream, where its concentrations are proportional to fat mass (Ahima and Flier, 2000). Leptin is rapidly transported across the blood-brain barrier in the mediobasal hypothalamus and other regions, and so has ready access to the CNS regions that regulate energy homeostasis. It binds to receptors in several brain regions, notably the ARC and other hypothalamic areas (Malik and Young, 1996).

When injected centrally in normal rodents, leptin inhibits eating and stimulates energy expenditure (via increased sympathetic stimulation), leading with repeated administration to loss of body weight and fat – hence its name, from 'leptos', the Greek for 'thin'. The loss of

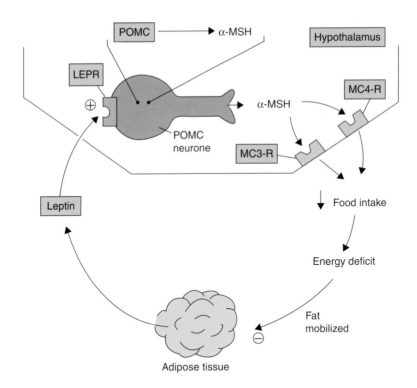

Figure 6.10 Leptin and the melanocortin neurones that are important mediators of its eating-inhibitory action. The diagram shows the sites of mutations in this control pathway that lead to rodent syndromes of hyperphagia and obesity.

leptin action in mutations affecting *lep*, *lepRb*, or downstream neural signalling molecules (see below) is responsible for the hyperphagia, reduced energy expenditure and obesity of several genetically-obese rodents (Figure 6.10) and in some extremely rare cases of human obesity (see Chapter 8) (O'Rahilly and Farooqi, in press). Both peripheral and ICV leptin administration reverses the hyperphagia, obesity and diabetes in *ob/ob* mice, which have no biologically active leptin because of the *ob* mutation. By contrast, *db/db* mice – whose LepRb are disabled by the *db* mutation and unable to bind leptin – show no response to leptin (Campfield *et al.*, 1995; Halaas *et al.*, 1995; Pelleymounter *et al.*, 1995). These effects were originally thought to be mediated primarily through the ARC, where LepRb density is high on neurones expressing the neuropeptides that act as downstream mediators of leptin: leptin inhibits the NPY neurones, which increase eating, while stimulating the POMC neurones, which inhibit eating. Recent evidence, however, indicates that the caudal brainstem is also important in mediating leptin's effect on eating (Grill *et al.*, 2002).

Any signal that controls body weight by changing food intake must modulate the frequency and/or size of single meals. Leptin reduces food intake mainly by decreasing meal size (Flynn *et al.*, 1998; Kahler *et al.*, 1998); conversely, the hyperphagia of both *ob/ob* and *db/db* mice is due to marked increases in meal size (Prins *et al.*, 1986; Strohmayer and Smith, 1987). Leptin also enhances the satiating effect of CCK (Emond *et al.*, 1999), an established physiological control of meal size (see above). Three possible mechanisms for this interaction have been described: (i) leptin may act on LepRb on ARC neurones that affect descending projections from the PVN to the NTS, where the CCK signal is processed (Morton *et al.*, 2005; Blevins, Schwartz and Baskin, 2004); (ii) leptin may act directly on LepRb on neurones in the NTS (Grill *et al.*, 2002); (iii) leptin may act on LepRb on abdominal vagal afferents involved in CCK signalling (Peters, Simasko and Ritter, 2006).

In normal, well-nourished humans, plasma leptin levels are proportional to body fat mass (see Figure 4.13). Thus, the increased leptin levels of obese patients appear inconsistent with a strong regulatory effect of leptin in energy homeostasis. This suggests either that obese people are 'resistant' to leptin, analogous to the insulin resistance of obesity, or that leptin is irrelevant to energy balance regulation in most humans.

Finally, under- or overeating causes acute changes in plasma leptin before any significant weight gain or loss occurs (Kolaczynski *et al.*, 1996; Lin *et al.*, 1998), suggesting that energy flux into and out of the adipocyte may regulate leptin synthesis and release. Thus, in addition to its putative long-term lipostatic function, leptin may correct short-term changes in energy intake by adjusting energy expenditure at a steady body weight. Leptin also has peripheral metabolic effects (Cohen *et al.*, 2002) that may contribute to its lipostatic function, and may explain certain links between body weight and reproductive (Ahima *et al.*, 1997) and immune functions (Gabay *et al.*, 2001).

Insulin

As with leptin, basal plasma and cerebrospinal insulin concentrations are correlated with body fat mass, insulin can enter the mediobasal hypothalamus and CSF by receptor-mediated processes (Woods *et al.*, 2003), and insulin receptors are present in the hypothalamus and elsewhere and their selective deletion in the hypothalamus increases food intake in female mice and body weight in both sexes (Bruning *et al.*, 2000) (Figure 6.12). The central actions of insulin on food intake and energy expenditure also are similar to those of leptin in many respects (Woods, Decke and Vasselli, 1974; Woods *et al.*, 2006; Woods and Seeley, 2001). Central administration of insulin, in amounts that have no peripheral effects, dose-dependently inhibits eating, while chronic central administration of insulin antibodies stimulates eating and increases body weight (McGowan *et al.*, 1992; Strubbe and Mein, 1977). Finally, transgenic mice with deletion of neuronal insulin receptors are hyperphagic and

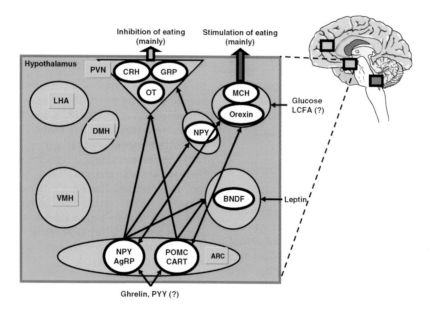

Figure 6.11 Principal hypothalamic areas implicated in the control of food intake. The diagram shows their neural interconnections, their hormone and metabolite sensitivities, and the signalling neuropeptides expressed in their neurones. Interconnections are depicted on one side only. Hypothalamic areas: ARC: arcuate nucleus; PVN: paraventricular nucleus; LHA: lateral hypothalamic area; VMH: ventromedial hypothalamic area. Neuropeptides: CRH: corticotropin releasing hormone; GRP: gastrin-releasing peptide; OT: oxytocin; NPY: neuropeptide Y; MCH: melanin-concentrating hormone; AgRP: agouti-related peptide; POMC: proopiomelanocortin; CART: cocaine- and amphetamine-related transcript; BDNF: brain-derived neurotropic factor. Metabolites: LCFA: long-chain fatty acids.

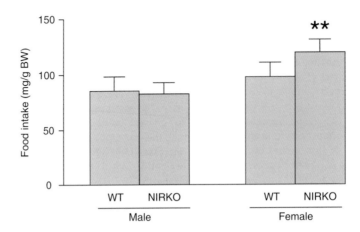

Figure 6.12 Evidence that insulin acts in the brain to decrease eating in transgenic mice with selective knock-out of neuronal insulin receptors (NIRKO) were hyperphagic and obese compared with wild-type controls (WT). From Bruning *et al.* (2000) Role of brain insulin receptor in control of body weight and reproduction. *Science,* **289**: 2122–5, with permission of the editor.

obese when fed a high-fat diet (Bruning *et al.*, 2000), indicating that insulin receptor signalling in the brain is important in restraining food intake and body weight (Figure 6.12).

Insulin apparently acts through the same hypothalamic neuropeptide systems as leptin, inhibiting the NPY neurones and stimulating the POMC neurones in the ARC (see Figure 6.11). ICV insulin also enhances the satiating effect of peri-pheral CCK (Riedy *et al.*, 1995), but unlike leptin, insulin also reduces nocturnal meal frequency, indicating some divergence in the mechanisms underlying the two hormones' effects.

Amylin

This 37-residue peptide, co-released with insulin by the β-cell, fulfils several criteria for an adiposity signal (Lutz, 2006; Woods *et al.*, 2006). Like insulin, its basal blood levels reflect total fat mass, and when injected centrally it inhibits eating. Amylin apparently acts in the AP in the caudal brainstem and indirectly affects neural signalling in the LHA, but does not target the ARC (Woods *et al.*, 2006). Peripheral and central chronic amylin administration reduces food intake, body weight and body adiposity, whereas blockade of central amylin receptors has the opposite effects (Rushing *et al.*, 2001). Consistent with this, mice lacking amylin gain weight more rapidly than controls (Lutz, 200).

Amylin is potentially of therapeutic interest in humans. An agonist, pramlintide, lowers glucose and is used to treat type 2 diabetes; it also slightly reduces food intake and body weight (Hollander *et al.*, 2004).

The neuroanatomy of eating regulation

In neurological terms, eating is a rhythmic behaviour produced by the lower motor neurones of cranial nerves V, VII, IX, X and XII in the caudal brainstem, which are controlled by central pattern generators that also reside in the caudal brainstem, various neural and endocrine feedback signals, and descending projections from the forebrain. These projections originate in an extensive, distributed neural network with nodes in the hypothalamus, NAc, amygdala and several other telencephalic sites. Of these, the hypothalamic networks are the best described (Figure 6.13).

The hypothalamus

The structure of the hypothalamus is broadly similar among mammals, including rats and humans. The hypothalamus contains a number of interconnected, microscopically defined nuclei and areas, many of which are involved in the control of eating (Figure 6.14). Fuelled by the revolution in molecular techniques,

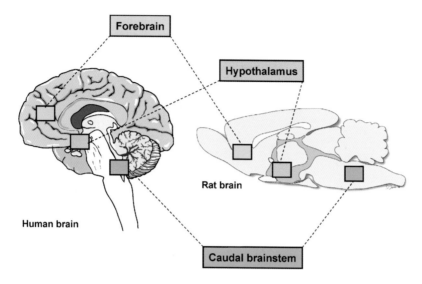

Figure 6.13 Principal brain areas implicated in the control of food intake and energy balance.

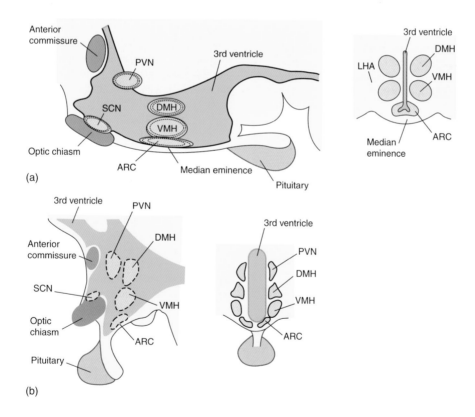

Figure 6.14 Anatomy of the hypothalamus in (a) the rat and (b) humans. Longitudinal sections are shown on the left, and coronal sections at the level of the arcuate nucleus on the right. ARC: arcuate nucleus (also known as (tubero)infundibular nucleus in humans); DMH: dorsomedial nucleus; LHA: lateral hypothalamic area; PVN: paraventricular nucleus; SCN: suprachiasmatic nucleus; VMH: ventromedial nucleus.

knowledge about the hypothalamic neuronal circuitry mediating eating has exploded in the last decade. Nevertheless, crucial aspects of the available methodologies for manipulating or measuring brain processes remain rather crude. Thus, the exact contributions of certain parts of the circuits described below remain to be determined.

Arcuate nucleus (ARC)

The ARC lies around the base of the third ventricle immediately above the median eminence. It contains two neuronal populations crucial for controlling food intake and regulating body weight (Berthoud, 2002; Cota et al., 2006; Cowley et al., 2003; Ellacott and Cone, 2004; Elmquist et al., 2005; Heisler et al., 2006; Hillebrand, de Wied and Adan, 2002; Simerly, 2004) (Figure 6.11). One expresses the orexigenic peptides, NPY and AgRP, and the other expresses the eating-inhibitory melanocortin, α-melanocyte stimulating hormone (α-MSH). The specialized blood- brain barrier of the ARC transports the hormones insulin, leptin and ghrelin to cognate receptors on one or both populations, so that these three hormones reciprocally regulate the NPY/AgRP and α-MSH neurones. ARC NPY/AgRP and α-MSH neurones project to most other hypothalamic areas implicated in eating, and in several neuroendocrine and autonomic functions. The ARC also has extensive reciprocal connections with the VMH, the dorsomedial hypothalamus (DMH) and especially LHA, where neurones expressing the eating-stimulating peptides, orexin A and melanin-concentrating hormone (MCH), receive NPY inputs.

The paraventricular nucleus (PVN)

The paraventricular nucleus (PVN) receives dense projections from Arc NPY and LHA α-MSH fibres, and its neurones express receptors for NPY and α-MSH as well as for eating-inhibitory peptides such as corticotrophin releasing factor (CRF), oxytocin, gastrin-releasing peptide (GRP), and thyrotrophin-releasing hormone (TRH) (Beck, 2006; Fan et al., 1997; Harrold, Widdowson and Williams, 1999; Mountjoy et al., 1994). These neurones also express receptors for other neurotransmitters that affect eating, including CCK (CCK-2R), orexin A (ORX-1R) and serotonin. In addition, the PVN also receives projections from several other hypothalamic and extra-hypothalamic sites (Figure 6.11).

The PVN appears to mediate the 'catabolic' effects of reducing feeding, increasing energy expenditure, and reducing body weight – consistent with the hyperphagia and obesity caused by experimental lesions of this nucleus. CRF, for example, is critical for mediating stress-induced decreases in eating. Another important function is apparently to communicate with the caudal brainstem areas that control eating. Oxytocin, CRF and GRP neurones all project to the NTS and nearby dorsal motor nucleus of the vagus (Blevins et al., 2003; Costello, Brown and Gray, 1991; Rinaman, 1998; Rogers et al., 1980; Sawchenko and Swanson, 1982). For example, the oxytocinergic projections are critical for mediating the effect of leptin on eating (Blevins, Schwartz and Baskin, 2004).

The ventromedial hypothalamic area (VMH)

This large hypothalamic area surrounds the ventromedial nucleus itself, receives projections from the ARC NPY and melanocortin neurones and has direct connections with the PVN and DMH. VMH efferents activate sympathetic outputs, including those that stimulate energy expenditure and gut motility.

The VMH contains neurones expressing high levels of LepRb. Leptin depolarizes and increases the firing rate of VMH neurones that express steroidogenic factor-1 (SF-1), while transgenic deletion of LepRb on these neurones leads to excessive weight gain (Dhillon et al., 2006). Other VMH neurones express CCK-2 receptors (whose physiological role is unclear) and brain-derived neurotrophic factor (BDNF), an eating-inhibitory peptide; transgenic knockdown of BDNF expression increases eating and body weight (Xu et al., 2003). Finally, VMH glucose-excited neurones may be involved in sensing falls in plasma glucose and initiating appropriate neuroendocrine responses to hypoglycaemia.

The dorsomedial hypothalamus (DMH)

The DMH contains NPY neurones that project to the PVN (see above). These are tonically inhibited via CCK-1 receptors activated by CCK released from neurones rather than derived from the circulation. Obesity in the OLETF rat, which has a mutation that disables the CCK-1 receptor, is accompanied by, and may be due to, over-expression of NPY in the DMH neurones (Moran and Bi, 2006). In addition, sustained exercise seems to cause tonic inhibition of these neurones (Moran and Bi, 2006).

The lateral hypothalamic area (LHA)

This anatomically diffuse area contains neurones that express predominantly orexigenic neurotransmitters, notably orexin A and MCH, and apparently functions overall to stimulate eating and body weight gain. The LHA also contains glucose-sensing neurones, some of which also express orexin, that may mediate 'glucoprivic' eating in response to marked hypoglycaemia. Other LHA neurones may also sense long-chain fatty acids as well as glucose.

LHA orexin and MCH neurones receive inputs from ARC NPY and melanocortin neurones and express NPY and melanocortin receptors, including the NPY Y5 receptor (Broberger et al., 1998; Chen et al., 1999; Elias et al., 1998); he orexin neurones also project back to ARC NPY and melanocortin neurones (van den Pol et al., 1998). Orexin's eating-stimulatory effect

appears to be in part related to its powerful effects on arousal (Saper, 2006).

The caudal brainstem

The caudal brainstem contains essential motor and sensory machinery contributing to the control of eating and regulation of energy homeostasis (Figure 6.15). It also receives neural inputs from the hypothalamus and telencephalon. Finally, many of the same neurotransmitters and receptors involved in hypothalamic eating-regulatory circuits are also expressed in the caudal brainstem, including receptors for NPY (Dumont et al., 1998) and melanocortins (Fodor et al., 1996; Mountjoy et al., 1994).

The integratory capacities of the caudal brainstem allow this region to control eating in its own right. This has been elegantly demonstrated in the chronic decerebrate rat; that is, with brain transections in the midbrain (Faulconbridge et al., 2003; Grill and Kaplan, 2002; Grill et al., 2002). These rats do not initiate meals unless food is presented into the mouth; when this is done by intraoral infusion, they exhibit facial and oropharyngeal movements indistinguishable

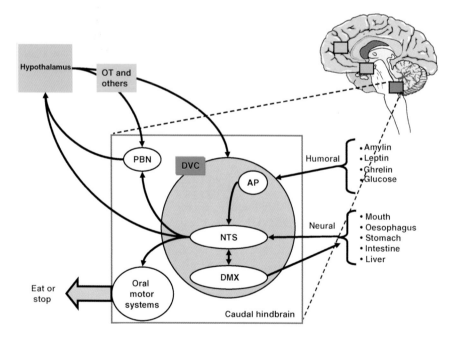

Figure 6.15 Principal caudal brainstem areas implicated in the control of food intake. The diagram shows their neural connections and peripheral inputs. OT: oxytocin; PBN: parabrachial nucleus; DVC: dorsal vagal complex; AP: area postrema; NTS: nucleus tractus solitarii; DMX: dorsal motor nucleus of the vagus.

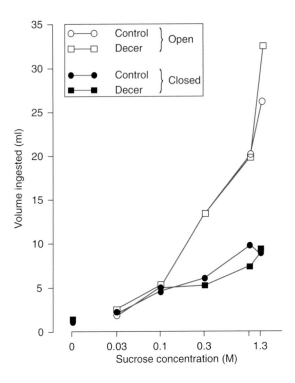

Figure 6.16 Chronic decerebrate rats show normal patterns of sucrose consumption. Various concentrations of sucrose were delivered by intraoral catheters so that rats could either ingest it or passively reject it (by allowing it to drip from the mouth). Decerebrate and normal rats showed closely similar concentration-related increases in sucrose ingestion ('closed' condition). Sucrose ingestion was dramatically increased in both decerebrate and normal rats by opening a gastric cannula to drain the stomach; again, the responses were remarkably similar. Decerebrate rats therefore preserve both the hyperphagic effect of increasing sucrose concentration, and its modulation by the inhibitory effect of normal postingestive food stimuli. From H.J. Grill and J.M. Kaplan (1992) 'Sham feeding in intact and chronic decerebrate rats'. *American Journal of Physiology*, **262**: R1070, with permission of the editor.

from those of normal rats. Moreover, they ingest well-defined meals that they terminate by the passive refusal of more food, and they increase or decrease meal size normally in response to taste and gastrointestinal feedback signals (Figure 6.16).

The nucleus of the solitary tract (nucleus tractus solitarii; NTS)

The NTS receives and integrates an impressive array of sensory information related to eating, including taste (but not olfactory) afferents as well as vagal and spinal afferents from the viscera. The NTS also contains glucose-sensing neurones and receptors for leptin, ghrelin and insulin, while the AP contains receptors for amylin (Berthoud, 2002; Grill and Kaplan, 2002).

Electrophysiological studies of second-order taste neurones in the NTS (i.e. neurones postsynaptic to primary gustatory afferents) show that their responses to taste are modulated by other eating-related factors, including plasma glucose and learned preferences or aversions for particular foods (Scott and Giza, 2000). Furthermore, studies of the expression of c-Fos protein (a nuclear transcription factor that indicates neuronal activation) indicate that eating or meal-related stimuli, such as gastric distension or CCK, dose-dependently activate NTS neurones and that the degree of activation can be up- or down-regulated by modulatory factors including leptin and oestradiol, with the c-Fos response in each case mirroring the synergistic effects of these manipulations on eating (Rinaman *et al.*, 1998; Asarian and Geary, 2007;

Thammacharoen *et al.*, 2008; Barrachina *et al.*, 1997; Emond *et al.*, 1999).

Leptin's influence on eating and on the responsivity of NTS neurones appears to be due in part to descending inputs from the hypothalamus. Koletsky rats that lack functional LepRb are less sensitive to the satiating effect of CCK, and show diminished CCK-induced c-Fos expression in the NTS (Morton *et al.*, 2005). Targeted adenoviral-vectored transfer of the *lepRb* gene restores LepRb expression in the ARC, and this normalizes both CCK's satiating action and c-Fos expression in the NTS. Leptin-sensitive ARC neurones presumably activate oxytocin neurones in the PVN, which project to the NTS, because these neurones are stimulated by leptin while oxytocin antagonists attenuate the ability of leptin to enhance CCK-induced c-Fos expression in the NTS (Morton *et al.*, 2005). The functional significance of this pathway remains uncertain, however, because, under other conditions, Koletsky rats show normal sensitivity to CCK's satiating effect (Wildman *et al.*, 2000).

The telencephalon

Food-related information is received and processed in many cortical and other areas of the telencephalon; that is, the part of the CNS anterior to the thalamus and hypothalamus. The huge anatomic and functional complexity of the telencephalon is a hallmark of human evolution; accordingly, the cognitive, emotional, motivational and social attributes of eating – both conscious and unconscious – remain poorly understood in humans (Berthoud, 2002).

One important telencephalic system, shared at least rudimentarily with lower mammals, is the reward system, which mediates the hedonic and self-reinforcing aspects of behaviours including eating. The main components of the telencephalic reward system are the nucleus accumbens (NAc), the amygdala (especially its central nucleus, CeA), and parts of the limbic, orbitofrontal, cingulate and insular cortical areas (Figure 6.17). Most of this system receives inputs from dopaminergic pathways (from the ventral tegmental area and substantia nigra),

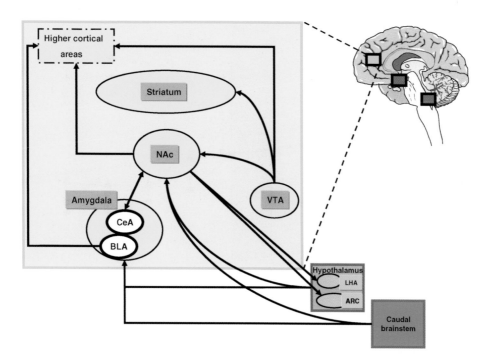

Figure 6.17 Principal forebrain brain areas implicated in the mediation of food reward, with their neural connections. NAc: nucleus accumbens; VTA: ventral tegmental area; CeA: central nucleus of the amygdala; BLA: basolateral nucleus of the amygdala; LHA: lateral hypothalamic area; ARC: arcuate nucleus.

noradrenergic (locus ceruleus) and serotonergic (rostral raphe nuclei). The NAc and the CeA, in particular, receive projections from the PVN and other hypothalamic areas and from the NTS. These ascending systems also provide important links among these areas and the brainstem and hypothalamus, as illustrated by the recent report that serotonin modulates the hypothalamic melanocortin pathway (Heisler *et al.*, 2006).

Food reward

As described above, orosensory pleasure is among the most powerful motivators of eating. The neural pathways mediating food reward overlap substantially with those serving other rewards, whether natural (e.g. sex, drinking water when thirsty) or unnatural (e.g. drugs of abuse) (Kelley, Baldo, Pratt and Will, 2005; Peciña, Smith and Berridge, 2006; Nestler and Carlezon, 2006; Berthoud, 2002; Berthoud, 2006). These pathways are extensively and reciprocally connected with those mediating more basic and reflexive

aspects of eating, suggesting that 'hedonic' and 'homeostatic' eating are too closely intertwined to be considered separately.

Several neurotransmitters including dopamine, opioids, endocannabinoids, acetylcholine and GABA have been implicated in food reward. Dopamine appears particularly important. In sham-feeding rats, dopamine release in the NAc mirrors the intake of palatable food, whether sucrose solution or corn-oil emulsion (Hajnal *et al.*, 2004; Liang, Hajnal and Norgren, 2006; Norgren *et al.*, 2006) (Figure 6.18). Among the implications of this work is that sensory information from two different sensory modalities (almost purely gustatory for sucrose; primarily olfactory and trigeminal for corn-oil) converge in the NAc. Other behavioural measures suggest that specific (and at least partly independent) neurotransmitters may serve different aspects of food reward (Berridge, 2004; Berridge and Robinson, 2003; Schultz, 2006; Wise, 2006). For example, within the NAc the affective or emotional impetus to eat (i.e. 'liking' and, presumably,

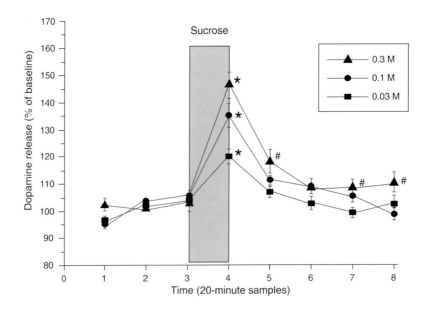

Figure 6.18 Evidence for the role of dopaminergic neurotransmission in the nucleus accumbens (NAc) in the orosensory reward of sweet taste. Various sucrose concentrations were presented to freely-feeding rats with open gastric cannulas to minimize the influence of postingestive satiety signals. Rats showed concentration-related increases in sucrose ingestion, and this was paralleled by dopamine release in the NAc (measured simultaneously using extracellular microdialysis). Data for 20-min periods are mean ± SEM of baseline. *$P < 0.01$; #$P < 0.05$ versus baseline. From A. Hajnal *et al.* (2004) Oral sucrose stimulation increases accumbens dopamine in the rat. *American Journal of Physiology*, **286**: R31, with permission of the editor.

conscious pleasure) may be mediated by opioids and GABA, while the motivational impetus ('wanting') may be mediated by dopamine (Berridge, 2004; Berridge and Robinson, 2003). Importantly, much evidence indicates a common basis for food reward in lower mammals and in humans (Berridge, 2004; Berridge and Robinson, 2003; Klein *et al.*, 2006; Nestler and Carlezon, 2006).

Opioids and endocannabinoids also contribute. Administration of μ-opioid agonists into the NAc preferentially stimulates ingestion of fat-rich foods and sucrose solutions, whereas injection of opioid antagonists selectively reduces ingestion of palatable foods (Zhang, Balmadrid and Kelley, 2003; Zhang and Kelley, 2000). In humans, opiate antagonists reduce food palatability but not subjective hunger (Yeomans *et al.*, 1990). Endocannabinoids act at brain CB1 receptors in both the NAc and hypothalamus to stimulate eating in rats, and endocannabinoid activity in these areas varies in relation to nutritional status and eating (Kirkham, 2005).

Connections between the NAc and other eating-related CNS areas also influence eating behaviour. Two important pathways involve the amygdala (Figure 6.17). A reciprocal connection between the CeA and the NAc is involved in opioid-mediated eating (Kim *et al.*, 2004), although it is not clear whether this pathway mediates selective reward processes or more general control over eating (Will, Franzblau and Kelley, 2004). Also, connections between the basolateral amygdala and forebrain cortical regions appear crucial in gauging food palatability (Balleine, Killcross and Dickinson, 2003). Links with lower centres also contribute. NAc manipulations that stimulate eating also activate NPY and inhibit melanocortin neurones in the ARC (Zheng *et al.*, 2003), while injection of a μ-opioid agonist into the NAc stimulates ingestion of palatable, high-fat food in satiated rats – but only if the Y1 receptor is intact (Berthoud, 2006). Reciprocal projections from the NAc to the LHA may also selectively stimulate consumption of palatable food (Stratford, Kelley and Simansky, 1999), possibly because activation of opioid neurones in the NAc releases the MCH and orexin neurones in the LHA from tonic inhibition (Kelley, Baldo and Pratt, 2005). Similarly, the stimulation of eating induced by NAc administration of a GABA(A) agonist was associated with increased activity of orexin neurones in the LHA (Zheng *et al.*, 2003).

The neuropharmacology of eating control

This section complements the preceding discussion by reviewing some of the CNS neurotransmitters most strongly implicated in the physiological control of eating and energy balance (Table 6.1). The expression patterns of some selected neurotransmitters and receptors are illustrated in Figure 6.19. Even though vast amounts of information have been acquired about CNS neuropharmacology related to eating, much remains to be learned, especially in regard to the normal physiological roles of the known players, and the contributions of newly reported and as yet undiscovered neurotransmitters.

Neuropeptide Y (NPY)

This 36-aminoacid peptide and its receptors are widely distributed throughout the CNS of mammals, including humans. ICV NPY administration potently stimulates eating, which is likely to be due to the contribution of NPY receptors in numerous brain sites. The NPY neurones most relevant to eating are those in the ARC, projecting to the PVN, as described above (Figure 6.20). However, NPY also induces hyperphagia when injected into the LHA or the fourth ventricle (in the caudal brainstem). NPY also reduces energy expenditure by inhibiting the sympathetic innervation of thermogenic tissues. Importantly, repeated administration results in obesity (Beck, 2006; Billington *et al.*, 1991; Stanley *et al.*, 1993) and, conversely, chronic inhibition of ARC NPY neurones by local injection of antisense NPY mRNA decreases food intake and body weight Reference ???. Interestingly, most mice with knockout of NPY or its receptors eat normally under basal conditions, presumably due to adaptive changes in other appetite-regulating systems; compensatory over-expression of AgRP (see below) by the ARC NPY/AgRP neurones may contribute.

The orexigenic effects of NPY appear to depend on the complicated interplay between postsynaptic Y1, Y4 and Y5 receptors (all of which stimulate eating under various conditions) and presynaptic Y2 receptors. Transgenic deletion of Y1 receptors, or the administration of Y1 receptor antagonists, reduces NPY- and fasting-induced eating (Ishigaki *et al.*, 2005;

Table 6.1 Some neurotansmitters and their receptors, implicated in the central control of eating behaviour.

Neurotransmitters	Site of production	Site of action	Receptors
Stimulate eating			
• Neuropeptide Y (NPY)	ARC	PVN, DMH, LHA	Y5, Y1, Y4
• Agouti gene related peptide (AgRP)	ARC (NPY neurones)	PVN, DMH	MC4-R (antagonist)
• Orexin A	LHA	LHA, PVN	OX-1R
• Melanin-concentrating hormone (MCH)	LHA	ARC, VMH	MCH-1R
• Opioids (eg. β–endorphin)	Hypothalamus	Various	μ opioid
• Endocannabinoids	Widespread	Hypothalamus, other	CB-1
Inhibit eating			
• α-melanocyte stimulating hormone (α-MSH)	ARC	PVN, DMH	MC4-R, MC3-R
• Corticotropin releasing factor (CRF)	PVN	NTS	CRF-2
• Cholecystokinin (CCK)	PVN	PVN, DMH	CCK-1 (CCK-2?)
• Oxytocin	PVN	NTS	OT-2
• Serotonin (5-HT)	Raphe nuclei	PVN	$5HT_{2c}$, $5HT_{1b}$
• Noradrenaline	CA nuclei of brainstem	PVN	α_2 adrenoceptor

Key: ARC: arcuate nucleus; CA: catecholaminergic nuclei; DMH: dorsomedial nucleus or hypothalamus; NTS: nucleus tractus solitarii; PVN: paraventricular nucleus; LHA: lateral hypothalamic area; VMH: ventromedial hypothalamic area.

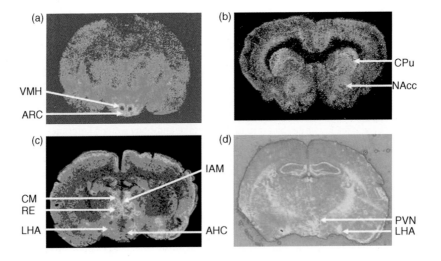

Figure 6.19 Hypothalamic expression patterns of selected neurotransmitters and their receptors that are implicated in the control of eating. Pseudocolour images of rat brain sections showing distributions of selected receptors that control food intake. (a) Melanocortin-3 and Melanocortin-4 receptors (MC3-, MC4-R); (b) Cannabinoid 1 receptors (CB1-R); (c) Neuropeptide Y (NPY) Y5 receptors; (d) ghrelin receptors. VMH: ventromedial hypothalamic nucleus; ARC: arcuate nucleus; CPu: caudate putamen; NAcc: nucleus accumbens; CM: central medial thalamic nucleus; RE: reuniens thalamic nucleus; LHA: lateral hypothalamic area; IAM: interanteromedial nucleus; AHC: anterior hypothalamic area; PVN: paraventricular nucleus.

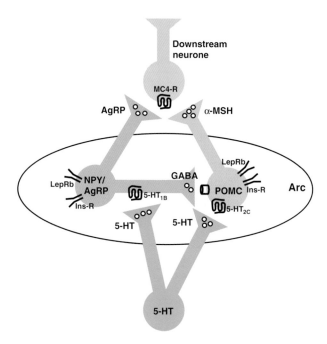

Figure 6.20 Current concepts of the principal inputs and outputs of neurones expressing orexigenic and anorexigenic neuropeptides in the hypothalamic arcuate nucleus (ARC). 5-HT: serotonin; 5-HT$_{1B}$ and 5-HT$_{2C}$: serotonin receptors; α-MSH: alpha-melanocyte-stimulating hormone; AgRP: agouti-related peptide; GABA: gamm-amino butyric acid; Ins-R: insulin receptor; LepRb: signalling form of the leptin receptor; MC4-R: melanocortin-4 receptor; NPY: neuropeptide Y; POMC: proopio-melanocortin.

Kanatani *et al.*, 2000). Y4 receptors, which are expressed by orexin neurones in the LHA, selectively recognize pancreatic polypeptide (PP) and their stimulation with PP stimulates eating (Campbell *et al.*, 2003). Y5 antagonists can reduce eating and body weight in rats fed palatable food but not ordinary chow (Ishihara *et al.*, 2006), and the long-term (10 h) but not short-term (2 h) eating response of rats to ICV NPY, suggesting that the Y5 receptor maintains the eating response to NPY rather than initiates it (Flynn *et al.*, 1999). Moreover, Y5 receptor knockout mice develop mild late-onset obesity rather than the expected weight loss (Marsh *et al.*, 1998). This may be due to adaptive responses following the deletion of a multi-function gene (Davey and MacLean, 2006). Y2 receptors are distinct from the others. They are autoceptors, carried by the ARC NPY neurones, and their activation (e.g. by PYY 3–36) inhibits NPY release (Batterham *et al.*, 2002; Beglinger and Degen, 2004). Consistent with this, Y2 knockout mice display hyperphagia and overweight (Naveilhan *et al.*, 1999).

NPY neurones also express AgRP, an endogenous antagonist of α-MSH at the MC4 receptors

(MC4-R). This represents one indirect mechanism by which the ARC NPY/AgRP neurones inhibit melanocortin action. Direct inhibition occurs by release of NPY and GABA from these neurones, which act respectively via Y1 and GABA(A) receptors on the melanocortin neurones (see Figure 6.20). The balance between ARC NPY/AgRP and melanocortin neurones appears critical to eating (Berthoud, 2002; Cota *et al.*, 2006; Cowley *et al.*, 2003; Ellacott and Cone, 2004; Elmquist *et al.*, 2005; Heisler *et al.*, 2006; Hillebrand, de Wied and Adan, 2002; Simerly, 2004). The various monogenic models of obesity in rodents, which are due to mutations that either delete leptin or disable leptin receptors (Table 6.2 and Figure 6.10), are also characterized by disinhibition of NPY/AgRP and inhibition of melanocortin neurones in the ARC; this causes hyperphagia and decreased thermogenesis, resulting in net energy gain and obesity.

Melanocortins

α-MSH is the main melanocortin implicated in eating control, although β-MSH may also contribute.

Table 6.2   Single gene mutations in rodent models of obesity.

Species	Model	Chromosome	Inheritance	Mutated Gene Product	Defect	Insulin resistance
Mouse	*ob/ob*	6	Recessive	Leptin	Loss of function	+++
	db/db	4	Recessive	Leptin receptor	Loss of function	+++
	fat/fat	8	Recessive	Carboxypeptidase E	Loss of function	−
	A^y	2	Dominant	Agouti	Overexpression in ectopic sites	+++
Rat	*fa/fa*	5	Recessive	Leptin receptor	Loss of function	+++
	cp/cp	5	Recessive	Leptin receptor	Loss of function	+++

Note: *fa db* and *cp* are alternative alleles of the leptin receptor (LepR)

Both act centrally to inhibit eating and stimulate energy expenditure, acting through MC4-R and MC3-R. Knockout of the MC4-R, or administration of synthetic MC4-R antagonists or of AgRP, leads to hyperphagia and obesity (Huszar *et al.*, 1997; Adan *et al.*, 2006).

The ARC melanocortin neurones projecting to the PVN appear to be crucial in restraining appetite and body fat mass in rodents, and also in humans (see below). They are stimulated by insulin and leptin and inhibited by ghrelin and by the ARC NPY/AgRP neurones (see above). They are therefore inhibited under conditions of energy deficit, which would help to increase hunger and feeding. The ARC melanocortin neurones also co-express and co-release another peptide, cocaine and amphetamine-related transcript (CART), which is described below.

Genetic studies indicate that the melanocortin system is important in human energy homeostasis. Obesity is associated with mutations that reduce melanocortin function by affecting the melanocortin precursor (POMC), the prohormone convertase-1 enzyme that cleaves α-MSH from POMC (and also insulin from proinsulin), or most commonly, the MC4-R (Mencarelli *et al.*, 2004; O'Rahilly and Farooqi, 2006). MC4-R mutations were identified in 5% of a group of patients with early-onset morbid obesity (Farooqi *et al.*, 2003) and in 2.5% of obese young adults (Larsen *et al.*, 2005) – making this by far the most common known monogenic cause of obesity. The high penetrance of MC4-R mutations in heterozygotes, as well as its lack of effect on reproductive function, presumably contributes to this high prevalence. The syndrome is characterized by hyperphagia, early-onset obesity with increased lean mass and height, and insulin resistance with marked hyperinsulinaemia – a similar phenotype to that of mice with knockout of MC4-R (Huszar *et al.*, 1997) (see Chapter 21).

Cocaine and amphetamine-related transcript (CART)

This peptide, whose expression is up-regulated by the eponymous substances, is co-expressed by the ARC melanocortin neurones. Initial studies reported that intracerebroventricular (ICV) administration of CART inhibited feeding, whereas CART-neutralizing antibodies injected ICV stimulated eating in rats (Lambert *et al.*, 1998) – suggesting a feeding-inhibitory function consistent with its co-localization in the melanocortin neurones (Figure 6.20). Further studies, however, suggest that non-specific motor effects may contribute to decreased food intake (Balkan and Li, 2000) and even that direct administration of CART into the ARC, PVN and other hypothalamic sites can stimulate eating. Its physiological role in eating therefore awaits clarification.

Orexins (Hypocretins)

Orexin A and B (also known as hypocretin −1 and −2) are 33- and 28-residue peptides, respectively. Orexins were originally named from the Greek for 'appetite' for their ability to stimulate eating, although only orexin A shows a robust and consistent hyperphagic action. Even this effect, however, is not sustained and repeated administration of orexin A does not lead to obesity (Haynes *et al.*, 1999; Sakurai, 2002).

Orexins are expressed by neurones in the LHA that project extensively throughout the CNS; in addition to reciprocal links with the ARC and other eating-regulatory regions (see above), there are extensive projections to areas involved in arousal and attention. Likewise, orexin receptors, OX-1R and OX-2R, are widely distributed in the hypothalamus and throughout the CNS (see Ohno and Sakurai, 2008). OX-1R, especially abundant in the VMH, is thought to mediate the stimulation of eating, while OX-2R is implicated in orexin's induction of arousal and wakefulness.

Orexin neurones may be directly and indirectly involved in sensing falls in glucose availability, and may trigger acute hunger and hyperphagia under glucoprivic conditions. Otherwise, a major role is in maintaining wakefulness: spontaneous mutations of the OX-2R in dogs, and experimental knockout of this receptor in mice, induce narcolepsy (Willie *et al.*, 2003). Orexin may stimulate eating in part secondarily to its powerful effects on arousal and sleep (Saper, 2006) and may serve to increase both hunger and arousal during starvation.

In humans, the relevance of orexins to eating is uncertain, but narcolepsy is often associated in some cases with loss (possibly autoimmune-mediated) of orexin neurones and reduced cerebrospinal fluid concentrations of the peptides (Zeitzer, Nishino and Mignot, 2006).

Melanin-concentrating hormone (MCH)

This cyclic 19-amino-acid peptide is expressed in LHA neurones, which also project widely throughout the brain. Two MCH receptors (MCH-1R and MCH-2R) are found especially in the ARC and the VMH. MCH administered centrally causes hyperphagia and can ultimately induce obesity (Qu *et al.*, 1996), while chronic administration of MCH-1R antagonists decreases food intake and body weight (Borowsky *et al.*, 2002). In addition, MCH knockout mice are lean and have an increased metabolic rate with reduced body fat, whereas transgenic over-expression of MCH leads to hyperphagia and obesity (Marsh *et al.*, 2002).

Monoamine neurotransmitters

Serotonin (5-hydroxytryptamine, 5-HT) is released from fibres that originate from neurones in the midbrain raphe nuclei. These projections innervate the ARC, PVN, VMH and LHA, where various subtypes of serotonin receptor are expressed. Serotonin neurones express leptin receptors, while the serotonin inputs to the ARC supply both NPY/AgRP and melanocortin neurones (which carry $5HT_{1B}$ and $5HT_{2C}$ receptors, respectively) and apparently act to enhance melanocortin activity over NPY (Figure 6.14).

Serotonin powerfully inhibits eating and stimulates energy expenditure, effects which have been exploited in various anti-obesity drugs such as fenfluramine (now obsolete) and sibutramine (see Chapter 17). The main receptor subtype mediating the eating-inhibitory effect in rats and humans is apparently $5HT_{2C}$.

As mentioned above, dopamine plays an important role in stimulating eating through the reward pathways.

Endocannabinoids

Endocannabinoids and their receptors are widely distributed in the gut and brain. The CB1 receptor is the principal CNS receptor, and its pharmacological manipulation has potent effects on a variety of reward processes in mammals, including eating. Endocannabinoids appear to increase the hedonic evaluation (i.e. 'liking') of food. The CB1 receptor antagonist, rimonabant, was introduced clinically to reduce appetite and treat obesity (Despres, Golay and Sjostrom, 2005; Van Gaal *et al.*, 2005; see Chapter 17). Information is awaited regarding the long-term influence of this compound on eating and its possible impact on other reward processes.

Modulating factors

The basic physiological controls of eating outlined above are influenced by a host of other factors, including environmental and cognitive variables, physiological and psychological stress, acute and chronic diseases, as well as reproductive function. This section offers a few perspectives related to two of these factors.

Acute infections and other immune challenges trigger a generalized host-defence reaction – the acute-phase response – in which anorexia is a prominent feature (Hart, 1988). Anorexia may be beneficial initially, but ultimately becomes deleterious (Murray and Murray, 1979). The most investigated experimental model is the widespread immune activation and anorexia induced by administration of lipopolysaccharide (LPS), a component of Gram-negative bacterial cell walls that is released during bacterial lysis and proliferation (Rietschel *et al.*, 1998). LPS provokes the release of pro-inflammatory cytokines such as IL-1, −2, and −6, tumour necrosis factor-α, interferon-γ and ciliary neurotrophic factor, together with prostanoids and other mediators (Asarian and Langhans, 2006; Lambert *et al.*, 2001; Langhans, 2004; Netea *et al.*, 2006; Plata-Salamàn, 1995). Cytokines actively cross the blood-brain barrier and could act on appetite-modulating pathways in the ARC or caudal brainstem. Also, cytokines may stimulate endothelial cells in the blood-brain barrier to produce prostaglandins such as PGE_2 (Lugarini *et al.*, 2002; Nadeau and Rivest, 1999; Nadjar *et al.*, 2005). PGE_2 is postulated to stimulate PG-EP3 receptors on serotonergic neurones in the median raphe nuclei – from where serotonergic projections to the hypothalamus would inhibit eating, possibly via enhanced melanocortin activity (Ericsson, Arias and Sawchenko, 1997; Heisler *et al.*, 2006; Nakamura *et al.*, 2001).

Sex and reproductive function have numerous complicated interactions with the control of energy balance, including sex differences in eating, growth, energy expenditure, nutrient partitioning and physical activity (Asarian and Geary, 2006; Blaak, 2001; Geary and Lovejoy, 2007). Knowledge is incomplete, partly because reproductive functions show extensive developmental and species variations. Marked sex differences affect many aspects of energy homeostasis, especially after puberty, and are mediated mainly by the gonadal steroid hormones, androgens, oestrogens and progestins. Detailed reviews in primates (Bruns and Kemnitz, 2004), rodents (Asarian and Geary, 2006) and humans (Geary and Lovejoy, 2007) are available. The physiological relevance of such sex differences in human energy homeostasis is underscored by several reports (i.e. Okura *et al.*, 2003; Tobias *et al.*, 2007) that polymorphisms of the oestrogen receptor (ER)-α gene are associated with increased adiposity.

Two well-characterized phenomena linked to reproductive function are the phasic decrease in food intake during the peri-ovulatory period of the ovarian cycle, and the lasting increase in food intake and resultant obesity when cycles are interrupted, for example by ovariectomy. Oestradiol is sufficient to explain both effects. Physiological, cyclical oestradiol replacement normalizes eating and body weight in ovariectomized rats (Geary and Asarian, 1999). In women (whose cycle is much longer), food intake may fall slightly throughout the follicular period and is clearly decreased during the peri-ovulatory phase. It is uncertain whether the menopause increases food intake in humans, but body adiposity increases, and body fat distribution changes from gluteo-femoral to abdominal. Again, this appears to be due to changes in oestradiol (Geary and Lovejoy, 2007; Matthews *et al.*, 2001; Wajchenberg *et al.*, 2000).

In rats, oestradiol acts in the NTS and perhaps also in the ARC and other hypothalamic sites to inhibit eating (Asarian and Geary, 2006). In the NTS, oestradiol acting via ER-α alters the neuronal processing of gut CCK-derived signals, resulting in an enhancement of its satiating action (Asarian and Geary, 2007; Thammacharoen *et al.*, 2008). Oestradiol also decreases the hyperphagic action of ghrelin (Clegg *et al.*, 2007) and may also enhance the appetite-inhibiting effects of glucagon, insulin and leptin (Asarian and Geary, 2006; Clegg *et al.*, 2006).

References

Abbott, C.R., Rossi, M., Wren, A.M. *et al.* (2001) Evidence of an orexigenic role for cocaine- and amphetamine-regulated transcript after administration into discrete hypothalamic nuclei. *Endocrinology*, **142**, 3457–63.

Adan, R.A., Tiesjema, B., Hillebrand, J.J. *et al.* (2006) The MC4 receptor and control of appetite. *British Journal of Pharmacology*, **149** (7), 815–27 Epub 2006 Oct 16.

Ahima, R.S. and Flier, J.S. (2000) Leptin. *Annual Review of Physiology*, **62**, 413–37.

Ahima, R.S., Dushay, J., Flier, S.N. *et al.* (1997) Leptin accelerates the onset of puberty in normal female mice. *Journal of Clinical Investigation*, **99**, 391–5.

Aja, S., Sahandy, S., Ladenheim, E.E. *et al.* (2001) Intracerebroventricular CART peptide reduces food intake and alters motor behavior at a hindbrain site. *American Journal of Physiology. Regulatory Integrative and Comparative Physiology*, **281**, R1862–7.

Akira, S. (2000) Toll-like receptors: lessons from knockout mice. *Biochemical Society Transactions*, 28(Part 5), 551–6.

An, J., Muoio, D.M., Shiota, M. *et al.* (2004) Hepatic expression of malonyl-CoA decarboxylase reverses muscle, liver and whole-animal insulin resistance. *Nature Medicine*, **10**, 268–74.

Anand, B.K. and Brobeck, J.R. (1951) Localization of a feeding center in the hypothalamus of the rat.

Proceedings of the Society for Experimental Biology and Medicine, **77**, 323–4.

Andersson, U., Filipsson, K., Abbott, C.R. *et al.* (2004) AMP-activated protein kinase plays a role in the control of food intake. *Journal of Biological Chemistry*, **279**, 12005–8.

Arnold, M., Mura, A., Langhans, W. and Geary, N. (2006) Gut vagal afferents are not necessary for the eating-stimulatory effect of intraperitoneally injected ghrelin in the rat. *Journal of Neuroscience*, **26**, 11052–60.

Asarian, L. and Geary, N. (2006) Modulation of appetite by gonadal steroid hormones. *Philosophical Transactions of the Royal Society. Series B, Biological Sciences*, **361**, 1251–63.

Asarian, l. and Geary, N. (2007) Estradiol enhances cholecystokinin-dependent lipid-induced satiation and activates estrogen receptor-alpha-expressing cells in the nucleus tractus solitarius of ovariectomized rats. *Endocrinology*, **148** (12), 5656–66.

Asarian, L. and Langhans, W. (2006) Current perspectives on behavioural and cellular mechanisms of illness anorexia. *International Review of Psychiatry*, **17**, 451–9.

Bady, I., Marty, N., Dallaporta, M. *et al.* (2006) Evidence from Glut2-null mice that glucose is a critical physiological regulator of feeding. *Diabetes*, **55**, 988–95.

Balkan, B. and Li, X. (2000) Portal GLP-1 administration in rats augments the insulin response to glucose via neuronal mechanisms. *American Journal of Physiology. Regulatory Integrative and Comparative Physiology*, **279**, R1449–54.

Balleine, B.W., Killcross, A.S. and Dickinson, A. (2003) The effect of lesions of the basolateral amygdala on instrumental conditioning. *Journal of Neuroscience*, **23**, 666–75.

Ballinger, A.B. and Clark, M.L. (1994) L-Phenylalanine releases cholecystokinin (CCK) and is associated with reduced food-intake in humans – evidence for a physiological role of CCK in control of eating. *Metabolism-Clinical and Experimental*, **43**, 735–8.

Banks, W.A. and Kastin, A.J. (1996) Passage of peptides across the blood-brain barrier: pathophysiological perspectives. *Life Sciences*, **59**, 1923–43.

Banks, W.A., Kastin, A.J., Huang, W. *et al.* (1996) Leptin enters the brain by a saturable system independent of insulin. *Peptides*, **17**, 305–11.

Barrachina, M.D., Martinez, V., Wang, L.X. *et al.* (1997) Synergistic interaction between leptin and cholecystokinin to reduce short-term food intake in lean mice. *Proceedings of the National Academy of Sciences of the United States of America*, **94**, 10455–60.

Bartoshuk, L.M., Duffy, V.B., Hayes, J.E. *et al.* (2006) Psychophysics of sweet and fat perception in obesity: problems, solutions and new perspectives. *Philosophical Transactions of the Royal Society. Series B, Biological Sciences*, **361**, 1137–48.

Basa, N.R., Wang, L.X., Arteaga, J.R. *et al.* (2003) Bacterial lipopolysaccharide shifts fasted plasma ghrelin to postprandial levels in rats. *Neuroscience Letters*, **343**, 25–8.

Batterham, R.L., Cowley, M.A., Small, C.J. *et al.* (2002) Gut hormone PYY3-36 physiologically inhibits food intake. *Nature*, **418**, 650–4.

Beck, B. (2006) Neuropeptide Y in normal eating and in genetic and dietary-induced obesity. *Philosophical Transactions of the Royal Society. Series B, Biological Sciences*, **361**, 1159–85.

Beglinger, C. and Degen, L. (2004) Fat in the intestine as a regulator of appetite – role of CCK. *Physiology & Behavior*, **83**, 617–21.

Beglinger, C. and Degen, L. (2006) Gastrointestinal satiety signals in humans – Physiologic roles for GLP-1 and PYY? *Physiology & Behavior*, **89**, 460–4.

Beglinger *et al.* (2001) Loxiglumide, a CCK-A receptor antagonist, stimulates calorie intake and hunger feedings in humans. *American Journal of Physiology*, **280**, R1149.

Benoit, S.C., Air, E.L., Coolen, L.M. *et al.* (2002) The catabolic action of insulin in the brain is mediated by melanocortins. *Journal of Neuroscience*, **22**, 9048–52.

Bernardis, L.L. and Bellinger, L.L. (1993) The lateral hypothalamic area revisited – neuroanatomy, body-weight regulation, neuroendocrinology and metabolism. *Neuroscience and Biobehavioral Reviews*, **17**, 141–93.

Berridge, K.C. (2004) Motivation concepts in behavioral neuroscience. *Physiology & Behavior*, **81**, 179–209.

Berridge, K.C. and Robinson, T.E. (2003) Parsing reward. *Trends in Neurosciences*, **26**, 507–13.

Berthoud, H.R. (2002) Multiple neural systems controlling food intake and body weight. *Neuroscience and Biobehavioral Reviews*, **26**, 393–428.

Berthoud, H.R. (2006) Homeostatic and non-homeostatic pathways involved in the control of food intake and energy balance. *Obesity*, **14**, 197–200.

Bi, S. and Moran, T.H. (2002) Actions of CCK in the controls of food intake and body weight: Lessons from the CCK-A receptor deficient OLETF rat. *Neuropeptides*, **36**, 171–81.

Bierhaus, A., Chen, J., Liliensiek, B. and Nawroth, P.P. (2000) LPS and cytokine-activated endothelium. *Seminars in Thrombosis and Hemostasis*, **26**, 571–87.

Billington, C.J., Briggs, J.E., Grace, M. and Levine, A.S. (1991) Effects of intracerebroventricular injection of neuropeptide Y on energy metabolism. *American Journal of Physiology*, **260**, R321–7.

Blaak, E. (2001) Gender differences in fat metabolism. *Current Opinion in Clinical Nutrition and Metabolic Care*, **4**, 499–502.

Blevins, J.E., Eakin, T.J., Murphy, J.A. *et al.* (2003) Oxytocin innervation of caudal brainstem nuclei activated by cholecystokinin. *Brain Research*, **993**, 30–41.

Blevins, J.E., Schwartz, M.W. and Baskin, D.G. (2004 (Jul) Evidence that paraventricular nucleus oxytocin neurons link hypothalamic leptin action to caudal brain stem nuclei controlling meal size. *American Journal of Physiology. Regulatory, Integrative and Comparative Physiology*, **287** (1), R87–96.

Borowsky, B., Durkin, M.M., Ogozalek, K. *et al.* (2002) Antidepressant, anxiolytic and anorectic effects of a melanin-concentrating hormone-1 receptor antagonist. *Nature Medicine*, **8**, 825.

Bowen, D.J. (1992) Taste and food preference changes across the course of pregnancy. *Appetite*, **19**, 233–42.

Brandt, K., Arnold, M., Geary, N. *et al.* (2006a) Beta-adrenergic-mediated inhibition of feeding by mercaptoacetate in food-deprived rats. *Pharmacology Biochemistry and Behavior*, **85**, 722–7.

Brandt, K., Geary, N., Langhans, W. and Leonhardt, M. (2006b) Mercaptoacetate fails to block the feeding-inhibitory effect of the beta3-adrenergic receptor agonist CGP 12177A. *Physiology & Behavior*, **89**, 128–32.

Broberger, C., Landry, M., Wong, H. *et al.* (1997) Subtypes Y1 and Y2 of the neuropeptide Y receptor are respectively expressed in pro-opiomelanocortin- and neuropeptide-Y-containing neurons of the rat hypothalamic arcuate nucleus. *Neuroendocrinology*, **66**, 393–408.

Broberger, C., De Lecea, L., Sutcliffe, J.G. and Hokfelt, T. (1998) Hypocretin/orexin- and melanin-concentrating hormone-expressing cells form distinct populations in the rodent lateral hypothalamus: Relationship to the neuropeptide Y and Agouti gene-related protein systems. *Journal of Comparative Neurology*, **402**, 460–74.

Bruning, J.C., Gautam, D., Burks, D.J. *et al.* (2000) Role of brain insulin receptor in control of body weight and reproduction. *Science*, **289**, 2122–5.

Bruns, C.M. and Kemnitz, J.W. (2004) Sex hormones, insulin sensitivity, and diabetes mellitus. *ILAR Journal*, **45**, 160–9.

Burcelin, R., Da Costa, A., Drucker, D. and Thorens, B. (2001) Glucose competence of the hepatoportal vein sensor requires the presence of an activated glucagon-like peptide-1 receptor. *Diabetes*, **50**, 1720–8.

Burdakov, D. (2007) K^+ channels stimulated by glucose: a new energy-sensing pathway. *Pflugers Archive: European Journal of Physiology*, **454**, 19–27.

Cai, X.J., Widdowson, P.S., Harrold, J. *et al.* (1999) Hypothalamic orexin expression – modulation by blood glucose and feeding. *Diabetes*, **48**, 2132–7.

Campbell, R.E., Smith, M.S., Allen, S.E. *et al.* (2003) Orexin neurons express a functional pancreatic polypeptide Y4 receptor. *Journal of Neuroscience*, **23**, 1487–97.

Campfield, L.A. and Smith, F.J. (2003) Blood glucose dynamics and control of meal initiation: a pattern detection and recognition theory. *Physiological Reviews*, **83**, 25–58.

Campfield, L.A., Smith, F.J., Guisez, Y. *et al.* (1995) Recombinant mouse Ob protein – evidence for a

peripheral signal linking adiposity and central neural networks. *Science*, **269**, 546–9.

Chapman, I., Parker, B., Doran, S. *et al.* (2005) Effect of pramlintide on satiety and food intake in obese subjects and subjects with type 2 diabetes. *Diabetologia*, **48**, 838–48.

Chaudri, O.B., Salem, V., Murphy, K.G. and Bloom, S.R. (2008) Gastrointestinal satiety signals. *Physiological Reviews*, **70**, 9.1–9.17.

Chen, C.T., Dun, S.L., Kwok, E.H. *et al.* (1999) Orexin A-like immunoreactivity in the rat brain. *Neuroscience Letters*, **260**, 161–4.

Chua, S.C., Chung, W.K., Wupeng, X.S. *et al.* (1996) Phenotypes of mouse diabetes and rat fatty due to mutations in the OB (leptin) receptor. *Science*, **271**, 994–6.

Clegg, D.J., Brown, L.M., Kemp, C.J. *et al.* (2007) Estradiol-dependent decrease in the orexigenic potency of ghrelin in female rats. *Diabetes*, **56**, 1051–8.

Clegg, D.J., Brown, L.M., Woods, S.C. and Benoit, S.C. (2006) Gonadal hormones determine sensitivity to central leptin and insulin. *Diabetes*, **55**, 978–87.

Cohen, M.A., Ellis, S.M., Le Roux, C.W. *et al.* (2003) Oxyntomodulin suppresses appetite and reduces food intake in humans. *The Journal of Clinical Endocrinology and Metabolism*, **88**, 4696–701.

Cohen, P., Miyazaki, M., Socci, N.D. *et al.* (2002) Role for stearoyl-CoA desaturase-1 in leptin-mediated weight loss. *Science*, **297**, 240–3.

Costello, J.F., Brown, M.R. and Gray, T.S. (1991) Bombesin immunoreactive neurons in the hypothalamic paraventricular nucleus innervate the dorsal vagal complex in the rat. *Brain Research*, **542**, 77–82.

Cota, D., Proulx, K., Smith, K.A. *et al.* (2006) Hypothalamic mTOR signaling regulates food intake. *Science*, **312**, 927–30.

Cowley, M.A., Cone, R.D., Enriori, P. *et al.* (2003) Electrophysiological actions of peripheral hormones on melanocortin neurons. *Melanocortin System*, **994**, 175–86.

Cowley, M.A. and Grove, K.L. (2004) Ghrelin-satisfying a hunger for the mechanism. *Endocrinology*, **145**, 2604–6.

Cowley, M.A., Smith, R.G., Diano, S. *et al.* (2003) The distribution and mechanism of action of ghrelin in the CNS demonstrates a novel hypothalamic circuit regulating energy homeostasis. *Neuron*, **37**, 649–61.

Craig, A.D. (2002) How do you feel? Interoception: the sense of the physiological condition of the body. *Nature Reviews Neuroscience*, **3**, 655–66.

Cummings *et al.* (2004) Plasma ghrelin levels and hunger scores in humans initiating meals voluntarily without time- and food-related cues. *American Journal of Physiology*, **287**, E297.

Cummings, D.E., Foster-Schubert, K.E. and Overduin, J. (2005) Ghrelin and energy balance: focus on current controversies. *Current Drug Targets*, **6**, 153–69.

Cummings, D.E. and Overduin, J. (2007) Gastrointestinal regulation of food intake. *Journal of Clinical Investigation*, **117**, 13–23.

Dahlstrom, A. and Fuxe, K. (1999) The autonomic nervous system and the histochemical fluorescence method for the microscopical localization of catecholamines and serotonin. *Brain Research Bulletin*, **50**, 365–7.

Davey, R.A. and MacLean, H.E. (2006) Current and future approaches using genetically modified mice in endocrine research. *American Journal of Physiology. Endocrinology and Metabolism*, **291**, E429–38.

DeFalco, J., Tomishima, M., Liu, H.Y. *et al.* (2001) Virus-assisted mapping of neural inputs to a feeding center in the hypothalamus. *Science*, **291**, 2608–13.

Degen, L., Oesch, S., Matzinger, D. *et al.* (2006) Effects of a preload on reduction of food intake by GLP-1 in healthy subjects. *Digestion*, **74** (2), 78–84.

Despres, J.P., Golay, A. and Sjostrom, L. (2005) Effects of rimonabant on metabolic risk factors in overweight patients with dyslipidemia. *New England Journal of Medicine*, **353**, 2121–34.

Dhillon, H., Zigman, J.M., Ye, C.P. *et al.* (2006) Leptin directly activates SF1 neurons in the VMH, and this action by leptin is required for normal body-weight homeostasis. *Neuron*, **49**, 191–203.

Dixit, V.D., Schaffer, E.M., Pyle, R.S. *et al.* (2004) Ghrelin inhibits leptin- and activation-induced proinflammatory cytokine expression by human monocytes and T cells. *Journal of Clinical Investigation*, **114**, 57–66.

Dobbins, R.L., Szczepaniak, L.S., Bentley, B. *et al.* (2001) Prolonged inhibition of muscle carnitine palmitoyltransferase-1 promotes intramyocellular lipid accumulation and insulin resistance in rats. *Diabetes*, **50**, 123–30.

Duggan, J.P. and Booth, D.A. (1986) Obesity, overeating, and rapid gastric-emptying in rats with ventromedial hypothalamic-lesions. *Science*, **231**, 609–11.

Dumont, Y., Fournier, A., Stpierre, S. and Quirion, R. (1995) Characterization of neuropeptide-Y binding-sites in rat-brain membrane preparations using [I-125] [Leu(31),Pro(34)]peptide YY and [I-125] peptide YY3-36 as selective Y-1 and Y-2 radioligands. *Journal of Pharmacology and Experimental Therapeutics*, **272**, 673–80.

Dumont, Y., Jacques, D., Bouchard, P. and Quirion, R. (1998) Species differences in the expression and distribution of the neuropeptide Y Y1, Y2, Y4, and Y5 receptors in rodents, guinea pig, and primates brains. *Journal of Comparative Neurology*, **402**, 372–84.

Eisen, S., Davis, J.D., Rauhofer, E. and Smith, G.P. (2001) Gastric negative feedback produced by volume and nutrient during a meal in rats. *American Journal of Physiology. Regulatory Integrative and Comparative Physiology*, **281**, R1201–14.

Eisen, S., Phillips, R.J., Geary, N. *et al.* (2005) Inhibitory effects on intake of cholecystokinin-8 and cholecystokinin-33 in rats with hepatic proper or common hepatic branch vagal innervation. *American Journal of Physiology. Regulatory Integrative and Comparative Physiology*, **289**, R456–62.

Elias, C.F., Saper, C.B., Maratos-Flier, E. *et al.* (1998) Chemically defined projections linking the mediobasal hypothalamus and the lateral hypothalamic area. *Journal of Comparative Neurology*, **402**, 442–59.

Ellacott, K.L.J. and Cone, R.D. (2004) The central melanocortin system and the integration of short- and long-term regulators of energy homeostasis. *Recent Progress in Hormone Research*, **59**, 395–408.

Elmquist, J.K., Coppari, R., Balthasar, N. *et al.* (2005) Identifying hypothalamic pathways controlling food intake, body weight, and glucose homeostasis. *Journal of Comparative Neurology*, **493**, 63–71.

Emond, M., Schwartz, G.J., Ladenheim, E.E. and Moran, T.H. (1999) Central leptin modulates behavioral and neural responsivity to CCK. *American Journal of Physiology. Regulatory Integrative and Comparative Physiology*, **276**, R1545–9.

Epstein, A.N. and Teitelbaum, P. (1967) Specific loss of hypoglycemic control of feeding in recovered lateral rats. *American Journal of Physiology*, **213**, 1159–67.

Ericsson, A., Arias, C. and Sawchenko, P.E. (1997) Evidence for an intramedullary prostaglandin-dependent mechanism in the activation of stress-related neuroendocrine circuitry by intravenous interleukin-1. *Journal of Neuroscience*, **17**, 7166–79.

Faggioni, R., Fuller, J., Moser, A. *et al.* (1997) LPS-induced anorexia in leptin-deficient (ob/ob) and leptin receptor-deficient (db/db) mice. *American Journal of Physiology. Regulatory Integrative and Comparative Physiology*, **42**, R181–6.

Fan, W., Boston, B.A., Kesterson, R.A. *et al.* (1997) Role of melanocortinergic neurons in feeding and the agouti obesity syndrome. *Nature*, **385**, 165–8.

Farooqi, I.S., Keogh, J.M., Yeo, G.S.H. *et al.* (2003) Clinical spectrum of obesity and mutations in the melanocortin 4 receptor gene. *New England Journal of Medicine*, **348**, 1085–95.

Faulconbridge, L.F., Cummings, D.E., Kaplan, J.M. and Grill, H.J. (2003) Hyperphagic effects of brainstem ghrelin administration. *Diabetes*, **52**, 2260–5.

Flynn, M.C., Scott, T.R., Pritchard, T.C. and Plata-Salamàn, C.R. (1998) Mode of action of OB protein (leptin) on feeding. *American Journal of Physiology. Regulatory Integrative and Comparative Physiology*, **44**, R174–9.

Flynn, M.C., Turrin, N.P., Plata-Salamàn, C.R. and ffrench-Mullen, J.M.H. (1999) Feeding response to neuropeptide Y-related compounds in rats treated with Y5 receptor antisense or sense phosphothio-oligodeoxynucleotide. *Physiology & Behavior*, **66**, 881–4.

Fodor, M., Sluiter, A., FrankhuijzenSierevogel, A. *et al.* (1996) Distribution of Lys-gamma(2)-melanocyte-stimulating hormone-(Lys-gamma(2)-MSH)-like immunoreactivity in neuronal elements in the brain and peripheral tissues of the rat. *Brain Research*, **731**, 182–9.

Friedman, M.I., Ramirez, I., Edens, N.K. and Granneman, J. (1985) Food-intake in diabetic rats – isolation of primary metabolic effects of fat feeding. *American Journal of Physiology*, **249**, R44–51.

Gabay, C., Dreyer, M.G., Pellegrinelli, N. *et al.* (2001) Leptin directly induces the secretion of interleukin 1 receptor antagonist in human monocytes. *Journal of Clinical Endocrinology and Metabolism*, **86**, 783–91.

Gabellec, M.M., Griffais, R., Fillion, G. and Haour, F. (1995) Expression of interleukin 1 alpha, interleukin 1 beta and interleukin 1 receptor antagonist mRNA in mouse brain: Regulation by bacterial lipopolysaccharide (LPS) treatment. *Molecular Brain Research*, **31**, 122–30.

Gardiner, J.V., Kong, W.M., Ward, H. *et al.* (2005) AAV mediated expression of anti-sense neuropeptide Y cRNA in the arcuate nucleus of rats results in decreased weight gain and food intake. *Biochemical and Biophysical Research Communications*, **327**, 1088–93.

Gautron, L., Mingam, R., Moranis, A. *et al.* (2005) Influence of feeding status on neuronal activity in the hypothalamus during lipopolysaccharide-induced anorexia in rats. *Neuroscience*, **134**, 933–46.

Gayle, D., Ilyin, S.E. and Plata-Salamàn, C.R. (1997) Interleukin-1 receptor type mRNA levels in brain regions from male and female rats. *Brain Research Bulletin*, **42**, 463–67.

Gayle, D.A., Desai, M., Casillas, E. *et al.* (2006) Gender-specific orexigenic and anorexigenic mechanisms in rats. *Life Sciences*, **79**, 1531–6.

Geary, N. (2001) Sex differences in disease anorexia. *Nutrition*, **17**, 499–507.

Geary, N. (2004) Endocrine controls of eating: CCK, leptin, and ghrelin. *Physiology & Behavior*, **81**, 719–33.

Geary, N. and Asarian, L. (1999) Cyclic estradiol treatment normalizes body weight and test meal size in ovariectomized rats. *Physiology & Behavior*, **67**, 141–7.

Geary, N., Asarian, L., Sheahan, J. and Langhans, W. (2004) Estradiol-mediated increases in the anorexia induced by intraperitoneal injection of bacterial lipopolysaccharide in female rats. *Physiology & Behavior*, **82**, 251–61.

Geary, N. and Lovejoy, J. (2007) Sex differences in energy metabolism, obesity and eating behavior, in *Sex on the Brain: From Genes to Behavior* (eds J. Becker, K.J. Berkley, N. Geary *et al.*), Oxford University Press, New York.

Gibbs, J., Young, R.C. and Smith, G.P. (1973) Cholecystokinin decreases food intake in rats. *Journal of Comparative and Physiological Psychology*, **84**, 488–95.

Gibson, E.L. and Brunstrom, J.M. (2007) Learned influences on appetite, food choice, and intake: Evidence in human beings, in *Appetite and Body Weight – Integrative Systems and the Development of Anti-Obesity Drugs*, (eds T.C. Kirkham and S.J. Cooper), Academic Press/Elsevier, Burlington, MA, pp. 271–300.

Grill, H.J. and Kaplan, J.M. (1992) Sham feeding in intact and chronic decerebrate rats. *American Journal of Physiology*, **262**, R1070–4.

Grill, H.J. and Kaplan, J.M. (2002) The neuroanatomical axis for control of energy balance. *Frontiers in Neuroendocrinology*, **23**, 2–40.

Grill, H.J., Schwartz, M.W., Kaplan, J.M. *et al.* (2002) Evidence that the caudal brainstem is a target for the inhibitory effect of leptin on food intake. *Endocrinology*, **143**, 239–46.

Grill, H.J. and Smith, G.P. (1988) Cholecystokinin decreases sucrose intake in chronic decerebrate rats. *American Journal of Physiology*, **254**, R853–6.

Grunfeld, C., Zhao, C., Fuller, J. *et al.* (1996) Endotoxin and cytokines induce expression of leptin, the ob gene product, in hamsters – A role for leptin in the anorexia of infection. *Journal of Clinical Investigation*, **97**, 2152–7.

Hajnal, A., Smith, G.P. and Norgren, R. (2004) Oral sucrose stimulation increases accumbens dopamine in the rat. *American Journal of Physiology. Regulatory Integrative and Comparative Physiology*, **286**, R31–7.

Halaas, J.L., Gajiwala, K.S., Maffei, M. *et al.* (1995) Weight-reducing effects of the plasma-protein encoded by the obese gene. *Science*, **269**, 543–6.

Harden, L.M., du Plessis, I., Poole, S. and Laburn, H.P. (2006) Interleukin-6 and leptin mediate lipopolysaccharide-induced fever and sickness behaviour. *Physiology & Behavior*, **89**, 146–55.

Harrold, J.A., Widdowson, P.S. and Williams, G. (1999) Altered energy balance causes selective changes in melanocortin-4 (MC4-R), but not melanocortin-3 (MC3-R), receptors in specific hypothalamic regions – further evidence that activation of MC4-R is a physiological inhibitor of feeding. *Diabetes*, **48**, 267–71.

Hart, B.L. (1988) Biological basis of the behavior of sick animals. *Neuroscience Biobehavioral Reviews*, **12**, 123–37.

Hataya, Y.J., Akamizu, T., Hosoda, H. *et al.* (2003) Alterations of plasma ghrelin levels in rats with lipopolysaccharide-induced wasting syndrome and effects of ghrelin treatment on the syndrome. *Endocrinology*, **144**, 5365–71.

Haynes, A.C., Jackson, B., Overend, P. *et al.* (1999) Effects of single and chronic intracerebroventricular administration of the orexins on feeding in the rat. *Peptides*, **20**, 1099–105.

Heisler, L.K., Jobst, E.E., Sutton, G.M. *et al.* (2006) Serotonin reciprocally regulates melanocortin neurons to modulate food intake. *Neuron*, **51**, 239–49.

Helmling, S., Maasch, C., Eulberg, D. *et al.* (2004) Inhibition of ghrelin action in vitro and in vivo by an RNA-Spiegelmer. *Proceedings of the National Academy of Sciences of the United States of America*, **101**, 13174–9.

Hetherington, A.W. and Ranson, S.W. (1940) Hypothalamic lesions and adiposity in the rat. *Anatomical Record*, **78**, 149–72.

Heymsfield, S.B., Greenberg, A.S., Fujioka, K. *et al.* (1999) Recombinant leptin for weight loss in obese and lean adults – a randomized, controlled, dose-escalation trial. *Journal of the American Medical Association*, **282**, 1568–75.

Hillebrand, J.J.G., de Wied, D. and Adan, R.A.H. (2002) Neuropeptides, food intake and body weight regulation: a hypothalamic focus. *Peptides*, **23**, 2283–306.

Hollander, P., Maggs, D.G., Ruggles, J.A. *et al.* (2004) Effect of pramlintide on weight in overweight and obese insulin-treated type 2 diabetes patients. *Obesity Research*, **12** (4), 661–8.

Holst, J.J. (2007) The physiology of glucagon-like peptide 1. *Physiological Reviews*, **87** (4), 1409–39.

Huszar, D., Lynch, C.A., Fairchild-Huntress, V. *et al.* (1997) Targeted disruption of the melanocortin-4 receptor results in obesity in mice. *Cell*, **88** (1), 131–41.

Ishigaki, Y., Katagiri, H., Yamada, T. *et al.* (2005) Dissipating excess energy stored in the liver is a potential treatment strategy for diabetes associated with obesity. *Diabetes*, **54**, 322–32.

Ishihara, A., Kanatani, A., Mashiko, S. *et al.* (2006) A neuropeptide Y Y5 antagonist selectively ameliorates body weight gain and associated parameters in diet-induced obese mice. *Proceedings of the National Academy of Sciences of the United States of America*, **103**, 7154–8.

Jambor de Sousa, U.L., Benthem, L., Arsenijevic, D. *et al.* (2006) Hepatic-portal oleic acid inhibits feeding more potently than hepatic-portal caprylic acid in rats. *Physiology & Behavior*, **89**, 329–34.

Kahler, A., Geary, N., Eckel, L.A. *et al.* (1998) Chronic administration of OB protein decreases food intake by selectively reducing meal size in male rats. *American Journal of Physiology. Regulatory Integrative and Comparative Physiology*, **44**, R180–5.

Kanatani, A., Ishihara, A., Asahi, S. *et al.* (1996) Potent neuropeptide Y Y1 receptor antagonist, 1229U91: Blockade of neuropeptide Y-induced and physiological food intake. *Endocrinology*, **137**, 3177–82.

Kanatani, A., Mashiko, S., Murai, N. *et al.* (2000) Role of the Y1 receptor in the regulation of neuropeptide Y-mediated feeding: Comparison of wild-type, Y1 receptor-deficient, and Y5 receptor-deficient mice. *Endocrinology*, **141**, 1011–6.

Kandel, E.R., Schwartz, J.H. and Jesel, T.M. (2000) *Principles of Neural Science*, McGraw-Hill, New York.

Kaplan, J.M.M. and Moran, T.H. (2004) Gastrointestinal signaling in the control of food intake, in *Handbook of Behavioral Neurobiology, volume 14, Neurobiology of Food and Fluid Intake*, 2nd edn (eds E.M. Stricker and S.C. Woods), Kluwer Academic/Plenum Publishers, New York, pp. 275–305.

Kelley, A.E., Baldo, B.A. and Pratt, W.E. (2005) A proposed hypothalamic-thalamic-striatal axis for the integration of energy balance, arousal, and food reward. *Journal of Comparative Neurology*, **493** (1), 72–85.

Kelley, A.E., Baldo, B.A., Pratt, W.E. and Will, M.J. (2005) Corticostriatal-hypothalamic circuitry and food motivation: Integration of energy, action and reward. *Physiology & Behavior*, **86**, 773–95.

Kim, E.M., Quinn, J.G., Levine, A.S. and O'Hare, E. (2004) A bi-directional mu-opioid-opioid connection between the nucleus of the accumbens shell and the central nucleus of the amygdala in the rat. *Brain Research*, **1029**, 135–9.

Kirchgessner, A.L. and Sclafani, A. (1988) PVN-hindbrain pathway involved in the hypothalamic hyperphagia-obesity syndrome. *Physiology & Behavior*, **42**, 517–28.

Kirkham, T.C. (2005) Endocannabinoids in the regulation of appetite and body weight. *Behavioural Pharmacology*, **16**, 297–313.

Klein, D.A., Schebendach, J.S., Devlin, M.J. *et al.* (2006) Intake, sweetness and liking during modified sham feeding of sucrose solutions. *Physiology & Behavior*, **87**, 602–6.

Kojima, M., Hosoda, H., Date, Y. *et al.* (1999) Ghrelin is a growth-hormone-releasing acylated peptide from stomach. *Nature*, **402**, 656–60.

Kolaczynski, J.W., Considine, R.V., Ohannesian, J. *et al.* (1996) Responses of leptin to short-term fasting and refeeding in humans – a link with ketogenesis but not ketones themselves. *Diabetes*, **45**, 1511–5.

Kringelbach, M.L. (2005) The human orbitofrontal cortex: Linking reward to hedonic experience. *Nature Reviews Neuroscience*, **6**, 691–702.

Kringelbach, M.L. (2007) Cortical systems involved in appetite and food consumption, in *Appetite and Body Weight* (eds T.C. Kirkham and S.J. Cooper), Elsevier, pp. 5–26.

Kurosawa, M., UvnasMoberg, K., Miyasaka, K. and Lundeberg, T. (1997) Interleukin-1 increases activity of the gastric vagal afferent nerve partly via stimulation of type A CCK receptor in anesthetized rats. *Journal of the Autonomic Nervous System*, **62**, 72–8.

La Fleur, S.E., Ji, H., Manalo, S.L. *et al.* (2003) The hepatic vagus mediates fat-induced inhibition of diabetic hyperphagia. *Diabetes*, **52**, 2321–30.

Laflamme, N. and Rivest, S. (2001) Toll-like receptor 4: the missing link of the cerebral innate immune response triggered by circulating gram-negative bacterial cell wall components. *FASEB Journal*, **15**, 155–63.

Lam, T.K., Schwartz, G.J. and Rossetti, L. (2005) Hypothalamic sensing of fatty acids. *Nature Neuroscience*, **8**, 579–84.

Lambert, P.D., Anderson, K.D., Sleeman, M.W. *et al.* (2001) Ciliary neurotrophic factor activates leptin-like pathways and reduces body fat, without cachexia or rebound weight gain, even in leptin-resistant obesity. *Proceedings of the National Academy of Sciences of the United States of America*, **98**, 4652–7.

Lambert, P.D., Couceyro, P.R., McGirr, K.M. *et al.* (1998) CART peptides in the central control of feeding and interactions with neuropeptide Y. *Synapse (New York, NY)*, **29**, 293–8.

Langhans, W. (1996) Metabolic and glucostatic control of feeding. *Proceedings of the Nutrition Society*, **55**, 497–515.

Langhans, W. (2004) Anorexia during disease, in *Handbook of Behavioral Neurobiology, volume 14, Neurobiology of Food and Fluid Intake*, 2nd edn (eds E.M. Stricker and S.C. Woods), Kluwer Academic/Plenum Publishers, New York, pp. 347–79.

Langhans, W. and Geary, N. (2006) Regulation of body weight, in *Obesity and Binge Eating Disorder* (eds S. Munsch and C. Beglinger), Karger, Basel, pp. 21–40.

Langhans, W., Grossmann, F. and Geary, N. (2001) Intrameal hepatic-portal infusion of glucose reduces spontaneous meal size in rats. *Physiology & Behavior*, **73**, 499–507.

Langhans, W., Zeiger, U., Scharrer, E. and Geary, N. (1982) Stimulation of feeding in rats by intraperitoneal injection of antibodies to glucagon. *Science*, **218** (4575), 894–6.

Larsen, L.H., Echwald, S.M., Sorensen, T.I.A. *et al.* (2005) Prevalence of mutations and functional analyses of melanocortin 4 receptor variants identified among 750 men with juvenile-onset obesity. *Journal of Clinical Endocrinology and Metabolism*, **90**, 219–24.

Le Sauter, J., Noh, U. and Geary, N. (1991 (Jul) Hepatic portal infusion of glucagon antibodies increases spontaneous meal size in rats. *The American Journal of Physiology*, **261** (1 Pt (2), R162–5.

Lee, J.Y., Sohn, K.H., Rhee, S.H. and Hwang, D. (2001) Saturated fatty acids, but not unsaturated fatty acids, induce the expression of cyclooxygenase-2 mediated through Toll-like receptor 4. *Journal of Biological Chemistry*, **276**, 16683–9.

Leibowitz, S.F. (1970) Reciprocal hunger-regulating circuits involving alpha-and beta-adrenergic receptors located, respectively, in ventromedial and lateral hypothalamus. *Proceedings of the National Academy of Sciences of the United States of America*, **67**, 1063–70.

Leibowitz, S.F. (1978) Paraventricular nucleus – Primary site mediating adrenergic-stimulation of feeding and drinking. *Pharmacology Biochemistry and Behavior*, **8**, 163–75.

Leonhardt, M. and Langhans, W. (2004) Fatty acid oxidation and control of food intake. *Physiology & Behavior*, **83**, 645–51.

Levin, B.E. (2002) Metabolic sensors: Viewing glucosensing neurons from a broader perspective. *Physiology & Behavior*, **76**, 397–401.

Levin, B.E. (2006) Metabolic sensing neurons and the control of energy homeostasis. *Physiology & Behavior*, **89**, 486–9.

Levin, B.E., Dunn-Meynell, A.A., McMinn, J.E. *et al.* (2003) A new obesity-prone, glucose-intolerant rat strain (F. DIO). *The American Journal of Physiology*, **285**, R1184–91.

Li, B., Xi, X.C., Roane, D.S. *et al.* (2003) Distribution of glucokinase, glucose transporter GLUT2, sulfonylurea receptor-1, glucagon-like peptide-1 receptor and neuropeptide Y messenger RNAs in rat brain by quantitative real time RT-PCR. *Molecular Brain Research*, **113**, 139–42.

Liang, N.C., Hajnal, A. and Norgren, R. (2006) Sham feeding corn oil increases accumbens dopamine in the rat. *American Journal of Physiology. Regulatory Integrative and Comparative Physiology*, **291**, R1236–9.

Licinio, J. and Wong, M.L. (1997) Pathways and mechanisms for cytokine signaling of the central nervous system. *Journal of Clinical Investigation*, **100**, 2941–7.

Lieverse, R.J., Jansen, J.B.M.J., Vandezwan, A. *et al.* (1993) Effects of a physiological dose of cholecystokinin on food-intake and postprandial satiation in man. *Regulatory Peptides*, **43**, 83–9.

Lin, X., Chavez, M.R., Bruch, R.C. *et al.* (1998) The effects of a high fat diet on leptin mRNA, serum leptin and the response to leptin are not altered in a rat strain susceptible to high fat diet-induced obesity. *Journal of Nutrition*, **128**, 1606–13.

LouisSylvestre, J. and LeMagnen, J. (1980) A fall in blood-glucose level precedes meal onset in free-feeding rats. *Neuroscience and Biobehavioral Reviews*, **4**, 13–5.

Lugarini, F., Hrupka, B.J., Schwartz, G.J. *et al.* (2002) A role for cyclooxygenase-2 in lipopolysaccharide-induced anorexia in rats. *American Journal of Physiology. Regulatory Integrative and Comparative Physiology*, **283**, R862–8.

Lugarini, F., Hrupka, B.J., Schwartz, G.J. *et al.* (2005) Acute and chronic administration of immunomodulators induces anorexia in Zucker rats. *Physiology & Behavior*, **84**, 165–73.

Lutz, T.A. (2005) Pancreatic amylin as a centrally acting satiating hormone. *Current Drug Targets*, **6** (2), 181–9.

Lutz, T.A. (2006) Amylinergic control of food intake. *Physiology & Behavior*, **89**, 465–71.

MacLagan, N. (1937) The role of appetite in the control of body weight. *Journal of Physiology (London)*, **90**, 385–94.

Malik, K.F. and Young, W.S. (1996) Localization of binding sites in the central nervous system for leptin (OB protein) in normal, obese (ob/ob), and diabetic (db/db) C57BL/6J mice. *Endocrinology*, **137**, 1497–1500.

Marsh, D.J., Hollopeter, G., Kafer, K.E. and Palmiter, R.D. (1998) Role of the Y5 neuropeptide Y receptor in feeding and obesity. *Nature Medicine*, **4**, 718–21.

Marsh, D.J., Weingarth, D.T., Novi, D.E. *et al.* (2002) Melanin-concentrating hormone 1 receptor-deficient mice are lean, hyperactive, and hyperphagic and have altered metabolism. *Proceedings of the National Academy of Sciences of the United States of America*, **99**, 3240–5.

Marty, N., Bady, I. and Thorens, B. (2006) Distinct classes of central GLUT2-dependent sensors control counterregulation and feeding. *Diabetes*, **55**, S108–113.

Matthews, K.A., Abrams, B., Crawford, S. *et al.* (2001) Body mass index in mid-life women: relative influence of menopause, hormone use, and ethnicity. *International Journal of Obesity*, **25**, 863–73.

Matzinger *et al.* (1999) Inhibition of food intake in response to intestinal lipid is mediated by cholecystokinin in humans. *American Journal of Physiology*, **277**, R1718.

McGowan, M.K., Andrews, K.M. and Grossman, S.P. (1992) Chronic intrahypothalamic infusions of insulin or insulin antibodies alter body weight and food intake in the rat. *Physiology & Behavior*, **51**, 753–66.

Melanson, K.J., Westerterp-Plantenga, M.S., Campfield, L.A. and Saris, W.H.M. (1999) Blood glucose and meal patterns in time-blinded males, after aspartame, carbohydrate, and fat consumption, in relation to sweetness perception. *British Journal of Nutrition*, **82**, 437–46.

Mencarelli, M., Maestrini, S., Tagliaferri, M. *et al.* (2004) *Identification of Three Novel Melanocortin-3 Receptor (MC3R) Gene Mutations in Patients with Morbid Obesity*, American Endocrine Society, New Orleans, Abstract OR45-1.

Mercer, J.G., Hoggard, N., Williams, L.M. *et al.* (1996) Coexpression of leptin receptor and preproneuropeptide Y mRNA in arcuate nucleus of mouse hypothalamus. *Journal of Neuroendocrinology*, **8**, 733–5.

Minokoshi, Y., Alquier, T., Furukawa, N. *et al.* (2004) AMP-kinase regulates food intake by responding to hormonal and nutrient signals in the hypothalamus. *Nature*, **428**, 569–74.

Monnikes, H., Helmling, S., Stengel, A. *et al.* (2005) Anti-ghrelin Spiegelmer NOX-B11 inhibits neurostimulatory and orexigenic effects of peripheral ghrelin in rats. *Gastroenterology*, **128**, A374.

Moran, T.H. (2006a) Gut peptide signaling in the controls of food intake. *Obesity*, **14**, 250–3.

Moran, T.H. (2006b) Neural and hormonal controls of food intake and satiety, in *Physiology of the gastrointestinal tract* (eds L.R. Johnson and M.A. Burlington), Elsevier Academic Press, pp. 877–94.

Moran, T.H. and Bi, S. (2006) Hyperphagia and obesity of OLETF rats lacking CCK1 receptors: Developmental aspects. *Developmental Psychobiology*, **48**, 360–7.

Moran, T.H. and Kinzig, K.P. (2004) Gastrointestinal satiety signals – II. Cholecystokinin. *American Journal of Physiology. Gastrointestinal and Liver Physiology*, **286**, G183–8.

Moran, T.H., Ameglio, P.J., Schwartz, G.J. and Mchugh, P.R. (1992) Blockade of type-A, not type-B, CCK receptors attenuates satiety actions of exogenous and endogenous CCK. *American Journal of Physiology*, **262**, R46–50.

Morton, G.J., Blevins, J.E., Williams, D.L. *et al.* (2005) Leptin action in the forebrain regulates the hindbrain response to satiety signals. *Journal of Clinical Investigation*, **115**, 703–10.

Mountjoy, K.G., Mortrud, M.T., Low, M.J. *et al.* (1994) Localization of the melanocortin-4 receptor (MC4-R) in neuroendocrine and autonomic control-circuits in the brain. *Molecular Endocrinology*, **8**, 1298–308.

Murphy, K.G. and Bloom, S.R. (2006) Gut hormones and the regulation of energy homeostasis. *Nature*, **444**, 854–9.

Murray, M.J. and Murray, A.B. (1979) Anorexia of infection as a mechanism of host defense. *American Journal of Clinical Nutrition*, **32**, 593–6.

Nadeau, S. and Rivest, S. (1999) Effects of circulating tumor necrosis factor on the neuronal activity and expression of the genes encoding the tumor necrosis factor receptors (p55 and p75) in the rat brain: A view from the blood-brain barrier. *Neuroscience*, **93**, 1449–64.

Nadjar, A., Bluthe, R.M., May, M.J. *et al.* (2005) Inactivation of the cerebral NF kappa B pathway inhibits interleukin-1 beta-induced sickness behavior and c-Fos expression in various brain nuclei. *Neuropsychopharmacology*, **30**, 1492–9.

Nakamura, K., Li, Y.Q., Kaneko, T. *et al.* (2001) Prostaglandin EP3 receptor protein in serotonin and catecholamine cell groups: A double immunofluorescence study in the rat brain. *Neuroscience*, **103**, 763–75.

Navarro, M., deFonseca, F.R., Alvarez, E.A. *et al.* (1996) Colocalization of glucagon-like peptide-1 (GLP-1) receptors, glucose transporter GLUT-2, and glucokinase mRNAs in rat hypothalamic cells: Evidence for a role of GLP-1 receptor agonists as an inhibitory signal for food and water intake. *Journal of Neurochemistry*, **67**, 1982–91.

Naveilhan, P., Hassani, H., Canals, J.M. *et al.* (1999) Normal feeding behavior, body weight and leptin response require the neuropeptide YY2 receptor. *Nature Medicine*, **5**, 1188–93.

Nestler, E.J. and Carlezon, W.A. (2006) The mesolimbic dopamine reward circuit in depression. *Biological Psychiatry*, **59**, 1151–9.

Netea, M.G., Joosten, L.A.B., Lewis, E. *et al.* (2006) Deficiency of interleukin-18 in mice leads to hyperphagia, obesity and insulin resistance. *Nature Medicine*, **12**, 650–6.

Niijima, A. (1969) Afferent impulse discharges from glucoreceptors in liver of guinea pig. *Annals of the New York Academy of Sciences*, **157**, 690–700.

Niijima, A. (1983) Glucose-sensitive afferent nerve-fibers in the liver and their role in food-intake and blood-glucose regulation. *Journal of the Autonomic Nervous System*, **9**, 207–20.

Niijima, A. (1996) The afferent discharges from sensors for interleukin-1beta in the hepatoportal system in the anesthetized rat. *Journal of the Autonomic Nervous System*, **61**, 287–91.

Norgren, R. and Grill, H.J. (1982) Brain-stem control of ingestive behaviour, in *The Physiological Mechanisms of Motivation* (ed. D. Pfaff), Springer, New York, pp. 99–132.

Norgren, R., Hajnal, A. and Mungarndee, S.S. (2006) Gustatory reward and the nucleus accumbens. *Physiology & Behavior*, **89**, 531–5.

O'Rahilly, S. and Farooqi, I.S. (2006) Genetics of obesity. *Philosophical Transactions of the Royal Society B. Series B, Biological Sciences*, **361**, 1095–105.

Obici, S., Feng, Z.H., Morgan, Y. et al. (2002) Central administration of oleic acid inhibits glucose production and food intake. *Diabetes*, **51**, 271–5.

Ohno, K. and Sakurai, T. (2008) Front neuroendocrinol. *Orexin neuronal circuitry: role in the regulation of sleep and wakefulness*, **29** (1), 70–87 Epub 2007, 29 Aug.

Okura, T., Koda, M., Ando, F. et al. (2003 (Sep)) Association of polymorphisms in the estrogen receptor alpha gene with body fat distribution. *International Journal of Obesity and Related Metabolic Disorders*, **27** (9), 1020–7.

Olney, J.W. (1969) Brain lesions obesity and other disturbances in mice treated with monosodium glutamate. *Science*, **164**, 719.

Peciña, S., Smith, K.S. and Berridge, K.C. (2006) Hedonic hot spots in the brain. *The Neuroscientist: A Review Journal Bringing Neurobiology, Neurology and Psychiatry*, **12** (6), 500–11.

Pelleymounter, M.A., Cullen, M.J., Baker, M.B. et al. (1995) Effects of the obese gene-product on body-weight regulation in Ob/Ob mice. *Science*, **269**, 540–3.

Peters, J.H., Simasko, S.M. and Ritter, R.C. (2006) Modulation of vagal afferent excitation and reduction of food intake by leptin and cholecystokinin. *Physiology & Behavior*, **89**, 477–85.

Phillips, R.J. and Powley, T.L. (1996) Gastric volume rather than nutrient content inhibits food intake. *American Journal of Physiology. Regulatory Integrative and Comparative Physiology*, **40**, R766–79.

Pieber, T.R., Roitelman, J., Lee, Y. et al. (1994) Direct plasma radioimmunoassay for rat amylin-(1–37): concentrations with acquired and genetic obesity. *The American Journal of Physiology*, **267**, E156–64.

Plata-Salamàn, C.R. (1995) Cytokines and feeding suppression: An integrative view from neurologic to molecular levels. *Nutrition*, **11**, 674–7.

Porter, M.H., Hrupka, B.J., Langhans, W. and Schwartz, G.J. (1998) Vagal and splanchnic afferents are not necessary for the anorexia produced by peripheral IL-1 beta, LPS, and MDP. *American Journal of Physiology. Regulatory Integrative and Comparative Physiology*, **44**, R384–9.

Powley, T.L. (1977) Ventromedial hypothalamic syndrome, satiety, and a cephalic phase hypothesis. *Psychological Review*, **84**, 89–126.

Prins, A.A., Dejongnagelsmit, A., Keijser, J. and Strubbe, J.H. (1986) Daily rhythms of feeding in the genetically-obese and lean Zucker rats. *Physiology & Behavior*, **38**, 423–6.

Qu, D.Q., Ludwig, D.S., Gammeltoft, S. et al. (1996) A role for melanin-concentrating hormone in the central regulation of feeding behaviour. *Nature*, **380**, 243–7.

Riedy, C.A., Chavez, M., Figlewicz, D.P. and Woods, S.C. (1995) Central insulin enhances sensitivity to cholecystokinin. *Physiology & Behavior*, **58**, 755–60.

Rietschel, E.T., Schletter, J., Weidemann, B. et al. (1998) Lipopolysaccharide and peptidoglycan: CD14-dependent bacterial inducers of inflammation. *Microbial Drug Resistance*, **4**, 37–44.

Rinaman, L. (1998) Oxytocinergic inputs to the nucleus of the solitary tract and dorsal motor nucleus of the vagus in neonatal rats. *Journal of Comparative Neurology*, **399**, 101–9.

Rinaman, L., Baker, E.A., Hoffman, G.E. et al. (1998) Medullary c-Fos activation in rats after ingestion of a satiating meal. *The American Journal of Physiology*, **275** (1 Pt 2), R262–8.

Ritter, R.C. (2004) Gastrointestinal mechanisms of satiation for food. *Physiology & Behavior*, **81**, 249–73.

Rogers, R.C., Kita, H., Butcher, L.L. and Novin, D. (1980) Afferent-projections to the dorsal motor nucleus of the vagus. *Brain Research Bulletin*, **5**, 365–73.

Rolls, B.J. (1986) Sensory-specific satiety. *Nutrition Reviews*, **44**, 93–101.

Rolls, B.J., Vanduijvenvoorde, P.M. and Rowe, E.A. (1983) Variety in the diet enhances intake in a meal and contributes to the development of obesity in the rat. *Physiology & Behavior*, **31**, 21–7.

Rolls, B.J., Gnizak, N., Summerfelt, A. and Laster, L.J. (1988) Food intake in dieters and nondieters after a liquid meal containing medium-chain triglycerides. *American Journal of Clinical Nutrition*, **48**, 66–71.

Rolls, E.T. (2006) Brain mechanisms underlying flavour and appetite. *Philosophical Transactions of the Royal Society B. Series B, Biological Sciences*, **361**, 1123–36.

Roseberry, A.G., Liu, H.Y., Jackson, A.C. et al. (2004) Neuropeptide Y-mediated inhibition of proopiomelanocortin neurons in the arcuate nucleus shows enhanced desensitization in ob/ob mice. *Neuron*, **41**, 711–22.

Rosenbaum, M., Goldsmith, R., Bloomfield, D. et al. (2005) Low-dose leptin reverses skeletal muscle, autonomic, and neuroendocrine adaptations to maintenance of reduced weight. *Journal of Clinical Investigation*, **115**, 3579–86.

Routh, V.H. (2002) Glucose-sensing neurons: Are they physiologically relevant? *Physiology & Behavior*, **76**, 403–13.

Rozin, P., Hanko, K. and Durlach, P. (2006) Self-prediction of hedonic trajectories for repeated use of body products and foods: poor performance, not improved by a full generation of experience. *Appetite*, **46**, 297–303.

Rushing, P.A., Hagan, M.M., Seeley, R.J. *et al.* (2001) Inhibition of central amylin signaling increases food intake and body adiposity in rats. *Endocrinology*, **142** (11), 5035.

Russek, M. (1963) Participation of hepatic glucoreceptors in control of intake of food. *Nature*, **197**, 79–80.

Sakurai, T. (2002) Roles of orexins in regulation of feeding and wakefulness. *Neuroreport*, **13**, 987–95.

Sanchez-Margalet, V., Martin-Romero, C., Santos-Alvarez, J. *et al.* (2003) Role of leptin as an immunomodulator of blood mononuclear cells: mechanisms of action. *Clinical and Experimental Immunology*, **133**, 11–9.

Saper, C.B. (2006) Staying awake for dinner: hypothalamic integration of sleep, feeding, and circadian rhythms. *Progress in Brain Research*, **153**, 243–52.

Savage, D.B., Choi, C.S., Samuel, V.T. *et al.* (2006) Reversal of diet-induced hepatic steatosis and hepatic insulin resistance by antisense oligonucleotide inhibitors of acetyl-CoA carboxylases 1 and 2. *Journal of Clinical Investigation*, **116**, 817–24.

Sawchenko, P.E. and Swanson, L.W. (1982) Immunohistochemical identification of neurons in the paraventricular nucleus of the hypothalamus that project to the medulla or to the spinal-cord in the rat. *Journal of Comparative Neurology*, **205**, 260–72.

Schmidt, P.T., Näslund, E., Grybäck, P. *et al.* (2003) Peripheral administration of GLP-2 to humans has no effect on gastric emptying or satiety. *Regulatory Peptides*, **116**, 21–5.

Schultz, W. (2006) Behavioral theories and the neurophysiology of reward. *Annual Review of Psychology*, **57**, 87–115.

Schutt, C., Bernheiden, M., Grunwald, U. *et al.* (1999) Implications for a general role of LPS-binding proteins (CD14, LBP) in combating bacterial infections. *Journal of Endotoxin Research*, **5**, 75–80.

Schwartz, M.W., Seeley, R.J., Campfield, L.A. *et al.* (1996) Identification of targets of leptin action in rat hypothalamus. *Journal of Clinical Investigation*, **98**, 1101–6.

Schwartz, M.W., Woods, S.C., Seeley, R.J. *et al.* (2003) Is the energy homeostasis system inherently biased toward weight gain? *Diabetes*, **52**, 232–8.

Sclafani, A. (2001) Psychobiology of food preferences. *International Journal of Obesity*, **25**, S13–5.

Scott, T.R. and Giza, B.K. (2000) Issues of gustatory neural coding: Where they stand today. *Physiology & Behavior*, **69**, 65–76.

Simerly, R.B. (2004) Anatomical substrates of hypothalamic integration, in *The Rat Nervous System* (ed. G. Paxinos), Elsevier, Amsterdam, pp. 335–68.

Smith, G.P., Jerome, C. and Norgren, R. (1985) Afferent axons in abdominal vagus mediate satiety effect of cholecystokinin in rats. *The American Journal of Physiology*, **249**, R638–41.

Stanley, B.G., Magdalin, W., Seirafi, A. *et al.* (1993) The perifornical area – the major focus of (a) patchy distributed hypothalamic neuropeptide Y-sensitive feeding system(s). *Brain Research*, **604**, 304–17.

Stanley, S., Wynne, K., McGowan, B. and Bloom, S. (2005) Hormonal regulation of food intake. *Physiological Reviews*, **85**, 1131–58.

Stellar, E. (1954) The physiology of motivation. *Psychological Review*, **61**, 5–22.

Strader, A.D. and Woods, S.C. (2005) Gastrointestinal hormones and food intake. *Gastroenterology*, **128**, 175–91.

Stratford, T.R., Kelley, A.E. and Simansky, K.J. (1999) Blockade of GABA(A) receptors in the medial ventral pallidum elicits feeding in satiated rats. *Brain Research*, **825**, 199–203.

Strohmayer, A.J. and Smith, G.P. (1987) The meal pattern of genetically-obese (Ob Ob) mice. *Appetite*, **8**, 111–23.

Strubbe, J.H. and Mein, C.G. (1977) Increased feeding in response to bilateral injection of insulin antibodies in the VMH. *Physiology & Behavior*, **19**, 309–13.

Stubbs, R.J. and Harbron, C.G. (1996) Covert manipulation of the ratio of medium- to long-chain triglycerides in isoenergetically dense diets: effect on food intake in ad libitum feeding men. *International Journal of Obesity and Related Metabolic Disorders*, **20**, 435–44.

Swanson, L.W. (1999) The neuroanatomy revolution of the 1970s and the hypothalamus. *Brain Research Bulletin*, **50**, 397.

Tang-Christensen, M., Larsen, P.J., Thulesen, J. *et al.* (2000) The proglucagon-derived peptide, glucagon-like peptide-2, is a neurotransmitter involved in the regulation of food intake. *Nature Medicine*, **6**, 802–7.

Tartaglia, L.A., Dembski, M., Weng, X. *et al.* (1995) Identification and expression cloning of a leptin receptor, OB-R. *Cell*, **83**, 1263–71.

Thammacharoen, S. Lutz, T.A. Geary, N. and Asarian, L. (2008) Hindbrain administration of estradiol inhibits feeding and activates ERα-expressing cells in the NTS of ovariectomized rats. *Endocrinology*, **149**, (4), 1609–17.

Tobias, J.H., Steer, C.D., Vilarino-Güell, C. and Brown, M.A. (2007) Effect of an estrogen receptor-alpha intron 4 polymorphism on fat mass in 11-year-old children. *The Journal of Clinical Endocrinology and Metabolism*, **92**, (6), 2286–91.

Tordoff, M.G. and Friedman, M.I. (1986) Hepatic portal glucose infusions decrease food-intake and increase food preference. *American Journal of Physiology*, **251**, R192–6.

Tordoff, M.G. and Friedman, M.I. (1988) Hepatic control of feeding – Effect of glucose, fructose, and mannitol infusion. *American Journal of Physiology*, **254**, R969–76.

Tordoff, M.G., Tluczek, J.P. and Friedman, M.I. (1989) Effect of hepatic portal glucose-concentration on food-intake and metabolism. *American Journal of Physiology*, **257**, R1474–80.

Tschop, M., Smiley, D.L. and Heiman, M.L. (2000) Ghrelin induces adiposity in rodents. *Nature*, **407**, 908–13.

Tso, P. and Liu, M. (2004) Apolipoprotein A-IV, food intake, and obesity. *Physiology & Behavior*, **83**, 631–43.

Turnley, A.M., Stapleton, D., Mann, R.J. *et al.* (1999) Cellular distribution and developmental expression of AMP-activated protein kinase isoforms in mouse central nervous system. *Journal of Neurochemistry*, **72** (4), 1707–16.

Turrin, N.P. and Rivest, S. (2004) Unraveling the molecular details involved in the intimate link between the immune and neuroendocrine systems. *Experimental Biology and Medicine*, **229**, 996–1006.

Turrin, N.P., Gayle, D., Ilyin, S.E. *et al.* (2001) Pro-inflammatory and anti-inflammatory cytokine mRNA induction in the periphery and brain following intraperitoneal administration of bacterial lipopolysaccharide. *Brain Research Bulletin*, **54**, 443–53.

Ueno, H., Yamaguchi, H, Kangawa, K. and Nakazato, M. (2005) Ghrelin: a gastric peptide that regulates food intake and energy homeostasis. *Regulatory Peptides*, **126**, 11–9.

Uher, R., Treasure, J., Heining, M. *et al.* (2006) Cerebral processing of food-related stimuli: Effects of fasting and gender. *Behavioural Brain Research*, **169**, 111–19.

Ungerstedt, U. (1971) Adipsia and aphagia after 6-hydroxydopamine induced degeneration of the nigro-striatal dopamine system. *Acta Physiologia Scandinavia Supplement*, **367**, 95–122.

van den Pol, A.N., Gao, X.B., Obrietan, K. *et al.* (1998) Presynaptic and postsynaptic actions and modulation of neuroendocrine neurons by a new hypothalamic peptide, Hypocretin/Orexin. *Journal of Neuroscience*, **18**, 7962–71.

Van Gaal, L.F., Rissanen, A.M., Scheen, A.J. *et al.* (2005) Effects of the cannabinoid-1 receptor blocker rimonabant on weight reduction and cardiovascular risk factors in overweight patients: 1-year experience from the RIO-Europe study. *Lancet*, **365**, 1389–97.

Velkoska, E., Morris, M.J., Burns, P. and Weisinger, R.S. (2003) Leptin reduces food intake but does not alter weight regain following food deprivation in the rat. *International Journal of Obesity*, **27**, 48–54.

von Meyenburg, C., Hrupka, B.H., Arsenijevic, D. *et al.* (2004) Role for CD14, TLR2, and TLR4 in bacterial product-induced anorexia. *American Journal of Physiology. Regulatory Integrative and Comparative Physiology*, **287**, R298–305.

Wajchenberg, B.L., Pereira, M.A.A., Medonca, B.B. *et al.* (2000) Adrenocortical carcinoma – Clinical and laboratory observations. *Cancer*, **88**, 711–36.

Wanders, R.J.A., Vreken, P., den Boer, M.E.J. *et al.* (1999) Disorders of mitochondrial fatty acyl-CoA beta-oxidation. *Journal of Inherited Metabolic Disease*, **22**, 442–87.

Wang, L.X., Basa, N.R., Shaikh, A. *et al.* (2006) LPS inhibits fasted plasma ghrelin levels in rats: role of IL-1 and PGs and functional implications. *American Journal of Physiology. Gastrointestinal and Liver Physiology*, **291**, G611–20.

Wang, S.P., Helmling, S., Stribling, D.S. *et al.* (2005) Ghrelin neutralization by an RNA-Spiegelmer yields body weight loss in diet-induced obese mice. *Obesity Research*, **13**, A32.

Widdowson, P.S. (1997) Regionally-selective down-regulation of NPY receptor subtypes in the obese Zucker rat. Relationship to the Y5 'feeding' receptor. *Brain Research*, **758**, 17–25.

Wildman, H.F., Chua, S., Leibel, R.L. and Smith, G.P. (2000) Effects of leptin and cholecystokinin in rats with a null mutation of the leptin receptor Lepr(fak). *American Journal of Physiology. Regulatory Integrative and Comparative Physiology*, **278**, R1518–23.

Will, M.J., Franzblau, E.B. and Kelley, A.E. (2004) The amygdala is critical for opioid-mediated binge eating of fat. *Neuroreport*, **15**, 1857–60.

Willie, J.T., Chemelli, R.M., Sinton, C.M. *et al.* (2003) Distinct narcolepsy syndromes in Orexin receptor-2 and Orexin null mice: molecular genetic dissection of non-REM and REM sleep regulatory processes. *Neuron*, **38** (5), 715–30.

Wise, R.A. (2006) Role of brain dopamine in food reward and reinforcement. *Philosophical Transactions of the Royal Society B. Series B, Biological Sciences*, **361**, 1149–58.

Wood, P.A. (2004) Genetically modified mouse models for disorders of fatty acid metabolism: Pursuing the nutrigenomics of insulin resistance and type 2 diabetes. *Nutrition*, **20**, 121–6.

Woods, S.C., Decke, E. and Vasselli, J.R. (1974) Metabolic hormones and regulation of body-weight. *Psychological Review*, **81**, 26–43.

Woods, S.C., Lutz, T.A., Geary, N. and Langhans, W. (2006) Pancreatic signals controlling food intake; insulin, glucagon and amylin. *Philosophical Transactions of the Royal Society B. Series B, Biological Sciences*, **361**, 1219–35.

Woods, S.C. and Seeley, R.J. (2001) Insulin as an adiposity signal. *International Journal of Obesity*, **25**, S35–8.

Woods, S.C., Seeley, R.J., Baskin, D.G. and Schwartz, M.W. (2003) Insulin and the blood-brain barrier. *Current Pharmaceutical Design*, **9**, 795–800.

Wortley, K.E., del Rincon, J.P., Murray, J.D. *et al.* (2005) Absence of ghrelin protects against early-onset obesity. *Journal of Clinical Investigation*, **115**, 3573–8.

Wu, C.D., Kang, J.E., Peng, L.J. *et al.* (2005) Enhancing hepatic glycolysis reduces obesity: Differential effects on lipogenesis depend on site of glycolytic modulation. *Cell Metabolism*, **2**, 131–40.

Xu, B.J., Goulding, E.H., Zang, K.L. *et al. (*2003) Brain-derived neurotrophic factor regulates energy balance downstream of melanocortin-4 receptor. *Nature Neuroscience*, **6**, 736–42.

Yeomans, M.R., Wright, P., Macleod, H.A. and Critchley, J.A.J.H. (1990) Effects of nalmefene on feeding in humans – Dissociation of hunger and palatability. *Psychopharmacology*, **100**, 426–32.

Zeitzer, J.M., Nishino, S. and Mignot, E. (2006) The neurobiology of hypocretins (orexins), narcolepsy and related therapeutic interventions. *Trends in Pharmacological Sciences*, **27** (7), 368–74.

Zellner, D.A., Garriga-Trillo, A., Centeno, S. and Wadsworth, E. (2004) Chocolate craving and the menstrual cycle. *Appetite*, **42**, 119–21.

Zhang, J., Matheny, M.K., Tumer, N. *et al.* (2007) Leptin antagonist reveals that the normalization of caloric intake and the thermic effect of food after high-fat feeding are leptin dependent. *American Journal of Physiology. Regulatory Integrative and Comparative Physiology*, **292**, R868–74.

Zhang, M., Balmadrid, C. and Kelley, A.E. (2003) Nucleus accumbens opioid, GABAergic, and dopaminergic modulation of palatable food motivation: Contrasting effects revealed by a progressive ratio study in the rat. *Behavioral Neuroscience*, **117**, 202–11.

Zhang, M. and Kelley, A.E. (2000) Enhanced intake of high-fat food following striatal mu-opioid stimulation: Microinjection mapping and Fos expression. *Neuroscience*, **99**, 267–77.

Zhang, Y., Proenca, R., Maffei, M. *et al.* (1994) Positional cloning of the mouse obese gene and its human homologue. *Nature*, **372**, 425–32.

Zhao, H.Y. (2005) Growth hormone secretagogue receptor antagonists as potential therapeutic agents for obesity. *Drug Development Research*, **65**, 50–4.

Zheng, H.Y., Corkern, M., Stoyanova, I. *et al.* (2003) Peptides that regulate food intake – Appetite-inducing accumbens manipulation activates hypothalamic orexin neurons and inhibits POMC neurons. *American Journal of Physiology. Regulatory Integrative and Comparative Physiology*, **284**, R1436–44.

Zigman, J.M., Nakano, Y., Coppari, R. *et al.* (2005) Mice lacking ghrelin receptors resist the development of diet-induced obesity. *Journal of Clinical Investigation*, **115**, 3564–72.

Energy Balance in Humans

Key points

- Obesity results from the failure of the homeostatic mechanisms that normally regulate energy intake and expenditure. An excess of intake over expenditure is stored as triglyceride, mainly in adipose tissue.

- Food intake in adult humans is generally 2000–2500 kcal/day. Human feeding is heavily influenced by psychological, social and economic factors. Very rarely, human obesity is due to hyperphagia resulting from mutations affecting the regulatory circuits that normally restrain appetite (e.g. leptin, leptin receptor, cholecystokinin receptor).

- Obese people expend more energy than lean, and at stable weight, must therefore consume more energy to maintain their higher weight. In general, obese subjects under-report their energy intake. Overconsumption of energy-dense food and drinks is an important factor in the spread of obesity.

- Energy as adenosine triphosphate (ATP) is generated by the oxidation of fats (yielding 9 kcal/g), carbohydrates and proteins (both yielding 4 kcal/g). The respiratory quotient (RQ) – the ratio of carbon dioxide produced to oxygen consumed during oxidation – varies between 1.0 for carbohydrate and 0.7 for fat, and can be used to determine the principal substrate being utilized.

- Total energy expenditure comprises resting energy expenditure (REE; about 60% of total), the thermic effect of food (i.e. the energy required for digestion and assimilation of ingested nutrients), and activity thermogenesis, which consists of both physical activity and non-exercise activity thermogenesis (NEAT).

- REE is determined mainly by fat-free mass, and 80% is due to the metabolic activity of the brain, heart, liver and kidneys; muscle contributes only 20%. In an average adult, REE is about 1.3 kcal/min.

- The contribution of physical activity is highly variable, accounting for less than 30% of total energy expenditure in sedentary subjects but 70% or more in highly-trained athletes or manual labourers.

- NEAT is involuntary, spontaneous physical activity, which varies widely between individuals. Subjects with low levels of NEAT may be more susceptible to obesity, whereas increases in NEAT may help to limit weight gain during overeating.

- Adaptive thermogenesis describes changes in energy expenditure that result from alterations in energy balance. Variations in this could partly determine susceptibility to obesity; differences in sympathetic-mediated thermogenesis for example in muscle or functional brown adipose tissue (BAT) could contribute, but its significance remains uncertain.

- Obesity could also develop through defects in fat oxidation, and there is evidence of decreased fat oxidation rates in some obese subjects (which can persist after weight loss) and in subjects who subsequently become obese.

Chapter 7 Energy Balance in Humans
Ellen E. Blaak

The maintenance of energy balance is one of the most vital processes for the survival of individuals and species. Elaborate mechanisms are in place to safeguard energy balance, even in primitive organisms. For example, the nematode worm, *Caenorhabditis elegans*, has been shown to possess 417 genes involved in regulating body fat, with 305 of these increasing and the remainder decreasing fat content (Ashrafi *et al.*, 2003). Major challenges for all species are how to prioritize food-seeking activity and regulate food intake, and how to avoid wasting any temporary energy excess, so that it can be stored efficiently in anticipation of future needs and rapidly mobilized as required.

Modern humans, especially in a westernized setting, are an exception to many of the fundamental rules that apply to lower species. The ready availability of energy-dense food, in addition to the social and other pressures that restrict physical activity, present important challenges to our regulatory mechanisms. Human obesity has a major genetic component, which varies markedly between individuals. In most cases, obesity is attributable to multiple genes, which individually have only small effects and which interact variably with environmental factors (Saunders *et al.*, 2007). Genetic adaptation to our environment occurs very slowly, perhaps over at least 25000 years; the dramatic increases in the prevalence of obesity over 50 years or less must be related primarily to changes in lifestyle, because the gene pool will barely have changed during this period. At the same time, however, many individuals have remained lean, suggesting that specific features of their energy homeostatic mechanisms and/or cognitive behaviour can effectively protect them against obesity.

This chapter will focus on the normal physiology of energy balance in non-obese humans, addressing the control of food intake and the various components of energy expenditure. The final section considers the influence of obesity on energy expenditure and overall energy balance.

Energy balance

It is self-evident that obesity results from a failure of homeostatic mechanisms that regulate body weight. Positive energy balance develops when energy intake exceeds its expenditure, and excess energy is then stored in the form of triglycerides, predominantly in adipose tissue.

The first law of thermodynamics states that energy can neither be created nor destroyed, but can only be transformed from one form into another. Although incontrovertible, this law describes the overall handling of energy. Understanding the complexities of human energy balance and obesity requires a more integrated and holistic approach. Various factors need to be considered, for example that both energy intake and expenditure may be influenced by changes in body energy stores; that voluntary energy intake may rise with increasing levels of physical activity; and that food intake itself may affect energy expenditure. These aspects are discussed below.

Energy intake

Humans, like rats and other mammals, are meal feeders. The amount of food ingested is generally 2000–2500 kcal/day (8.5–10.7 MJ/day), but may range between 0 and 5000 kcal/day (21 MJ/day), depending on the degree of hyperphagia and physical activity. Research on food intake in humans is complicated because habitual intake is not easily measured. It is now well recognized that energy and especially fat intake is under-reported, in particular by obese people (Goris, Westerterp-Plantenga and Westerterp, 2000). This systematic bias in self-reported food intake data can invalidate studies that rely solely on these measures

Obesity: Science to Practice   Edited by Gareth Williams and Gema Frühbeck
© 2009 John Wiley & Sons, Ltd

(see Chapter 3). The extent of this is highlighted by the report on Diet Nutrition and the Prevention of Chronic Diseases from the WHO FAO (Food and Agriculture Organization) (WHO/FAO, 2003). This showed that edible fat production (and thus available food energy) has risen steadily over the past decades – for example the available fat per capita in the USA increased from 117 to 143 g/day between 1967 and 1997. During the same period, the average self-reported fat intake, as estimated from questionnaires and interviews, hardly changed; although wastage of food has increased significantly, it is unlikely to account for the increase in production, and the discrepancy is most likely to be explained by under-reporting.

It is reasonable to conclude that, at a population level, overconsumption of food occurs and this is likely to contribute to the spread of obesity. This, and the important role of the high energy density of westernized foods and drinks, is discussed further in Chapter 8.

At an individual level, human feeding behaviour is heavily influenced by psychological, economic and social factors (see Chapter 8). In modern society, these effectively override the physiological mechanisms in the brain and periphery that have been shown to regulate energy balance in rodents and other mammals. Nevertheless, cases of human obesity (albeit rare) have recently been identified who have specific genetic defects affecting some of these mechanisms, indicating that these pathways also serve a basic regulatory function in humans (see Chapter 8). Some of these conditions are described below, and in more detail in Chapter 6. Novel factors implicated in appetite control in rodents, and which have at least some relevance to humans, include the gut peptide, ghrelin (Otto *et al.*, 2005), the hypothalamic peptide, orexin A (Dhillo, 2007), and the endogenous cannabinoids (Harrold and Williams, 2003).

Control of energy intake

The main brain areas responsible for regulating energy balance are the hypothalamus and brain stem (see Chapter 6). These receive numerous central and peripheral inputs, including nutritional signals from the body that convey information about current energy stores and fat mass.

There have been many developments in recent years in understanding the central control of food intake. Much of our knowledge derives from experiments in laboratory animals, including the ablation or stimulation of specific areas in the hypothalamus and other key brain regions

(Hillebrand, de Wied and Adan, 2002; Dulloo, 2005). A long-standing proposal is that specific hypothalamic centres are crucial to the control of feeding behaviour, with the ventromedial hypothalamus (VMH) implicated in satiety, the lateral hypothalamic area (LHA) involved in initiating feeding, and the paraventricular nucleus (PVN) acting as an integrating centre that is important in terminating feeding. These centres serve to analyse and integrate a wide range of afferent sensory signals, both neural (especially from the gut, via the vagus nerve) and circulating nutrients or hormones (such as leptin, insulin and ghrelin). These centres are undoubtedly important, but many other hypothalamic and extrahypothalamic areas are now known to be involved in the control of food intake and energy balance.

Molecular and genetic studies over the past decade have led to significant advances in understanding the neurochemical basis of some of these pathways (see Table 7.1). Orexigenic pathways, which stimulate food intake, include specific hypothalamic neuronal populations that express neuropeptide Y (NPY) and agouti-related peptide (AgRP), and others that express melanin concentrating hormone (MCH) and orexin A. The endocannabinoids, lipids synthesized in the brain and gut, also stimulate feeding (Hillebrand, de Wied and Adan, 2002; Dulloo, 2005; Trayhurn, 2005). By contrast, anorexigenic pathways, which decrease feeding, have also been defined. The most important appears to be the hypothalamic neurones expressing the melanocortin precursor, POMC; others include neurones producing corticotrophin-releasing factor (CRF) (Hillebrand, de Wied and Adan, 2002; Dulloo, 2005; Bhattacharya *et al.*, 2005; Larsen and Hunter, 2006). Much effort is currently being directed towards defining these networks, their interactions, and the operational hierarchies that govern overall energy homeostasis.

Several peripheral signals that influence these central pathways have been identified (see Chapters 4 and 6). The best characterized is leptin, a cytokine peptide that is secreted principally by white adipose tissue. Leptin secretion and plasma concentrations increase broadly in proportion to body fat mass in mammals, including humans; leptin can therefore signal the body's energy stores to the brain, although its secretion is also regulated by other short-term nutritional and endocrine factors (see below). In rodents, leptin has been shown to act via receptors in the hypothalamus to reduce food intake (Arch, 2005). In addition, leptin increases energy

Table 7.1 Some important orexigenic (appetite-stimulating) and anorexigenic (appetite-suppressing) neurotransmitters that influence feeding behaviour in rodents.

	Site of production	Site of action	Receptors
Orexigenic neurotransmitters:			
• Neuropeptide Y (NPY)	Hypothalamus	Hypothalamus	Y5, Y1
• Melanin-concentrating hormone (MHC)	Hypothalamus	Hypothalamus	MCH-1R, MCH-2R
• Orexin A	Hypothalamus	Hypothalamus	OX-1R
• Endocannabinoids	Hypothalamus and elsewhere	Hypothalamus and elsewhere	CB-1
Anorexigenic neurotransmitters:			
• α-MSH	Hypothalamus	Hypothalamus	MC-4R, MC-3R
• CRF	Hypothalamus	Hypothalamus	CRF-2
• Serotonin (5HT)	Raphe nuclei	Hypothalamus	$5HT_{1A}$, $5HT_{2c}$

expenditure in rodents by increasing the activity of the sympathetic nervous system (SNS) outflow to thermogenic tissues and by stimulating locomotor activity (Hukshorn and Saris, 2004).

Leptin affects food intake through its interactions with various orexigenic and anorexigenic pathways in the hypothalamus and elsewhere (Trayhurn, 2005; Trayhurn and Bing, 2006; see Chapter 6) (Figure 7.1). Thus, the NPY/AgRP, MCH, orexin A and endocannabinoid systems are each reported to be inhibited by leptin, whereas the anorexigenic systems (POMC and CRF) are up-regulated by the hormone. These combined effects of leptin lead to the powerful suppression

of feeding and the mobilization of body fat stores—experimental actions which originally led to its being named 'leptin' (from the Greek for 'thin').

Leptin is not the only signal that indicates the extent of the body's triglyceride stores to the hypothalamus. There has been a resurgence of interest in the role of insulin as a potential adiposity signal and central regulator of food intake and energy balance. Insulin is secreted by the pancreatic β cells in response to glucose and numerous other stimuli, and its basal circulating levels are generally proportional to body fat mass. Like leptin, insulin enters the hypothalamus and

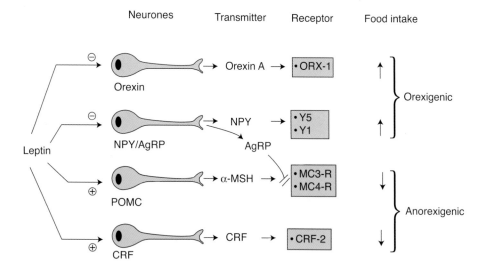

Figure 7.1 The role of leptin in regulating food intake and energy balance. Leptin decreases feeding through its central effects on the hypothalamus and other brain regions, where it inhibits orexigenic (appetite-stimulating) neuronal pathways and stimulates anorexigenic (appetite-suppressing) pathways. See also Table 7.1.

other regulatory brain regions, where it interacts with autonomic circuits that control feeding and meal size; similarly, it inhibits NPY/AgRP neurones while stimulating the anorexigenic POMC system. In rodents, selective knockout of insulin receptors in the brain leads to overeating and weight gain, indicating that insulin also acts tonically to limit food intake and adiposity; in humans, its role remains speculative (see Chapter 6).

Leptin and insulin levels are broadly correlated with body fat mass, but show rapid falls during starvation and early increases during re-feeding, suggesting that their circulating concentrations are not regulated solely by changes in body fat content. Indeed, these circulating levels may be a function of changes in the flux of energy intake and in fat mobilization and storage, rather than a classical 'lipostatic' signal that simply reflects the degree of repletion or depletion of fat stores (Dulloo, 2005).

Shorter-term signals also influence food intake. Postprandial satiety and hunger are not apparently mediated primarily by leptin. Instead, neural and endocrine signalling from the gut is believed to be important in the short-term regulation of appetite (Chapter 6). The progression of food through the stomach and small intestine initiates a sequence of peripheral satiety signals that are thought to control and ultimately terminate the feeding episode, as well as preparing for the interval before the next meal.

These satiety signals are both neural and endocrine (Figure 7.2). Mechanoreceptors, stretch and chemoreceptors that respond to the products of digestion (sugars, fatty acids, amino acids and peptides) in the gastrointestinal tract signal through the vagus nerve to the brain stem (the nucleus of the solitary tract (NTS)), and thence to the hypothalamus. These neural signals are integrated centrally with various hormones released by the gut and its associated structures, notably the pancreas. These gut hormones may either stimulate ascending vagal pathways from the gut to the brain stem (e.g. cholecystokinin, CCK), or travel in the bloodstream to act directly on target neurones in the brain. The endocrine signals generated by the gut that are believed to play important roles on food intake in rodents include:

- Cholecystokinin, released from the small intestine into the circulation in response to luminal fatty acids, and which in turn decreases meal size by acting on vagal sensory endings in the

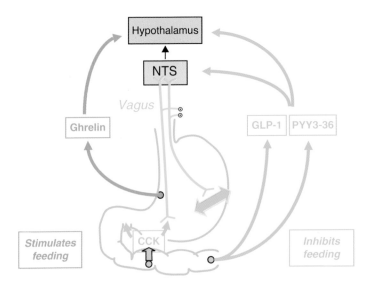

Figure 7.2 Signals generated by the gut that influence feeding in rodents and humans. Vagal afferent nerves convey both gastric distension (sensed by mechanoreceptors in the stomach wall) and satiety signals from cholecystokinin (CCK), released when food enters the duodenum. Vagal afferents synapse in the nucleus of the solitary tract (NTS) in the hindbrain, an important integrating centre for neural and circulating information about nutritional state, which projects to the hypothalamus. Ghrelin, released by the stomach between meals, stimulates hunger, whereas GLP-1 and PYY$_{3-36}$ are released from the small intestine after eating and induce satiety. See Chapter 6 for further details.

gut. CCK receptor mutations are a rare cause of human obesity, implying that the peptide serves a physiological role in mediating satiety in humans (Chapters 6 and 8).

- Peptides that are released postprandially and have been shown to reduce appetite in humans as well as rodents, including gastric inhibitory peptide (GIP), glucagon-like peptide-1 (GLP-1), and PYY_{3-36}.
- The growth hormone secretagogue, ghrelin, released into the circulation from the stomach, which increases sensations of hunger and food intake in humans.

These gut hormones and their significance in human obesity are reviewed in more detail by Murphy and Bloom (2006), and in Chapter 6.

Energy expenditure

Definition and components

The chemical processes that underlie life and bodily functions require the continuous provision of energy, which is supplied by the high-energy bonds within adenosine triphosphate (ATP). ATP levels and availability are maintained mainly by the oxidation of the major fuels, glucose and fatty acids, to carbon dioxide and water. In the short term, fuel utilization and ATP production may occur anaerobically (e.g. by the production of lactate from glucose), but the capacity of this source and therefore its duration of supply are limited.

The conversion of available food energy is not an efficient process; indeed, about 75% of the chemical energy contained in foods may ultimately be dissipated as heat because of inefficiencies in the intermediary metabolic processes that transform food energy into ATP. The chemical energy obtained from food may be used for chemical work (i.e. the synthesis of new macromolecules), for the mechanical work of muscular contraction, or for electrical work such as maintaining ionic gradients across cell membranes (Figure 7.3).

The overall process through which fuel energy is converted to ATP and subsequently used in various metabolic processes, or is lost as heat, is referred to as energy expenditure. Because of the close relationship of energy expenditure to the body's metabolic processes, the terms 'energy expenditure' and 'metabolic rate' are used synonymously (Farshchi *et al.*, 2005).

Energy content of macronutrients

There are important differences in the amount of oxygen used and in the energy released when different macronutrients are used as metabolic fuels (Table 7.2). The oxidation of fat yields over twice as much energy (9 kcal/g) as the oxidation of carbohydrates or proteins (4 kcal/g). Furthermore, for a given amount of energy expenditure, more oxygen is needed when using fat as a substrate, as compared with carbohydrate or protein. Moreover, the ratio of carbon dioxide produced to oxygen consumed – the respiratory quotient

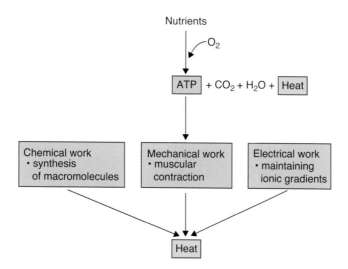

Figure 7.3 Ultimate uses and fate of chemical energy generated by the oxidation of food.

Table 7.2 Products of the oxidation of macro-nutrients. Adapted from Frayn and Macdonald (1997)

Glucose

1 g of glucose + 0.747 L O_2 = 0.747 L of CO_2 + 0.6 g H_2O + 15.15 kJ

- RQ = 1.0
- Energy content = 15.15 kJ/g (3.57 kcal/g)
- Energy release = 20.83 kJ (4.90 kcal) per L O_2

Triglyceride

1 g of fat + 2.023 L O_2 = 1.436 L CO_2 + 1.07 g H_2O + 39.63 kJ

- RQ = 0.71
- Energy content = 39.63 kJ/g (9.32 kcal/g)
- Energy release = 19.59 kJ (4.60 kcal) per L O_2

Protein

1 g of protein + 1.031 L O_2 = 0.859 L CO_2 + 0.403 g H_2O + (urea, ammonia and creatinine) + 19.72 kJ/g

- RQ = 0.833
- Energy content = 19.72 kJ/g (4.61 kcal/g)
- Energy release = 19.13 kJ (4.51 kcal) per L O_2

(RQ) – differs between the macronutrient substrates, being highest (1.0) for carbohydrate, and lowest (0.7) for fat.

Measurement of respiratory gas exchange by indirect calorimetry enables energy expenditure to be estimated, while the RQ value provides an indication of the principal substrates used (Murgatroyd, Shetty and Prentice, 1993; see Chapter 3). Note that an RQ of >1.0 indicates net lipogenesis, whereas an RQ of <0.7 occurs in ketogenesis.

Components of energy expenditure

Total energy expenditure (TEE) comprises three main components (Figure 7.4):

- Resting energy expenditure (REE) is that required for core body functions, and is measured at complete rest after an overnight fast and in a thermoneutral environment.
- The thermic effect of food, which is the energy required to digest, absorb and assimilate ingested nutrients.
- Activity thermogenesis, that is the energy expended by skeletal muscle contraction,

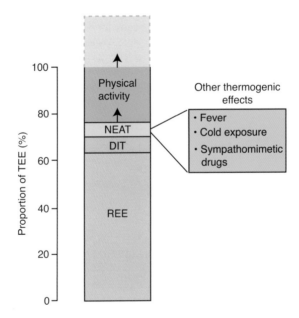

Figure 7.4 Components of energy expenditure in humans. Resting energy expenditure (REE) normally accounts for about two-thirds of total energy expenditure (TEE). Physical activity is the most variable component, while non-exercise activity thermogenesis (NEAT) comprises involuntary activities such as maintaining posture and fidgeting. Thermogenesis can be increased by various factors, including sympathomimetic drugs and catecholamines, fever and cold exposure.

which can be divided into exercise and non-exercise activity thermogenesis (NEAT).

The proportion of energy spent on physical activity depends on the type, intensity and duration of the various activities. In sedentary, non-obese people, the energy expended through physical activity accounts for only 20–40% of the daily total. In addition, energy expenditure can be increased further by thermogenic drugs (e.g. sympathomimetic agents), diseases such as thyrotoxicosis (which enhances sympathetic activity) and febrile illnesses, and by cold exposure. Conversely, energy expenditure falls in hypothyroidism, even subclinical.

Total energy expenditure rises as BMI increases (Figure 7.5), largely because REE is related to body size and specifically fat-free mass (FFM), which also increases in obesity. Therefore, energy expenditure is greater in obese than in lean subjects, and at stable weight, energy intake in the obese must also be greater than in the lean in order to maintain the higher weight (see Chapter 3).

Resting energy expenditure (REE)

In most individuals, REE is the major component of energy expenditure, accounting for about 60% of the total in a sedentary person. The REE is measured after an overnight fast and 30 minutes of supine rest; it is more convenient and appropriate as an assessment of the basal level of metabolism than the basal metabolic rate (BMR), which is measured under stricter and more demanding conditions (see Chapter 3) and is of limited value when considering energy expenditure in relation to obesity. REE includes the expenditure of energy to maintain membrane potentials, resting cardiorespiratory function, basal protein turnover and body temperature.

Body size, in particular FFM, is the main predictor of REE, and explains 60–85% of the variance in energy expenditure (Nelson et al., 1992). FFM is in turn influenced by weight, height, age and gender. Most, but not all, of the variance in REE disappears after correcting for FFM, but FFM is dominated by highly metabolically active organs (see below) and so tends to overestimate REE to a variable degree.

The brain, liver, heart and kidneys are collectively responsible for most (70–80%) of the total REE, even though they comprise only 7% of total body weight (Gallagher et al., 1998). Indeed, the brain's basal glucose consumption (as its primary metabolic fuel under normal conditions) accounts for about 80% of the body's total glucose requirement of 6.5–7.5 g/h in the resting, fasted state. There are strong correlations between the metabolic rate of these organs and total energy expenditure (McClave and Snider, 2001). By contrast, muscle mass generally accounts for almost 90% of the total organ mass and 45% of the FFM, but for only 20% of the REE (Weinsier, Schutz and Bracco, 1992). Although adipose tissue has a relatively high mass (15–30% of body weight), its contribution to whole-body energy expenditure is only 3–5% (Elia, 1996) (Table 7.3). Different studies have variously shown that the individual variance in REE correlates most closely with the combined mass of brain and skeletal muscle (Gallagher et al., 1998),

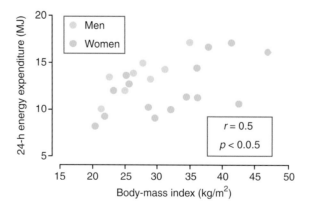

Figure 7.5 Energy expenditure increases with rising BMI. REE is largely determined by fat-free mass (FFM), which rises in parallel with fat mass in obesity. From Ravussin et al. (1982) *American Journal of Clinical Nutrition*, **35**: 566–73, with kind permission of the editor.

Table 7.3 Contribution of organs and tissues to resting energy expenditure and body weight of a non-obese man.

Tissue	Tissue metabolic rate (% of REE)	Tissue weight (% of total body weight)
Adipose	4	21.4
Muscle	22	40.0
Liver	21	2.6
Brain	22	2.0
Heart	9	0.5
Kidneys	8	0.5
Other (includes bone, skin, intestine and glands)	16	33.1

From: Elia (1996) 'Fuel of the tissues', in J.S. Garrow, W.P.T. James and A. Ralph (eds), *Human Nutrition and Dietetics*, 10th edn. Churchill Livingstone, Edinburgh, pp. 37–59.

or skeletal muscle and liver (Illner *et al.*, 2000), or the liver alone (Sparti *et al.*, 1997). These apparent discrepancies are probably explained by technical differences in measuring organ mass, and in individual variability due to age, sex and size.

In general, fasting REE is approximately 0.021 kcal per kg of FFM per minute. Thus, a typical subject weighing 75 kg with an FFM of 63 kg (corresponding to a fat mass of 16% of body weight) will have a fasting REE of approximately 1.3 kcal/min (5.5 kJ/min). Some variation in the metabolic activity of FFM occurs due to individual differences in the composition of the tissue. The above factors do not wholly account for variance in REE, which may also be partly genetically determined (Bogardus *et al.*, 1986).

Some representative levels of energy expenditure, for a healthy but generally sedentary adult undertaking various activities, are shown in Table 7.4.

Thermic effect of food

The ingestion of food is associated with increases in oxygen consumption and in energy expenditure, which with normal diets, amounts to 8–10% of total energy intake. This phenomenon, first observed over 200 years ago by Lavoisier, has been given various terms; the most appropriate are the 'thermic effect of food' (TEF) (Weaver *et al.*, 2006), and 'diet-induced thermogenesis'. TEF can be divided into an obligatory component, related to the energy costs of the absorption and metabolic processing of nutrients, and a facultative component

that may be partly due to the sensory aspects of foods (smell and taste) and partly to stimulation of the SNS.

The major determinant of TEF is the energy content and particularly the protein content of the test meal (Reed and Hill, 1996; Donahoo, Levine and Melanson, 2004). Also, a high-carbohydrate meal produces a higher TEF than an isoenergetic meal high in fat. It has been shown that administration of glucose (orally or intravenously) stimulates energy expenditure by the equivalent of 7–10% of the amount of glucose stored (Thiebaud *et al.*, 1983), whereas triglyceride infusion increases energy expenditure by only an amount equivalent to 2% of the fat stored (Thiebaud *et al.*, 1983). However, these effects

Table 7.4 Energy costs of various physical activities.

Activity	Energy expenditure	
	kJ/min	kcal/min
Sleeping	4.5	1.1
Sitting	5.0	1.2
Standing	6.0	1.4
Brisk walking (6.4 km/h)	30	7.1
Running (8 km/h)	43	10.0
Cycling (16 km/h)	30	7.1
Swimming (25 m/min)	28	6.7
Shovelling snow	67	15.7

Values are for a non-obese 70-kg individual. Adapted from (Dulloo, 2005).

are not always clearly demonstrated when foods are ingested (Kinabo and Durnin, 1990).

The type of fat and carbohydrate may also have significant effects on TEF. Ingestion of fructose or sucrose produces a higher thermogenic response than glucose (Blaak and Saris, 1996). A meal containing medium-chain fatty acids has a greater TEF than one containing long-chain fatty acids or saturated fat (Ogawa *et al.*, 2007; Scalfi, Coltorti and Contaldo, 1991).

In addition, the type of meal affects TEF, with solid food producing a greater response than homogenized liquids (Leblanc, 1985). This has been attributed to solid food being more palatable and therefore producing a stronger hedonic response that activates the SNS; however, some studies have not reported a higher SNS response after solid food as compared with a liquid test meal (Farshchi *et al.*, 2005). Large meals may increase the thermogenic response for several hours, which makes it difficult to measure their total impact.

Cold exposure

In lower mammals, chronic exposure to cold is associated with an increase in energy expenditure. In the cold-exposed rat, energy expenditure is initially increased through shivering, but is soon replaced by non-shivering thermogenesis due to SNS-induced activation of brown adipose tissue (BAT) and other heat-producing tissues (see Chapter 4). Present-day humans rarely need to increase their heat production for the purposes of thermal regulation, because they can wear appropriate clothing or seek a warmer environment. As with energy intake, large inter-individual differences in energy expenditure in the response to cold have been reported. After a 24-h exposure to a temperature of 16 °C (from a baseline of 22 °C), total daily energy expenditure increased on average by 190 kcal (0.82 MJ); however, individuals ranged between 35 and 340 kcal/day (0.15 and 1.45 MJ/day) (van Marken Lichtenbelt *et al.*, 2002). Similar results have been found on decreasing ambient temperature from 28 to 22 °C (Warwick and Busby, 1990).

A recent study in humans indicated that the variability in cold-induced thermogenesis is highly correlated with that in diet-induced thermogenesis, suggesting that there are common underlying mechanisms (Wijers, Saris and van Marken Lichtenbelt, 2007). These could include, in both humans and small mammals, uncoupling of oxidative phosphorylation in mitochondria, protein turnover, 'futile' cycling within metabolic pathways, and non-exercise activity thermogenesis (NEAT). It is also clear that the SNS plays an important role in this adaptive thermogenesis.

Activity thermogenesis

Non-exercise activity thermogenesis (NEAT)

NEAT describes the low level of involuntary physical activity, which is spontaneous and subconscious, and is distinct from voluntary exercise; these activities including maintaining posture and muscle tone, and fidgeting. Several factors affect NEAT, such as occupation, age, genetic background, body composition and seasonal variations.

NEAT varies widely among subjects, and the difference can amount to 300 kcal or more of total daily energy expenditure – enough to influence susceptibility to long-term weight gain. Indeed, variations in NEAT have been reported to account for differences in fat gain between individuals, with the suggestion that NEAT is activated when humans overeat and thus helps to dissipate excess energy, whereas subjects who fail to increase NEAT will gain weight (Frühbeck, 2007).

The importance of NEAT in weight regulation is highlighted by findings that, even when subjects are confined to a metabolic chamber, the 24-h energy expenditure attributed to NEAT (as assessed by radar systems) was found to vary between 94 and 700 kcal (0.4 and 3 MJ), and also predicted subsequent weight gain in the longer term. In one study, where 12 pairs of twins were overfed by 1000 kcal per day, differences in NEAT were implicated in the fourfold variation in the weight gain that followed (Bouchard *et al.*, 1990). When positive energy balance is imposed through overfeeding, NEAT increases, and may account for more than 60% of the rise in total daily energy expenditure; again, the change in NEAT was found to be the most significant predictor of increase in fat mass (Levine, Eberhardt and Jensen, 1999). Those who do not increase their NEAT with overfeeding gain the most fat (Figure 7.6). It should, however, be emphasized that NEAT could also reflect post-exercise or post-activity stimulation of thermogenesis. Further studies are warranted to investigate the underlying mechanisms for NEAT and its overall relevance to human energy balance.

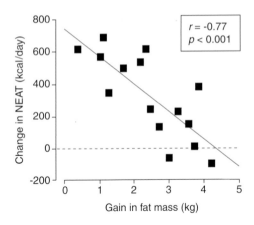

Figure 7.6 Inverse relationship between NEAT and gain in fat mass during experimental overfeeding in humans. From C. Bouchard, A. Tremblay, J.P. Després *et al.* (1990) 'The response to long-term overfeeding in identical twins'. *New England Journal of Medicine*, **322**(21): 1477–82, with kind permission of the editor.

Energy expenditure through physical activity

Physical activity makes a highly variable contribution to daily energy expenditure, representing up to 70% of the total for competitive athletes or for those involved in heavy manual labour. However, most individuals in developed populations are now so sedentary that physical activity accounts for less than 30% of total daily energy expenditure. The decline in physical activity has undoubtedly contributed to the rising prevalence of obesity, and low levels of physical activity are also an independent risk factor for the development of diabetes and cardiovascular disease (see Chapters 8 and 10).

Attempts to increase physical activity are an important strategy in public health efforts to reduce obesity and diabetes (Knowler *et al.*, 2002; Tuomilehto *et al.*, 2001; Mensink *et al.*, 2003; see Chapter 22). A recent study has indicated that the positive effects of enhanced physical activity extend beyond the improvements in fitness and fatness, in that increased physical activity reduced fasting triglyceride and insulin concentrations and postprandial glucose, independent of changes in fat mass (Ekelund *et al.*, 2007).

The energy spent on physical activity depends on its type, intensity and duration. Physical activity is often considered to be synonymous with muscular work, which has a strict definition in physics (i.e. force x distance), where work is performed on the environment. During muscular work, muscle produces three times more heat than mechanical energy, and this considerably increases the total energy costs of exercise. There is wide variation in the energy costs for given activities between and within individuals, partly due to differences in body size and the speed with which the activity is performed. Any weight-bearing activity (such as walking, running or climbing) demands energy expenditure that is proportional to body weight at the speed of movement. By contrast, activities such as swimming, rowing and to some extent cycling, are less affected by body weight.

To adjust for differences in body size, energy expended during physical activities is commonly expressed as multiples of REE (Durnin, 1991). During moderate exercise, energy expenditure generally increases by up to fivefold, but can reach values of 10- to 14-fold during intense exercise. With learning and training, the efficiency of movements improves, so that the energy expenditure required for a given activity declines; however, this effect is small and unlikely to change overall energy expenditure by more than a small percentage (Dulloo, 2005).

The 'physical activity level' (PAL) is the standard method for expressing the overall impact of exercise on total daily energy expenditure, and is defined as: PAL = TEE/REE. PAL generally ranges from 1.4 for a sedentary person to 2.0 for someone who is physically active. Measurements of energy expenditure during rest and exercise are described in Chapter 3.

Mechanisms for adaptive thermogenesis

Adaptive thermogenesis describes changes in energy expenditure that occur in response to alterations in energy balance. In theory, individual differences in adaptive thermogenesis could contribute to susceptibility to obesity.

Ever since studies into the mechanisms of diet-induced thermogenesis (DIT) began in 1960, attention has focused on the SNS, which plays an important role in energy expenditure and substrate utilization in mammals, including humans (van Baak, 2001). The catecholamines, noradrenaline and adrenaline, are crucial in the regulation of energy expenditure. This is because they increase cellular oxygen uptake and stimulate the conversion of complex fuels into readily available substrates through the processes of lipolysis, glycogenolysis and gluconeogenesis.

Both catecholamines have been shown to be potent stimuli for increasing metabolic rate (Blaak, Saris and van Baak, 1993). Moreover, in some circumstances the β-adrenoceptor antagonist propranolol may reduce the thermogenic response due to glucose (Thorin et al., 1986) or to food, and can reduce resting energy expenditure (Welle, Schwartz and Statt, 1991), suggesting that several components of energy expenditure may be partly controlled by the SNS (Farshchi et al., 2005). However, data are not entirely consistent, because β-adrenoceptor blockade does not always reduce the TEF response (Nacht et al., 1987).

The site of sympathetically-mediated thermogenesis is still debated. In rats, brown adipose tissue (BAT) has been shown to be an important source site of heat production, through 'uncoupling' of mitochondrial respiration (i.e. oxidizing free fatty acids, but without producing ATP) via uncoupling protein-1 (UCP-1) (Dulloo, Seydoux and Jacquet, 2004). As described in Chapter 4, BAT receives a dense sympathetic innervation, and noradrenaline acts on β_3 adrenoceptors to up-regulate UCP-1 and hormone-sensitive lipase, thus increasing the supply of fatty acids for oxidation. Sympathetic stimulation also enhances BAT blood flow, thus dissipating the heat generated.

Studies in humans have shown that skeletal muscle may be an important thermogenic tissue, explaining over 50% of the increase in oxygen consumption during sympathetic stimulation (Blaak et al., 1994). BAT is present in the human neonate but its relevance in most adult humans has been believed to be marginal (Chapter 4). Interestingly, recent studies using PET scanning have indicated that metabolically active BAT may also be present in adults ((Nedergaard, Bengtsson and Cannon, 2007); see Figure 7.7). However, the functional significance of these small depots remains to be determined.

Other mitochondrial uncoupling proteins have recently been discovered, notably UCP2 and UCP3. However, these uncoupling proteins may not be a significant site for adaptive thermogenesis in tissues other than BAT (Dulloo, Seydoux and Jacquet, 2004). In addition to uncoupling of mitochondrial respiration from ATP production,

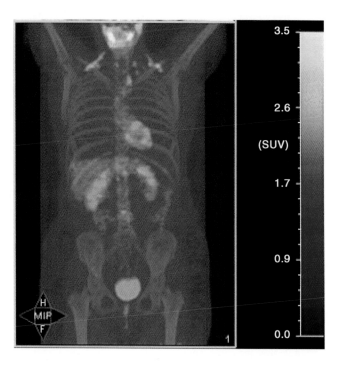

Figure 7.7 PET scan of a normal adult, showing discrete areas of increased metabolic activity in the fat of the upper thorax and neck, which are thought to correspond to functionally active brown adipose tissue (BAT). Other organs with high metabolic activity are the heart, kidneys and liver; residual isotope (fluorodeoxyglucose) is also seen in the bladder. Images courtesy of Dr MJ García Velloso, Department of Nuclear Medicine, Clínica Universitaria de Navarra, Pamplona, Spain.

there are numerous other thermogenic mechanisms – including futile cycling and increased sodium pump activity – which may contribute to sympathetically-mediated thermogenesis.

It is of interest that not all nutrients produce thermogenic responses in the same tissues or organs. Infusion of amino acids increases whole-body energy expenditure by 19%, with half of this increase occurring in the splanchnic tissues (Aksnes *et al.*, 1995). By contrast, the stimulation of energy expenditure due to ingestion of glucose or fructose has no contribution from the splanchnic tissues (Brundin and Wahren, 1993), but may take place mostly in skeletal muscle (Blaak *et al.*, 1992).

Altered sympathetic activity in obesity

Since the demonstration by Landsberg and Young (1978) and Young (2006) of reduced sympathetic activity in rats during fasting, there has been great interest in the possibility that decreased sympathoadrenal activity might contribute to the development of obesity. Conversely, the use of sympathomimetic drugs to stimulate energy expenditure has been explored as a possible therapeutic approach in obesity (see Chapter 17).

The level of sympathetic activity in obese subjects remains controversial. It is widely held that certain aspects of sympathetic activity are increased in obesity and could contribute to abnormalities such as hypertension and insulin resistance. Overall, however, roughly similar numbers of studies have shown reduced, unchanged or increased SNS activity in obese people as compared with lean subjects (Macdonald, 1995). Additionally, a reduction in sympathetically-mediated thermogenesis has been demonstrated in some obese subjects, although data are not entirely consistent (van Baak, 2001). As discussed in Chapter 8, some studies suggest that a low REE may predict excessive weight gain, but the contribution of SNS activity to this is uncertain.

There is some evidence for a link between SNS activity and the TEF response to a meal in younger subjects but this may not apply to older subjects (Schwartz, Jaeger and Veith, 1990). Diet composition may affect indices of sympathetic activity such as fasting noradrenaline concentrations, with sucrose-rich diets producing greater responses than high-fat or high-starch diets; in parallel, an increase in energy expenditure was observed with the high-sucrose diets (Raben, Macdonald and Astrup, 1997). Further studies will be necessary to clarify the impact of diet composition on SNS activity and related energy expenditure.

Obesity and adaptive thermogenesis

There is ongoing debate about whether obesity is associated with an increased efficiency of cellular metabolism and thus reduced energy expenditure, and the extent to which this might contribute to a positive energy balance and the development or maintenance of excessive adipose tissue stores.

An important cause of controversy in this context concerns the components of energy expenditure that might be affected by changes in metabolic efficiency and hence contribute to adaptive thermogenesis. Some studies of heat production in the resting state suggest that changes in fat-free mass and fat mass may not fully account for alterations in energy expenditure following weight change, and this may be an indication of adaptive thermogenesis (Major *et al.*, 2007).

Also, part of the thermic effect of food may not be explained by the obligatory costs of food absorption and nutrient assimilation, and may instead be due to a component that has been referred to as 'facultative thermogenesis'. A defect in this component of heat production could, in theory, predispose to obesity. The literature is replete with studies on the thermic effects of food in obesity. de Jonge and Bray (2002) evaluated 49 studies that compared TEF between obese and lean subjects. Of the 29 studies in which obese subjects had a significantly higher BMI than the lean but were well matched for age, 22 reported a significantly lower TEF in obesity. Granata and Brandon (2002) endorse the theory that TEF is reduced in obesity, yet discrepant findings persist in the literature, and numerous flaws have been uncovered in the methods used to measure and calculate TEF. These discrepancies may be explained, at least in part, by failing to control for age differences, the degree of obesity and the difference in BMI between obese and control groups, the presence of insulin resistance and the subjects' habitual diet composition.

Variations in the macronutrient composition of the test meal may also contribute.

It has been suggested that diet composition may affect thermogenic responses; in one study, no differences were found in glucose or fat-induced thermogenesis between lean and obese subjects, but fat-induced thermogenesis was reduced in obese subjects (Swaminathan et al., 1985). This finding was confirmed in a recent study, which also showed that reduced fat-induced thermogenesis in obese subjects was independent of body composition, age, gender or REE (Blaak et al., 2007). In addition, insulin resistance, habitual physical activity, postprandial triglyceride and insulin levels were all independently positively related to the magnitude of fat-induced thermogenesis.

Differences in heat production through non-exercise activity thermogenesis (NEAT) are more difficult to quantify. The most direct evidence that NEAT might contribute to adaptive thermogenesis comes from studies in the eight men and women who participated in the Biosphere-2 experiment, a self-contained ecologic 'mini-world' and prototype planetary habitat built in Arizona. As result of an unexpected shortage of food, the subjects lost 8–25% of body weight over a 2-year period, and this was found to be accompanied by significant reductions in adjusted 24-h energy expenditure (by 6%) and spontaneous activity (45%). Six months after exit and returning to a free diet, body weight had increased to pre-entry levels, while adjusted 24-h energy expenditure and spontaneous physical activity were still significantly reduced as compared with control subjects (Weyer et al., 2000). These findings may have implications for the obese individual, in that weight loss may be accompanied by metabolic alterations (e.g. decreased NEAT) that make it difficult to maintain the lower weight.

A study by Leibel, Rosenbaum and Hirsch (1995), also performed under circumstances of marked manipulation of energy intake and weight change, contributed significantly to the concept of adaptive thermogenesis. This study defined the changes in energy expenditure as a result of 10% weight gain or of 10–20% weight loss, in obese and non-obese subjects. The differences between predicted and measured energy expenditure were calculated at each weight plateau and were found to be significant. Here, obese subjects showed adaptive thermogenesis, defined as (observed − predicted TEE), which averaged −1025 kcal/day

and −1264 kJ/day following 10 and 20% body weight loss, respectively. Thus, maintenance of a reduced or elevated body weight is associated with compensatory changes in energy expenditure, which opposes the maintenance of a body weight that is different from usual weight.

Furthermore, clinical studies during weight-reduction programmes have shown that a decrease in daily energy intake averaging 470–700 kcal (2000–3000 kJ) can induce a greater fall in energy expenditure than is expected from the loss of weight. These and other studies, reviewed extensively by Major et al. (2007), suggest that the adaptive decrease in energy expenditure could be a factor that complicates long-term maintenance of weight loss. Such compensatory changes may also contribute to the poor long-term efficacy of dietary and pharmacological treatments for obesity.

Substrate oxidation and predisposition to obesity

The traditional concept of energy homeostasis implies that weight gain develops as result of a chronic positive energy imbalance. According to a model proposed by Flatt (1988; 1995), the long-term stability of body weight requires not only that energy expenditure equals intake, but also that the relative proportions of fuels oxidized are the same as those consumed. Protein and carbohydrate stores in the body are limited, and they tend to be modulated by an autoregulatory process that allows their oxidation rate to increase in response to their own oxidation (Flatt, 1988; 1995). By contrast, fat oxidation is not tightly regulated by the fat stores, and fat oxidation rises only slowly as an adaptive response to an increase in dietary fat intake. The failure to adjust fat oxidation to a high-fat diet will lead to a depletion of the body's glycogen stores by increasing carbohydrate oxidation, and it is believed that this glycogen depletion may act as a signal to increase energy intake (Flatt, 1988). Human intervention trials have shown that a greater proportion of excess energy is stored as fat during high-fat overfeeding, compared with high-carbohydrate overfeeding, and that this is due to the minimal enhancement of fat oxidation and energy expenditure during the high-fat diet (Horton et al., 1995).

Flatt and colleagues have argued that one of the mechanisms for adapting to a high-fat diet is an increase in fat mass, which rises until a new equilibrium is reached at which fat oxidation equals intake. Several studies demonstrate a positive correlation between fat mass and 24-h fat oxidation (Blaak *et al.*, 2006), although this relationship has not been confirmed in all studies (Nagy *et al.*, 1996). The interpretation of this concept of nutrient balance is that food intake may be controlled by both (short-term) 'glycogenic' and (long-term) 'lipostatic' mechanisms and that glycogen stores and fat mass both act as regulatory signals (see Chapter 6). Stubbs (1995), however, challenged this nutrient balance theory on the grounds that appetite does not increase in people who were fed a very low carbohydrate diet (high-fat) diet to deplete the glycogen stores, and that fat oxidation increased to meet energy needs. Furthermore, according to Frayn (1995), it is too simplistic to argue that protein, carbohydrate and fat balance can be considered separately, or that the complex relationship between fat and other constituents of foods in the control of energy balance can be ignored.

Despite this, there is increasing evidence that a reduced ability to use fat as a fuel may predispose some people towards developing obesity. A subgroup of obese subjects shows a blunted fat oxidation in response to a high-fat load (Blaak *et al.*, 2006; see Figure 7.8). Moreover, obese subjects adapt more slowly to a chronic high-fat diet as compared with lean individuals (Thomas *et al.*, 1992). Additionally, 'post-obese' women (i.e. who have lost weight, having previously been obese) (Astrup *et al.*, 1994), or women predisposed to develop obesity (Raben, Macdonald and Astrup, 1994), have lower postprandial and 24-h fat oxidation rates as compared with lean controls who have never been obese. Consistent with this notion, longitudinal studies in Pima Indians in Arizona have shown that those with low fat oxidation rates have a greater risk of gaining body weight over time, compared with high-fat oxidizers (Zurlo *et al.*, 1990).

A reduced ability to adjust fat oxidation to homeostatic signals, which has been defined as metabolic inflexibility of substrate oxidation, is an important characteristic of obesity and insulin resistance and may possibly be associated with reductions in mitochondrial content and/or function (Ukropcova *et al.*, 2007). Thus, the impaired ability to oxidize fat may translate into a positive energy balance over time, possibly by affecting thermogenesis and/or by affecting energy intake. Further studies will be needed to clarify the underlying mechanisms.

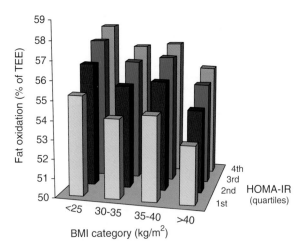

Figure 7.8 Postprandial fat oxidation (expressed as a percentage of energy expenditure) after a high fat load, in groups of subjects stratified according to BMI category and quartiles of insulin sensitivity (estimated by HOMA). All values represent means, adjusted for gender, fat mass and distribution, dietary intake, physical activity and fasting fat oxidation rate. Data are from the EU-NUGENOB study of 814 subjects across Europe (Blaak *et al.*, 2006). E.E. Blaak, G.C. Hul, Verdich *et al.* (2006) 'Fat oxidation before and after a high fat load in the obese insulin-resistant state'. *Journal of Clinical Endocrinology and Metabolism*, **91**(4): 1462–9. Reproduced with kind permission of the editor.

References

Aksnes, A.K., Brundin, T., Hjeltnes, N. and Wahren, J. (1995) Metabolic, thermal and circulatory effects of intravenous infusion of amino acids in tetraplegic patients. *Clinical Physiology*, **15** (4), 377–96.

Arch, J.R. (2005) Central regulation of energy balance: inputs, outputs and leptin resistance. *Proceedings of the Nutrition Society*, **64** (1), 39–46.

Ashrafi, K., Chang, F.Y., Watts, J.L. et al. (2003) Genome-wide RNAi analysis of *Caenorhabditis elegans* fat regulatory genes. *Nature*, **421** (6920), 268–72.

Astrup, A., Buemann, B., Christensen, N.J. and Toubro, S. (1994) Failure to increase lipid oxidation in response to increasing dietary fat content in formerly obese women. *The American Journal of Physiology*, **266** (4 Pt 1), E592–9.

Bhattacharya, A., Rahman, M.M., Sun, D. et al. (2005) The combination of dietary conjugated linoleic acid and treadmill exercise lowers gain in body fat mass and enhances lean body mass in high fat-fed male Balb/C mice. *The Journal of Nutrition*, **135** (5), 1124–30.

Blaak, E.E., Hul, G., Verdich, C. et al. (2006) Fat oxidation before and after a high fat load in the obese insulin-resistant state. *The Journal of Clinical Endocrinology and Metabolism*, **91** (4), 1462–9.

Blaak, E.E., Hul, G., Verdich, C. et al. (2007) Impaired fat-induced thermogenesis in obese subjects: the NUGENOB study. *Obesity (Silver Spring)*, **15** (3), 653–63.

Blaak, E.E. and Saris, W.H. (1996) Postprandial thermogenesis and substrate utilization after ingestion of different dietary carbohydrates. *Metabolism: Clinical and Experimental*, **45** (10), 1235–42.

Blaak, E.E., Saris, W.H. and van Baak, M.A. (1993) Adrenoceptor subtypes mediating catecholamine-induced thermogenesis in man. *International Journal of Obesity and Related Metabolic Disorders*, **17** (Suppl 3), S78–81; discussion S82.

Blaak, E.E., Van Baak, M.A., Kemerink, G.J. et al. (1994) Beta-adrenergic stimulation of energy expenditure and forearm skeletal muscle metabolism in lean and obese men. *The American Journal of Physiology*, **267** (2 Pt 1), E306–15.

Blaak, E.E., Van Baak, M.A., Kempen, K.P. and Saris, W.H. (1992) Effect of hand heating by a warm air box on O2 consumption of the contralateral arm. *Journal of Applied Physiology (Bethesda, Md: 1985)*, **72** (6), 2364–8.

Bogardus, C., Lillioja, S., Ravussin, E. et al. (1986) Familial dependence of the resting metabolic rate. *The New England Journal of Medicine*, **315** (2), 96–100.

Bouchard, C., Tremblay, A., Despres, J.P. et al. (1990) The response to long-term overfeeding in identical twins. *The New England Journal of Medicine*, **322** (21), 1477–82.

Brundin, T. and Wahren, J. (1993) Whole body and splanchnic oxygen consumption and blood flow after oral ingestion of fructose or glucose. *The American Journal of Physiology*, **264** (4 Pt 1), E504–13.

de Jonge, L. and Bray, G.A. (2002) The thermic effect of food is reduced in obesity. *Nutrition Reviews*, **60** (9), 299–300.

Dhillo, W.S. (2007) Appetite regulation: an overview. *Thyroid*, **17** (5), 433–45.

Donahoo, W.T., Levine, J.A. and Melanson, E.L. (2004) Variability in energy expenditure and its components. *Current Opinion in Clinical Nutrition and Metabolic Care*, **7** (6), 599–605.

Dulloo, A. (2005) Energy balance and body weight homeostasis, in *Clinical Obesity*, 2nd edn (eds Kopelman, P.G., Caterson, I.D. and Dietz, W.H.), Blackwell, pp. 67–80.

Dulloo, A.G., Seydoux, J. and Jacquet, J. (2004) Adaptive thermogenesis and uncoupling proteins: a reappraisal of their roles in fat metabolism and energy balance. *Physiology and Behavior*, **83** (4), 587–602.

Durnin, J.V. (1991) Practical estimates of energy requirements. *The Journal of Nutrition*, **121** (11), 1907–13.

Ekelund, U., Franks, P.W., Sharp, S. et al. (2007) Increase in physical activity energy expenditure is associated with reduced metabolic risk independent of change in fatness and fitness. *Diabetes Care*, **30** (8), 2101–6.

Elia, M., (1996) Fuel of the tissues, in *Human Nutrition and Dietetics*, 10th edn (eds J.S. Garrow, W.P.T. James and A. Ralph), Churchill Livingstone. pp. 37–59.

Farshchi, H.R., Taylor, M.A. and Macdonald, I.A. (2005) Chapter 11. Energy expenditure in humans: the influence of activity, diet and the sympathetic nervous system, in *Clinical Obesity*, 2nd edn (eds P.G. Kopelman, I.D. Caterson and W.H. Dietz), Blackwell, pp. 149–60.

Flatt, J.P. (1988) Importance of nutrient balance in body weight regulation. *Diabetes-Metabolism Reviews*, **4** (6), 571–81.

Flatt, J.P. (1995) Body composition, respiratory quotient, and weight maintenance. *The American Journal of Clinical Nutrition*, **62** (5 Suppl), 1107S–17S.

Frayn, K.N. (1995) Physiological regulation of macronutrient balance. *International Journal of Obesity and Related Metabolic Disorders*, **19** (Suppl 5), S4–10.

Frühbeck, G.F. (2005) Does a NEAT difference in energy expenditure lead to obesity? *Lancet*, **366**, 615–6.

Gallagher, D., Belmonte, D., Deurenberg, P. et al. (1998) Organ-tissue mass measurement allows modeling of REE and metabolically active tissue mass. *The American Journal of Physiology*, **275** (2 Pt 1), E249–58.

Goris, A.H., Westerterp-Plantenga, M.S. and Westerterp, K.R. (2000) Undereating and underrecording of habitual food intake in obese men: selective underreporting of fat intake. *The American Journal of Clinical Nutrition*, **71** (1), 130–4.

Granata, G.P. and Brandon, L.J. (2002) The thermic effect of food and obesity: discrepant results and methodological variations. *Nutrition Reviews*, **60** (8), 223–33.

Harrold, J.A. and Williams, G. (2003) The cannabinoid system: a role in both the homeostatic and hedonic control of eating? *The British Journal of Nutrition*, **90** (4), 729–34.

Hillebrand, J.J., de Wied, D. and Adan, R.A. (2002) Neuropeptides, food intake and body weight regulation: a hypothalamic focus. *Peptides*, **23** (12), 2283–306.

Horton, T.J., Drougas, H., Brachey, A. *et al.* (1995) Fat and carbohydrate overfeeding in humans: different effects on energy storage. *The American Journal of Clinical Nutrition*, **62** (1), 19–29.

Hukshorn, C.J. and Saris, W.H. (2004) Leptin and energy expenditure. *Current Opinion in Clinical Nutrition and Metabolic Care*, **7** (6), 629–33.

Illner, K., Brinkmann, G., Heller, M. *et al.* (2000) Metabolically active components of fat free mass and resting energy expenditure in nonobese adults. *American Journal of Physiology. Endocrinology and Metabolism*, **278** (2), E308–15.

Kinabo, J.L. and Durnin, J.V. (1990) Thermic effect of food in man: effect of meal composition, and energy content. *The British Journal of Nutrition*, **64** (1), 37–44.

Knowler, W.C., Barrett-Connor, E., Fowler, S.E. *et al.* (2002) Reduction in the incidence of type 2 diabetes with lifestyle intervention or metformin. *The New England Journal of Medicine*, **346** (6), 393–403.

Landsberg, L. and Young, J.B. (1978) Fasting, feeding and regulation of the sympathetic nervous system. *The New England Journal of Medicine*, **298** (23), 1295–301.

Larsen, P.J. and Hunter, R.G. (2006) The role of CART in body weight homeostasis. *Peptides*, **27** (8), 1981–6.

Leblanc, J. (1985) Thermogenesis in relation to feeding and exercise training. *International Journal of Obesity*, **9** (Suppl 2), 75–9.

Leibel, R.L., Rosenbaum, M. and Hirsch, J. (1995) Changes in energy expenditure resulting from altered body weight. *The New England Journal of Medicine*, **332** (10), 621–8.

Levine, J.A., Eberhardt, N.L. and Jensen, M.D. (1999) Role of nonexercise activity thermogenesis in resistance to fat gain in humans. *Science*, **283**, 212–4.

Macdonald, I.A. (1995) Advances in our understanding of the role of the sympathetic nervous system in obesity. *International Journal of Obesity and Related Metabolic Disorders*, **19** (Suppl 7), S2–7.

Major, G.C., Doucet, E., Trayhurn, P. *et al.* (2007) Clinical significance of adaptive thermogenesis. *International Journal of Obesity (London)*, **31** (2), 204–12.

McClave, S.A. and Snider, H.L. (2001) Dissecting the energy needs of the body. *Current Opinion in Clinical Nutrition and Metabolic Care*, **4** (2), 143–7.

Mensink, M., Blaak, E.E., Corpeleijn, E. *et al.* (2003) Lifestyle intervention according to general recommendations improves glucose tolerance. *Obesity Research*, **11** (12), 1588–96.

Murgatroyd, P.R., Shetty, P.S. and Prentice, A.M. (1993) Techniques for the measurement of human energy expenditure: a practical guide. *International Journal of Obesity and Related Metabolic Disorders*, **17** (10), 549–68.

Murphy, K.G. and Bloom, S.R. (2006) Gut hormones and the regulation of energy homeostasis. *Nature*, **444** (7121), 854–9.

Nacht, C.A., Christin, L., Temler, E. *et al.* (1987) Thermic effect of food: possible implication of parasympathetic nervous system. *The American Journal of Physiology*, **253** (5 Pt 1), E481–8.

Nagy, T.R., Goran, M.I., Weinsier, R.L. *et al.* (1996) Determinants of basal fat oxidation in healthy Caucasians. *Journal of Applied Physiology (Bethesda, Md: 1985)*, **80** (5), 1743–8.

Nedergaard, J., Bengtsson, T. and Cannon, B. (2007) Unexpected evidence for active brown adipose tissue in adult humans. *American Journal of Physiology. Endocrinology and Metabolism*, **293** (2), E444–52.

Nelson, K.M., Weinsier, R.L., Long, C.L. and Schutz, Y. (1992) Prediction of resting energy expenditure from fat-free mass and fat mass. *The American Journal of Clinical Nutrition*, **56** (5), 848–56.

Ogawa, A., Nosaka, N., Kasai, M. *et al.* (2007) Dietary medium- and long-chain triacylglycerols accelerate diet-induced thermogenesis in humans. *Journal of Oleo Science*, **56** (6), 283–7.

Otto, B., Spranger, J., Benoit, S.C. *et al.* (2005) The many faces of ghrelin: new perspectives for nutrition research? *The British Journal of Nutrition*, **93** (6), 765–71.

Raben, A., Andersen, H.B., Christensen, N.J. *et al.* (1994) Evidence for an abnormal postprandial response to a high-fat meal in women predisposed to obesity. *The American Journal of Physiology*, **267** (4 Pt 1), E549–59.

Raben, A., Macdonald, I. and Astrup, A. (1997) Replacement of dietary fat by sucrose or starch: effects on 14 d ad libitum energy intake, energy expenditure and body weight in formerly obese and never-obese subjects. *International Journal of Obesity and Related Metabolic Disorders*, **21** (10), 846–59.

Ravussin, E., Burnand, B., Schutz, Y., *et al.* (1982) Twenty-four-hour energy expenditure and resting metabolic rate in obese, moderately obese, and control subjects. *American Journal of Clinical Nutrition*, **35**, 566–73.

Reed, G.W. and Hill, J.O. (1996) Measuring the thermic effect of food. *The American Journal of Clinical Nutrition*, **63** (2), 164–9.

Saunders, C.L., Chiodini, B.D., Sham, P. *et al.* (2007) Meta-analysis of genome-wide linkage studies in BMI and obesity. *Obesity (Silver Spring)* **15** (9), 2263–75.

Scalfi, L., Coltorti, A. and Contaldo, F. (1991) Postprandial thermogenesis in lean and obese subjects after meals supplemented with medium-chain and long-chain triglycerides. *The American Journal of Clinical Nutrition*, **53** (5), 1130–3.

Schwartz, R.S., Jaeger, L.F. and Veith, R.C. (1990) The thermic effect of feeding in older men: the importance of the sympathetic nervous system. *Metabolism: Clinical and Experimental*, **39** (7), 733–7.

Sparti, A., DeLany, J.P., de la Bretonne, J.A. *et al.* (1997) Relationship between resting metabolic rate and the composition of the fat-free mass. *Metabolism: Clinical and Experimental*, **46** (10), 1225–30.

Stubbs, R.J. (1995) Macronutrient effects on appetite. *International Journal of Obesity and Related Metabolic Disorders*, **19** (Suppl 5), S11–9.

Swaminathan, R., King, R.F., Holmfield, J. *et al.* (1985) Thermic effect of feeding carbohydrate, fat, protein and mixed meal in lean and obese subjects. *The American Journal of Clinical Nutrition*, **42** (2), 177–81.

Thiebaud, D., Acheson, K., Schutz, Y. *et al.* (1983) Stimulation of thermogenesis in men after combined glucose-long-chain triglyceride infusion. *The American Journal of Clinical Nutrition*, **37** (4), 603–11.

Thiebaud, D., Schutz, Y., Acheson, K. *et al.* (1983) Energy cost of glucose storage in human subjects during glucose-insulin infusions. *The American Journal of Physiology*, **244** (3), E216–21.

Thomas, C.D., Peters, J.C., Reed, G.W. *et al.* (1992) Nutrient balance and energy expenditure during ad libitum feeding of high-fat and high-carbohydrate diets in humans. *The American Journal of Clinical Nutrition*, **55** (5), 934–42.

Thorin, D., Golay, A., Simonson, D.C. *et al.* (1986) The effect of selective beta adrenergic blockade on glucose-induced thermogenesis in man. *Metabolism: Clinical and Experimental*, **35** (6), 524–8.

Trayhurn, P. (2005) The biology of obesity. *Proceedings of the Nutrition Society*, **64** (1), 31–8.

Trayhurn, P. and Bing, C. (2006) Appetite and energy balance signals from adipocytes. *Philosophical Transactions of the Royal Society of London. Series B, Biological Sciences*, **361** (1471), 1237–49.

Tuomilehto, J., Lindstrom, J., Eriksson, J.G. *et al.* (2001) Prevention of type 2 diabetes mellitus by changes in lifestyle among subjects with impaired glucose tolerance. *The New England Journal of Medicine*, **344** (18), 1343–50.

Ukropcova, B., Sereda, O., de Jonge, L. *et al.* (2007) Family history of diabetes links impaired substrate switching and reduced mitochondrial content in skeletal muscle. *Diabetes*, **56** (3), 720–7.

van Baak, M.A. (2001) The peripheral sympathetic nervous system in human obesity. *Obesity Reviews*, **2** (1), 3–14.

van Marken Lichtenbelt, W.D., Schrauwen, P., van De Kerckhove, S. and Westerterp-Plantenga, M.S. (2002) Individual variation in body temperature and energy expenditure in response to mild cold. *American Journal of Physiology. Endocrinology and Metabolism*, **282** (5), E1077–83.

Warwick, P.M. and Busby, R. (1990) Influence of mild cold on 24h energy expenditure in 'normally' clothed adults. *The British Journal of Nutrition*, **63** (3), 481–8.

Weaver, H.A., Stern, S.A., Mutchler, M.J. *et al.* (2006) Discovery of two new satellites of Pluto. *Nature*, **439** (7079), 943–5.

Weinsier, R.L., Schutz, Y. and Bracco, D. (1992) Reexamination of the relationship of resting metabolic rate to fat-free mass and to the metabolically active components of fat-free mass in humans. *The American Journal of Clinical Nutrition*, **55** (4), 790–4.

Welle, S., Schwartz, R.G. and Statt, M. (1991) Reduced metabolic rate during beta-adrenergic blockade in humans. *Metabolism: Clinical and Experimental*, **40** (6), 619–22.

Weyer, C., Walford, R.L., Harper, I.T. *et al.* (2000) Energy metabolism after 2 y of energy restriction: the biosphere 2 experiment. *The American Journal of Clinical Nutrition*, **72** (4), 946–53.

WHO/FAO (2003) Diet Nutrition and the prevention of chronic diseases, Technical report series.

Wijers, S.L., Saris, W.H. and van Marken Lichtenbelt, W.D. (2007) Individual thermogenic responses to mild cold and overfeeding are closely related. *The Journal of Clinical Endocrinology and Metabolism*, **92** (11), 4299–305.

Young, J.B. (2006) Developmental origins of obesity: a sympathoadrenal perspective. *International Journal of Obesity (London)*, **30** (Suppl 4), S41–9.

Zurlo, F., Lillioja, S., Esposito-Del Puente, A. *et al.* (1990) Low ratio of fat to carbohydrate oxidation as predictor of weight gain: study of 24-h RQ. *The American Journal of Physiology*, **259** (5 Pt 1), E650–7.

Chapter 8

Aetiology of Human Obesity

Key points

- Over 95% of cases of human obesity are due to the impact of an obesogenic lifestyle (over-consumption of energy and/or insufficient energy expenditure) on a variable background of genetic susceptibility. Causes of secondary obesity include certain drugs, endocrine disorders and monogenic syndromes.

- The rapid spread of obesity within two generations indicates that environmental factors are mainly responsible for the global obesity epidemic. However, individual susceptibility to obesity is predominantly inherited, with family studies suggesting that 50–70% of total variance in BMI is genetically determined. Obesity also spreads through social networks.

- Susceptibility to common, lifestyle-related obesity is polygenic, determined by the cumulative effect of many minor genes. Putative obesity susceptibility genes include *FTO* ('fused toe'), *INSIG-2* (insulin-induced gene 2) and *GAD2* (an isoform of glutamic acid decarboxylase). Their roles in energy balance regulation are yet to be determined.

- Certain aspects of energy intake are partly genetically determined, including the total energy consumed at a meal and 'restraint' (the ability to stop eating). Candidate genes include those encoding CNS neurotransmitters that regulate appetite.

- A relatively low energy expenditure may predispose to obesity and this may be partly genetically determined. Candidate genes include the β_3 adrenoceptor receptor involved in thermogenesis, although its overall importance remains uncertain.

- The persistence of obesity genes has been attributed to the survival value of 'thrifty' genes (promoting food intake and energy storage) during human evolution. An alternative suggestion is that body weight has been subject to random genetic drift for 2 million years, since overweight individuals would have been 'released from predation risk'.

- Population-wide increases in obesity can be largely explained by overconsumption of food and sweetened drinks. Factors shown to favour overconsumption include high energy density of food, larger portions, greater dietary variety, snacking, eating outside the home, and 'social facilitation', that is, increased consumption when eating with company.

- Reduced energy expenditure may also contribute to the spread of obesity, consistent with increases in the use of labour-saving devices, car ownership and sedentary pursuits; however, direct evidence is lacking. The obesogenic effect of watching television is explained by the associated overeating.

- Numerous drugs increase adiposity, by stimulating appetite (e.g. glucocorticoids, antipsychotic and anti-epileptic drugs), decreasing energy expenditure (β adrenoceptor blockers), or promoting lipogenesis (insulin, sulphonylureas) or adipocyte differentiation (thiazolidinediones). Weight can increase by several kilograms with glucocorticoids, insulin, atypical antipsychotics and anti-epileptic agents.

- Hypothyroidism decreases energy expenditure and causes weight gain, but overt obesity is rare. Central and visceral obesity, due mainly to hyperphagia, are characteristic of Cushing syndrome and hypothalamic damage. Polycystic ovarian syndrome is commonly associated with obesity.

- Over 30 Mendelian syndromes include obesity; the most common is Prader-Willi syndrome, with early-onset hyperphagia and morbid obesity, short stature and mental retardation. Other monogenic causes of human obesity, mostly extremely rare, include mutations affecting leptin, the leptin receptor and the melanocortin-4 receptor (MC4-R); the latter may account for 5% of morbid obesity that begins in early childhood.

Chapter 8 Aetiology of Human Obesity

John R. Speakman and David A. Levitsky

Obesity is widely agreed to be due to a prolonged period of energy imbalance. Given this fact, two questions that arise are the extent to which obesity results from genetic or environmental factors, and the roles played by overconsumption of calories, or the under-expenditure of energy, particularly due to low physical activity (e.g. Prentice and Jebb, 1995).

Relatively few cases of obesity, totalling less than 5%, are secondary to factors such as drug treatment, specific endocrine disorders or defined monogenic syndromes (Table 8.1). The remaining 95% of obesity results from differences in energy intake or expenditure that are due to multiple minor genetic (polygenic) effects, and/or to environmentally mediated differences in lifestyle. This is referred to here as 'lifestyle-related' obesity.

This chapter describes the causes of human obesity, focusing on the issues of genetic versus environmental factors and the roles of energy intake and expenditure, referring where necessary to informative animal data.

Lifestyle-related obesity

It is useful to break down the aetiology of lifestyle-related obesity into two distinct issues (O'Rahilly and Farooqi, 2006). The first concerns the massive global expansion in the prevalence of overweight and obese individuals in modern times (WHO, 1998). Demographic studies suggest that this began in Western societies at the beginning of the twentieth century (Dubois, 1936), but was halted during the 1940s by the Second World War. Since then, sustained peace throughout most of Europe, Asia and North America has been accompanied by a progressive rise in the prevalence of obesity in these countries. By the end of the 1990s, the obesity epidemic was spreading to involve South America and Africa (Flegal et al., 2002; Ogden et al., 2006). The speed of this progression, over a period spanning only two generations, strongly indicates that the epidemic is due to a change in environmental factors rather than due to standard demographic processes of survival and mortality altering the genetic make-up of the population.

The second issue relates to the fact that individuals differ in their susceptibility to become obese. Hence, any subpopulation will consist of a mix of obese, overweight and lean individuals. Because these individuals will be potentially exposed to broadly the same environmental factors, the major factor influencing whether a person becomes obese or stays slim in that environment will be predominantly genetic.

Therefore, the answer to the question 'Is obesity due to environmental or genetic factors?' depends on which aspect is being addressed. When considering differences between individuals within a population the answer is 'predominantly genetic', but 'predominantly environmental' when considering the increase in prevalence over recent times. Overall, the interaction between genetics and environment is of key importance.

Individual susceptibility to obesity

Family studies have been informative in determining the magnitude of the genetic component involved in individual variation in susceptibility. The review by Maes et al. (1997) systematically examined the correlation coefficients of BMI between spouses, parents and siblings. The key findings are shown in Figure 8.1(a). First, correlation coefficients of BMI between blood relatives (parents and offspring, and siblings) were significantly higher than those between spouses. This strongly suggests that BMI has a high genetic component because parents share half of their genetic material with their offspring – as do siblings – whereas spouses are usually

Obesity: Science to Practice   Edited by Gareth Williams and Gema Frühbeck
© 2009 John Wiley & Sons, Ltd

Table 8.1 Causes of human obesity.

---

*Common or lifestyle-related obesity
(>95% of cases)*

- genetic susceptibility (polygenic)
- obesogenic environment (overconsumption of
  energy and/or decreased expenditure)

Obesogenic drugs (see Table 8.3)

Endocrine disorders

- Hypothyroidism
- Cushing syndrome
- Polycystic ovarian syndrome
- Hypothalamic disease
- Pituitary disorders: panhypopituitarism, growth
  hormone deficiency

Inherited syndromes (see Table 21.2)

- Prader–Willi syndrome
- Bardet–Biedl syndrome
- Alström syndrome
- Fragile X syndrome

Monogenic disorders due to mutations affecting:

- Leptin (*LEP*)
- Leptin receptor (*LEPR*)
- Proopiomelanocortin (*POMC*)
- Prohormone convertase-1 (*PC-1*)
- Melanocortin-3 receptor (*MC3-R*)
- Melanocortin-4 receptor (*MC4-R*)

---

genetically unrelated. Also, the correlation between the BMI of siblings was higher than that between parents and offspring; this suggests that siblings share a more similar environment, and that this contributes more to the determination of BMI than the environmental factors that are common to them and their parents. This finding contrasts with many other genetic analyses, which concluded that the environment shared by relatives contributes little to variations in body weight or BMI (Hunt *et al.*, 1989; Maes, Neale and Eaves, 1997).

The genetic contribution to individual variation in BMI is demonstrated more clearly by studies that compare monozygotic with dizygotic twins. Monozygotic (identical) twins share all their genes, whereas dizygotic twins share only 50%. Although there is a tendency for identical twins to be treated more similarly than non-identical ones (Joseph, 1998), phenotypic differences between dizygotic and monozygotic twins are most likely to be explained by their differing genetic makeup. In the studies reviewed by Maes *et al.* (1997), the average correlation coefficient for BMI between monozygotic twins was 0.7, whereas that between dizygotic twins was only 0.3 – which is comparable to that in non-twin siblings (Figure 8.1(b)). Subsequent studies of twins have yielded broadly consistent findings. Overall, correlation coefficients (r) of between 0.7 and 0.95 have been found for BMI between monozygotic twins, suggesting that the variance (r^2) attributable to genetic factors is between 50 and 90% of the total. This demonstrates that most of the individual variation in susceptibility to obesity is genetic. Interestingly, the correlation of BMI between twins decreases with age in both monozygotic and dizygotic twins, representing an increasing influence of environmental factors on energy balance as people age (Hewitt, 1997). The 'heritability' of BMI (a measure of the extent to which BMI is genetically determined) also declines with age.

Although genetic factors are the most important determinants of BMI, environmental factors account for the remaining 10–50% of the variance in BMI. These environmental factors can be divided into 'shared' (i.e. common to both siblings) and 'non-shared' (unique to each individual) factors. Perhaps against expectation, several large-scale studies have found that non-shared environmental factors account for about 20% of the variance in BMI, whereas almost none is attributable to shared factors (Grilo and Pogue-Geile, 1991; Hewitt, 1997; Maes, Neale and Eaves, 1997). The consistent lack of effect of shared environmental factors has been confirmed in a longitudinal study of genetic and environmental influences on BMI (Fabsitz, Carmelli and Hewitt, 1992), and has also been demonstrated in adolescent twins (Bodurtha *et al.*, 1990) and adopted children (Cardon, 1994, 1995). These data appear to contradict the commonly-held belief that the home environment is important in determining long-term eating and exercise patterns in children.

Obesity susceptibility genes

The above studies establish that genetic factors play a major role in the individual susceptibility to obesity, but they do not tell us anything about the actual genes, or even how many these

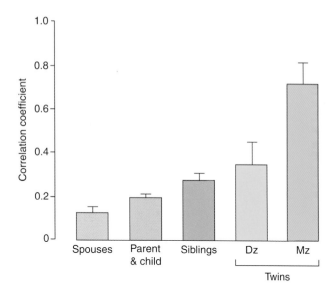

Figure 8.1 Correlation coefficients of BMI, between spouses, parent and child, siblings and dizygotic (Dz) and monozygotic (Mz) twins. From Maes *et al.* (1997), with permission of the editor of *Behavior Genetics*.

are. There could be relatively few genes with large effects, or obesity could result from the actions of a large number of genes that each have only a minor contribution. Specific genetic disorders have long been know that include obesity as part of the phenotype – for example, the Prader-Willi syndrome, which is characterized by short stature, hypogonadism, mental retardation, and obesity. The Mendelian nature of inheritance of Prader-Willi syndrome indicates that it is caused by disruption of a single gene (or small number of genes); the locus lies on chromosome 15, but the gene(s) have not yet been specifically identified. To date, over 30 clinically different Mendelian disorders have been recognized; some are described in detail in Chapter 21.

Overall, however, studies of common human obesity indicate very strongly that genetic susceptibility is generally not 'monogenic' – that is, the consequence of single genes with large effects – but is a 'polygenic' trait due to the cumulative action of many genes, each of which has a relatively minor effect. The identity and nature of the specific genes that determine susceptibility to obesity have generated much interest. Several strategies have been used to identify obesity susceptibility genes, made possible by the sequencing of the mouse and human genomes in 2002 and 2003, respectively.

Quantitative trait loci (QTL) mapping

In QTL mapping, a statistical association is made between the phenotype and genotype of an individual as compared with the phenotypes and genotypes of its parents or other relatives. In animals, this is generally performed by taking inbred strains of mice that exhibit either an obese or a lean phenotype. These are then crossed to generate a heterozygous F1 population, which is then intercrossed to generate an F2 population, which is phenotyped for the trait of interest – in this case obesity. By using markers along the genome of these F2 individuals, it is possible to identify whether a given segment of the genome came from the original obese line or the lean line. Consequently, if all the obese mice in the F2 generation consistently have a segment of their genome inherited from the original obese line, it can be inferred that a gene (or genes) responsible for obesity resides in that region of the genome – called a quantitative trait locus, or QTL. It is important to recognize that identifying a QTL is not the same as identifying a gene that has significant polymorphic variation linked to obesity. In mice, QTL analyses have yielded many regions that segregate with obesity (Perusse *et al.*, 2005).

In humans, the task is more laborious; unlike mice, humans cannot be bred to order. Nevertheless, QTL mapping in humans has identified

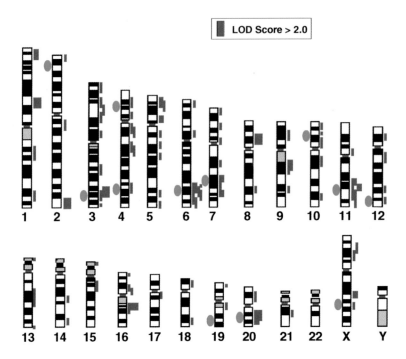

Figure 8.2 Obesity susceptibility loci in the human genome, identified by quantitative trait loci (QTL) mapping. The red bars indicate regions that have been replicated in several studies with a LOD score of >2.0. The blue spots indicate the regions that have been identified in linkage studies performed in cohorts with extreme obesity phenotypes.

253 different QTLs that may be involved in susceptibility to obesity (Rankinen *et al.*, 2006) (Figure 8.2 indicates regions that have been replicated in several studies conditions.) A QTL contains multiple genes, and depending on the separation of the markers used, a QTL could include hundreds of genes. Certain 'candidate' genes – encoding factors known to be involved in controlling energy balance and whose position is known from the annotated maps of the mouse and humans genomes (Rance *et al.*, 2005, 2007) – can be identified within some of these QTLs. Some appear intuitive, such as the region of chromosome 1 (region 1p31) containing the *LEPR* (leptin receptor) gene, which has been identified in several independent studies. Moreover, important genes can be missed, either because they have not yet been discovered or implicated in energy homeostasis, or because key mutations may affect introns rather than the coding regions of genes (see below).

Single nucleotide polymorphism (SNP) mapping is a different approach that relates phenotypic features to specific SNPs in the genome. This is, theoretically, more productive because specific genes and their obesogenic variants can be identified rather than the much wider QTLs. However, the task is potentially enormous. The human genome contains about 3.5 billion base pairs, with SNPs at about 10 million loci; a genome-wide search for associations of all these SNPs with obesity would require 10 million genotyping reactions in about 1000 obese and 1000 lean subjects.

Fortunately, the process can be abbreviated because SNPs located close together tend to be inherited together in so-called 'linkage disequilibrium'. The inter-relationships between the various SNPs have been clarified by the International HAPMAP Consortium (2007), and this allows a reasonably comprehensive genome-wide association study (GWAS) to be performed by genotyping only 500 000 SNPs. These key SNPs can now be incorporated onto a single DNA 'chip', which can be used to identify the genotype at each of the 500 000 loci. Genotyping the 2000 subjects stipulated above would now cost $1 million, compared with over $20 billion, as was estimated for all the SNPs in 2002.

Several genome-wide association studies have now been completed and have identified links between polymorphic variation at specific SNPs and obesity. These include SNPs in the *INSIG*-2 (the insulin-induced gene 2) (Herbert *et al.*, 2006) and *GAD2*, encoding an isoform of glutamic acid decarboxylase that generates GABA (Boutin *et al.*, 2003). Attempts to replicate these findings, and to implicate variants of these genes in obesity, have met with variable success. In 2007, a GWAS that linked obesity to a common variant in a key SNP was conducted in over 1900 type 2 diabetic subjects and 2900 controls, and this association was subsequently replicated in 13 different cohorts totalling 39 000 individuals (Frayling *et al.*, 2007). Homozygosity for the A variant of the gene (A/A) increased the probability of developing obesity by 30%, and A/A subjects weighed an average of 3 kg more than those carrying the T/T genotype; A/T carriers had an intermediate BMI. The gene containing this SNP is called *FTO*, because its locus corresponds to that for a mutation that cases fused toes in the mouse (Petersen *et al.*, 2002) – although this latter effect may actually be due to deletion of a neighbouring gene. The function of *FTO* remains unknown, although recent studies have implicated it in variations in food intake rather than in energy expenditure. The SNP in question is located in one of the gene's introns, not in the coding region, and is in linkage disequilibrium with 9 other SNPs (Figure 8.3). The true obesity

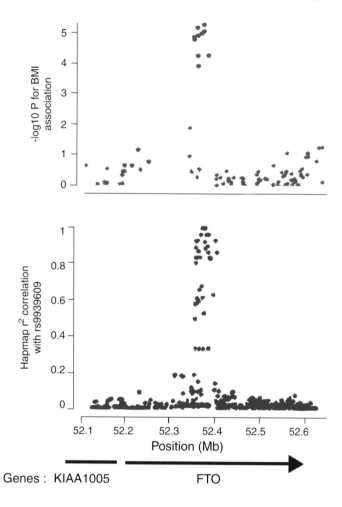

Figure 8.3 Upper panel: associations of single nucleotide polymorphisms (SNPs) in the *FTO/KIA1005* region of chromosome 16 with BMI in adults with type 2 diabetes. Lower panel: linkage disequilibrium (r^2) between an associated SNP (designated rs9939609) and all other SNPs in HapMap data from Caucasian European populations. From (Frayling *et al.* 2007).

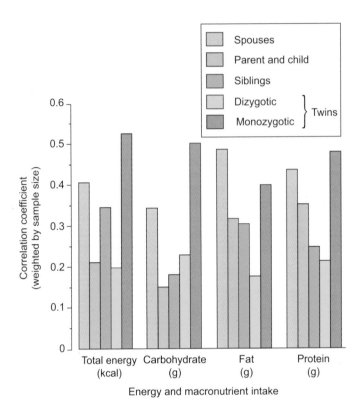

Figure 8.4 Correlation coefficients for total energy and macronutrient intakes, between spouses, parent and child, siblings and dizygotic and monozygotic twins. From Maes *et al.* (1997), with permission of the editor of *Behavior Genetics*.

susceptibility gene may therefore prove to be one of its neighbours. This highlights the limitations of searching for SNPs in candidate obesity genes, which are selected for known involvement in energy homeostasis.

Although our understanding of the genetic basis of individual susceptibility is increasing, the exact functions of most of the QTL and genes identified by association studies, and of the *INSIG-2*, *GAD-2* and *FTO* genes identified by GWAS, remain unknown – as is their impact on energy intake and expenditure.

Genetic determinants of energy intake

Numerous family studies have examined the inherited basis that determines an individual's consumption of macronutrients and total energy intake (Laskarzewski *et al.*, 1980; Mitchell *et al.*, 2003; Park, Yim and Cho, 2004; Perusse *et al.*, 1988; Vauthier *et al.*, 1996). Unlike BMI, all the correlations for macronutrient and total energy intake were higher between spouses than

between parents and children (Figure 8.4). This may indicate that the environment affects behaviour more than genetic factors, or perhaps that spouses are attracted to each other by similar lifestyles. However, as with BMI, nutrient and energy intake was more highly correlated among monozygotic than dizygotic twins.

Almost all these studies estimated nutrient and energy intake from self-completed, 3–5 day food diaries, which are subject to systematic bias because food intake is generally underreported by the obese and over-reported by the thin (Johansson *et al.*, 2001; Schoeller, 1990; see Chapter 3). When food intake was measured under laboratory conditions, correlations of energy intake among all three groups of family members were generally higher than when calculated from food records, but with less marked differences between monozygotic and dizygotic twins (Faith *et al.*, 1999).

de Castro (2004a, 2004b) performed sophisticated genetic analyses of eating behaviour in twins, and also examined the influence and interaction of environmental factors. His find-ings suggest that genetic factors influence the selection of energy-dense foods (to about the same degree as environmental factors), as well as restraint (a psychological measure indicating active inhibition of eating), and the total volume or energy content of the food consumed at a meal. Intriguingly, genetic fac-tors also significantly influence the number of people with whom one eats — which has been shown to be positively related to the amount of food consumed at a meal (see below and Figure 8.8 on page 197). Both genetic and environmental factors affect the slope of the relationship between the amount of food consumed at a meal and the number of other people present (see Figure 8.8), as well as the cyclicity of meal patterns. Finally, heredity dominates the selection of foods according to their energy density, but has no apparent role in determining how energy density influences total food intake.

Thus, key aspects of eating behaviour that might lead to overeating and thus obesity have a genetic basis, and these can modulate envi-ronmental influences that also determine energy balance. Candidate genes that influence appetite and food intake could include those encoding the CNS transmitters that regulate feeding, such as the melanocortin-4 receptor (*MC4-R*; see below and Chapter 6).

Genetic determinants of energy expenditure

The importance of reduced energy expenditure in causing human obesity, and the extent to which this might be genetically determined, have been controversial. This is partly because the accurate and reproducible measurement of energy expenditure is technically difficult (see Chapter 3). Also, there have been relatively few longitudinal studies of sufficient precision and statistical power to detect small deficits in energy expenditure that could lead to obesity over several years and which have followed up subjects for long enough to determine an impact on body weight.

Once established, obesity is associated with increased total energy expenditure, because lean tissue, which is the most metabolically active, increases in proportion to fat mass (see Chapters 3 and 7). It is possible, however, that a relative decrease in energy expenditure might contribute to the development of obesity, and there is some evidence that any such deficit might be partly genetically determined. This issue has been controversial, because different studies have reported discrepant findings.

In Pima Indians, Ravussin et al. (1988) found that a low daily total energy expenditure (TEE) predicted greater weight gain over a 4-year period; subjects with a TEE in the lowest quartile gained the most weight, and those whose TEE was 200 kcal/day (0.8 MJ/day) below average had a fourfold higher risk of gaining over 7.5 kg. More-over, in this study, values of TEE varied widely between families, but were more closely segre-gated within families, suggesting that heredity is a significant determinant of TEE (Figure 8.5). A role for decreased energy expenditure in pre-disposing to obesity is also supported by the findings of Roberts et al. (1988) in infants during the first year of life. TEE, measured by the doubly-labelled water technique (see Chapter 3), at 3 months of age was on average 20% lower in babies who went on to become overweight at 1 year, compared with those whose weight remained normal. Most of the overweight babies were born to obese mothers, again pointing to an inherited predisposition. Moreover, Tataranni et al. (2003) found that individual differences in resting metabolic rate (RMR), adjusted appro-priately for body size, were inversely associated with weight gain over 4.7 years of follow-up, while physical activity level (PAL) showed no such relationship, in a cohort of non-diabetic Pima Indians. By contrast, Goran et al. (1998) found that weight gain among a group of children was completely unrelated to various components of energy expenditure.

The possible causal role of reduced energy ex-penditure in obesity has also been investigated in previously obese subjects who have lost their excess weight. Early studies in such 'post-obese' individuals suggested that TEE was lower than in controls of comparable weight who had never been obese (Geissler et al., 1987). However, no such defect in TEE was found in studies using the rigorous doubly-labelled water technique (Prentice et al., 1986).

As mentioned above, variations in energy intake could compensate for, or overcome, any inherited differences in energy expenditure. The studies by Goran et al. (1998) and Tataranni et al. (2003) suggest that individuals might overeat to compensate for increased energy expenditure

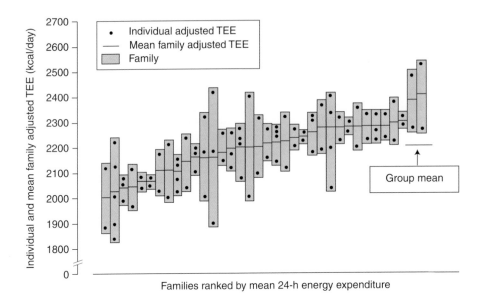

Figure 8.5 Clustering of total energy expenditure (TEE) within families of Pima Indians. Data are from 94 subjects, from 36 families. Variability is wide between families, but relatively low among family members. In this study, individuals whose initial TEE fell in the lowest quartile gained the most weight over four years. From Ravussin *et al.* (1988), with permission of the editor of the *New England Journal of Medicine*.

through exercise, but that this compensation is less effective for differences in RMR. By contrast, studies in animals have tended to suggest that variations in RMR are not linked to subsequent weight gain (Johnston *et al.*, 2007). Moreover, a recent review of the human literature suggested that changes in energy intake do not normally compensate for increases in energy expenditure due to acute exercise (King *et al.*, 2007), although Westerterp (1998) has suggested that the modest changes in body weight of individuals training over a period of months for a half-marathon can be accounted for only by a compensatory increase in food intake.

Candidate obesity susceptibility genes that operate by decreasing energy expenditure could theoretically include any of the components of the thermogenic processes described in Chapters 5 and 7. A point mutation has been identified in the β_3 adrenoceptor, which in mammals mediates the thermogenic effects of catecholamines and sympathetic nerve activity in brown adipose tissue (BAT; see Chapter 4). In humans, the β_3 adrenoceptor is expressed in visceral fat and skeletal muscle and increases heat production in those tissues. The mutation is a Trp→Arg substitution at amino acid position 64, a key functional site in the first intracellular loop of this

7-transmembrane domain receptor (Figure 8.6). The mutation has been associated with a tendency to decreased RMR and enhanced weight gain (Clément *et al.*, 1995) as well as an earlier age of onset of type 2 diabetes in Pima Indians (Walston *et al.*, 1995). However, these associations are relatively weak and their significance remains uncertain. Other candidates could include components of the leptin-CNS circuit, which as well as restraining food intake in rodents also stimulates the sympathetic nervous outflow to thermogenic tissues and thus energy expenditure.

Differences between individuals in their levels of activity may be an important factor influencing individual susceptibility to obesity. Recent studies suggest that habitual levels of physical activity appear to have a strong genetic component (Joosen *et al.*, 2007), perhaps also contributing to the genetic susceptibility to obesity. One previously neglected factor is the energy expended on minor 'non-exercise' movements, including fidgeting and subconscious and spontaneous muscular activity, such as that related to maintaining posture. This has been called 'non-exercise activity thermogenesis' (NEAT). NEAT appears to have a genetic component, but also depends on age and occupation; it varies widely between individuals and may account

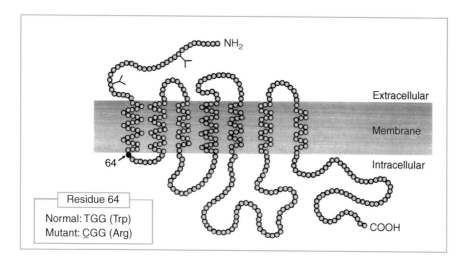

Figure 8.6 Structure of the human β₃ adrenoceptor, showing the Trp→Arg SNP at residue 64 that has been associated with an increased risk of developing obesity. From Walston *et al.* (1995), with permission of the editor of the *New England Journal of Medicine*.

for differences of as much as 300 kcal (1.3 MJ) in total daily energy expenditure. Some studies report that subjects who do not increase NEAT gain more weight when overfed under experimental conditions (Levine, Eberhardt and Jensen, 1999) (Figure 8.7). However, other studies have failed to observe such an effect (Riumallo *et al.*, 1989). Overall, NEAT is a potentially important factor in susceptibility to obesity, but its true significance requires further clarification.

Evolutionary context of obesity susceptibility

The fact that humans have genes that predispose to obesity is beyond question; why we possess these genes is less certain, although most agree that the reasons are rooted in our evolutionary history.

The 'thrifty gene' hypothesis, first proposed by Neel in the early 1960s, suggests that food

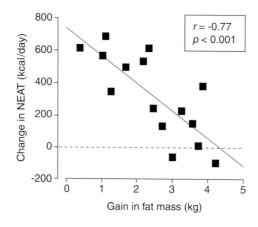

Figure 8.7 Non-activity thermogenesis (NEAT) and susceptibility to weight gain during experimental overfeeding of normal subjects. There was a significant inverse correlation between the increase in NEAT and weight gain. From Levine *et al.* (1999), Role of nonexercise activity thermogenesis in resistance to fat gain in humans. *Science*, **283**, 212 with permission of the editor.

supplies were tenuous throughout most of our history and that individuals possessing genes that encouraged the collection of food and the storage of excess energy as fat would tend to survive better during periods of famine (Neel, 1962). These advantageous 'thrifty' genes would be positively selected through thousands of generations; their persistence into modern and affluent societies, where food is readily and continuously available, will continue to promote the deposition of fat and hence obesity. Obesity shortens life expectancy, but most obese people survive into and beyond the reproductive years, so there is no selection pressure against the thrifty genes under present-day conditions.

The thrifty gene hypothesis has dominated thinking for over 50 years, but has recently been challenged (Benyshek and Watson, 2006; Speakman, 2004, Speakman, 2007). It is argued that major famines are a comparatively recent phenomenon (since the spread of organized agriculture), and they are rare events (every 150 years, in most populations) and kill relatively few people. Consequently, famine might not have a sufficiently powerful or long-lasting selection impact to cause the widespread acquisition of thrifty genes. Modern hunter-gatherers, such as the !kung san tribe from Cameroon do not become obese between periods of famine (Speakman, 2007). Moreover, the distribution of BMI in modern populations indicates that there exists a subgroup who remain lean despite the prevailing obesogenic environment (Flegal et al., 2002; Ogden et al., 2006). This begs the question as to why the intense positive selection for thrifty genes has somehow spared these individuals.

Speakman (2007) has suggested a radical alternative, namely the 'release from predation' hypothesis. This proposes that body weight ranges between a lower limit, imposed by the risk of starvation, and an upper limit that relates to the risk of being killed by predators. Ancient hominids such as Australopithecus (2–6 million years ago) lived among large predators, and overweight individuals might not have survived. The development of social behaviour, fire and weapons is postulated to have removed the threat of predation and thus the ceiling on body weight – when weight, freed from selection pressure, would be subject to random genetic drift. This hypothesis is supported by mathematical modelling of the distribution of BMI in modern populations following 2 million years of genetic drift: the predicted distribution is close to that in present-day USA (Speakman, 2007).

Changes in the prevalence of obesity over time

As already mentioned, environmental factors rather than population-level genetic change must explain the steady climb in BMI over the last 30 years, which has been seen in many populations (see Chapter 2). Environmental factors include numerous societal and other changes that tend to encourage overconsumption of food and/or decrease energy expenditure, primarily through reduced physical activity. As discussed below, 'assortative mating' – that is, the tendency of obese people to select obese partners – may have augmented the effects of obesogenic environmental factors.

The importance of social contacts in facilitating the spread of obesity has been highlighted by recent data from the Framingham Heart Study. The changing pattern of obesity was mapped within neighbourhoods over several years. Obesity developed in clusters and appeared to spread within social networks, especially among groups of individuals who are linked by friendship and family ties – with the chances of close friends and family members of an obese person also becoming obese increasing by 40–60% (see Figure 8.8). By contrast, immediate neighbours were unaffected, arguing against local environmental influences. This implies that social contacts are important in propagating obesogenic behaviours.

The relative importance of decreased physical activity versus increased food intake has been much discussed; both may contribute to the spread of obesity, to degrees that vary with time and between populations. Numerous methodological difficulties have clouded this issue.

Increased food intake

Several early studies, notably the influential 'gluttony and sloth' paper by Prentice and Jebb (1995), found that population levels of food intake had apparently remained stable or even fallen while obesity was becoming more common. It was therefore concluded that reduced energy expenditure, especially through decreased physical activity, was responsible. However, food intake was assessed largely from

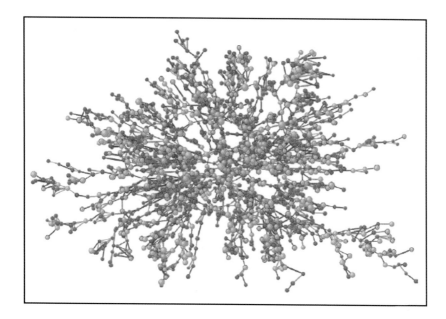

Figure 8.8 Obesity spreads through social contacts: distribution of obesity within a social network of over 2000 people in the Framingham Heart Study population. Each circle represents an individual. Blue and red borders respectively denote females and males, while a yellow fill indicates obesity (BMI >30 kg/m²; size proportional to BMI) and green a non-obese subject. Purple lines indicate non-genetic ties (friendship or marital) between individuals, and orange lines a familial tie. From (Christakis and Fowler, *New England Journal of Medicine* (2007), 370–9), with kind permission of the editor of the *New England Journal of Medicine*. An animation showing the spread of obesity through the social networks with time can be downloaded at www.nejm.org.

self-reported recall records, which are now known to be subject to systematic bias, in that obese subjects consistently under-report their food consumption (Goldberg *et al.*, 1991; see Chapter 3). Accordingly, these surveys cannot conclusively determine whether energy intake increased or not.

Numerous environmental factors affect human eating behaviour, ranging from the nature of food itself to the societal setting (Table 8.2).

Energy density

Humans given food whose energy density is increased by adding fat do not decrease the total amount that they eat to compensate for the increased energy intake, and thus gain weight (Kendall *et al.*, 1991; Levitsky, 2002). Conversely, decreasing the energy density by adding water or air to food does not cause any compensatory over-eating, and weight will be lost (Osterholt, Roe and Rolls, 2007; Rolls,

Table 8.2 Environmental factors affecting human eating behaviour.

Factors	Effect on energy intake
Properties of food	
• Increased energy density	• Increased
• Larger portion size	• Increased
• Greater dietary variety	• Increased
Social context and eating patterns	
• Number of people also eating	• Increased in proportion
• Eating outside the home	• Increased
• Snacking between meals	• Increased

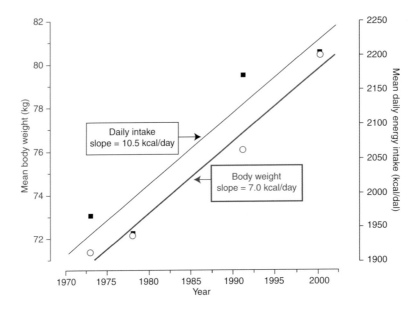

Figure 8.9 Increases in mean body weight (blue symbols and plot line, shown against left-hand y-axis) and mean energy intake (black symbols and plot, right-hand y-axis), of the US population between 1973 and 2000. Data are corrected for age, gender and ethnicity. From Zhang and Wang (2004) and Kant and Graubard (2006), using data from NHANES.

Bell and Waugh, 2000). Several studies have reported a direct correlation between energy density of the diet and BMI (Kant and Graubard, 2005; Ledikwe et al., 2006), although others have not (Cuco et al., 2001; de Castro, 2004a). The Continuing Survey of Food Intakes by Individuals (CSFII) survey found that the dietary energy density for obese subjects (1.95 kcal/g) was significantly higher than that for the lean (1.87 kcal/g) (Ledikwe et al., 2006). The energy density of food in the US has increased steadily since 1970; as the impact of energy density on consumption appears to be totally determined by the environment (de Castro, 2004a, 2004b), it is likely that this has contributed to the obesity epidemic.

Though small, this small energy difference from ingesting foods of lower energetic density can have a cumulative effect, as exemplified by vegetarianism. In a recent review of vegetarian diets and weight status (Berkow and Barnard, 2006), 43 out of 45 comparisons between groups of vegetarians and non-vegetarians showed vegetarians to have a significantly lower BMI than non-vegetarians. The mean difference in body weight was 5.4 kg – which is comparable to the average weight gained by the US

population during the obesity epidemic, from the early 1970s until 2000 (see Figure 8.9). The reason for the weight difference is clear – vegetarians consume fewer calories than do vegetarians (Nieman et al., 1989; Thorogood et al., 1990; Appleby et al., 1998; Kennedy et al., 2001; Sabate, 2003), because their diet is energetically less dense than the typical omnivorous diet as it contains less fat (Resnicow et al., 1991; Alexander, Ball and Mann, 1994; Appleby et al., 1999; Kennedy et al., 2001) and more fibre (Fraser, 1999; Haddad et al., 1999; Larsson and Johansson, 2002; Haddad and Tanzman, 2003).

Portion size is also related to total energy intake. Increasing size of portions (meal servings, sandwiches or even packages) leads to higher energy consumption, by as much as 50% at a given meal (Levitsky and Youn, 2004; Rolls et al., 2004; Wansink and Kim, 2005). In addition, people who eat larger portions have higher BMI (Rolls, Roe, Kral et al., 2004).

Dietary variety increases food consumption, whether offered at a meal (Spiegel and Stellar, 1990; McCrory et al., 1999a; Levitsky, 2005; Norton, Anderson and Hetherington, 2006), over courses served within a meal (Rolls et al., 1981), or at sequential meals (Meiselman, DeGraaf and Lesher, 2000; Stubbs *et al.*, 2001). The long-term effects on food intake of varying the diet are unknown, but people with a high BMI appear to eat a greater variety of foods than do lean subjects (Lyles *et al.*, 2006).

Various conditions surrounding the consumption of food can also affect energy intake, notably *social facilitation*. This describes the phenomenon whereby the amount eaten at a meal is increased in proportion to the number of other people present, which can markedly raise food intake at a meal by as much as 400 kcal (1.6 MJ) (Figure 8.10). This effect is robust (de Castro 1990; Edelman *et al.*, 1986; Klesges *et al.*, 1984), and the increase in food intake is enhanced when the others present are friends rather than strangers and are eating more (Levitsky, 2005). Social facilitation can contribute to the higher energy consumption when people eat outside the home (Clemens, Slawson and Klesges, 1999). As yet, however, there is no evidence that the social facilitation effect is associated with increased BMI.

Eating outside the home, and especially in fast-food outlets, has been an increasing trend over the last 30 years in the USA and other countries (Briefel and Johnson, 2004). Since 1977–1978, the change to eating more outside the home has resulted in a net increase in energy intake of nearly 300 kcal/day (1.2 MJ/day) (Figure 8.11). The effect is probably due to

a combination of social facilitation and greater variety, together with higher energy density and larger portion sizes – in many fast-food outlets, a served meal frequently contains over 1000 kcal (4.3 MJ) (Malouf and Colaguiri, 1995; Chanmugam *et al.*, 2003; Satia, Galanko and Siega-Riz, 2004). Eating out regularly (at least twice per week) is associated with an average increase in daily energy intake of some 400 kcal (1.7 MJ) (Clemens, Slawson and Klesges, 1999). Not surprisingly, those who eat out regularly have a higher BMI than those who eat mainly at home (Duffey *et al.*, 2007; McCrory *et al.*, 1999b).

Missing breakfast and snacking between meals are also associated with increasing weight (Kant and Graubard, 2006). On its own, missing breakfast is not compensated for by increased food consumption later in the day, and total daily energy intake falls by about 200 kcal (Cho *et al.*, 2003; Levitsky, 2005). Paradoxically, BMI is higher in those who miss breakfast – but probably because this is one of the initial ploys used by overweight people when attempting to lose weight (Serdula *et al.*, 1999; Williamson *et al.*, 1992). Snacking does not lead to compensatory decreases in subsequent meals eaten more than 30 minutes later – at least under laboratory conditions (Rolls *et al.*, 1991) – and so would be expected to increase weight. Some older epidemiological studies (Bellisle, Mcdevitt and Prentice, 1997)

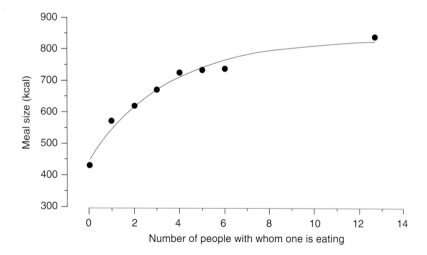

Figure 8.10 Social facilitation of eating behaviour: an individual's food intake increases as a function of the number of people present at the meal. The effect can increase energy intake at a single meal by up to 400 kcal. From de Castro and Brewer (1992), with permission of the editor of *Physiology & Behavior*.

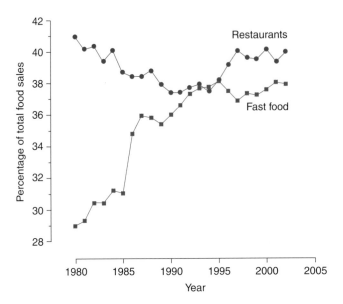

Figure 8.11 Mean percentage of total food sales consumed outside the home (at restaurants and fast-food establishments), between 1980 and 2003. Data are adjusted for age, gender and socioeconomic variables. Adapted from Steward *et al.* (2004).

suggest that a higher frequency of eating is associated with a lower BMI, but these conclusions are invalidated by the under-reporting bias (especially for snacks) in the obese (Prentice *et al.*, 1986; Heitmann and Lissner, 1995). With stringently-validated data, the total number of eating episodes, including snacks, is related to both total daily energy intake and to BMI (Kant *et al.*, 1995; Summerbell *et al.*, 1996) (Figure 8.12).

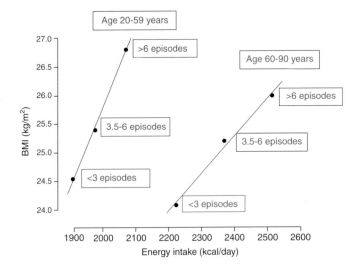

Figure 8.12 Total number of eating episodes (including snacks) each day (indicated in the boxes) is related to total energy intake and to BMI. This applies to individuals aged 20–59 years and to those aged 60–90 years, but the slope of the relationship is steeper in the younger age group. For energy intake, all points are significantly different from each other in each group; the trend for BMI is significant ($p < 0.01$) in each group. Adapted from Howarth *et al.* (2007), with permission of the editor of *International Journal of Obesity (London)*.

When close exclusion criteria are used for the acceptance of self-reported dietary intake, clear and reasonable relationships are expressed between eating frequency, total daily intake and BMI. Although the amount of snacking does not correlate with BMI (Howarth *et al.*, 2007), the total number of eating episodes does. Thus, it is not the amount of food consumed at a particular snack nor the number of daily snacks that is related to total daily intake and to body weight, but rather it is the number of eating occasions and whether it is a meal or a snack, that is correlated with intake and body weight.

Energy expenditure

The most variable component of energy expenditure is due to physical exercise, which can differ by several hundred kcal/day between sedentary and active individuals. The importance of exercise, and also of NEAT, is discussed in detail in Chapter 7.

The last half-century has seen enormous social changes, many of which have resulted in population-wide decreases in physical activity and thus in total energy expenditure. Examples include the spread of car ownership and labour-saving devices, which have discouraged everyday active transport (walking or cycling) and routine physical activity in the home. Car ownership in the UK has risen from 20% of families during the 1950s to over 60% now, and has replaced walking or cycling to work, school and shopping. The development of out-of-town supermarkets and the advent of home freezers have further reduced the traditional activities of frequent shopping trips on foot and carrying purchases home. In the home, numerous labour-saving devices have substantially reduced manual and physical activities, ranging from washing to clearing fireplaces.

It is important to recognize, however, that all these changes in physical activity patterns are anecdotal and that there is no direct evidence that they have led to changes in daily energy demands. Studies using the doubly-labelled water technique suggest that total energy expenditure has declined little if at all between the 1980s and the present day (Westerterp and Speakman, 2008). but the absence of accurate measurements of energy expenditure before the early 1980s makes the crucial comparison with the 1950s impossible. In an attempt to overcome this problem Hayes *et al.* (2005) compared levels of expenditure in modern humans with those of wild mammals. They concluded humans do have much lower energy demands than wild mammals. However this analysis is flawed by the failure to account adequately for the effects of ambient temperature on energy expenditure, which dominate the demands of most wild mammals (Speakman, 2000).

Perhaps the most spectacular changes have been in the pervasive spread of television, video and computer games. In the 1950s, the UK had a single television channel, which only broadcast from the late afternoon (and was interrupted for one hour each evening to allow families to eat together); now, 50 or more television channels are available around the clock. Most homes have multiple television sets, including in children's bedrooms. During the 1990s, the average American child watched television for 6 hours each day; current viewing times are less, but only because television has been supplanted by other, equally sedentary, entertainments such as videos and computer games.

Most studies examining the impact of television on weight have found that the duration of viewing is positively related to BMI, especially in children (Dietz and Gortmaker, 1985; Crespo *et al.*, 2001; Jeffery and French 1998; Kaur *et al.*, 2003; Utter *et al.*, 2003); however, others found only a weak or no relationship (Gorely, Marshall and Biddle, 2004; Hancox, Milne and Poulton, 2004; Marshall *et al.*, 2004). The effect of television viewing is complicated and not explained simply by a decrease in physical activity (Gorely, Marshall and Biddle, 2004; Katzmarzyk *et al.*, 2002; Marshall *et al.*, 2004) or in total daily energy expenditure (Buchowski and Sun, 1996; Dietz *et al.*, 1994). Perhaps unexpectedly, it is due to an increase in total daily energy intake (Blass *et al.*, 2006; Crespo *et al.*, 2001; Wiecha *et al.*, 2006) (Figure 8.13). Indeed, it has been estimated that people increase their energy intake by over 160 kcal for each hour of television viewing (Wiecha *et al.*, 2006) – enough to account for much of the population increase in overweight and obesity. Energy intake is increased in several ways, including consumption of sugar-rich drinks (Rajeshwari *et al.*, 2005; Nielsen *et al.*, 2002) and fast foods (Coon *et al.*, 2001; Matheson *et al.*, 2004) while viewing, and exposure to televised food commercials have been shown to increase eating (Blass *et al.*, 2006; Halford *et al.*, 2004; Halford *et al.*, 2007).

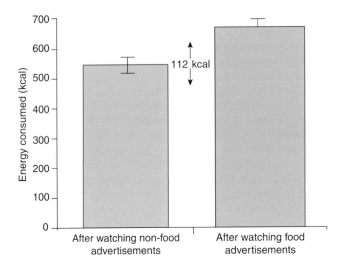

Figure 8.13 Television viewing is associated in children with increased energy intake, especially after watching advertisements for foods. From (Halford *et al.*, 2007).

Children asked to watch television commercials ate over 100 kcal (0.4 MJ) more when these advertised foods (Halford *et al.*, 2004; Halford *et al.*, 2007). Finally, watching television may distract from internal satiety signals that normally terminate eating Blass *et al.*, 2006; Temple *et al.*, 2001).

Assortative mating

Although it is widely accepted that genetic factors have probably not caused the trends in obesity over recent times, a genetic effect might arise because of the impact of assortative mating – that is when people choose partners non-randomly with regard to a particular trait. Assortative mating is well described for many traits, such as height, race, religion and social class. Recent studies have shown that assortative mating may also apply to obesity, in that overweight people tend to select overweight partners (Allison *et al.*, 1996; Hebebrand *et al.*, 2000; Speakman *et al.*, 2007).

Assortative mating would only contribute to the obesity epidemic if it had become more prevalent over time. Theoretical models show that this may have a significant contributory effect, but cannot explain the entire scale of the current obesity epidemic. An increase in assortative mating may be occurring because people now marry and have children later, but become fatter younger – which would make the identification of a similarly obese potential partner much easier now than it would have been in the 1950s.

Drug-induced obesity

Many drugs cause increases in body fat, arising through various mechanisms. Some important examples are shown in Table 8.3. Clinical aspects of drug-induced obesity are covered in Chapter 19.

Glucocorticoids

Glucocorticoids commonly cause weight gain, especially with long-term administration of high dosages. Weight gain is due mainly to increased fat mass, together with sodium and water retention from mineralocorticoid actions.

Increased adiposity is multifactorial. Appetite is increased, especially at high dosages, possibly due to inhibition of the anorexigenic CRF neurones in the paraventricular nucleus of the hypothalamus; stimulation of the orexigenic NPY neurones in the hypothalamic arcuate nucleus may also contribute (see Chapter 6). In addition, the expression of uncoupling proteins in various tissues is decreased, thus potentially reducing energy expenditure. Finally, glucocorticoids act in visceral fat depots to stimulate the differentiation of pre-adipocytes into mature adipocytes, thus favouring the selective expansion of visceral fat and leading to the characteristic central obesity.

Table 8.3   Drugs that induce obesity, and their mechanisms of action.

Class and drug	Increased appetite	Decreased energy expenditure	Other obesogenic effects
Glucocorticoids	++	+	• ↑ Adipocyte differentiation
Antidiabetic drugs			
• Insulin	±	−	• Anabolic effects
• Sulphonylureas	±	−	• Abolish glycosuria
• Thiazolidinediones	−	−	• ↑ Adipocyte differentiation
Antipsychotic drugs			
• 'Atypical' e.g. clozapine	++	+	−
• Classical e.g. haloperidol	++	+	−
Antidepressants			
• Tricyclics	++	+	−
Antiepileptic drugs			
• Carbamazepine	++	−	−
• Gabapentin	++	−	−
β-blockers			
• Propranolol	−	++	−
Endocrine drugs			
• Progestagens	+	−	−
• Tamoxifen	?	?	?
Miscellaneous	+	+	−
• Antihistamines	++	−	−
• Cyproheptadine	++	−	−
• Pizotifen	+	−	−
• Flunarizine	?	?	?
• Cyclophosphamide	?	?	?
• 5-Fluorouracil			

Antidiabetic drugs

Insulin treatment, especially if intensive, can cause weight gain in both type 1 and type 2 diabetic subjects. In type 1 diabetes, this is partly explained initially by the reversal of the catabolic processes triggered by insulin deficiency, with restoration of normal body fat and protein reserves, and by reduced energy losses through glycosuria (which can amount to several hundred kcal/day). Hyperinsulinaemia, which is inevitable with therapeutic insulin regimens, also promotes lipogenesis and fat accumulation and can cause hypoglycaemia; the latter induces intense hunger and, if recurrent, can significantly increase food intake.

Sulphonylureas and *meglitinide analogues*, which are insulin secretagogues, act similarly. *Thiazolidinediones* cause weight gain through increased subcutaneous fat accumulation (PPARγ activation promotes differentiation of preadipocytes in this depot). Sodium and water retention also occur, sometimes with clinical oedema; importantly, these drugs can precipitate cardiac failure.

By contrast, drugs such as exenatide that enhance or mimic the action of GLP-1 (an insulin secretagogue that also induces satiety) are less likely to increase body fat. Metformin does not cause weight gain.

Psychoactive drugs

Antipsychotic agents can cause significant increases in body fat and weight, which may take several months to reach a plateau. The main culprits are certain 'atypical' (second generation) neuroleptics such as olanzepine and clozapine, and 'classical' neuroleptics including chlorpromazine, thioridazine and haloperidol. Suggested mechanisms include increased appetite through blockade of anorexigenic serotonin, dopamine and histamine receptors, together with decreased physical activity due to their sedative effects.

Antidepressants

Tricyclic antidepressants such as amitriptyline and imipramine may cause mild hyperphagia and a decrease in energy expenditure, resulting in weight gain. By contrast, most selective serotonin reuptake inhibitors (SSRIs) do not cause weight gain, presumably because their central actions are dominated by the anorexigenic effects of increased serotonin availability (see Chapter 17).

Antiepileptic drugs

Some widely-used drugs, notably carbamazepine and gabapentin, cause weight gain that can reach 15 kg over a few months; this is largely due to increased appetite. By contrast, topiramate can induce significant weight loss (its side effects preclude its use to treat obesity *per se*).

Beta-adrenoceptor blockers

Non-selective β*-blockers* (e.g. propranolol) induce modest but sustained weight gain, attributed to decreased energy expenditure, perhaps involving both inhibition of sympathetically-mediated thermogenesis and reduced physical activity (see Chapter 7).

Miscellaneous drugs

Progestagen contraceptives such as megestrol acetate cause weight gain, related mainly to increased appetite. Hormone replacement therapy containing progestagens can also increase weight. *Tamoxifen*, the partial agonist at the oestrogen receptor, may induce weight gain despite its anorectic effect, through unknown mechanisms.

Antihistamines such as chlorpheniramine stimulate appetite, and may also decrease physical activity through their sedative effects; newer non-sedating antihistamines (e.g. loratidine and astemizole) cause less weight gain.

Cyproheptadine and *pizotifen* both initially stimulate appetite (probably due to inhibition at central serotonin and histamine receptors) and produce modest weight gain. *Flunarizine*, a calcium antagonist used for migraine prophylaxis, induces a dose-dependent rise in weight during the first few months of treatment, attributed to increased appetite.

Cyclophosphamide and *fluorouracil* are reported to cause weight gain, through unknown mechanisms.

Endocrine causes of obesity

Hypothyroidism causes weight gain in two-thirds of cases, due to a fall in basal metabolic rate (basal thyroid hormone levels are required for catecholamines to exert their full thermogenic effect) and in physical activity. However, overt obesity is unusual. Population-wide, only a small percentage of the variance in BMI is attributable to variations in TSH, and even profound hypothyroidism does not cause massive weight gain. Nevertheless, hypothyroidism is relatively common – with an overall prevalence of about 4% in most adult populations – and it should be actively excluded as a cause of weight gain, especially in women of middle age or older. Weight is lost when thyroid replacement is started, but is often not substantial. In children, hypothyroidism may present with continuing weight gain but arrest of vertical growth; the latter resumes with thyroxine replacement.

Cushing syndrome

Central obesity is a classical feature of glucocorticoid excess, whether due to therapeutic corticosteroids (by far the most common cause), ACTH hypersecretion from a pituitary adenoma or ectopic source, or primary overproduction of cortisol by an adrenocortical tumour. Obesity is due partly to hyperphagia (high glucocorticoid levels may inhibit the anorexigenic CRF neurones in the hypothalamus) and partly to enhanced differentiation of preadipocytes into mature adipocytes. The latter effect is most marked in visceral fat depots, which partly explains the characteristic central obesity. Successful treatment of Cushing syndrome, or withdrawal of therapeutic corticosteroids, leads to loss of weight and reductions in central obesity and facial rounding.

Polycystic ovarian syndrome (PCOS)

This is associated with obesity in up to 50% of cases, but the nature of the relationship remains uncertain. Insulin resistance is common and often accompanied by glucose intolerance (including type 2 diabetes in up to 10% of cases) and the characteristic skin lesion, acanthosis nigricans (Figures 13.7 and 21.11). Insulin resistance and hyperinsulinaemia are implicated in the raised androgen levels of PCOS.

Panhypopituitarism and *growth hormone deficiency* are often accompanied by obesity, which may be due to loss of the lipolytic effect of growth hormone. Other features, notably growth arrest in children, may dominate the clinical picture.

Hypothalamic lesions, especially those damaging the ventromedial region, can cause severe hyperphagia and obesity. This is probably due to loss of the POMC neurones in the arcuate (tuberoinfundibular) nucleus, which are crucial in mediating the appetite-suppressing action of leptin (see Chapter 6). Common causes include tumours (e.g. craniopharyngioma or invasive pituitary macroadenomas), infiltration with tuberculosis or histiocytosis X, or damage following pituitary surgery or radiotherapy.

Insulinomas can induce overall hyperphagia and eventual weight gain through hypoglycaemia-induced hunger, possibly enhanced by the anabolic effects of high circulating insulin concentrations.

Specific genetic disorders

Specific genetic syndromes that include overweight or obesity in their phenotype have long been recognized, especially in children. To date, 36 distinct Mendelian disorders of 'syndromic' obesity have been recognized. Most of these also involve short stature and mental retardation. The most common is the Prader-Willi syndrome, characterized by insatiable hyperphagia from early childhood, leading to early-onset morbid obesity, accompanied by muscular hypotonia, short stature, hypogonadism and mental retardation (see Chapter 21).

All these conditions are rare, accounting in total for less than 1% of unselected cases of obesity in adults. The prevalence is higher among children, especially those with early-onset morbid obesity and those referred to specialist centres for investigation and management of obesity (Figure 8.15).

Elucidation of the causes of genetic obesity in rodents has led to the identification of several genes that are crucial to energy homeostasis, and mutations in some of the human analogues of these genes have now been shown to cause obesity in humans; reviews of animal models of obesity can be found in West and York (1998) and Speakman *et al.* (2008). Several genetic obesity syndromes in rodents are due to mutations affecting leptin and its target neurones in the central nervous system (CNS). These are illustrated in Figure 8.14 and Table 8.4, and are described further in Chapter 6.

The *ob/ob* mouse develops overeating and obesity (accompanied by type 2 diabetes) due to a mutation of the *ob* gene that encodes leptin, the adipocyte-derived hormone that acts on the hypothalamus and other CNS regions to reduce feeding and decrease fat mass (Zhang *et al.*, 1994). Mutations of the leptin receptor in the *db/db* mouse and the *fa/fa* Zucker rat produce a similar phenotype, because the CNS neurones that normally respond to leptin and reduce feeding are unable to recognize the hormone (Tartaglia *et al.*, 1995). Crucial to mediating leptin's anorectic effect are neurones in the hypothalamic arcuate nucleus that express proopiomelanocortin (POMC). These neurones release the POMC derivative, α-MSH, which acts via melanocortin receptors 3 and 4 (MC4-R and MC3-R) to inhibit feeding; POMC neurones carry leptin receptors and are stimulated by leptin (see Chapter 6). Obesity in the yellow obese (Aʸ) mouse is due to a mutation that causes widespread overexpression of a protein termed 'agouti', which acts as an endogenous antagonist of α-MSH at melanocortin receptors. In the hypothalamus, agouti over-expression causes hyperphagia and obesity, while antagonism of α-MSH in hair follicles prevents melanin formation and leaves the fur yellow.

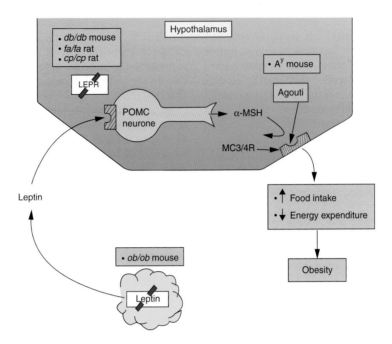

Figure 8.14 Genetic obesity syndromes in rodents related to leptin and the proopiomelanocortin (POMC) neurones in the hypothalamus, which are important in mediating leptin's appetite-suppressing action.

Very rare causes of human obesity have been related to mutations in the human analogues of these and other appetite-regulating genes (Figure 8.15 and Table 8.4). Most obese humans have raised leptin levels in proportion to their increased fat mass (Considine *et al.*, 1996; see Figure 4.13), but a small number of extremely obese children have been identified who have no circulating leptin. The first two cases had a mutation that introduced a premature stop codon in the leptin gene (*LEP*) and thus produced a truncated peptide with no biological activity (Montague *et al.*, 1997). Other families have subsequently been identified with various loss of function

mutations in *LEP*. These children have an insatiable appetite and early-onset morbid obesity from soon after weaning, with severe insulin resistance and hypogonadism; all these abnormalities were reversed by prolonged treatment with recombinant human leptin (see Chapter 21; Figure 8.16). Mutations of the leptin receptor (*LEPR*, analogous to *db*) have also been identified in a consanguineous family with early-onset obesity (Clément *et al.*, 1998). This confirms that basal levels of leptin are required to restrain appetite and prevent obesity in humans, although the relevance of physiological and supraphysiological leptin levels to human energy balance remains uncertain.

Table 8.4 Monogenic obesity syndromes in rodents, and their human counterparts.

Mutation affecting:	Rodent syndrome	Human counterpart
• Leptin	*ob/ob* mouse	*LEP*
• Leptin receptor	*db/db* mouse, *fa/fa, cp/cp* rats	*LEPR*
• Agouti (overexpression)	A[y] mouse	–
• Proopiomelanocortin	–	*POMC*
• Prohormone convertase 1	–	*PC-1*
• Melanocortin-3 receptor	–	*MC3-R*
• Melanocortin-4 receptor	–	*MC4-R*
• CCK1R receptor	OLETF rat	*CCK1R*

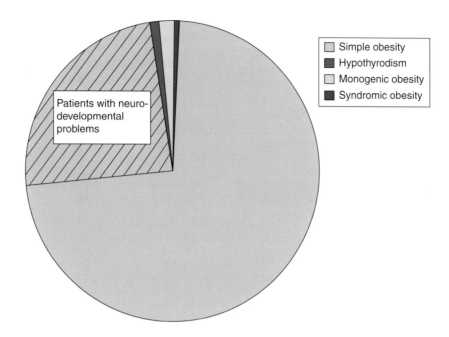

Figure 8.15 Genetic obesity syndromes in humans related to the leptin-POMC axis.

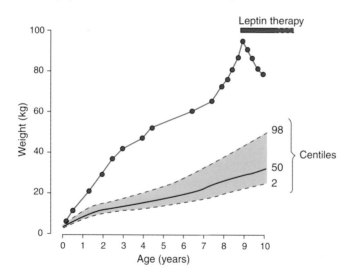

Figure 8.16 Body weight curve in a child with a leptin mutation, showing early-onset morbid obesity. Body weight and fat fell rapidly during treatment with recombinant human leptin. From Farooqi *et al.* (1999), with kind permission of the editor of the *New England Journal of Medicine*.

Mutations affecting CNS targets of leptin and other signals of energy balance have also been linked to human obesity – which typically in these cases begins early in childhood and is accompanied by hyperphagia (Table 8.4). These include mutations of POMC, the α-MSH precursor (Krude *et al.*, 1998; Challis *et al.*, 2002); the enzyme prohormone convertase 1 (PC-1) that is responsible for cleaving α-MSH from POMC (Jackson *et al.*, 1997, 2003) and the melano-cortin receptor MC4-R (Challis *et al.*, 2002; Yeo *et al.*, 1998; Vaisse *et al.*, 2000; Farooqi *et al.*, 2000, 2003). The MC4-R gene in particular is highly polymorphic, with several 'hot spots' for mutations that cause variable loss of function. Such MC4-R mutations are the most common of the monogenic defects yet identified, affecting perhaps up to 5% of morbidly obese subjects whose overweight began in childhood (Farooqi *et al.*, 2003). The other syndromes are extremely rare, with perhaps 200–300 affected individuals so far identified worldwide (Rankinen and Bouchard, 2006; Farooqi and O'Rahilly, 2006, 2007). Very rare cases have also been found with mutations that disable the CCK1 (CCK$_A$) receptor, which mediates the satiating effect of the gut peptide, cholecystokinin (CCK) (see Chapter 6).

References

Alexander, D., Ball, M.J. and Mann, J. (1994) Nutrient intake and haematological status of vegetarians and age-sex matched omnivores. *European Journal of Clinical Nutrition*, **48**, 538–46.

Allison, D.B., Neale, M.C., Kezis, M.I., Alfonso, V.C., Heshka, S. and Heymsfield, S.B. (1996). Assortative mating for relative weight: genetic implications. *Behavior Genetics* **26**,103–11.

Appleby, P.N., Thorogood, M., Mann, J.I. and Key, T.J. (1998) Low body mass index in non-meat eaters: the possible roles of animal fat, dietary fibre and alcohol. *International Journal of Obesity and Related Metabolic Disorders*, **22**, 454–60.

Appleby, P.N., Thorogood, M., Mann, J.I. and Key, T.J. (1999) The Oxford Vegetarian Study: an overview. *The American Journal of Clinical Nutrition*, **70**, 525S–31S.

Bellisle, F., Mcdevitt, R. and Prentice, A.M. (1997) Meal frequency and energy balance. *The British Journal of Nutrition*, **77** (Suppl 1), S57–70.

Benyshek, D.C. and Watson, J.T. (2006) Exploring the thrifty genotype's food-shortage assumptions: a cross-cultural comparison of ethnographic accounts of food security among foraging and agricultural societies. *American Journal of Physical Anthropology*, **131**, 120–6.

Berkow, S.E. and Barnard, N. (2006) Vegetarian diets and weight status. *Nutrition Reviews*, **64**, 175–88.

Black, A.E., Coward, W.A., Cole, T.J. and Prentice, A.M. (1996) Human energy expenditure in affluent societies: an analysis of 574 doubly-labelled water measurements. *European Journal of Clinical Nutrition*, **50**, 72–92.

Blass, E.M., Anderson, D.R., Kirkorian, H.L. *et al.* (2006) On the road to obesity: Television viewing increases intake of high-density foods. *Physiology & Behavior*, **88** (4–5), 597–604.

Bodurtha, J.N., Mosteller, M., Hewitt, J.K. *et al.* (1990) Genetic analysis of anthropometric measures in 11-year-old twins: the Medical College of Virginia Twin Study. *Pediatric Research*, **28** (1), 1–4.

Boutin, P., Dina, C., Vasseur, F. *et al.* (2003) GAD2 on chromosome 10p12 is a candidate gene for human obesity. *PLOS Biology*, **1**, 361–71.

Buchowski, M.S. and Sun, M. (1996) Energy expenditure, television viewing and obesity. *International Journal of Obesity* **20**, 236–244.

Cardon, L. (1994) Height, weight, and obesity, in *Nature and Nurture During Middle Childhood* (eds J. DeFries, R. Plomin and D. Fulker), Blackwell, London.

Cardon, L. (1995) Genetic influences on body mass index in early childhood, in *Behavior Genetic Approaches in Behavioral Medicine* (eds J. Turner, L. Cardon and J. Hewitt), Plenum, New York, pp. 133–43.

Challis, B.G., Pritchard, L.E., Creemers, J.W. *et al.* (2002) A missense mutation disrupting a dibasic prohormone processing site in proopiomelanocortin (POMC) increases susceptibility to early-onset obesity through a novel molecular mechanism. *Human Molecular Genetics*, **11**, 1997–2004.

Chanmugam, P., Guthrie, J.F., Cecilio, S. *et al.* (2003) Did fat intake in the United States really decline between 1989–1991 and 1994–1996? *Journal of the American Dietetic Association*, **103**, 867–72.

Cho, S., Dietrich, M., Brown, C.J. *et al.* (2003) The effect of breakfast type on total daily energy intake and body mass index: results from the Third National Health and Nutrition Examination Survey (NHANES III). *Journal of the American College of Nutrition*, **22** (4), 296–302.

Clemens, L.H., Slawson, D.L. and Klesges, R.C. (1999) The effect of eating out on quality of diet in premenopausal women. *Journal of the American Dietetic Association*, **99**, 442–4.

Clément, K., Ruiz, J., CassardDoulcier, A.M., Bouillaud, F., Ricquier, D., Basdevant, A, GuyGrand, B. and Froguel, P. (1995) Additive effect of A->G (-3826) variant of the uncoupling protein gene and the Trp64Arg mutation of the beta 3-adrenergic receptor gene on weight gain in morbid obesity. *International Journal of Obesity*, **20**, 1062–6.

Clément, K., Vaisse, C., Lahlou, N. *et al.* (1998) A mutation in the human leptin receptor gene causes obesity and pituitary dysfunction. *Nature*, **392**, 398–401.

Considine, R.V. *et al.* (1996) Serum immunoreactive leptin concentrations in normal-weight and obese humans. *New England Journal of Medicine*, **334**, 292–5.

Coon, K.A., Goldberg, J., Rogers, B.L. and Tucker, K.L. (2001) Relationships between use of television during meals and children's food consumption patterns. *Pediatrics*, **107**, e7.

Crespo, C.J., Smit, E., Troiano, R.P., Bartlett, S.J. *et al.* (2001) Television watching, energy intake, and obesity in US children: results from the third National Health and Nutrition Examination Survey 1988–1994. *Archives of Pediatrics & Adolescent Medicine*, **155**, 360–5.

Cuco, G., Arija, V., Marti-Henneberg, C. and Fernandez-Ballart, J. (2001) Food and nutritional profile of high energy density consumers in an adult Mediterranean population. *European Journal of Clinical Nutrition*, **55** (3), 192–9.

de Castro, J.M. and Brewer, E.M (1992). The amount eaten in meals by humans is a power function of the number of people present, *Physiology & Behavior*, **51**, 121–25.

de Castro, J.M. (2004a) Dietary energy density is associated with increased intake in free-living humans. *The Journal of Nutrition*, **134** (2), 335–41.

de Castro, J.M. (2004b) Genes, the environment and the control of food intake. *The British Journal of Nutrition*, **92** (Suppl 1), S59–62.

Dietz, W.H., Jr. and Gortmaker, S.L. (1985) Do we fatten our children at the television set? Obesity and television viewing in children and adolescents. *Pediatrics*, **75**, 807–12.

Dietz, W.H., Bandini, L.G., Morelli, J.A., Peers, K.F. and Ching, P.L.Y.H. (1994) Effect of sedentary activities on resting metabolic-rate. *American Journal of Clinical Nutrition*, **59**, 556–9.

Dubois, E.F. (1936) *Basal Metabolism in Health and Disease*, 3rd edn, Lea and Febiger, Philadelphia.

Duffey, K.J., Gordon-Larsen, P., Jacobs, D.R., Jr. *et al.* (2007) Differential associations of fast food and restaurant food consumption with 3-y change in body mass index: the Coronary Artery Risk Development in Young Adults Study. *The American Journal of Clinical Nutrition*, **85**, 201–8.

Edelman, B., Engell, D., Bronstein, P. and Hirsch, E. (1986) Environmental-effects on the intake of overweight and normal-weight men. *Appetite*, **7**, 71–83.

Fabsitz, R.R., Carmelli, D. and Hewitt, J.K. (1992) Evidence for independent genetic influences on obesity in middle age. *International Journal of Obesity and Related Metabolic Disorders*, **16** (9), 657–66.

Faith, M.S., Rha, S.S., Neale, M.C. and Allison, D.B. (1999) Evidence for genetic influences on human energy intake: results from a twin study using measured observations. *Behavior Genetics*, **29** (3), 145–54.

Farooqi *et al.* (1999) Effects of recombinant human leptin therapy in a child with congenital leptin deficiency. *New England Journal of Medicine*, **341**, 879–84.

Farooqi, I.S. and O'Rahilly, S. (2006) Monogenic human obesity syndromes. *Hypothalamic Integration of energy metabolism*, **153**, 119–25.

Farooqi, I.S. and O'Rahilly, S. (2007) Genetic factors in human obesity. *Obesity Reviews*, **8**, 37–40.

Farooqi, I.S., Keogh, J.M., Yeo, G.S. *et al.* (2003) Clinical spectrum of obesity and mutations in the melanocortin 4 receptor gene. *The New England Journal of Medicine*, **348**, 1085–95.

Farooqi, I.S., Yeo, G.S., Keogh, J.M. *et al.* (2000) Dominant and recessive inheritance of morbid obesity associated with melanocortin 4 receptor deficiency. *The Journal of Clinical Investigation*, **106**, 271–9.

Flegal, K.M. *et al.* (2002) Prevalence and trends in obesity among US adults, 1999–2000. *Journal of the American Medical Association* **288**, 1723–7.

Fraser, G.E. (1999) Associations between diet and cancer, ischemic heart disease, and all-cause mortality in non-Hispanic white California Seventh-day Adventists. *The American Journal of Clinical Nutrition*, **70**, 532S–8S.

Frayling, T.M. *et al.* (2007) A common variant in the FTO gene is associated with body mass index and predisposes to childhood and adult obesity. *Science* **316**, 889–94.

Geissler, C.A., Miller, D.S. and Shah, M. (1987) The daily metabolic-rate of the post-obese and the lean. *American Journal of Clinical Nutrition*, **45**, 914–20.

Goldberg, G., Black, A., Jebb, S., Cole, T., Murgatroyd P., Coward, W. and Prentice A. (1991) Critical evaluation of energy intake data using fundamental principles of energy physiology: 1. Derivation of cut-off limits to identify under-recording. *European Journal of Clinical Nutrition*, **45**, 569–81.

Goran, M.I., Shewchuk, R., Gower, B.A. *et al.* (1998) Longitudinal changes in fatness in white children: no effect of childhood energy expenditure. *The American Journal of Clinical Nutrition*, **67**, 309–16.

Gorely, T., Marshall, S.J. and Biddle, S.J. (2004) Couch kids: correlates of television viewing among youth. *International Journal of Behavioral Medicine*, **11**, 152–63.

Grilo, C.M. and Pogue-Geile, M.F. (1991) The nature of environmental influences on weight and obesity: a behavior genetic analysis. *Psychological Bulletin*, **110** (3), 520–37.

Haddad, E.H., Berk, L.S., Kettering, J.D. *et al.* (1999) Dietary intake and biochemical, hematologic, and immune status of vegans compared with nonvegetarians. *The American Journal of Clinical Nutrition*, **70**, 586S–93S.

Haddad, E.H. and Tanzman, J.S. (2003) What do vegetarians in the United States eat? *The American Journal of Clinical Nutrition*, **78**, 626S–32S.

Halford, J.C., Boyland, E.J., Hughes, G. *et al.* (2007) Beyond-brand effect of television (TV) food advertisements/commercials on caloric intake and food choice of 5–7-year-old children. *Appetite*, **49** (1), 263–7.

Halford, J.C., Gillespie, J., Brown, V. *et al.* (2004) Effect of television advertisements for foods on food consumption in children. *Appetite*, **42** (2), 221–5.

Hancox, R.J., Milne, B.J. and Poulton, R. (2004) Association between child and adolescent television viewing and adult health: a longitudinal birth cohort study. *Lancet*, **364**, 257–62.

Hayes, M., Chustek, M., Heshka, S. *et al.* (2005) Low physical activity levels of modern Homo sapiens among free-ranging mammals. *International Journal of Obesity*, **29**, 151–6.

Hebebrand, J., Wulftange, H., Goerg, T., Ziegler, A., Hinney, A., Barth, N., Mayer, H., and Remschmidt, H. (2000). Epidemic obesity: are genetic factors involved via increased rates of assortative mating? *International Journal of Obesity* **24**, 345–53.

Heitmann, B.L. and Lissner, L. (1995) Dietary underreporting by obese individuals – is it specific or nonspecific? *British Medical Journal (Clinical research edition)*, **311**, 986–9.

Herbert, A., Gerry, N.P., McQueen, M.B. *et al.* (2006) A common genetic variant is associated with adult and childhood obesity. *Science*, **312**, 279–83.

Hewitt, J.K. (1997) The genetics of obesity: what have genetic studies told us about the environment. *Behavior Genetics*, **27** (4), 353–8.

Howarth, N.C., Huang, T.T., Roberts, S.B. *et al.* (2007) Eating patterns and dietary composition in relation to BMI in younger and older adults. *International Journal of Obesity (London)*, **31**, 675–84.

Hunt, S.C., Hasstedt, S.J., Kuida, H. *et al.* (1989) Genetic heritability and common environmental components of resting and stressed blood pressures, lipids, and body mass index in Utah pedigrees and twins. *American Journal of Epidemiology*, **129** (3), 625–38.

International HAPMAP Consortium (2007) A second generation human haplotype map of over 3.1 million SNPs. *Nature*, **449**, 851–U3.

Jackson, R.S., Creemers, J.W., Farooqi, I.S. *et al.* (2003) Small-intestinal dysfunction accompanies the complex endocrinopathy of human proprotein convertase 1 deficiency. *The Journal of Clinical Investigation*, **112** (10), 1550–60.

Jackson, R.S., Creemers, J.W., Ohagi, S. *et al.* (1997) Obesity and impaired prohormone processing associated with mutations in the human prohormone convertase 1 gene. *Nature Genetics*, **16**, 303–6.

Jeffery, R.W. and French, S.A. (1998) Epidemic obesity in the United States: are fast foods and television viewing contributing? *American Journal of Public Health*, **88**, 277–80.

Johansson, G., Wikman, A., Ahren, A.M. *et al.* (2001) Underreporting of energy intake in repeated 24-hour recalls related to gender, age, weight status, day of interview, educational level, reported food intake, smoking habits and area of living. *Public Health Nutrition*, **4** (4), 919–27.

Johnston, S.L., Bell, L.M., Murray, S.J., Tolkamp, B.J., Yearsley, J., Kyriazakis, I., Illius, A.W. and Speakman, J.R. (2007) Intake compensates for resting metabolic rate variation in female C57BL/6J mice fed high-fat diets. *Obesity*, **15**, 600–6.

Joosen, A.M.C.P., Geilen, M., Vlietinck, R. and Westerterp, K.R. (2007) Genetic analysis of physical activity in twins. *American Journal of Clinical Nutrition*, **82**, 1253–9.

Joseph, J. (1998) The equal environment assumption of the classical twin method: a critical analysis. *Journal of Mind and Behavior*, **19** (3), 325–58.

Kant, A.K. and Graubard, B.I. (2005) Energy density of diets reported by American adults: association with food group intake, nutrient intake, and body weight. *International Journal of Obesity (London)*, **29**, 950–6.

Kant, A.K. and Graubard, B.I. (2006) Secular trends in patterns of self-reported food consumption of adult Americans: NHANES 1971–1975 to NHANES 1999–2002. *American Journal of Clinical Nutrition*, **84**, 1215–23.

Kant, A.K., Schatzkin, A., Graubard, B.I. and Ballard-Barbash, R. (1995) Frequency of eating occasions and weight change in the NHANES I Epidemiologic Follow-up Study. *International Journal of Obesity and Related Metabolic Disorders*, **19**, 468–74.

Katzmarzyk, P.T. (2002) The Canadian obesity epidemic: an historical perspective. *Obesity Research*, **10** (7), 666–74.

Kaur, H., Choi, W.S., Mayo, M.S. and Harris, K.J. (2003) Duration of television watching is associated with increased body mass index. *The Journal of Pediatrics*, **143**, 506–11.

Kendall, A., Levitsky, D.A., Strupp, B.J. and Lissner, L. (1991) Weight loss on a low-fat diet: consequence of the imprecision of the control of food intake in humans. *The American Journal of Clinical Nutrition*, **53** (5), 1124–9.

Kennedy, E.T., Bowman, S.A., Spence, J.T. *et al.* (2001) Popular diets: correlation to health, nutrition, and obesity. *Journal of the American Dietetic Association*, **101**, 411–20.

King, N.A., Caudwell, P., Hopkins, M. *et al.* (2007) Metabolic and behavioral compensatory responses to exercise interventions: barriers to weight loss. *Obesity (Silver Spring)*, **15**, 1373–83.

Klesges, R.C., Bartsch, D., Norwood, J.D. *et al.* (1984) The effects of selected social and environmental variables on the eating behavior of adults in the natural environment. *International Journal of Eating Disorders*, **3**, 35–41.

Krude, H., Biebermann, H., Luck, W. *et al.* (1998) Severe early-onset obesity, adrenal insufficiency and red hair pigmentation caused by POMC mutations in humans. *Nature Genetics*, **19**, 155–7.

Larsson, C.L. and Johansson, G.K. (2002) Dietary intake and nutritional status of young vegans and omnivores in Sweden. *The American Journal of Clinical Nutrition*, **76**, 100–6.

Laskarzewski, P., Morrison, J.A., Khoury, P. *et al.* (1980) Parent-child nutrient intake interrelationships in school children ages 6 to 19: the Princeton School District Study. *The American Journal of Clinical Nutrition*, **33** (11), 2350–5.

Ledikwe, J.H., Blanck, H.M., Khan, L.K. *et al.* (2006) Dietary energy density is associated with energy intake and weight status in US adults. *American Journal Of Clinical Nutrition*, **83**, 1362–8.

Levine, J.A., Eberhardt, N.L. and Jensen, M.D. (1999) Role of nonexercise activity thermogenesis in resistance to fat gain in humans. *Science*, **283**, 212–4.

Levitsky, D.A. (2002) Putting behavior back into feeding behavior: a tribute to George Collier. *Appetite*, **38**, 143–8.

Levitsky, D.A. and Youn, T. (2004) The more food young adults are served the more they overeat. *Journal of Nutrition*, **134**, 2546–9.

Levitsky, D.A. (2005) The non-regulation of food intake in humans: hope for reversing the epidemic of obesity. *Physiology & Behavior*, **86**, 623–32.

Maes, H.H., Neale, M.C. and Eaves, L.J. (1997) Genetic and environmental factors in relative body weight and human adiposity. *Behavior Genetics*, **27** (4), 325–51.

Malouf, N. and Colaguiri, S. (1995) The effects of McDonalds, Kentucky Fried Chicken and Pizza Hut meals on recommended diets. *Asia Pacific Journal of Clinical Nutrition*, **4**, 265–9.

Marshall, S.J., Biddle, S.J., Gorely, T. *et al.* (2004) Relationships between media use, body fatness and physical activity in children and youth: a meta-analysis. *International Journal of Obesity and Related Metabolic Disorders*, **28**, 1238–46.

Matheson, D.M., Killen, J.D., Wang, Y., Varady, A., Robinson, T.N. (2004) Children's food consumption during television viewing. *American Journal of Clinical Nutrition*, **79**, 1088–94.

McCrory, M.A., Fuss, P.J., McCallum, J.E. *et al.* (1999a) Dietary variety within food groups: association with energy intake and body fatness in men and women. *The American Journal of Clinical Nutrition*, **69**, 440–7.

McCrory, M.A., Fuss, P.J., Hays, N.P. *et al.* (1999b) Overeating in America: Association between restaurant food consumption and body fatness in healthy adult men and women ages 19 to 80. *Obesity Research*, **7**, 564–71.

McCrory, M.A., Suen, V.M.M. and Roberts, S.B. (2002) Biobehavioral influences on energy intake and adult weight gain. *Journal of Nutrition*, **132**, 3830–34S.

Meiselman, H.L., DeGraaf, C. and Lesher, L.L. (2000) The effects of variety and monotony on food acceptance and intake at a midday meal. *Physiology & Behavior*, **70**, 119–25.

Mitchell, B.D., Rainwater, D.L., Hsueh, W.C. *et al.* (2003) Familial aggregation of nutrient intake and physical activity: results from the San Antonio Family Heart Study. *Annals of Epidemiology*, **13** (2), 128–35.

Montague, C.T. *et al.* (1997) Congenital leptin deficiency is associated with severe early-onset obesity in humans. *Nature*, **387**, 903–8.

Neel, J.V. (1962) Diabetes mellitus: a 'thrifty' genotype rendered detrimental by 'progress'? *American Journal of Human Genetics*, **14**, 352–3.

Nielsen, S.J., Siega-Riz, A.M. *et al.* (2002) Trends in energy intake in U.S. between 1977 and 1996: similar shifts seen across age groups. *Obesity Research*, **10** (5), 370–8.

Nieman, D.C., Underwood, B.C., Sherman, K.M. *et al.* (1989) Dietary status of Seventh-Day Adventist vegetarian and non-vegetarian elderly women. *Journal of the American Dietetic Association*, **89**, 1763–9.

Norton, G.N.M., Anderson, A.S. and Hetherington, M.M. (2006) Volume and variety: relative effects on food intake. *Physiology & Behavior*, **87**, 714–22.

O'Rahilly, S. and Farooqi, I.S. (2006) Genetics of obesity. *Philosophical Transactions of the Royal Society*, **361**, 1095–105.

Ogden, C.L., Carroll, M.D., Curtin, L.R. *et al.* (2006) Prevalence of overweight and obesity in the United States, 1999–2004. *Journal of the American Medical Association* **295**, 1549–55.

Osterholt, K.M., Roe, L.S. and Rolls, B.J. (2007) Incorporation of air into a snack food reduces energy intake. *Appetite*, **48**, 351–8.

Park, H.S., Yim, K.S. and Cho, S.I. (2004) Gender differences in familial aggregation of obesity-related phenotypes and dietary intake patterns in Korean families. *Annals of Epidemiology*, **14** (7), 486–91.

Perusse, L., Tremblay, A., Leblanc, C. *et al.* (1988) Familial resemblance in energy intake: contribution of genetic and environmental factors. *The American Journal of Clinical Nutrition*, **47** (4), 629–35.

Perusse, L., Rankinen, T., Zuberi, A., Chagnon, Y.C., Weisnagel, S.J., Argyropoulos, G., Walts, B., Snyder, E.E. and Bouchard, C. (2005) The Human obesity gene map: the 2004 update. *Obesity research*, **13**, 381–490.

Peters, T., Ausmeier, K., Dildrop, R. and Ruther, U. (2002) The mouse Fused toes (Ft) mutation is the result of a 1.6-Mb deletion including the entire Iroquois B gene cluster. *Mammalian genome* **13**, 186–8.

Prentice, A.M., Black, A.E., Coward, W.A. *et al.* (1986) High levels of energy expenditure in obese women. *British Medical Journal (Clinical research edition)*, **292**, 983–7.

Prentice, A.M. and Jebb, S.A. (1995) Obesity in Britain: gluttony or sloth? *British Medical Journal*, **311**, 437–9.

Rajeshwari, R., Yang, S.J., Nicklas, T.A. and Berenson, G.S. (2005) Secular trends in children's sweetened-beverage consumption (1973 to 1994): the Bogalusa Heart Study. *Journal of the American Dietetic Association*, **105**, 208–14.

Rance, K.A., Hambly, C., Dalgleish, D., Fustin, J.M., Bünger, L. and Speakman, J.R. (2007) Quantitative Trait Loci for total and regional adiposity in mouse lines divergently selected for food intake. *Obesity*, **15**, 2994–3004.

Rance, K.A., Fustin, J.M., Dalgleish, G., Hambly, C., Bünger, L. and Speakman, J.R.(2005) A Paternally imprinted QTL for mature body mass on mouse chromosome 8. *Mammalian genome*, **16**, 567–77.

Rankinen, T. and Bouchard, C. (2006) Genetics of food intake and eating behaviour phenotypes in humans. *Annual Review of Nutrition*, **26**, 413–34.

Rankinen, T., Zuberi, A., Chagnon, Y.C. *et al.* (2006) The human obesity gene map: the 2005 update. *Obesity*, **14**, 529–644.

Ravussin, E., Lillioja, S., Knowler, W.C. *et al.* (1988) Reduced rate of energy expenditure as a risk factor for body-weight gain. *The New England Journal of Medicine*, **318**, 467–72.

Resnicow, K., Barone, J., Engle, A. *et al.* (1991) Diet and serum lipids in vegan vegetarians: a model for risk reduction. *Journal of the American Dietetic Association*, **91**, 447–53.

Riumallo, J.A., Schoeller, D., Barrera, G. *et al.* (1989) Energy expenditure in underweight free-living adults: impact of energy supplementation as determined by doubly labeled water and indirect calorimetry. *The American Journal of Clinical Nutrition*, **49**, 239–46.

Roberts, S.B., Savage, J., Coward, W.A., Chew, B. and Lucas, A. (1988) Energy-expenditure and intake in infants born to lean and overweight mothers. *New England Journal of medicine*, **318**, 461–6.

Rolls, B.J., Bell, E.A. and Waugh, B.A. (2000) Increasing the volume of a food by incorporating air affects satiety in men. *The American Journal of Clinical Nutrition*, **72**, 361–8.

Rolls, B.J., Kim, S., McNelis, A.L., Fischman, M.W., Foltin, R.W. and Moran, T.H. (1991) Time course of effects of preloads high in fat or carbohydrate on food-intake and hunger ratings in humans. *American Journal of Physiology*, **260**, R756–63.

Rolls, B.J., Roe, L.S., Meengs, J.S. and Wall, D.E. (2004) Increasing the portion size of a sandwich increases energy intake. *Journal of the American Dietetic Association*, **104**, 367–72.

Rolls, B.J., Rowe, E.A., Rolls, E.T. *et al.* (1981) Variety in a meal enhances food intake in man. *Physiology & Behavior*, **26**, 215–21.

Sabate, J. (2003) The contribution of vegetarian diets to health and disease: a paradigm shift? *The American Journal of Clinical Nutrition*, **78**, 502S–7S.

Satia, J.A., Galanko, J.A. and Siega-Riz, A.M. (2004) Eating at fast-food restaurants is associated with dietary intake, demographic, psychosocial and behavioural factors among African Americans in North Carolina. *Public Health Nutrition*, **7**, 1089–96.

Schoeller, D.A. (1990) How accurate is self-reported dietary energy intake? *Nutrition Reviews*, **48** (10), 373–9.

Serdula, M.K., Mokdad, A.H., Williamson, D.F. *et al.* (1999) Prevalence of attempting weight loss and strategies for controlling weight. *Journal of the American Medical Association* **282** (14), 1353–8.

Speakman, J.R. (2000) The cost of living: factors influencing the daily energy demands of small mammals. *Advances in Ecological Research*, **30**, 177–297.

Speakman, J.R. (2004) Obesity: the integrated roles of environment and genetics. *Journal of Nutrition*, **134**, 2090–2105S

Speakman, J.R. (2007) A novel non-adaptive scenario explaining the genetic pre-disposition to obesity: the 'predation release' hypothesis. *Cell metabolism*, **6**, 5–11.

Speakman, J.R., Djafarian, K., Stewart, J. and Jackson, D.M. (2007) Assortative mating for obesity. *American Journal of Clinical Nutrition*, **86**, 316–23.

Speakman, J.R., Hambly, C., Mitchell, S.E. and Krol, E. (2008) The contribution of animal models to the study of obesity Laboratory Animals, (in press).

Spiegel, T.A. and Stellar, E. (1990) Effects of variety on food intake of underweight, normal-weight and overweight women. *Appetite*, **15**, 47–61.

Steward, H., Blisard, N., Bhuyan, S. and Nayga, R. (2004). *The demand for food away from home: full-service or fast food?* Agricultural Economic Service, United States Department of Agriculture, 829.

Stubbs, R.J., Johnstone, A.M., Mazlan, N. *et al.* (2001) Effect of altering the variety of sensorially distinct foods, of the same macronutrient content, on food intake and body weight in men. *European Journal of Clinical Nutrition*, **55**, 19–28.

Summerbell, C.D., Moody, R.C., Shanks, J. *et al.* (1996) Relationship between feeding pattern and body mass index in 220 free-living people in four age groups. *European Journal of Clinical Nutrition*, **50**, 513–9.

Tartaglia, L.A., Dembski, M., Weng, X. *et al.* (1995) Identification and expression cloning of a leptin receptor, OB-R. *Cell*, **83**, 1263–71.

Tataranni, P.A., Harper, I.T., Snitker, S. *et al.* (2003) Body weight gain in free-living Pima Indians: effect of energy intake vs expenditure. *International Journal of Obesity*, **12**, 1578–83.

Temple, N.J., Steyn, K., Hoffman, M. *et al.* (2001) The epidemic of obesity in South Africa: a study in a disadvantaged community. *Ethnicity and Disease*, **11** (3), 431–7.

Thorogood, M., Roe, L., McPherson, K. and Mann, J. (1990) Dietary intake and plasma lipid levels: lessons from a study of the diet of health conscious groups. *British Medical Journal*, **300**, 1297–1301.

Utter, J., Neumark-Sztainer, D., Jeffery, R. and Story, M. (2003) Couch potatoes or french fries: are sedentary behaviors associated with body mass index, physical activity, and dietary behaviors among adolescents? *Journal of the American Dietetic Association*, **103**, 1298–1305.

Vaisse, C., Clement, K., Durand, E. *et al.* (2000) Melanocortin-4 receptor mutations are a frequent and heterogeneous cause of morbid obesity. *The Journal of Clinical Investigation*, **106**, 253–62.

Walston, J., Silver K., Bogardus C. (1995) Time of onset of non-insulin-dependent diabetes mellitus and genetic variation in the β_3 adrenergic receptor. *New England Journal of medicine*, **333**, 348–51.

Walston, J., Silver, K., Bogadus, C., Knowler. W.C., Celi, F.S., Austin, S., Manning, B., Strosberg, A.D., Stern, M.P., Raben, N., Sorkin, J.D., Roth, J. and Shuldiner, A.R (1995) Time of onset of non-insulin-dependent diabetes-mellitus and genetic-variation in the beta(3)-adrenergic-receptor gene. *New England Journal of medicine*, **333**, 343–7.

Wansink, B. and Kim, J. (2005) Bad popcorn in big buckets: portion size can influence intake as much as taste. *Journal of Nutrition Education and Behavior*, **37**, 242–5.

West, D.B. and York, B. (1998) Dietary fat, genetic predisposition, and obesity: lessons from animal models. *The American Journal of Clinical Nutrition*, **67**, 505S–12S.

Westerterp, K.R. (1998) Alterations in energy balance with exercise. *The American Journal of Clinical Nutrition*, **68**, 970S–4S.

WHO (1998) Obesity: preventing and managing a global epidemic. Geneva.

Wiecha, J.L., Peterson, K.E., Ludwig, D.S. *et al.* (2006) When children eat what they watch: impact of television viewing on dietary intake in youth. *Archives of Pediatrics & Adolescent Medicine*, **160** (4), 436–42.

Williamson, D.F., Serdula, M.K., Anda, R.F. *et al.* (1992) Weight loss attempts in adults: goals, duration, and rate of weight loss. *American Journal of Public Health*, **82** (9), 1251–7.

Yeo, G.S., Farooqi, I.S., Aminian, S. *et al.* (1998) A frameshift mutation in MC4R associated with dominantly inherited human obesity. *Nature Genetics*, **20**, 111–2.

Zhang, Y., Proenca, R., Maffei, M. *et al.* (1994) Positional cloning of the mouse obese gene and its human homologue. *Nature*, **372**, 425–32.

Health Hazards of Obesity: An Overview

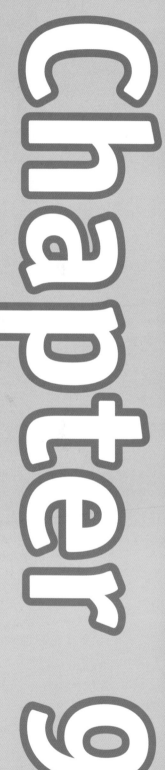

Key points

- Obesity predisposes to various comorbid conditions and may account for a substantial proportion of the risk (10–60% of total) of developing disorders such as type 2 diabetes, hypertension, coronary heart disease, several cancers, osteoarthritis and gall-bladder disease.

- Obesity significantly shortens life expectancy, especially in men. The risk of premature death from all causes rises progressively as BMI increases above normal, to a two- to fourfold excess at BMI $\geq 30\,kg/m^2$. Physical inactivity further increases excess mortality; the combination of overweight or obesity (BMI $\geq 25\,kg/m^2$) and low activity may account for 30% of all premature deaths worldwide.

- Mortality risk also increases at low BMI ($<20\,kg/m^2$), largely because of the confounding effects of smoking and co-existent chronic diseases that cause weight loss and shorten life.

- Cardiovascular disease is the main cause (50–70%) of excess obesity-related deaths. Central obesity especially predisposes to cardiovascular disease. Waist circumference and waist:hip ratio predict cardiovascular disease and mortality more powerfully than BMI; risk increases significantly above waist circumference levels of 94–102 cm in men and 80–88 cm in women. Overall, the cardiac risk related to obesity is higher in men, lower in certain ethnic groups (e.g. African-Americans) and is mitigated by good physical fitness.

- Central obesity is commonly associated with hyperglycaemia, hypertension, dyslipidaemia and other features of the metabolic syndrome, a clustering of risk factors that increases the risk of atherosclerosis and cardiovascular disease, including myocardial infarction and death. The aetiological links between obesity and the syndrome's other features remain uncertain. The co-existence of obesity amplifies the cardiovascular impact of other risk factors, such as diabetes, hypertension and smoking.

- Obesity, especially central, is a powerful predictor of hypertension, increasing the risk from 40% to threefold at BMI $\geq 30\,kg/m^2$. Although weight reduction is associated with a lowering of blood pressure, by about 1 mm Hg diastolic for each 1 kg of weight loss, the effect of weight reduction on cardiovascular outcomes remains to be confirmed.

- Obesity is specifically linked with congestive cardiac failure, perhaps related to myocardial fat deposition in addition to the deleterious effects of coronary artery disease. Prognosis is worse in patients with severe heart failure who also have a low BMI, probably because of increased catabolism ('cardiac cachexia').

- Central obesity predisposes strongly to type 2 diabetes, and accounts for up to 60% of also total risk. Some populations (e.g. Pima Indians and Asians) are particularly susceptible. Weight gain in adult life and low levels of physical activity and fitness also predispose.

- Obesity contributes to the risk for several malignancies, including cancers of the endometrium (30% of total risk), colon, oesophagus and breast, and lymphoma. Suggested mechanisms include dietary factors and physical inactivity (colorectal cancer), gastro-oesophageal reflux (oesophageal cancer) and cirrhosis complicating fatty liver disease (hepatocellular carcinoma). Overall, overweight and obesity may account for 14% of all cancer-related deaths in men and 20% in women.

Chapter 9

Health Hazards of Obesity: An Overview

Ronald C.W. Ma, Gary T.C. Ko, and Juliana C.N. Chan

Obesity has long been linked with various diseases and with premature death. Associations are well recognized with type 2 diabetes, hypertension, dyslipidaemia and vascular disease – commonly grouped together as the 'metabolic syndrome' – and with osteoarthritis, sleep apnoea and the polycystic ovarian syndrome (PCOS). Obesity has also been implicated as a risk factor for many other diseases, including several malignancies and chronic renal failure (see Table 9.1). Wolf and Colditz (1998) and James *et al.* (2004) have estimated the proportion of total risk of developing several major diseases that can be attributed to obesity. There are some discrepancies between the two reports, probably due to differences in the study populations and sampling periods (Wolf and Colditz used only American data from the 1988 and 1994 National Health Interview Survey). Overall, however, obesity appears to contribute about 60% of the total risk for type 2 diabetes, up to 40% of that for hypertension and endometrial carcinoma, 20–30% of the risk for coronary heart disease, stroke, osteoarthritis and gall-bladder disease, and about 10% for carcinoma of the breast and colon (Figure 9.1). The relationship between risk and BMI varies considerably among these diseases, with the risk for type 2 diabetes rising particularly sharply as BMI increases above the normal range (Figure 9.2, and Figure 9.9 on page 226).

This chapter reviews the key epidemiological evidence linking obesity to its main comorbidities and premature death, and touches on some of the possible aetiological mechanisms. We shall also discuss the predictive value of the various measures of obesity, and how risk is modulated by factors such as gender, ethnic origin, physical fitness and smoking. Detailed accounts of the pathophysiology, clinical features and management of the major comorbidities can be found elsewhere in this book, namely type 2 diabetes and its metabolic complications (Chapter 10), liver disease (Chapter 11), cardiovascular disease (Chapter 12) and other diseases (Chapter 13).

Measures of obesity as predictors of morbidity and mortality

Epidemiological studies have established numerous links between obesity and various diseases and premature death, but the strength of the reported associations varies considerably. This is due partly to inconsistencies in defining and measuring obesity, as well as to differences in study design and populations.

Obesity can be quantified in many ways, ranging from simple anthropometric measurements suitable for large-scale 'field' studies to complicated (and expensive) laboratory techniques (see Chapter 3). Most epidemiological studies have used simple measurements such as weight, BMI, waist circumference, waist-hip ratio (WHR) and skin-fold thickness. Increasingly, more sophisticated indices of adiposity (e.g. body fat mass, measured by bioimpedance) and of body fat distribution (e.g. using DEXA scanning) are being employed. Some of these measures are more informative than others in revealing associations with morbidity or mortality. In particular, imaging techniques that quantify regional fat distribution have helped to clarify the health hazards of central obesity and to identify possible aetiological mechanisms.

As discussed below there is considerable ethnic variation in body fat distribution, which can affect the relationship between measures of obesity and risk of comorbidities. Accordingly, anthropometric definitions of obesity are being redrawn for Asian and other populations.

Obesity: Science to Practice Edited by Gareth Williams and Gema Frühbeck
© 2009 John Wiley & Sons, Ltd

Table 9.1   Diseases for which obesity is a risk factor.

Metabolic:	Type 2 diabetes and other states of glucose intolerance
	Dyslipidaemia
	Gout
Cardiovascular:	Hypertension
	Cardiac failure
	Arrhythmias, including sudden death
	Coronary artery disease, including acute myocardial infarction
	Stroke
	Peripheral vascular disease
	Pulmonary hypertension
Malignancies:	Endometrial carcinoma
	Colorectal carcinoma
	Hepatocellular carcinoma
	Breast carcinoma
	Lymphoma and haematological malignances
Gastrointestinal:	Fatty liver disease, including cirrhosis
	Gall-bladder disease
	Gastro-oesophageal reflux
Respiratory:	Obstructive sleep apnoea
	Obesity-hypoventilation syndrome
Renal:	Obesity-related glomerulopathy
	Chronic renal failure
Endocrine:	Polycystic ovarian syndrome
	Infertility
Musculoskeletal:	Osteoarthritis of weight-bearing joints and hands
Psychiatric:	Depression

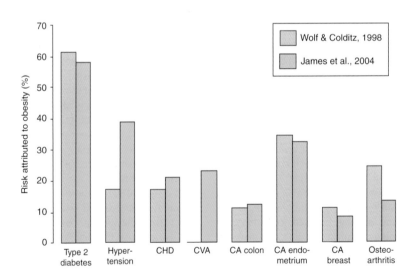

Figure 9.1 Percentage of risk attributed to obesity in developing certain diseases in North American and global populations, as estimated by Wolf and Colditz (1998) and James *et al.* (2004) respectively. Both reports used a BMI risk threshold of 30 kg/m². Risk for stroke was not available in Wolf's report.

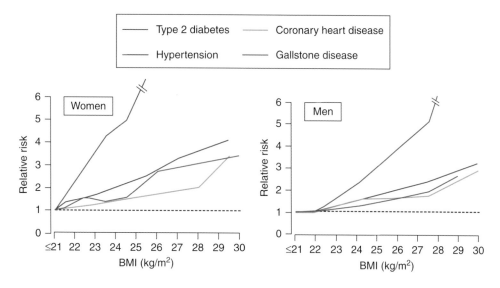

Figure 9.2 Relationships between BMI and the risk of developing certain diseases, in women (left panel) and men (right panel). From Willett *et al.* (1999).

Obesity and premature mortality

It has been recognized for centuries that obese people are more likely to die prematurely. For the methodological reasons mentioned above, the overall importance of obesity as a cause of mortality, and the ways in which it leads to death, have been much debated. Here, we review initially the impact of obesity on overall (all-cause) mortality, and then focus on the contributions of obesity to the major comorbidities of cardiovascular disease, diabetes and malignancy.

All-cause mortality

Early studies using various measures of adiposity indicated that obesity carries significant risks of dying prematurely. In the late 1970s, a longitudinal observational survey of 750000 subjects showed that those who were ≥40% above the cohort's average weight had a nearly twofold risk of dying during the ten years of follow up (Lew and Garfinkel, 1979). Increased skin-fold thickness was also found to predict premature mortality (Noppa *et al.*, 1980). However, BMI was found to be a better predictor (Noppa *et al.*, 1980; Menotti *et al.*, 1993) and has been widely used to stratify health risk (Chapter 3).

Many studies using BMI have reported either a U- or J- shaped relationship with mortality, with

increases at the lowest as well as the highest extremes of BMI. An example is the NHANES-III follow up study (Flegal *et al.*, 2005). This effect is partly due to incomplete adjustment for confounders such as cardiovascular risk factors and co-existent conditions that reduce weight while increasing mortality (Sjöström, 1992). Of particular importance is smoking, which generally reduces weight by approximately 3–5 kg (Albanes *et al.*, 1987; Nemery *et al.*, 1983), partly because smoking suppresses appetite (Chen *et al.*, 2006; Miyata *et al.*, 1999). Conversely, smokers who stop the habit tend to gain weight – up to 13 kg in some studies (Levine *et al.*, 2007). Other potential factors that could explain increased mortality at low BMI may include 'cachexia' due to undetected malignancy and other co-existent conditions (see below).

When careful allowance is made for the effects of smoking and other confounders, the effect of BMI in increasing mortality is clearly revealed (Bender *et al.*, 1998; Stevens *et al.*, 1998; Calle *et al.*, 1999; Calle *et al.*, 2003; Flegal *et al.*, 2005; Gu *et al.*, 2006; Park, Song and Cho, 2006). An example is one of the largest US prospective cohorts (900000 subjects) followed up for 14 years by (Calle *et al.*, 2003). The BMI nadir for mortality among subjects who had never smoked was 23.5–24.9 kg/m² in men and 22.0–23.4 kg/m² in women; above these values, mortality rose progressively and more steeply in men, reaching relative risks of premature death of

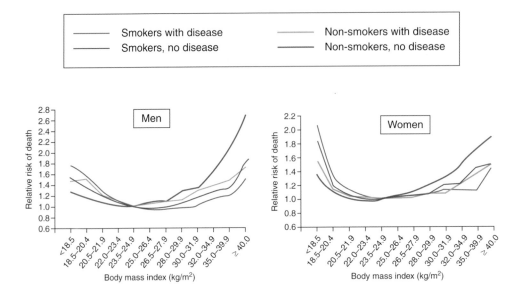

Figure 9.3 Relationships between BMI and relative risk of death, in men (left panel) and women (right panel). The impact of smoking (current or previous) and co-existence of chronic diseases in increasing relative risk at low BMI is evident in both sexes. The reference population (relative risk = 1.0) comprised subjects with BMI 23.5–24.9 kg/m² who had never smoked and had no co-existent diseases. From Calle *et al.* (1999).

2.6 for men and 1.8 for women, at BMI >40 kg/m² (Figure 9.3). There remained a slight excess mortality at BMI <20 kg/m² in subjects of either sex who had never smoked, but this was greatly increased – effectively restoring a clear U-shaped relationship – when current and ex-smokers and subjects with known co-existent diseases were included.

Broadly similar findings have emerged from other studies that excluded potential bias from smoking and co-existent chronic diseases. A large US study of 500 000 50-year old men and women showed that the risk of premature death increased two- to threefold among both men and women with BMI > 30 kg/m², and by 20–30% in those with BMI 25–29.9 kg/m², as compared with normal-weight subjects (Adams *et al.*, 2006). The Cancer Prevention Study I followed up 62 000 men and 262 000 women who had never smoked and had no cardiovascular disease, cancer or recent weight loss, from 1960 to 1972 (Stevens *et al.*, 1998). This study found a steady increase in mortality as BMI rose from <19 kg/m² to >32 kg/m², with a 3.5-fold increase for both sexes at BMI > 32 kg/m². A similar pattern was seen in the 16-year US Nurses' Health Study, with the lowest mortality in women who weighed at least 15% below the average for age-matched women (Manson *et al.*, 1995). Among non-smokers with stable weight, as BMI increased from <19 kg/m² to ≥32 kg/m², the risk of death after four years rose progressively from 120 to 220% of that in subjects with a BMI of 25 kg/m². Some other studies, however, have found a U-shaped relationship between BMI and mortality, especially in women, which persisted after adjustment for smoking (Rissanen *et al.*, 1991; Lindsted and Singh, 1997).

BMI shows considerable ethnic variation and is an imperfect surrogate for the degree of adiposity (see page 240 and Chapter 3). Body fat mass may be a more powerful predictor of premature death. A prospective Swedish study of 787 men aged 60 years, followed for 22 years, found a significant correlation between fat mass (estimated by ⁴⁰K measurements) and all-cause mortality (Heitmann *et al.*, 2000). Similarly, the Malmö Diet and Cancer Study (10 900 men and 16 800 women followed up for mean 5.7 years) found that fat mass was more strongly associated than BMI with premature death in both sexes, with the impact of excess body fat being most striking in young women (Lahmann *et al.*, 2002).

Central obesity specifically increases the risks of developing type 2 diabetes, the metabolic syndrome and cardiovascular disease, as described below. Moreover, central obesity, as measured by waist circumference or WHR, is in general, a better predictor of all-cause as well as cardiovascular mortality, as compared with the generalized obesity measure of BMI (Folsom *et al.*, 2000; Kanaya *et al.*, 2003).

Factors modulating effects of obesity on all-cause mortality

Gender

Some studies (e.g. Calle *et al.*, 1999) suggest that the obesity-associated risk of dying prematurely rises more steeply in men (see Figure 9.3). In addition, the Charleston Heart Study, a prospective 25-year follow up of 1400 African-Americans, found that BMI and waist circumference were associated with all-cause (and coronary heart disease related) mortality in men, but not in women (Stevens *et al.*, 1992a, 1992b). The effect of age in decreasing the impact of BMI on all-cause mortality also appears to favour women (see below and Figure 9.4).

Gender may have confounding effects on the prognostic significance of particular anthropometric measurements. An Australian study of 3300 men and 3600 women reported that high values of BMI (kg/m^2) and kg/m both predicted early mortality in men, whereas only kg/m (and not BMI) predicted cardiovascular mortality in women (Welborn, Knuiman and Vu, 2000).

Age

Obesity appears to increase the risk of all-cause mortality across adult life and into old age. The Cancer Prevention Study, for example, demonstrated this effect in men and women up to 75 years of age (Stevens *et al.*, 1998). Interestingly, however, this study showed that the relative risk associated with a standard increment of BMI *decreases* with increasing age. For each 1 kg/m^2 increment in BMI, the relative risk of death fell progressively from 1.07 at age 30–44 years to 1.01 at age >85 years (Figure 9.4). Other studies have shown the same effect. In a German prospective study of 6000 obese subjects followed for 15 years, obesity-related excess mortality was found to decrease with age at all levels of obesity. Standardized mortality fell progressively and significantly in both sexes: in men, from 2.46 at 18–29 years to 1.31 at 50–74 years, and in women from 1.81 to 1.26 at the same ages (Bender *et al.*, 1999). This phenomenon may be explained by the increasing likelihood of death with increasing age, which would diminish any specific impact of obesity.

Ethnicity

There is considerable ethnic variation in the relationship between adiposity and the sequelae of obesity, and these can confound the attribution of risk to measures such as BMI and waist circumference. Of particular note is the higher risk of type 2 diabetes in Asian and American

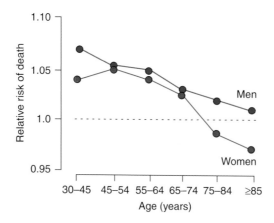

Figure 9.4 Effect of age on the excess all-cause mortality conferred by a 1-kg/m^2 increment in BMI, in men and women. Data from the Cancer Prevention Study (Stevens, 1992a,b).

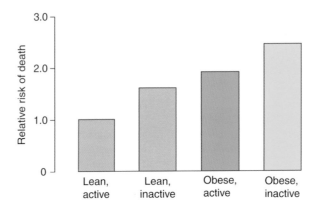

Figure 9.5 Impact of obesity alone and in combination with physical activity on all-cause mortality in women. The reference population (risk = 1.0) comprised women with BMI <25 kg/m² who spent ≥3.5 hours per week in physical exercise. Data from Hu *et al.* (2004).

ethnic populations at BMI levels that do not increase risk in Caucasians. Conversely, the cardiovascular risk associated with obesity appears to rise more slowly with BMI in some diabetes-prone ethnic groups, compared with Caucasians. This is discussed further below and in Chapters 2, 10 and 12.

This diversity complicates the interpretation of the impact of obesity on all-cause mortality among different populations. The Cancer Prevention Study II found that the relative risk of obesity-associated mortality was lower in African-Americans than in White populations (Stevens, 2000) – even though susceptibility to obesity-related diabetes is increased. Moreover, the San Antonio Heart Study showed that Mexican-Americans were more likely to be overweight than non-Hispanic whites, but that their age-specific and age-adjusted mortality rates were no higher (Stern *et al.*, 1990). Similar findings have been reported in other diabetes-prone populations, including Pima Indians (Pettitt *et al.*, 1982) and Pacific Islanders (Hodge *et al.*, 1996).

The apparent protection against premature death in these populations, especially given the increased prevalence of diabetes, is unexplained.

Physical activity and general health

Physical fitness is an important factor that can confound the relationships between obesity, morbidity and mortality (Barlow *et al.*, 1995). The risk of premature death conferred by physical

inactivity, and its synergistic interaction with obesity, is clearly illustrated in Figure 9.5, based on data from a 24-year prospective study of 117 000 women who were initially free from cardiovascular disease and cancer (Hu *et al.*, 2004). From these findings, the authors estimate that the combination of overweight and inactivity may account for up to 31% of premature all-cause mortality.

General health status also seems to modulate the effect of BMI on mortality. A 4-year prospective study stratified 54 000 elderly Chinese subjects into five groups according to baseline health status, defined by a comprehensive 12-item index covering illnesses, medication, frailty and smoking. Within the healthiest group, obese people (BMI > 25 kg/m²) had a 54% higher mortality than normal-weight subjects, whereas in the least healthy group, obese subjects had a 45% lower mortality than those with normal body weight (Schooling *et al.*, 2006). These data suggest that other factors – notably co-existing diseases and catabolic states causing weight loss – carry mortality risks that modulate and can indeed outweigh those of obesity.

Causes of death in obese subjects

Cardiovascular disease constitutes the major cause of premature mortality attributable to obesity, and is estimated to account for 50–70% of all excess obesity-related deaths in various populations (Drenick *et al.*, 1980; Bender *et al.*, 2006; McGee, 2005). Other important causes of obesity-related death include malignancy and renal failure, especially related to diabetic nephropathy.

Cardiovascular disease

Cardiovascular disease, notably myocardial infarction, is the most common cause of premature death in obese people. Conversely, obesity is a major contributor to cardiovascular death – indeed, the combination of obesity with inactivity may explain up to 60% of premature cardiovascular mortality, and has been estimated to be the third most important cause of death worldwide (Hu *et al.*, 2004) (see Figure 9.12 on page 228).

Coronary heart disease (CHD), notably myocardial infarction but also including heart failure, is the major immediate cause (50–80%) of premature cardiovascular death in obese subjects (McGee, 2005; Bender *et al.*, 2006; Poirier *et al.*, 2006). Cerebrovascular accidents (CVA) account for about 20%, with the remainder due mainly to peripheral vascular disease and its complications.

Importance of central obesity

Various studies, such as Stevens *et al.* (1998), have found that cardiovascular disease and mortality increase with BMI (Figure 9.6). However, of the various measures of obesity, those relating to central and especially visceral adiposity are the most powerful predictors of cardiovascular outcomes. Possible aetiological links between abdominal fat and cardiovascular disease are explored in Chapter 12.

The original observation of this association is generally credited to Vague (1956), who noted an increased risk of cardiovascular disease in subjects with 'upper body' obesity in the abdominal or 'android' distribution characteristic of males, as compared with the 'lower body' or 'gynoid' fat deposition around the hips typified by women. However, Kahn and Williamson (1994) have pointed out that an American actuarial study performed over 50 years before Vague's reported the particular risks of central adiposity among overweight men: those whose abdominal girth exceeded that of the expanded chest had higher mortality than similarly overweight men without abdominal obesity.

Several large-scale prospective studies have confirmed the strong cardiovascular risk associated with central obesity (measured as WHR or waist circumference) and various CHD end-points (Rexrode *et al.*, 1998; Folsom *et al.*, 1993; Thompson *et al.*, 1991; Kanaya *et al.*, 2003; Freedman *et al.*, 1995; Kannel *et al.*, 1991; Yusuf *et al.*, 2005). The CHD end-points included acute myocardial infarction (Yusuf *et al.*, 2005) and sudden death (Albert *et al.*, 2003; Empana *et al.*, 2004). Various studies have identified threshold values above which cardiovascular risk increases

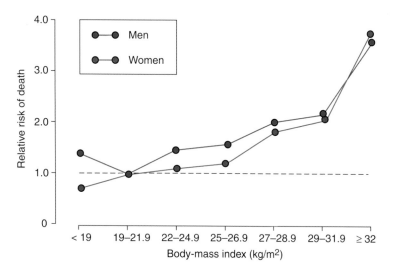

Figure 9.6 Relationship between BMI and risk of death from cardiovascular disease, in men and women. Data from the Cancer Prevention Study (Stevens *et al.*, 1998).

steeply: commonly used cut-off values are a WHR of 0.95 in men and 0.8 in women (Björntorp, 1987; Dowse *et al.*, 1991; Han and Morrison, 1995), and a waist circumference of ≥94–102 cm in men and ≥80–88 cm in women (Han *et al.*, 1995; Seidell and Flegal, 1997; Molarius *et al.*, 1999) (see Chapter 3).

Perhaps the most compelling evidence comes from the INTERHEART Survey, a massive case-control study that recruited over 12 000 cases and 14 000 controls from 52 countries (Yusuf *et al.*, 2005). This demonstrated that the risk of acute myocardial infarction rose progressively with increasing WHR and waist circumference; that this effect operated across a wide range of BMI; and that the influence of WHR and waist-circumference was considerably greater than that of BMI (see Figure 9.7). The population-attributable risk (PAR) for myocardial infarction was increased by 27% in the two highest quintiles of WHR, while the two highest quintiles of BMI increased risk by only 8%. After adjusting for all confounding variables, including BMI, the highest quintile of waist circumference was associated with a 77% higher odds ratio for myocardial infarction than the lowest quintile.

Also consistent with a dominant effect of central obesity, increased WHR (but not BMI) was found to predict a twofold increased risk of cardiovascular mortality in a prospective cohort of subjects undergoing coronary angiography (Hoefle *et al.*, 2005).

Obesity, the metabolic syndrome and cardiovascular risk

Obesity (especially central) is frequently associated with one or more cardiovascular risk factors, notably hyperglycaemia, hypertension, dyslipidaemia, and prothrombotic and proinflammatory changes (Table 9.2). This variable clustering of vascular risk factors is termed the metabolic syndrome (Eckel, Grundy and Zimmet, 2005) and is strongly associated with cardiovascular disease. Using current definitions for the metabolic syndrome, the PAR for cardiovascular disease is estimated at 12–17% overall in a recent meta-analysis (Ford, 2005), and in the Framingham Heart Offspring Study at 34% for men and 16% for women (Wilson *et al.*, 2005).

As discussed in Chapter 10, the definition, nature and significance of the metabolic syndrome have provoked much debate (Kahn *et al.*, 2006; Grundy, 2007; Reaven, 2006). Also uncertain is the extent to which obesity itself contributes to cardiovascular disease, and how much of this effect is mediated through its influences on other components of the syndrome.

The issue is clouded by methodological difficulties, including inconsistencies in the definitions of metabolic syndrome and of central obesity. One approach, focusing on measures of central obesity, has identified the threshold levels for cardiovascular risk mentioned above.

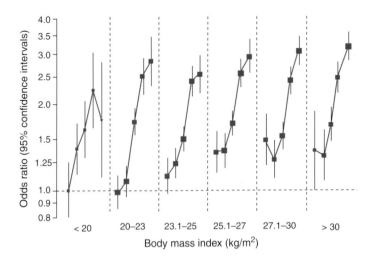

Figure 9.7 Relationship between waist-hip ratio (WHR expressed in quintiles) and risk of myocardial infarction, within defined ranges of BMI. Within each BMI range above a BMI of 20 kg/m², risk increased consistently with increasing quintiles of WHR; there was little overall increase in risk attributable to high BMI alone. Overall, the risk associated with high WHR was about threefold higher than with high BMI. Data from the INTERHEART Study (Yusuf *et al.*, 2005).

Table 9.2 Features of the metabolic syndrome. Note that precise definitions of the 'syndrome' vary (see Table 15.6).

Central (especially visceral) obesity

Hyperglycaemia

- Type 2 diabetes
- Impaired glucose tolerance (IGT)
- Impaired fasting glucose (IFG)

Dyslipidaemia

- Raised triglycerides
- Raised LDL cholesterol (with increased small dense LDL)
- Decreased HDL cholesterol

Hypertension

Non-alcoholic fatty liver disease

- Steatosis (fatty liver)
- Steatohepatitis
- Fibrosis and cirrhosis

Hyperuricaemia

- Gout

Prothrombotic changes

- Raised plasminogen activator inhibitor-1 (PAI-1)

Proinflammatory changes

- Raised acute-phase proteins

Criteria for IGT and IFG are described in Chapter 3.

On the other hand, mathematical modelling suggests that this multi-faceted 'syndrome' is made up of distinct components – raised blood pressure, lipids and inflammatory factors – which frequently overlap and are variably linked with obesity (Chan *et al.*, 1996; Meigs *et al.*, 1997; Anderson *et al.*, 2001; Hanley *et al.*, 2004).

These uncertainties undoubtedly contribute to the discrepancies in the literature. Some studies have demonstrated either an independent effect of obesity, or significant interactions with other risk factors that enhance cardiovascular risk. For example, Yan *et al.* (2006) found that obesity (BMI $\geq$ 30 kg/m^2) in both men and women increased by two- to fourfold the risk of CHD-related death or hospitalization, as compared with normal-weight subjects (BMI $\leq$ 25 kg/m^2); this effect was seen across all risk categories defined by the number of co-risk factors (i.e. smoking, hypertension and hypercholesterolaemia) and persisted after adjustment for blood pressure and cholesterol levels. Similarly, the Lipid Research Clinics Study found that BMI was independently associated with cardiovascular mortality in men, after adjustment for the confounding effects of other cardiovascular risk factors such as smoking, blood pressure and dyslipidaemia (Wilcosky *et al.*, 1990). Moreover, Bengtsson *et al.* (1993) found that both WHR and triglyceride levels were independent predictors of cardiovascular (and total) mortality, whereas the association of BMI with cardiovascular mortality was lost after adjustment for initial blood lipid levels. By contrast, Kanaya *et al.* (2003) reported that the associations of both waist circumference and BMI with premature cardiovascular risk disappeared after adjustment for diabetes, hypertension and dyslipidaemia. Similarly, the Framingham Heart Offspring Study (Wilson *et al.*, 2005) found that hypertension and decreased HDL-cholesterol were the most powerful predictors of cardiovascular disease, having PAR values of 22% and 25% respectively; obesity had only a minor residual effect.

Many studies indicate that the presence of obesity amplifies the impact of co-existent cardiovascular risk factors – smoking, dyslipidaemia, hypertension and diabetes – and that morbidity and mortality increased step-wise with the number of risk factors. Pelkonen *et al.* (1977) found that the risk of cardiovascular death in Finnish men was highest in those who were obese, smoked and had hypertriglyceridaemia. In the Lipids Research Clinic Study, the co-existence of obesity increased cardiovascular mortality due to either smoking or hypertension (Wilcosky *et al.*, 1990).

Obesity and hypertension

Obesity has long been regarded as a powerful predictor and potential cause of hypertension, and recent work has specifically implicated central fat deposition (see Chapter 12). Hypertension is several-fold more common in obese subjects, the overall prevalence increasing from 15% in men and women with BMI $\leq$ 22 kg/m^2, to 40% at BMI $\geq$ 30 kg/m^2. However, the relationship of BMI with serious cardiovascular outcomes (myocardial infarction, death and stroke) in hypertension is less clear; for example, premature death rates were higher in hypertensive subjects whose BMI was 26–29 kg/m^2 than in those with BMI $\leq$ 22 kg/m^2. These points are discussed further in Chapter 12.

Focusing on central obesity reveals an even stronger relationship with blood pressure across various populations, even at 'lean' values of

BMI. Bengali Hindu men showed an 83% increase in risk of hypertension when their waist circumference (WC) exceeded 80 cm (Bose et al., 2003), while American adults whose WC exceeded 90 cm and 101 cm had prevalences of hypertension of 72% and 78%, respectively (Vanhala et al., 1998). A Finnish study also reported that hypertension increased from 4% in non-obese control subjects to 18% in those with central obesity (WHR ≥ 1.00 in men and ≥ 0.88 in women) and a BMI < 30 kg/m² (de Simone et al., 2005). Among Italian men with a WC of ≥ 102 cm, the odds ratios for hypertension was approximately three times that of men with WC < 94 cm, while women with WC ≥ 88 cm had a risk of hypertension twice that of women with WC < 80 cm (Guagnano et al., 2001).

Possible pathophysiological mechanisms to explain how blood pressure is increased by a high fat mass, especially in a central distribution, are discussed in Chapter 12.

The importance of obesity in maintaining hypertension, and the benefit of weight loss in its practical management, are underlined by a large meta-analysis, which concluded that diastolic blood pressure falls overall by 1 mm Hg for each 1 kg of weight loss (Neter et al., 2003).

Obesity and heart failure

Central obesity has been specifically linked with an increased risk of congestive cardiac failure, possibly related to myocardial fat deposition and insulin resistance (Kenchaiah et al., 2002; McGavock et al., 2006). This is discussed further in Chapters 11 and 12. The effect is difficult to distinguish from general myocardial ischaemia due to coronary artery disease; current estimates are that the risk of heart failure increases by 5% in men and 7% in women for each increment of 1 kg/m² in BMI (Kenchaiah et al., 2002). This consequence of obesity is of potential importance in type 2 diabetic patients treated with thiazolidinediones (notably rosiglitazone and pioglitazone), which can precipitate heart failure.

Intriguingly, several studies have reported that a low BMI – variably defined as < 20.7 kg/m² (Horwich et al., 2001) or < 18.5 kg/m² (Gustafsson et al., 2005) or the lowest quartile (Fonarow et al., 2007) – predicts a particularly poor prognosis in patients with heart failure. This 'obesity paradox' suggests that the catabolic state associated with severe heart failure ('cardiac cachexia')

may increase mortality while reducing weight. This effect could also contribute to the low extreme of the U-shaped relationship between BMI and mortality (see Figure 9.3).

Factors modulating cardiovascular risk in obesity

Gender

Many studies have found that the risk association with CHD is particularly strong in men (Calle et al., 1999; Hubert et al., 1983; Carmelli, Zhang and Swan, 1997; Jousilahti et al., 1996; Stevens et al., 1992b). For example, in the 25-year long Charleston Heart Study of African Americans, BMI and waist circumference predicted CHD-related deaths in men but not women (Stevens et al., 1992b). On the other hand, the relationship between BMI and cardiovascular death reported by Stevens et al. (1998) in the US Cancer Prevention Study I was very similar in men and women (Figure 9.6).

Ethnicity

As mentioned above, some populations appear to be relatively protected against cardiovascular disease, even in the face of high prevalences of obesity and increased susceptibility to type 2 diabetes. These include various American ethnic groups (Mexicans, Africans and Pima Indians) and Pacific Islanders (Stern et al., 1990; Pettitt et al., 1982; Hodge et al., 1996). This paradox is unexplained.

Physical Fitness

As with all-cause mortality, physical fitness is a major determinant of the cardiovascular impact of obesity. The 8-year longitudinal study of nearly 22 000 men reported by Blair and Jackson (1999) found that low levels of physical fitness (measured by maximal exercise testing) increased cardiovascular mortality in both lean and obese groups, with an effect comparable to that of conventional risk factors such as smoking, diabetes, hypertension and hypercholesterolaemia. Moreover, risk was higher in lean, unfit men than in those who were fit and obese. The Aerobic Centre Longitudinal Study of 26 000 men confirmed that low cardio-respiratory fitness

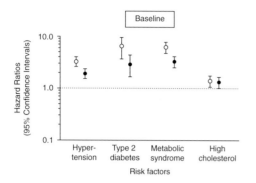
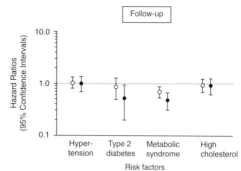

Figure 9.8 Effects of physical fitness on the risk (hazard ratio) of developing hypertension, diabetes, the metabolic syndrome and hypercholesterolaemia. Low physical fitness at baseline (measured by exercise testing) significantly increased the risk of both hypertension and the metabolic syndrome (left panel). Among subjects followed up after seven years, those whose fitness level had improved showed a significant reduction in the risk of developing the metabolic syndrome (right panel). Note the logarithmic scale of the y-axis. Multifactorial analysis showed that the effects of fitness were largely attributable to the difference in BMI at baseline and weight change over seven years. Data from Carnethon *et al.* (2003).

was a strong and independent predictor of cardiovascular disease, and was of comparable significance to traditional cardiovascular risk factors, namely smoking, hypercholesterolaemia, diabetes and hypertension (Wei *et al.*, 1999). Low physical fitness increased by three- to six-fold the risks of developing hypertension and the metabolic syndrome, whereas a subsequent improvement in fitness over a 7-year period substantially reduced this excess risk (Carnethon *et al.*, 2003) (Figure 9.8). Poor physical fitness may largely account for the increased cardiovascular risk in subjects with the metabolic syndrome (Katzmarzyk *et al.*, 2005).

Overall, Hu *et al.* (2004) have estimated that the combination of obesity and physical inactivity may account for nearly 60% of cardiovascular deaths in the general population.

Type 2 diabetes

Diabetes is arguably the most important health consequence of obesity, and one that is set to tax the world's healthcare resources. Obesity has long been recognized as a potential risk factor for type 2 diabetes, and this accounts for the vast majority of cases of diabetes attributable to obesity. Type 2 diabetes is due to a combination of tissue insulin resistance and failure of insulin secretion by the islet β cells; the mechanisms through which increased fat

mass, especially visceral, can exacerbate these processes are discussed in Chapter 10. There is also evidence that obesity can hasten the auto-immune-mediated β-cell destruction that leads to type 1 diabetes, but this disease is rarer and contributes little to the global burden of obesity-associated diabetes.

General relationship with obesity

Numerous studies have established firm links between obesity and diabetes. Particularly clear associations have emerged from circumscribed ethnic groups with high susceptibility to diabetes. A classic example is the Pima Indians of Arizona, whose adult prevalence rates of obesity and diabetes are respectively 60 and 40%. In a 23-year longitudinal study of over 3000 Pima Indians, preceding obesity was strongly associated with increased incidence of diabetes, even in subjects with no family history of the disease (Knowler *et al.*, 1991).

Unselected populations also show strong associations. The much-cited study of Colditz *et al.* (1995) reported that the risk of men developing diabetes over a 14-year period rose steeply as BMI increased above a surprisingly low value of 25 kg/m². The risk for those aged 40–49 years whose BMI was >35 kg/m² was almost 80 times higher than in those with a BMI of <22 kg/m², while those aged 50–59 had a 40-fold increased risk at BMI > 35 kg/m²

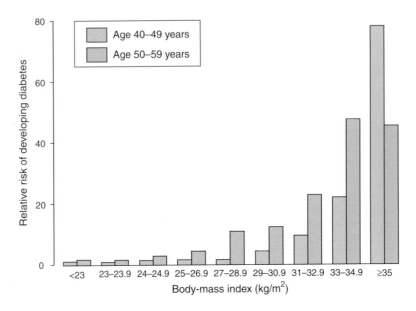

Figure 9.9 Relationship of BMI with risk of developing diabetes over five years, in American men aged 40–49 and 50–59 years. Risk is relative to a reference population of men aged 40–49 years with BMI <23 kg/m². Data from the Health Professionals' Follow-up Study of American men (Chan *et al.*, 1994).

(Figure 9.9). These levels of risk equate with a lifetime probability of developing diabetes of about 50%. The Nurses' Health Study also found a strong continuous relationship between BMI and risk of diabetes. Although less dramatic at high BMI levels, the excess risk even at 'normal' BMI was confirmed: women with a BMI of 23–24 kg/m² had a 3.6-fold higher risk of developing diabetes, compared with those whose BMI was <22 kg/m² (Colditz *et al.*, 1990).

Duration of obesity and duration of weight gain during adult life are also important determinants of diabetes risk. Among Pima Indians, those with obesity (BMI > 30 kg/m²) for >10 years had twice the incidence of diabetes as those who had been obese for <5 years (Everhart *et al.*, 1992). The British Regional Heart Study confirmed the importance of the duration of weight gain in men: compared with subjects whose BMI was <25 kg/m², the risk of diabetes was increased by threefold and fivefold, respectively, among those who had been overweight for <5 years and >5 years (Wannamethee and Shaper, 1999). Moreover, women in the Nurses' Health Study who gained 5–8 kg during early adulthood had a twofold higher risk of developing diabetes compared with those whose weight had remained stable, whereas women who lost ≥5 kg reduced their risk by 50% (Colditz

et al., 1995). Similarly, the Health Professionals Follow-up Study (Chan *et al.*, 1994) found that men who gained 6–7 kg after 21 years of age had twice the risk of diabetes, as compared with those who gained <2 kg (see Figure 9.10).

Nutritional status early in life may also be important. People with low birth weight, attributed to malnutrition *in utero*, have an increased risk of developing type 2 diabetes, possibly due to 'programmed' defects in tissue insulin sensitivity and in β-cell function. In these subjects, the development of obesity during adult life further increases the risk of type 2 diabetes (Yajnik, 2002; Barker *et al.*, 1993).

Importance of central and visceral fat

As for cardiovascular disease, abdominal and especially visceral adiposity confers the greatest risk of diabetes. This has been demonstrated by numerous studies, many of which have adjusted for confounders such as BMI and conventional risk factors (Ohlson *et al.*, 1985; Carey *et al.*, 1997; Boyko *et al.*, 2000). This effect, and its synergistic interaction with BMI, is illustrated in Figure 9.11.

Interestingly, a recent Receiver Operator Characteristics (ROC) analysis of the Health

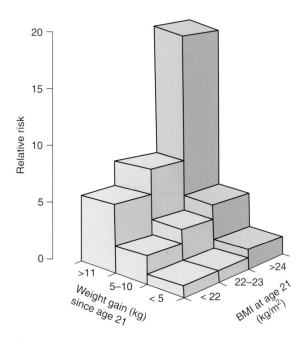

Figure 9.10 Effect of weight gain since age 21 years of age, and its interaction with BMI at age 21, on the relative risk of developing diabetes by age 40–49 years. Weight gain and initial BMI are expressed as tertiles; risk is relative to the group with the lowest tertile for both variables. Data from the Health Professionals' Follow-up Study of American men (Chan *et al.*, 1994).

Professionals Follow-up Study has indicated that waist circumference and also BMI are better predictors of type 2 diabetes than WHR (Figure 9.12). The cumulative proportions of cases identified in men incorporating BMI, waist circumference and WHR into the ROC curve were, respectively, 83, 84 and 74% (Wang *et al.*, 2005).

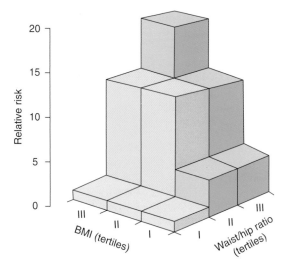

Figure 9.11 Synergistic interaction between increasing WHR and BMI (both expressed as tertiles) in conferring risk for the development of diabetes in men.

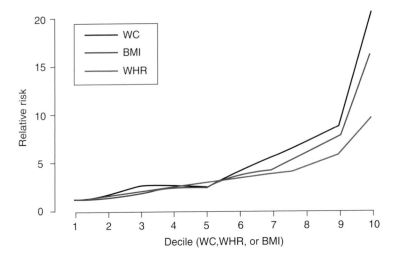

Figure 9.12 Comparison of the ability of waist circumference (WC), WHR and BMI to predict the risk of developing type 2 diabetes in men from the US Health Professionals Follow-Up Study. This Receiver Operator Characteristics (ROC) analysis indicates that WC is a more powerful predictor than both WHR and BMI. Data from Wang *et al.* (2005).

Factors modulating effects of obesity on diabetes risk

Ethnicity

Some ethnic groups, notably the Pima Indians and Pacific Islanders, are especially prone to both obesity and type 2 diabetes. In addition, Asian, Hispanic and black populations have a 1.5 to 2-fold higher risk of developing diabetes than Caucasians, after adjusting for confounders including BMI. The diabetogenic risk of obesity is especially increased in Asians: for each 5-kg weight gain, the risk of developing diabetes increased by 37% in Caucasians, but by 84% in Asians, 44% in Hispanics and 38% in blacks. Ethnic differences in the relationships between fat mass and BMI, and in their ability to predict risks of diabetes and cardiovascular disease, are discussed further below.

Physical activity and fitness

Physical activity and fitness appear to protect against diabetes, whereas inactivity and poor fitness predispose to the disease and enhance the diabetogenic effect of obesity. In a 15-year follow up of US men and women aged 18–39 years, subjects with fitness in the lowest quintile were threefold more likely to develop diabetes than those whose fitness was in the highest two quintiles. Adjusting for baseline BMI significantly reduced the strength of this association (Carnethon *et al.*, 2003).

Malignancy

Obesity has been firmly linked with various malignancies. As already mentioned, Wolf and Colditz (1998) estimated that obesity may have significant contributions to the overall prevalence of cancers of the colon (11%), endometrium (34%) and breast (11%) (see Figure 9.2). These conclusions derive from various source studies in diverse populations. In the Whitehall prospective cohort study of 18 403 middle-aged government employees in London followed up for a median of 28 years, obese or overweight men showed excess deaths from carcinoma of the colon, rectum, liver (hepatocellular carcinoma), bladder and lymphoma, following adjustment for covariates including socio-economic status and physical activity (Batty *et al.*, 2005). In the US prospective study of over 900 000 adults followed for 16 years, Calle *et al.* (2003) found that BMI was significantly associated with risk of death from cancers of the gut (including hepatocellular carcinoma), genitourinary tract, breast and haematological malignancies including non-Hodgkin lymphoma and multiple myeloma. Overall, subjects with BMI ≥ 40 kg/m^2 had a 50–60% increased risk of malignancies compared with those of normal weight. From these data, the authors estimated that obesity and overweight might account for up to 14% of all cancer-related deaths in men and 20% in women.

Links between obesity and cancer are only partly explained by body weight. It has been estimated that the risk of colorectal cancer increases by 7% for every $2 kg/m^2$ increase in BMI, or by around 4% for every 2 cm increase in waist circumference (Moghaddam, Woodward and Huxley, 2007). In two large prospective cohort studies, obesity in women (BMI > $29 kg/m^2$) or central obesity in men (WHR ≥ 0.99) conferred an approximately 1.5-fold increased risk of developing colorectal cancer relative to subjects with normal weight (Martinez et al., 1997; Giovannucci et al., 1995). Colorectal cancer has been attributed to dietary factors in around 75% of sporadic cases in Western countries, while high physical activity levels seem to protect against the disease. Proposed mechanisms include metabolic stress and chronic low-grade inflammation, perhaps compounded by adverse dietary factors such as red and processed meat and loss of the protective effects of dietary fibre and n-3 polyunsaturated fatty acids (Johnson and Lund, 2007). Obesity has also been shown to be associated with the presence of adenomatous polyps in the colon, which are believed to be premalignant lesions in the development of colorectal cancer (Bird et al., 1998).

Obesity now explains a significant proportion of new cases of oesophageal adenocarcinoma possibly by causing gastro-oesophageal reflux, a risk factor for the premalignant changes of Barrett's oesophagus (Pisegna et al., 2004; Corley, 2007; see Chapter 13).

The association with hepatocellular carcinoma appears to be explained by progression of non-alcoholic fatty liver (a common finding in obesity) to cirrhosis, which in about 7% of cases becomes complicated by the development of this tumour (see Chapter 11).

Other malignancies linked with obesity include gall-bladder cancer, pancreatic carcinoma, renal cell carcinoma, non-Hodgkin lymphoma and multiple myeloma. In addition, Calle et al. (2003) noted increased risk of death from prostate and stomach carcinoma in obese men and breast and endometrial carcinoma in obese women. In the Nurses' Health Study, it was noted that weight gain after 18 years of age was associated with an increased risk of postmenopausal breast cancer. It was calculated that 15% of breast cancer cases in this population could be attributed to weight gain of ≥ 2 kg since age 18, and 4.4% to weight gain of ≥ 2 kg after the menopause (Eliassen et al., 2006). One possible explanation of the increased risk of endometrial and breast cancer in obese women is the increased production of oestrogens through the conversion of androstenedione to oestrone (which is then reduced to oestradiol in peripheral tissues), under the action of the aromatase enzyme in adipose tissue (see Chapter 13).

Overall, approximately 5% of all cancers in Europe can be attributed to excess body weight. The highest attributable proportions were for cancers of the endometrium (39%), kidney (25%) and gall bladder (24%), while the greatest attributable number of cases was colorectal cancer (21 500 cases per year). Reducing the prevalence of overweight and obesity in Europe by half could potentially lead to a reduction of 36 000 in cases of cancer per year (Bergstrom et al., 2001).

Gall-bladder disease

The prevalence of cholesterol gallstones is increased in obese men and women. The risk is highest among those with the highest BMI, who may have up to a fivefold increased risk compared to subjects with normal weight (Stampfer et al., 1992; Willett, Dietz and Colditz, 1999; Erlinger, 2000). Women with a BMI of over $30 kg/m^2$ had an annual incidence of gallstones that exceeded 1% (Stampfer et al., 1992). The increased prevalence of stones is mostly due to supersaturation of bile with cholesterol, a consequence of increased synthesis by the liver and secretion into bile. Saturation is further increased during weight loss, which explains the increased risk associated with weight loss following bariatric surgery (Erlinger, 2000).

Osteoarthritis

Obesity is associated with increased risk of osteoarthritis, which accounts for a significant proportion of the health costs relating to obesity. In the Nurses' Health Study, women with BMI ≥ $35 kg/m^2$ had a twofold increased risk of total hip replacement due to hip osteoarthritis, as compared with women with BMI ≤ $22 kg/m^2$ (Karlson et al., 2003). A population-based twin study of middle-aged women reported a significant increase of 9–13% in risk of osteoarthritis per kg increase in body weight (Cicuttini, Baker and Spector, 1996). In a population-based case-control study performed in the UK, it was estimated that 24% of surgical cases of knee osteoarthritis might be avoided if overweight and obese people reduced their weight by 5 kg (Coggon et al., 2001).

Interestingly, increased body weight is associated with increased risk of osteoarthritis in non weight-bearing joints. In a longitudinal study of 588 males and 688 females conducted in the US, baseline obesity (measured here by an index of relative weight) was significantly associated with the 23-year incidence of osteoarthritis of the hands among subjects who were initially disease-free. Furthermore, higher baseline body weight was associated with greater severity of osteoarthritis of the hands on follow-up (Carman et al., 1994). This suggests that obesity may lead to changes in cartilage and bone metabolism independently of excess weight-bearing (see Chapter 13).

Chronic renal failure

There is growing evidence that the metabolic syndrome and its components predict increased risk for chronic renal disease (Chen et al., 2004). Among 320 000 adult members of a US healthcare delivery system, followed-up for a median of 21 years, higher baseline BMI was found to be an independent predictor for end-stage renal disease (ESRD), even after adjustment for baseline blood pressure and presence of diabetes (Hsu et al., 2006). Obesity itself, independently of diabetes, is associated with a specific glomerulopathy and proteinuria (Kambham et al., 2001) and is often overlooked as a factor in the progression of renal impairment (see Chapter 13).

Hyperinsulinaemia, even before the onset of hyperglycaemia, has been observed in numerous studies to correlate with microalbuminuria and to exert effects on the renovascular system (Mykkanen et al., 1998). Multiple structural and functional mechanisms have been proposed to explain obesity-related renal dysfunction, including an excessive excretory load (by virtue of greater body mass and hence tissue turnover), lipotoxicity of the renal tubular cells from heavy exposure to albumin-bound free fatty acid with proteinuria, and hyperinsulinaemia-induced glomerular hypertension (Bagby, 2004). This complication will be of increasing concern as obesity affects ever younger people, and especially in Asian populations who are generally more susceptible to renal disease (Karter et al., 2002; Roglic et al., 2005).

Ethnic differences in obesity-related predictors of disease

It has become clear that there is considerable variation between different populations in the relationships between measures of obesity and outcomes such as diabetes and cardiovascular disease. In particular, conventional anthropometric thresholds derived from Caucasians consistently underestimate cardiovascular and diabetes risk for Asian populations (Ko et al., 1999; Deurenberg-Yap, Chew and Deurenberg, 2002). This probably relates to ethnic variations in body composition and fat distribution. There is strong evidence that Asian people have more visceral fat than other populations, for the same BMI (Yajnik and Yudkin, 2004) or subcutaneous fat content (Tanaka, Horimai and Katsukawa, 2003); this is illustrated in Japanese subjects in Figure 9.13. A meta-analysis has concluded that for the same age, gender and level of body fat, the BMI of Chinese, Indonesians and Thais were effectively 1.9, 3.2 and 2.9 kg/m² lower than that in Caucasians; in blacks, BMI was effectively 1.3 kg/m² lower (Deurenberg, Yap and van Staveren, 1998).

It follows that a substantial number of Asian people are at increased risk of diabetes and cardiovascular disease, even though their BMI falls below the conventional, Caucasian-derived levels defining obesity (30 kg/m²) and overweight (25 kg/m²). This has led to the proposed redefinition of obesity in Asian populations, based on increased risk of comorbidity. According to the suggested criteria, obesity is defined as: BMI ≥ 25 kg/m², or a waist circumference ≥90 cm in men and ≥80 cm in women (WHO/IASO/IOTF, 2000). These thresholds should be compared with those in Caucasian populations in Figures 2.2 and 2.3.

These relatively low limits tally with recent ROC analyses in Chinese and Japanese populations, showing that waist circumference values of 80–90 cm in women and 87–90 cm in men were optimal cut-off levels for predicting clustering of

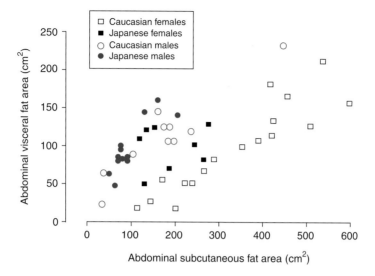

Figure 9.13 Relationship between subcutaneous and visceral fat contents in Japanese and Caucasian men and women. Japanese subjects tend to have higher relative amounts of visceral fat, compared with Caucasians. Fat content was measured as cross-sectional area of the visceral fat depots using CT scanning. Data from a meta-analysis by Tanaka, Horimai and Katsukawa (2003).

comorbid risk factors (Tokunaga *et al.*, 1983; Jia *et al.*, 2003; Hayashi *et al.*, 2007) (Figure 9.14). For Pacific Islanders, by contrast, corresponding levels for defining overweight and obesity are proposed to be BMI of 26 kg/m² and 32 kg/m², respectively (Swinburn *et al.*, 1999). Research is actively under way to test and refine these working definitions in various populations.

Conclusions

A recent World Health Organization report (World Health Organization, 2005) estimated that one billion people worldwide are obese or overweight, and this number is set to rise steeply over the coming decades. The burdens

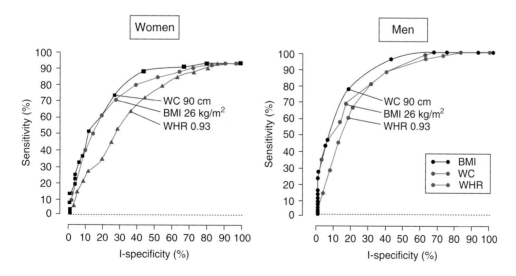

Figure 9.14 Comparison of the ability of various measures of adiposity (WC, WHR and BMI) to predict abdominal obesity (defined as a visceral fat area of ≥100 cm²), in Chinese men and women. This ROC analysis shows that the best predictor is a WC of 90 cm. Data from Jia *et al.* (2003).

of ill health and premature death that will affect these people are of growing concern for the medical and scientific communities, healthcare providers and the general public. The impact will be particularly grave in developing countries, and especially among young and middle-aged inhabitants (Wild *et al.*, 2004; Yoon *et al.*, 2006). For example, of the 17 million people who die from stroke or heart disease each year worldwide, 11 million are from developing countries (World Health Organization, 2003). Thus, the countries that will see the most dramatic increases in obesity include many which can ill afford the cost of obesity-related disease, disability, lost productivity and early death.

References

Adams, K.F., Schatzkin, A., Harris, T.B. *et al.* (2006) *The New England Journal of Medicine*, **355**, 763–78.

Albanes, D., Jones, D.Y., Micozzi, M.S. and Mattson, M.E. (1987) *American Journal of Public Health*, **77**, 439–44.

Albert, C.M., Chae, C.U., Grodstein, F. *et al.* (2003) *Circulation*, **107**, 2096–101.

Anderson, P.J., Critchley, J.A., Chan, J.C. *et al.* (2001) *International Journal of Obesity and Related Metabolic Disorders*, **25**, 1782–8.

Bagby, S.P. (2004) *Journal of the American Society of Nephrology*, **15**, 2775–91.

Barker, D.J.P., Hales, C.N., Fall, C.D. *et al.* (1993) *Diabetologia*, **36**, 62–7.

Barlow, C.E., Kohl, H.W., Gibbons, L.W. and Blair, S.N. (1995) *International Journal of Obesity and Related Metabolic Disorders*, **19** (Suppl 4), S41–4.

Batty, G.D., Shipley, M.J., Jarrett, R.J. *et al.* (2005) *International Journal of Obesity (London)*, **29**, 1267–74.

Bender, R., Jockel, K.H., Trautner, C. *et al.* (1999) *Journal of the American Medical Association*, **281**, 1498–1504.

Bender, R., Trautner, C., Spraul, M. and Berger, M. (1998) *American Journal of Epidemiology*, **147**, 42–8.

Bender, R., Zeeb, H., Schwarz, M. *et al.* (2006) *Journal of Clinical Epidemiology*, **59**, 1064–71.

Bengtsson, C., Bjorkelund, C., Lapidus, L. and Lissner, L. (1993) *BMJ*, **307**, 1385–8.

Bergstrom, A., Pisani, P., Tenet, V. *et al.* (2001) *International Journal of Cancer*, **91**, 421–30.

Bird, C.L., Frankl, H.D., Lee, E.R. and Haile, R.W. (1998) *American Journal of Epidemiology*, **147**, 670–80.

Björntorp, P. (1987) *The American Journal of Clinical Nutrition*, **45**, 1120–25.

Bose, K., Ghosh, A., Roy, S. and Gangopadhyay, S. (2003) *Journal of Physiological Anthropology and Applied Human Science*, **22**, 169–73.

Boyko, E.J., Fujimoto, W.Y., Leonetti, D.L. and Newell-Morris, L. (2000) *Diabetes Care*, **23**, 465–71.

Calle, E.E., Rodriguez, C., Walker-Thurmond, K. and Thun, M.J. (2003) *The New England Journal of Medicine*, **348**, 1625–38.

Calle, E.E., Thun, M.J., Petrelli, J.M. *et al.* (1999) *The New England Journal of Medicine*, **341**, 1097–105.

Carey, V.J., Walters, E.E., Colditz, G.A. *et al.* (1997) *American Journal of Epidemiology*, **145**, 614–9.

Carman, W.J., Sowers, M., Hawthorne, V.M. and Weissfeld, L.A. (1994) *American Journal of Epidemiology*, **139**, 119–29.

Carmelli, D., Zhang, H. and Swan, G.E. (1997) *Epidemiology*, **8**, 378–83.

Carnethon, M.R., Gidding, S.S., Nehgme, R. *et al.* (2003) *Journal of American Medical Association*, **290**, 3092–100.

Chan, J.C.N., Cheung, J.C.K., Lau, E.M.C. *et al.* (1996) *Diabetes Care*, **19**, 953–9.

Chan, J.M., Rimm, E.B., Colditz, G.A. *et al.* (1994) *Diabetes Care*, **17**, 961–9.

Chen, H., Hansen, M.J., Jones, J.E. *et al.* (2006) *American Journal of Respiratory and Critical Care Medicine*, **173**, 1248–54.

Chen, J., Muntner, P., Hamm, L.L. *et al.* (2004) *Annals of Internal Medicine*, **140**, 167–74.

Cicuttini, F.M., Baker, J.R. and Spector, T.D. (1996) *The Journal of Rheumatology*, **23**, 1221–6.

Coggon, D., Reading, I., Croft, P. *et al.* (2001) *International Journal of Obesity and Related Metabolic Disorders*, **25**, 622–7.

Colditz, G.A., Willett, W.C., Rotnitzky, A. and Manson, J.E. (1995) *Annals of Internal Medicine*, **122**, 481–6.

Colditz, G.A., Willett, W.C., Stampfer, M.J. *et al.* (1990) *American Journal of Epidemiology*, **132**, 501–13.

Corley, D.A. (2007) *Gut*, **56**, 1493–4.

de Simone, G., Devereux, R.B., Kizer, J.R. *et al.* (2005) *The American Journal of Clinical Nutrition*, **81**, 757–61.

Deurenberg-Yap, M., Chew, S.K. and Deurenberg, P. (2002) *Obesity Reviews*, **3**, 209–15.

Deurenberg, P., Yap, M. and van Staveren, W.A. (1998) *International Journal of Obesity and Related Metabolic Disorders*, **22**, 1164–71.

Dowse, G.K., Zimmet, P.Z., Gareeboo, H. *et al.* (1991) *Diabetes Care*, **14**, 271–82.

Drenick, E.J., Bale, G.S., Seltzer, F. and Johnson, D.G. (1980) *Journal of the American Medical Association*, **243**, 443–5.

Eckel, R.H., Grundy, S.M. and Zimmet, P.Z. (2005) *Lancet*, **365**, 1415–28.

Eliassen, A.H., Colditz, G.A., Rosner, B. *et al.* (2006) *Journal of the American Medical Association*, **296**, 193–201.

Empana, J.P., Ducimetiere, P., Charles, M.A. and Jouven, X. (2004) *Circulation*, **110**, 2781–5.

Erlinger, S. (2000) *European Journal of Gastroenterology and Hepatology*, **12**, 1347–52.

Everhart, J.E., Pettitt, D.J., Bennett, P.H. and Knowler, W.C. (1992) *Diabetes*, **41**, 235–40.

Flegal, K.M., Graubard, B.I., Williamson, D.F. and Gail, M.H. (2005) *Journal of the American Medical Association*, **293**, 1861–7.

Folsom, A.R., Kaye, S.A., Sellers, T.A. *et al.* (1993) *Journal of the American Medical Association*, **269**, 483–7.

Folsom, A.R., Kushi, L.H., Anderson, K.E. *et al.* (2000) *Archives of Internal Medicine*, **160**, 2117–28.

Fonarow, G.C., Srikanthan, P., Costanzo, M.R. *et al.* (2007) *American Heart Journal*, **153**, 74–81.

Ford, E.S. (2005) *Diabetes Care*, **28**, 1769–78.

Freedman, D.S., Williamson, D.F., Croft, J.B. *et al.* (1995) *American Journal of Epidemiology*, **142**, 53–63.

Giovannucci, E., Ascherio, A., Rimm, E.B. *et al.* (1995) *Annals of Internal Medicine*, **122**, 327–34.

Grundy, S.M. (2007) *Journal of Clinical Endocrinology and Metabolism*, **92**, 399–404.

Gu, D., He, J., Duan, X. *et al.* (2006) *Journal of the American Medical Association*, **295**, 776–83.

Guagnano, M.T., Ballone, E., Colagrande, V. *et al.* (2001) *International Journal of Obesity and Related Metabolic Disorders*, **25**, 1360–4.

Gustafsson, F., Kragelund, C.B., Torp-Pedersen, C. *et al.* (2005) *European Heart Journal*, **26**, 58–64.

Han, T.S., van Leer, E.M., Seidell, J.C. and Lean, M.E. (1995) *BMJ*, **311**, 1401–5.

Hanley, A.J., Festa, A., D'Agostino, R.B.J. *et al.* (2004) *Diabetes*, **53**, 1773–81.

Hayashi, T., Boyko, E.J., McNeely, M.J. *et al.* (2007) *Diabetes Care*, **30**, 120–7.

Heitmann, B.L., Erikson, H., Ellsinger, B.M. *et al.* (2000) *International Journal of Obesity and Related Metabolic Disorders*, **24**, 33–7.

Hodge, A.M., Dowse, G.K., Collins, V.R. and Zimmet, P.Z. (1996) *American Journal of Epidemiology*, **143**, 442–55.

Hoefle, G., Saely, C.H., Aczel, S. *et al.* (2005) *International Journal of Obesity (London)*, **29**, 785–91.

Horwich, T.B., Fonarow, G.C., Hamilton, M.A. *et al.* (2001) *Journal of the American College of Cardiology*, **38**, 789–95.

Hsu, C.Y., McCulloch, C.E., Iribarren, C. *et al.* (2006) *Annals of Internal Medicine*, **144**, 21–8.

Hu, F.B., Willett, W.C., Li, T. *et al.* (2004) *The New England Journal of Medicine*, **351**, 2694–703.

Hubert, H.B., Feinleib, M., McNamara, P.M. and Castelli, W.P. (1983) *Circulation*, **67**, 968–77.

James, W., Jackson-Leach, R., Ni Mhurchu, C. *et al.* (2004) *Comparative Quantification of Health Risks: Global and Regional Burden of Disease Attributable to Selected Major Risk Factors, Vol. 1* (eds M. Ezzati, A. Lopez, A. Rogers and C. Murray,), WHO, Geneva, pp. 495–596.

Jia, W.P., Lu, J.X., Kiang, K.S. *et al.* (2003) *Biomedical Environmental Science*, **2003**, 206–11.

Johnson, I.T. and Lund, E.K. (2007) *Alimentary Pharmacology and Therapeutics*, **26**, 161–81.

Jousilahti, P., Tuomilehto, J., Vartiainen, E. *et al.* (1996) *Circulation*, **93**, 1372–9.

Kahn, R., Buse, J., Ferrannini, E. and Stern, M. (2006) American Diabetes Association and European Association for the Study of Diabetes. *Diabetes Care*, **28**, 2289–304.

Kahn, H.S. and Williamson, D.F. (1994) *International Journal of Obesity and Related Metabolic Disorders*, **18**, 686–91.

Kambham, N., Markowitz, G.S., Valeri, A.M. *et al.* (2001) *Kidney International*, **59**, 1498–509.

Kanaya, A.M., Vittinghoff, E., Shlipak, M.G. *et al.* (2003) *American Journal of Epidemiology*, **158**, 1161–170.

Kannel, W.B., Cupples, L.A., Ramaswami, R. *et al.* (1991) *Journal of Clinical Epidemiology*, **44**, 183–90.

Karlson, E.W., Mandl, L.A., Aweh, G.N. *et al.* (2003) *The American Journal of Medicine*, **114**, 93–8.

Karter, A., Ferrara, A., Liu, J. *et al.* (2002) *Journal of American Medical Association*, **287**, 2519–27.

Katzmarzyk, P.T., Church, T.S., Janssen, I. *et al.* (2005) *Diabetes Care*, **28**, 391–7.

Kenchaiah, S., Evans, J.C., Levy, D. *et al.* (2002) *The New England Journal of Medicine*, **347**, 305–13.

Knowler, W.C., Pettitt, D.J., Saad, M.F. *et al.* (1991) *The American Journal of Clinical Nutrition*, **53**, 1543S–51S.

Ko, G.T., Chan, J.C., Cockram, C.S. and Woo, J. (1999) *International Journal of Obesity and Related Metabolic Disorders*, **23**, 1136–42.

Lahmann, P.H., Lissner, L., Gullberg, B. and Berglund, G. (2002) *Obesity Research*, **10**, 361–9.

Lean, M.E., Han, T.S. and Morrison, C.E. (1995) *British Medical Journal*, **311**, 158–61.

Lee, C.D., Blair, S.N. and Jackson, A.S. (1999) *The American Journal of Clinical Nutrition*, **69**, 373–80.

Levine, M.D., Kalarchian, M.A., Courcoulas, A.P. *et al.* (2007) *Addictive Behaviors*, **32**, 2365–71.

Lew, E.A. and Garfinkel, L. (1979) *Journal of Chronic Diseases*, **32**, 563–76.

Lindsted, K.D. and Singh, P.N. (1997) *American Journal of Epidemiology*, **146**, 1–11.

Manson, J.E., Willett, W.C., Stampfer, M.J. *et al.* (1995) *The New England Journal of Medicine*, **333**, 677–85.

Martinez, M.E., Giovannucci, E., Spiegelman, D. *et al.* (1997) *Journal of the National Cancer Institute*, **89**, 948–55.

McGavock, J.M., Victor, R.G., Unger, R.H. and Szczepaniak, L.S. (2006) *Annals of Internal Medicine*, **144**, 517–24.

McGee, D.L. (2005) *Annals of Epidemiology*, **15**, 87–97.

Meigs, J.B., D'Agostino, R.B.S., Wilson, P.W. *et al.* (1997) *Diabetes*, **46**, 1594–1600.

Menotti, A., Descovich, G.C., Lanti, M. *et al.* (1993) *Preventive Medicine*, **22**, 293–303.

Miyata, G., Meguid, M.M., Fetissov, S.O. *et al.* (1999) *Surgery*, **126**, 255–63.

Moghaddam, A.A., Woodward, M. and Huxley, R. (2007) *Cancer Epidemiology, Biomarkers and Prevention: A Publication of the American Association for*

Cancer Research, Cosponsored by the American Society of Preventive Oncology, **16**, 2533–47.

Molarius, A., Seidell, J.C., Sans, S. et al. (1999) International Journal of Obesity and Related Metabolic Disorders, **23**, 116–25.

Mykkanen, L., Zaccaro, D.J., Wagenknecht, L.E. et al. (1998) Diabetes, **47**, 793–800.

Nemery, B., Moavero, N.E., Brasseur, L. and Stanescu, D.C. (1983) British Medical Journal (Clinical research edition), **286**, 249–51.

Neter, J.E., Stam, B.E., Kok, F.J. et al. (2003) Hypertension, **42**, 878–84.

Noppa, H., Bengtsson, C., Wedel, H. and Wilhelmsen, L. (1980) American Journal of Epidemiology, **111**, 682–92.

Ohlson, L.O., Larsson, B., Svardsudd, K. et al. (1985) Diabetes, **34**, 1055–8.

Park, H.S., Song, Y.M. and Cho, S.I. (2006) International Journal of Epidemiology, **35**, 181–7.

Pelkonen, R., Nikkila, E.A., Koskinen, S. et al. (1977) British Medical Journal, **2**, 1185–7.

Pettitt, D.J., Lisse, J.R., Knowler, W.C. and Bennett, P.H. (1982) American Journal of Epidemiology, **115**, 359–66.

Pisegna, J., Holtmann, G., Howden, C.W. et al. (2004) Alimentary Pharmacology and Therapeutics, **9** (Suppl 20), 47–56.

Poirier, P., Giles, T.D., Bray, G.A. et al. (2006) Circulation, **113**, 898–918.

Reaven, G.M. (2006) American Journal of Clinical Nutrition, **83**, 1237–47.

Rexrode, K.M., Carey, V.J., Hennekens, C.H. et al. (1998) Journal of the American Medical Association, **280**, 1843–8.

Rissanen, A., Knekt, P., Heliovaara, M. et al. (1991) Journal of Clinical Epidemiology, **44**, 787–95.

Roglic, G., Unwin, N., Bennett, P. et al. (2005) Diabetes Care, **28**, 2130–5.

Schooling, C.M., Lam, T.H., Li, Z.B. et al. (2006) Archives of Internal Medicine, **166**, 1498–1504.

Seidell, J.C. and Flegal, K.M. (1997) British Medical Bulletin, **53**, 238–52.

Sjöström, L.V. (1992) The American Journal of Clinical Nutrition, **55**, 516S–23S.

Stampfer, M.J., Maclure, K.M., Colditz, G.A. et al. (1992) The American Journal of Clinical Nutrition, **55**, 652–8.

Stern, M.P., Patterson, J.K., Mitchell, B.D. et al. (1990) International Journal of Obesity, **14**, 623–9.

Stevens, J. (2000) Nutrition Reviews, **58**, 346–53.

Stevens, J., Cai, J., Pamuk, E.R. et al. (1998) The New England Journal of Medicine, **338**, 1–7.

Stevens, J., Keil, J.E., Rust, P.F. et al. (1992a) Body mass index and body girths as predictors of mortality in black and white women. Archives of Internal Medicine, **152**, 1257–62.

Stevens, J., Keil, J.E., Rust, P.F. et al. (1992b) Body mass index and body girths as predictors of mortality in black and white men. American Journal of Epidemiology, **135**, 1137–46.

Swinburn, B.A., Ley, S.J., Carmichael, H.E. and Plank, L.D. (1999) International Journal of Obesity and Related Metabolic Disorders, **23**, 1178–83.

Tanaka, S., Horimai, C. and Katsukawa, F. (2003) Acta Diabetologia, **40**, S302–4.

Thompson, C.J., Ryu, J.E., Craven, T.E. et al. (1991) Arteriosclerosis and Thrombosis: a Journal of Vascular Biology/American Heart Association, **11**, 327–33.

Tokunaga, K., Matsuzawa, Y., Ishikawa, K. and Tarui, S. (1983) International Journal of Obesity, **7**, 437–45.

Vague, J. (1956) The American Journal of Clinical Nutrition, **4**, 20–34.

Vanhala, M.J., Pitkajarvi, T.K., Kumpusalo, E.A. and Takala, J.K. (1998) International Journal of Obesity and Related Metabolic Disorders, **22**, 369–74.

Wang, Y., Rimm, E.B., Stampfer, M.J. et al. (2005) The American Journal of Clinical Nutrition, **81**, 555–63.

Wannamethee, S.G. and Shaper, A.G. (1999) Diabetes Care, **22**, 1266–72.

Wei, M., Kampert, J.B., Barlow, C.E. et al. (1999) Journal of the American Medical Association, **282**, 1547–53.

Welborn, T.A., Knuiman, M.W. and Vu, H.T. (2000) International Journal of Obesity and Related Metabolic Disorders, **24**, 108–15.

WHO/IASO/IOTF (2000) Redefining obesity and its treatment. A report from the International Diabetes Institute, regional office for the Western Pacific (WPRO), the World Health Organization, the International Study of Obesity and the International Obesity Task Force.

Wilcosky, T., Hyde, J., Anderson, J.J. et al. (1990) Journal of Clinical Epidemiology, **43**, 743–52.

Wild, S., Roglic, G., Green, A. et al. (2004) Diabetes Care, **27**, 1047–53.

Willett, W.C., Dietz, W.H. and Colditz, G.A. (1999) Guidelines for healthy weight. The New England Journal of Medicine, **341**, 427–34.

Wilson, P.W., D'Agostino, R.B., Parise, H. et al. (2005) Circulation, **112**, 3066–72.

Wolf, A.M. and Colditz, G.A. (1998) Obesity Research, **6**, 97–106.

World Health Organization (2005) Preventing chronic diseases: a vital investment. http://www.who.int/chp/chronic_disease_report/en/index.html, last accessed 1 June 2006.

World Health Organization (2003) The World Health Report 2003. Shaping the future. World Health Organization, pp. 83–99.

Yajnik, C. and Yudkin, J. (2004) Lancet, **363**, 163.

Yajnik, C.S. (2002) Obesity Reviews, **3**, 217–24.

Yan, L.L., Daviglus, M.L., Liu, K. et al. (2006) Journal of the American Medical Association, **295**, 190–8.

Yoon, K.H., Lee, J.H., Kim, J.W. et al. (2006) Lancet, **368**, 1681–8.

Yusuf, S., Hawken, S., Ounpuu, S. et al. (2005) Lancet, **366**, 1640–9.

Metabolic Complications of Obesity

Key points

- Obesity accounts for 80–85% of the overall risk of developing type 2 diabetes, and underlies the current global spread of the disease. However, up to 50% of morbidly obese individuals do not develop type 2 diabetes, while 20% of type 2 diabetic subjects are not obese.

- The risk of type 2 diabetes increases steadily as BMI rises above 24 kg/m^2, to an 80-fold increase at BMI >35 kg/m^2. Weight gain of over 5 kg in early adult life doubles risk, which also increases with the duration of obesity. Central (and especially visceral) obesity is specifically associated with type 2 diabetes, and the risk of high waist circumference synergises with that of high BMI.

- Obesity-associated diabetes risk is higher in certain ethnic groups, such as Pima (Native American) Indians, Black and Asian populations. Risk thresholds for both BMI and waist circumference are lower than in Caucasians. Higher body fat content in non-Caucasians may contribute.

- Obesity is associated in the metabolic syndrome with insulin resistance, glucose intolerance (including type 2 diabetes), hypertension, gout and pro-inflammatory and pro-coagulant changes. Up to 10% of adults in developed countries are affected. Fatty liver, glomerulopathy, polycystic ovarian syndrome and sleep apnoea are also associated.

- Obesity induces insulin resistance, which worsens with rising BMI and especially increasing visceral abdominal fat mass. Possible mediators include high free fatty acid (FFA) levels generated by overactive lipolysis in fat, and disturbances in adipokines produced by adipose tissue, such as adiponectin and leptin, which both improve insulin sensitivity in peripheral tissues. Adiponectin levels fall in obesity, while obese subjects may become resistant to leptin's actions.

- High FFA levels interfere with glucose utilization in muscle and liver (the glucose-fatty acid, or Randle cycle), and with insulin signalling. Muscle glucose uptake decreases, while hepatic gluconeogenesis and glucose production are enhanced, thus opposing insulin's glucose-lowering actions.

- Ectopic triglyceride deposition occurs in muscle, liver, β cells and other tissues in obesity. High FFA levels contribute to reduced adiponectin levels and leptin resistance. Both adipokines activate AMP kinase, resulting in the clearing of intracellular trigylceride. Intracellular triglyceride deposition impairs insulin action and causes various functional abnormalities ('lipotoxicity'), including steatohepatitis, impaired insulin secretion and perhaps heart failure.

- Obesity predisposes to type 2 diabetes by causing both insulin resistance and β-cell dysfunction. The latter may be due to high FFA levels and intracellular triglyceride deposition, which may lead to β-cell apoptosis through oxidative damage and perhaps amyloid formation from aggregated amylin. Substantial weight loss, for example following bariatric surgery, may improve or even reverse glucose intolerance, including established type 2 diabetes.

- Obesity and the metabolic syndrome are accompanied by dyslipidaemia, typically with high triglyceride levels throughout the day and low HDL cholesterol. Hepatic production of very low density lipoprotein (VLDL) cholesterol (fuelled by high FFA levels) is increased, whereas VLDL clearance by lipoprotein lipase (an insulin-sensitive enzyme) is decreased.

- High triglyceride levels favour the formation of small dense low density lipoprotein (LDL), which is taken up by subendothelial macrophages to form foam cells. Small dense high density lipoprotein (HDL) also forms, which is readily catabolized, thus lowering levels of anti-atherogenic HDL cholesterol. The dyslipidaemia is therefore atherogenic.

Chapter 10 Metabolic Complications of Obesity

Ronald Ma and Juliana Chan

Obesity is strongly associated with type 2 diabetes and lipid disorders, which are widely regarded as components of a broader 'metabolic syndrome'. This chapter reviews the nature and possible causes of these associations, including the ways in which obesity could lead to insulin resistance, viewed by some as the core defect of the metabolic syndrome. Other important comorbidities of the metabolic syndrome are covered in Chapter 11 (obesity-associated liver disease) and Chapter 12 (cardiovascular diseases).

Type 2 diabetes

Type 2 diabetes is one of the top four killer diseases identified by the World Health Organization which, collectively, accounted for over 35 million deaths (60% of the total worldwide) in 2005 (World Health Organization, 2006). Diabetes will become increasingly important, with the global number of sufferers predicted to rise from 150 million in 2005 to 220 million by 2010, and 300 million by 2025. Over 95% of cases will be type 2 diabetes, and will include an increasing proportion of children (Roglic et al., 2005). Most new cases will come from developing countries, notably the Asia-Pacific region (Figure 10.1); these countries will find the economic burden of diabetes and obesity particularly hard to bear (Zimmet, Alberti and Shaw, 2001). A recent United Nations Resolution has recognized diabetes as a chronic, debilitating and costly disease that poses a severe threat to global health, and that will demand concerted national policies to prevent and manage the disease (International Diabetes Federation, 2006).

Obesity is estimated to account for 80–85% of the overall risk of developing type 2 diabetes, and is the main factor driving the worldwide epidemic of the disease (see Chapter 2). It may also be a risk factor for the rare 'atypical' diabetes, described especially in Chinese and Black populations, which presents acutely with ketosis but subsequently resembles type 2 diabetes in its clinical course (Tan et al., 2000; Banerji et al., 1994). Obesity does not apparently make an important contribution to the risk of developing autoimmune type 1 diabetes or the rare monogenic types of the disease such as maturity-onset diabetes of the young (MODY) and the mitochondrial mutation syndromes (Mathis et al., 2001; Cho et al., 2007; Liou et al., 2007; Vaxillaire and Froguel, 2008). However, as discussed below, there is evidence that obesity impairs β-cell function and so could unmask a β-cell defect at an earlier age.

Epidemiological links

Numerous longitudinal studies have demonstrated that obesity predisposes strongly to type 2 diabetes in both sexes and that the anatomical distribution and time course of adiposity are important determinants of risk (see Chapter 9). Nonetheless, type 2 diabetes is multifactorial in origin and obesity is not the sole determinant: 20–50% of morbidly obese individuals do not become diabetic, while up to 20% of subjects with type 2 diabetes are not obese by conventional criteria.

Body mass index (BMI) shows a strong continuous relationship with the risk of developing diabetes in both men and women (see Figure 9.9). In men, the Health Professionals' Follow-Up Study found that the risk rose rapidly once BMI exceeded $24 \, kg/m^2$, reaching an 80-fold increase for subjects initially aged 40–49 years who had a BMI of $\geq 35 \, kg/m^2$; this level of risk equates to a life-time probability of about 50% of becoming diabetic (Chan et al., 1994). The American Nurses' Health Study (Colditz et al., 1990) also found that risk increased

Obesity: Science to Practice   Edited by Gareth Williams and Gema Frühbeck
© 2009 John Wiley & Sons, Ltd

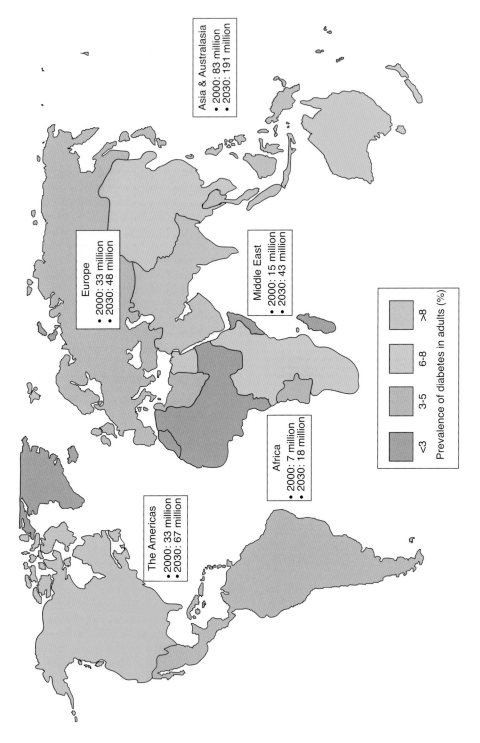

Figure 10.1 Estimates of the regional and global prevalence of diabetes in 2030. Data from the International Diabetes Federation (Roglic *et al.*, 2005).

rapidly with BMI, and from a surprisingly low threshold: women who initially had a 'normal' BMI of only 23–24 kg/m² had a nearly fourfold increased risk of developing diabetes during the 20 years of follow up, as compared with those whose BMI was <22 kg/m². Among the Pima Indians, who have a particularly high prevalence of both obesity and type 2 diabetes, preceding obesity in either sex is also strongly associated with a higher incidence of diabetes, independently of a family history (Knowler *et al.*, 1991).

The age of onset and duration of overweight are also important. Follow up of the Nurses' Health Study cohort showed that women who gained 5–7.9 kg during early adulthood had a twofold higher risk of developing diabetes after 20 years, compared with those whose weight remained stable. Conversely, those who lost ≥5 kg reduced their risk by 50% or more (Colditz *et al.*, 1995). Weight gain showed a synergistic interaction with BMI in determining diabetes risk (see Figure 9.10). Similarly, in the Health Professionals' Follow-Up Study, men who gained 6–7 kg from the age of 21 years had twice the risk of those who had gained <2 kg (Chan *et al.*, 1994).

The progressive rise in obesity prevalence among younger subjects in many populations has made it possible to examine the effects of the duration of obesity. Pima Indians who had a BMI of ≥30 kg/m² for over ten years had a twofold higher prevalence of diabetes than those who had been similarly obese for less than five years (Everhart *et al.*, 1992). The British Regional Heart Study also found that, compared with men whose BMI was <25 kg/m², the risk of diabetes was increased almost threefold in subjects whose BMI had been 28–29 kg/m² for less than five years and fivefold in those who were overweight for over five years (Wannamethee and Shaper, 1999).

Central obesity is an especially powerful predictor of type 2 diabetes in both sexes, as suggested by Vague over 50 years ago and confirmed by numerous studies using various measures of abdominal and visceral adiposity (Carey *et al.*, 1997; Unwin *et al.*, 1997; Boyko *et al.*, 2000; Wat *et al.*, 2001; Wang *et al.*, 2005). The importance of central obesity, and its synergistic interaction with BMI, is illustrated in Figure 10.2. In the Health Professionals' Follow-Up Study, although BMI remained the overall dominant risk factor for diabetes, the disease was strongly predicted by having a waist circumference in the top 20% of the cohort or a waist:hip ratio (WHR) in the top 5% (Chan *et al.*, 1994).

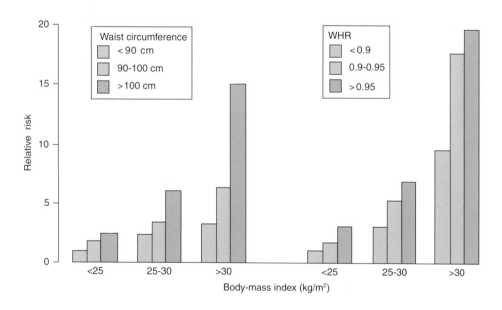

Figure 10.2 Synergistic effects on the risk of developing type 2 diabetes of increasing BMI and measures of central obesity, namely waist circumference (left) and waist:hip ratio (WHR; right). Subjects were women in the Nurses' Health Study (Carey *et al.*, 1997). Age, physical activity, smoking and alcohol and cereal fibre intakes were adjusted for using Cox models.

The dominant effect of central obesity is seen in all populations.

As discussed in Chapter 2, certain populations – including Asians and Native and other American ethnic groups – are particularly susceptible to the diabetogenic effects of obesity. This is shown clearly by the Nurses' Health Study (Shai *et al.*, 2006), in which the overall 20-year incidence of diabetes (adjusted for BMI) was substantially higher in Black, Hispanic and especially Asian subjects than in Caucasians, with Asians having over twice the risk (Figure 10.3). Moreover, for each 5-unit increment in BMI, the relative risk of diabetes, compared with Caucasians, rose to 1.6 in Blacks, 2.2 in Hispanics and 2.4 in Asians. The additional risk among Asians is probably explained by their higher percentage of body-fat content at the same level of adiposity (whether measured by BMI, waist circumference or WHR), as compared with their Caucasian counterparts (Jia *et al.*, 2003; Deurenberg, Deurenberg-Yap and Guricci, 2002; Yajnik and Yudkin, 2004; Tanaka, Horimai and Katsukawa, 2003; He *et al.*, 2001). Accordingly, the risk thresholds for measures of obesity are lower than in Caucasians (see Chapter 2). For example, the waist circumference cut-off values for high cardio-metabolic risk have been set for Asian women and men at 80 and 90 cm, respectively, compared with 88 and 102 cm for Caucasian women and men (NCEP, 2001; Alberti, Zimmet and Shaw, 2005). Other factors may include the higher prevalence of chronic infections such as hepatitis B and C (Lao *et al.*, 2003) and of smoking (Sawada *et al.*, 2003; Corrao *et al.*, 2000) and low socio-economic status (Ko, Chan and Cockram, 2001), in Asian populations (Table 10.1).

The diabetogenic effect of obesity generally increases with age, as illustrated by Figure 9.9. This may be related to declining levels of physical activity and to age-related endocrine and metabolic changes that tend to worsen insulin resistance. The latter include reduced levels of sex hormone-binding globulin (SHBG), growth hormone and IGF-1 in both genders; relatively elevated androgen and reduced oestrogen in women; declining testosterone concentrations in men; and increasing body fat and reduced muscle mass in both sexes (Chan, Tong and Critchley, 2002; Swerdloff and Wang, 1993; Björntorp, 1991; Muller *et al.*, 2005; Blouin *et al.*, 2005; Tong *et al.*, 2005; Laaksonen *et al.*, 2004).

Physical inactivity (itself an important contributor to obesity) and poor physical fitness are independent predictors of the risk of developing diabetes (Sawada *et al.*, 2003; Connolly *et al.*, 2000; Carnethon *et al.*, 2003; Hubert, Snider and Winkleby, 2005), and also of cardiovascular disease (Li *et al.*, 2006; Hancox, Milne and Poulton, 2004) and premature death (Hu *et al.*, 2004). The effect of inactivity is weaker than that of obesity, but interacts synergistically with it, as demonstrated by data from

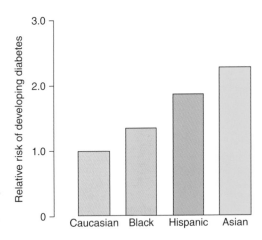

Figure 10.3 Risk of developing diabetes is higher in Asian and other ethnic populations than in Caucasians. The graph shows the 20-year relative risk (set at 1.0 for Caucasians), after adjusting for BMI. From Shai *et al.*, 2006.

Table 10.1 Common risk factors for type 2 diabetes.

Family history (type 2 diabetes in first-degree relatives)

Non-Caucasian ethnic origin

Obesity, especially central

Low birth weight (especially with adult obesity)

Obesogenic lifestyle

- Physical inactivity and low physical fitness
- Watching television for >2 h per day
- Overconsumption of energy-dense foods and drinks
- Rapid acculturation in non-Western populations

High alcohol consumption

Tobacco use

Previous gestational diabetes

Chronic low-grade infections (e.g. hepatitis B and C)

Socio-economic factors

- Low socio-economic status (in developed countries)
- High income and low education level (in developing countries)

women in the Nurses' Health Study (Rana *et al.*, 2007) shown in Figure 10.4. In both the Finnish and US Diabetes Prevention Programs, weight loss (even relatively modest) was the most important determinant for reducing the risk of subjects with impaired glucose tolerance going on to develop diabetes; increased physical activity conferred additional benefits (Hamman *et al.*, 2006; Kubaszek *et al.*, 2003). These findings suggest that enhancing physical activity alone might not be enough to mitigate the adverse metabolic effects of obesity (Weinstein *et al.*, 2004).

The overall importance of obesity, and the potential reversibility of the sequence of events culminating in type 2 diabetes, is highlighted by the finding that substantial weight loss through bariatric surgery can cause many patients with type 2 diabetes to revert to normal glycaemia (see below).

The metabolic syndrome

In the 1920s, Kylin described an association of hypertension, hyperglycaemia and gout (Kylin, 1923). In 1988, Reaven (1988) drew attention to the clustering of hypertension, diabetes, dyslipidaemia and cardiovascular disease in obese subjects, an association initially referred to as the 'insulin resistance' syndrome or 'syndrome X' (Reaven, 1988; DeFronzo and Ferrannini, 1991) (Figure 10.5). The term 'metabolic syndrome' was first used in a WHO document in 1999 to highlight the increased risk of cardiovascular disease, as well as microvascular complications, in type 2 diabetes (World Health Organization, 1999).

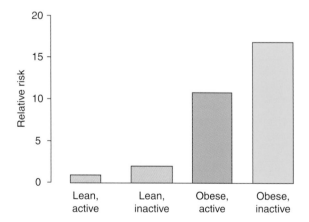

Figure 10.4 Synergistic interaction between obesity and physical inactivity in predicting type 2 diabetes in women. Relative risk is compared with that in lean women (BMI <25 kg/m²) taking ≥21.8 MET hours per week (i.e. moderate) exercise (RR = 1.0). Data from the Nurses' Health Study (Rana *et al.*, 2007).

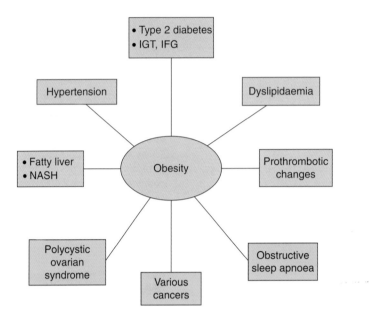

Figure 10.5 Features of the metabolic syndrome and some other disorders associated with obesity and insulin resistance. Those generally accepted as components of the metabolic syndrome are shown in blue.

Definitions

The precise definition of the metabolic syndrome remains undecided. Insulin resistance, initially suggested as the central defect, is hard to measure in clinical practice and does not relate consistently to hypertension or other features of the syndrome (Saad *et al.*, 1991; Cheal *et al.*, 2004). Various bodies have proposed definitions of the syndrome, including the WHO (World Health Organization, 1999), the European Group for the Study of Insulin Resistance (EGIR) (Balkau and Charles, 1999), the National Cholesterol Education Program (NCEP) (NCEP, 2001) and the International Diabetes Federation (IDF) (Alberti, Zimmet and Shaw, 2005). These definitions are shown in Table 10.2.

Epidemiology

Irrespective of the definition used, the metabolic syndrome affects 10% of adults in most developing and developed countries after age and sex adjustments (Sundstrom *et al.*, 2006; The DECODA Study Group, 2006). In the third US National Health and Nutrition Examination Survey (NHANES III), the metabolic syndrome was present in 5% of those with normal weight,

22% of overweight, and 60% of obese subjects (Park *et al.*, 2003).

Debate continues regarding the validity of these definitions and their clinical utility and it has even been argued that the 'syndrome' is not a distinct entity, but merely the coincidental co-occurrence of factors that are relatively common in westernized populations (Kahn *et al.*, 2006; Reaven, 2006; Grundy, 2007). However, the metabolic syndrome may have value for health awareness and surveillance, risk prediction and stratification, and possibly monitoring and intervention (Després and Lemieux, 2006; Meigs *et al.*, 2004), and may add to traditional cardiovascular risk factors such as those defined by the Framingham Study (age, gender, smoking, cholesterol and hypertension). Furthermore, results from epidemiological studies (Malik *et al.*, 2004; Isomaa *et al.*, 2001), genetic analysis (Ng *et al.*, 2004; Hong *et al.*, 1997; Li *et al.*, 2006) and statistical modelling (Chan *et al.*, 1996; Oh *et al.*, 2004; Anderson *et al.*, 2001; Wang *et al.*, 2004; Meigs *et al.*, 1997) all strongly suggest that the various components of the metabolic syndrome (hyperglycaemia, dyslipidaemia, inflammation and hypertension) behave as distinct entities (albeit with some overlap) that show strong familial clustering and are linked to particular chromosomal regions. Specific genes are yet to be identified (Figure 10.6).

Table 10.2 Different definitions of the metabolic syndrome.

WHO (1999)	EGIR (1999)	NCEP-ATPIII (2001)	IDF (2004)
• Diabetes, IFG, IGT or insulin resistance (i.e. lowest quartile of glucose uptake during clamp study)	• Insulin resistance (i.e. highest quartile of fasting insulin)		• Central obesity (increased waist circumference (WC) according to race/ethnic threshold)
Plus any 2 [or 3] or more of the following:	Plus any 2 [or 3] or more of the following:	Any 3 or more of the following:	Any 3 or more of the following:
• Obesity: (BMI >30 kg/m²) or central obesity (WHR >0.9 (M) or >0.85 (F),	• Central obesity (WC ≥94 cm (M), ≥80 cm (F),	• Central obesity (WC >102 cm (M) or >88 cm (F),	
• TG ≥1.7 mmol/l	• TG >2.0 mmol/l	• TG ≥1.7 mmol/l	• TG ≥1.7 mmol/l or treatment
• Low HDL (<0.9 mmol/l (M), <1.0 (F),	• Low HDL <1.0 mmol/l	• Low HDL (<1.0 mmol/l (M), <1.3 (F),	• Low HDL (<1.0 mmol/l (M), <1.3 (F), or treatment for low HDL)
• Hypertension (BP ≥140/90 mmHg)	• Hypertension (BP ≥ 140/90 or on medication)	• Hypertension (BP ≥130/85 for NCEP-ATPIII or on medication)	• Hypertension (SBP >130, DBP >80 for IDF (2004), or on medication)
	• Hyperglycaemia (fasting plasma glucose ≥6.1 mmol/l)	• Hyperglycaemia (fasting plasma glucose ≥6.1 mmol/l)	• Hyperglycaemia (fasting plasma glucose ≥5.6 mmol/l, or previously diagnosed type 2 diabetes)
Additional features			
• Microalbuminuria ≥20 μg/min			
	Excludes known diabetes mellitus		

*The AHA/NHLBI definition is based on the NCEP-ATP III criteria and includes drug treatment of raised TG and reduced HDL-C as diagnostic criteria with a fasting plasma glucose of ≥5.6 mmol/l. TG: triglycerides; WC: waist circumference.

Health risks

Various other disorders are associated with obesity and insulin resistance, and have been suggested as components of the metabolic syndrome (Figure 10.5). These include pro-coagulant and pro-inflammatory changes in the blood (Van Gaal, Mertens and De Block, 2006), endothelial dysfunction (Jiang et al., 1999; Rask-Madsen and King, 2007), glomerulopathy and chronic renal impairment (Sarafidis and Ruilope, 2006), non-alcoholic fatty liver disease (Medina et al., 2004), polycystic ovarian syndrome (PCOS) (Dunaif, 1997) and sleep apnoea (Vgontzas et al., 2000). These conditions are discussed in detail in Chapters 11 and 13.

Of particular note are the intertwining relationships between obesity, diabetes, cardiovascular disease and renal impairment (Sarnak et al., 2003). Renal dysfunction, including microalbuminuria and chronic renal failure, is a powerful and independent predictor of cardiovascular morbidity and mortality in both non-diabetic and diabetic populations (Chen et al., 2004; Tanaka et al., 2006; Chen et al., 2007; Go et al., 2004; So et al., 2006). Possible underlying mechanisms include increased oxidative stress, vascular inflammation, arterial calcification and anaemia (Pecoits-Filho, Lindholm and Stenvinkel, 2002). These associations contribute to the health risks associated with the metabolic syndrome, which carries a two-to fivefold increased

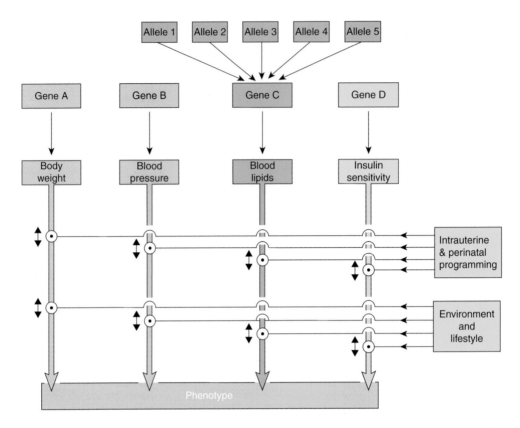

Figure 10.6 Hypothetical interactions between genes and environment, determining heterogeneity in the phenotype of the metabolic syndrome. The effects of polymorphisms at the hypothetical 'gene C', encoding a protein that influences lipid metabolism, are illustrated.

risk of diabetes, cardiovascular disease and all-cause mortality (Ford, 2005; Dekker *et al.*, 2005). Coronary-heart disease (CHD) remains the main cause of death among affected Caucasian subjects, whereas non-Caucasians, notably Asian diabetic patients, are more likely to die from stroke or renal failure (Morrish *et al.*, 2001). With type 2 diabetes affecting ever-younger subjects, and the greater propensity of non-Caucasians to develop renal disease (Wu *et al.*, 2005; Karter *et al.*, 2002), the spread of obesity may be followed in many developing countries by an epidemic of cardiac, vascular and renal disease.

Obesity and insulin resistance

Insulin resistance and/or the compensatory increase in plasma insulin levels that it causes, has been suggested to underlie many features of the metabolic syndrome. In particular, insulin resistance – together with failure of

the β cell to secrete enough insulin to overcome it – is a critical factor in the development of type 2 diabetes. Obesity causes insulin resistance, and this largely explains how it predisposes to type 2 diabetes. Some other abnormalities of the metabolic syndrome, such as dyslipidaemia and hypertension, may also be due at least in part to obesity-related insulin resistance.

This section describes the relationship between obesity and insulin resistance, the possible underlying mechanisms, and how obesity is thought to contribute to the development of type 2 diabetes.

Obesity induces insulin resistance

'Insulin resistance' describes reduced sensitivity of insulin's target tissues to the hormone's actions. It is commonly measured as the loss of insulin's ability to enhance glucose uptake into peripheral tissues, and thus to lower blood glucose concentrations – the basis of the hyperinsulinaemic-euglycaemic clamp and other techniques described in Chapter 3. However, insulin has many diverse actions – ranging from lipid and protein metabolism to arterial tone, sympathetic nervous system activation and appetite control – and measurements of insulin resistance in one system do not necessarily reflect other aspects of insulin action or sensitivity elsewhere in the body.

Numerous studies have demonstrated that obese subjects tend to be less sensitive than lean controls to the glucose-lowering action of insulin. For example, Figure 10.7 shows an inverse relationship in non-diabetic subjects between BMI and whole-body glucose uptake, measured using the clamp technique. Although the overall correlation is highly significant, it is apparent that insulin sensitivity varies widely among subjects with a given BMI; indeed, individual values of insulin sensitivity in non-diabetic subjects may overlap with those in some patients with type 2 diabetes.

Importance of visceral fat

Evidence summarized above and in Chapters 3 and 9 points to the importance of abdominal, and especially visceral, adipose tissue in the association of obesity with type 2 diabetes and the metabolic syndrome (Liu *et al.*, 2006; Liu *et al.*, 2003). Various measures of abdominal fat,

notably the visceral (intra-abdominal) fat mass, are inversely related to insulin sensitivity, as illustrated in Figure 10.8. In this study, there was no significant correlation between subcutaneous fat cross-sectional area and insulin sensitivity.

The greater propensity of abdominal and especially visceral adipose tissue to induce whole-body insulin resistance may be explained by particular properties of this fat depot. Adipocytes in mesenteric and omental depots show higher basal rates of lipolysis than subcutaneous, and lipolysis is less readily suppressed by insulin; enhanced sensitivity of this depot to catecholamines and sympathetic stimulation may be partly responsible (see Chapter 4). This would liberate larger amounts of FFA, which are likely mediators of insulin resistance in the liver, muscle and other tissues (see below). As visceral fat drains into the portal vein, the high FFA levels would impact directly on the liver, theoretically exerting more potent effects. However, it appears that FFA derived from visceral fat probably account for only 10% of total FFA reaching the liver, and that subcutaneous abdominal fat contributes more than visceral fat to the excess in circulating FFA levels that occur in obesity (Martin and Jensen, 1991). Nonetheless, increased FFA delivery to the liver is convincingly implicated in the loss of insulin's ability to inhibit hepatic gluconeogenesis and thus glucose production, and in the increased secretion of VLDL that occurs in obesity.

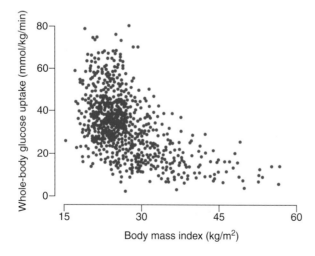

Figure 10.7 Insulin sensitivity (measured as whole-body glucose uptake during the hyperinsulinaemic-euglycaemic clamp) declines as BMI increases. Subjects were non-diabetic. Data from the European Group for the Study of Insulin Resistance (EGIR) database, with kind permission of Professor Ele Ferrannini.

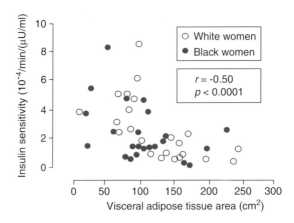

Figure 10.8 Insulin sensitivity (measured using the hyperinsulinaemic-euglycaemic clamp) declines as visceral fat cross-sectional area (at the standard anatomical level, L4/L5) increases. Subjects were White and Black obese, non-diabetic women. From Albu *et al.* (1997) *Diabetes Care* 46: 456–62.

High FFA delivery also leads to the accumulation of 'ectopic' triglyceride in the liver, which leads to fatty change and worsening hepatic insulin resistance.

Regional differences in the amounts of secreted adipokines – cytokines and other proteins released by adipose tissue – may also contribute to the adverse metabolic impact of visceral fat (Kershaw and Flier, 2004). Visceral fat expresses and secretes higher levels of adiponectin, interleukin-1β (IL-1 β), IL-8 and plasminogen activator inhibitor-1 (PAI-1), as compared with subcutaneous fat, which releases relatively more leptin. These cytokines are described in detail in Chapter 4 and below.

Adiponectin exerts various beneficial metabolic benefits, including improved insulin sensitivity. When given experimentally to rodents, adiponectin enhances whole-body insulin sensitivity, reduces hepatic gluconeogenesis and clears ectopic triglyceride from liver and muscle (Berg *et al.*, 2001). Strikingly, adiponectin secretion and plasma concentrations fall in obesity in animals and humans. Adiponectin levels are decreased in mouse models of obesity and lipoatrophy, and are directly implicated in the development of insulin resistance (Yamauchi *et al.*, 2001). In humans, plasma adiponectin levels are reduced in obesity and type 2 diabetes, and are inversely correlated with indices of insulin resistance (Weyer *et al.*, 2001). Thus, declining adiponectin secretion as the visceral fat mass expands could contribute to hepatic insulin resistance.

IL-1β and IL-8 are pro-inflammatory cytokines and, if released in excess from an enlarged visceral fat depot, could contribute to the chronic inflammatory state that occurs in obesity and is thought to worsen both insulin resistance and cardiovascular risk. Enhanced release of the pro-coagulant PAI-1 would also tend to favour thrombosis and arterial disease (see Chapter 12).

Leptin, familiar for its role in regulating appetite and body fat (Chapter 6), is now known to have important peripheral actions that largely improve insulin sensitivity. Specifically, it promotes lipolysis and stimulates fatty acid oxidation, while inhibiting lipogenesis; the net effect is therefore to clear ectopic deposits of triglyceride that accumulate in liver, muscle and other tissues of obese subjects and are thought to interfere with insulin action and other functions (Unger, 2003; Minokoshi *et al.*, 2002; see below).

Thus, selective increases in visceral fat, leading to relative falls in both adiponectin and leptin, which promote insulin sensitivity and help to clear ectopic lipid deposits, would tend to aggravate insulin resistance. It has also been suggested that obese people become 'resistant' or insensitive to the actions of leptin (Caro *et al.*, 1996). Theoretically, leptin resistance could worsen insulin sensitivity in peripheral tissues.

Possible mediators of insulin resistance in obesity

Several mechanisms have been suggested to explain how obesity induces insulin resistance.

The main candidates are increased levels of FFA, ectopic lipid deposition in insulin-sensitive tissues other than adipocytes, and various adipokines and other products secreted by fat.

Free fatty acids (FFA)

FFA are a valuable energy substrate for many organs, but sustained high levels can induce insulin resistance and damage tissues ('lipotoxicity'). FFA are cleaved from circulating triglyceride (either chylomicrons, from dietary triglyceride in the gut, or VLDL secreted by the liver), under the action of lipoprotein lipase (LPL). In adipose tissue, LPL is activated by insulin, thus favouring FFA uptake into adipocytes and their storage as triglyceride. Eventually, FFA are liberated by lipolysis of triglyceride stored in adipocytes, and secreted into the bloodstream. The rate of lipolysis is regulated by hormone-sensitive lipase, which is activated especially by catecholamines (and by growth hormone, thyroxine and cortisol), and powerfully inhibited by insulin. These processes are described in detail in Chapter 4.

As already mentioned, obese subjects and those with type 2 diabetes have generally high FFA levels, due to enhanced lipolysis, the rate increasing as fat mass rises. High FFA levels persist throughout the day and in diabetic patients, are proportionate to the degree of hyperglycaemia, and are sustained despite high insulin levels, indicating failure of insulin to suppress lipolysis in adipose tissues (Fraze *et al.*, 1985; Swislocki *et al.*, 1987). Increased sympathetic activity and/or enhanced sensitivity to catecholamines may be responsible (Anderson *et al.*, 1997; Lee *et al.*, 2001; Kaaja and Poyhonen-Alho, 2006), and mesenteric adipocytes are particularly susceptible (Richelsen *et al.*, 1991).

Raised FFA levels may exert various deleterious metabolic and other effects (Table 10.3). Direct metabolic actions in muscle and liver result in impairment of aspects of insulin action. Randle and co-workers first proposed, from observations in heart muscle, that increased utilization of FFA competes with glucose utilization and decreased glucose uptake – the 'glucose-fatty acid' (or Randle) cycle (Randle *et al.*, 1963). The cycle is illustrated in Figure 10.9.

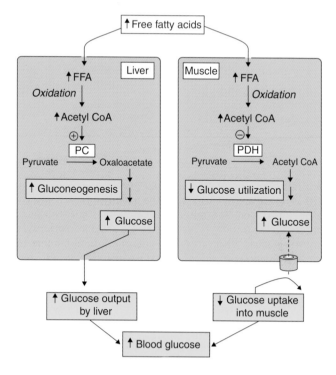

Figure 10.9 The glucose-fatty acid (Randle) cycle. Raised FFA levels inhibit glucose utilization in muscle and liver, leading to decreased uptake into muscle and enhanced hepatic glucose production from gluconeogenesis. These effects antagonize two important glucose-lowering actions of insulin. PC: pyruvate carboxylase; PDH: pyruvate dehydrogenase.

Table 10.3   Detrimental effects of FFA (lipotoxicity) in obesity and the metabolic syndrome.

Skeletal muscle

- Inhibits glucose utilization
- Inhibits glucose uptake   } Insulin resistance
- Triglyceride deposition

Liver

- Inhibits glucose utilization
- Increases hepatic glucose output   } Insulin resistance
- Triglyceride deposition
- Inflammation and fibrosis

β cell

- Triglyceride deposition
- Amyloid deposition (?)   } • Impaired insulin secretion
- Apoptosis   • β-cell damage and death

Heart

- Inhibits glucose utilization
- Triglyceride deposition   } Insulin resistance
- Contractile dysfunction

Arteries

- Triglyceride deposition
- Endothelial dysfunction

Kidney

- Glomerular dysfunction

In muscle, FFA are oxidized to produce acetyl CoA, and this inhibits pyruvate dehydrogenase, thus decreasing glucose utilization. This raises the intracellular glucose concentration, reducing the transmembrane gradient that drives glucose into the cell, and so decreases glucose uptake. In liver, raised acetyl CoA levels inhibit pyruvate carboxylase and stimulate gluconeogenesis and glycogen breakdown (Björntorp, 1991; Magnusson *et al.*, 1992; DeFronzo, Simonson and Ferrannini, 1982). Gluconeogenesis is the main source of hepatic glucose output, and an important target of insulin's action to prevent the liver from producing glucose.

Studies in humans have confirmed that high FFA concentrations impair insulin-mediated glucose disposal (Ferrannini *et al.*, 1983), but the underlying mechanisms now appear to involve various signal-transduction pathways that mediate insulin's actions (see Figure 10.10). Following insulin binding to its receptor in a target cell, the insulin receptor substrate-1 (IRS-1) protein is phosphorylated, and then activates phosphatidylinositol 3 kinase (PI3 kinase); this in turn activates a cascade of kinases, culminating in the activation of protein kinase B (Akt). This causes the GLUT4 glucose transporters to be translocated from around the nucleus to the cell membrane, possibly by remodelling the cell's actin cytoskeleton. Insertion of GLUT4 into the membrane increases glucose entry into the cell, where it

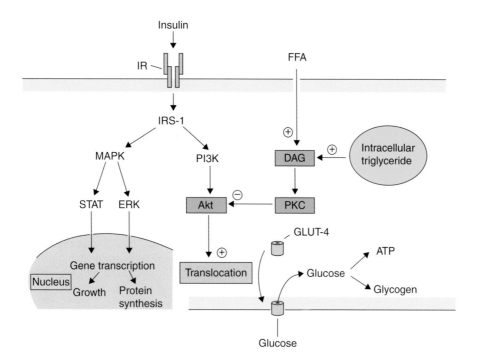

Figure 10.10 Insulin signalling pathways, showing possible points of interference by high FFA levels, leading to impaired insulin action. DAG: diacylglycerol; IR: insulin receptor; PKC: protein kinase C.

is oxidized to produce ATP or stored as glycogen (Figure 10.10). Insulin-receptor binding also activates the MAP kinase pathway which leads to expression of genes regulating protein synthesis and cell growth (Niswender and Schwartz, 2003; Griffin *et al.*, 1999; Liu *et al.*, 2006).

High FFA levels interfere with these processes at various levels. In subjects with or without type 2 diabetes, intravenous triglyceride infusion (which raises FFA levels) has been shown to reduce glucose oxidation (Boden, 2002) and glycogen synthesis (Shulman *et al.*, 1990) in muscle, and to enhance glycogenolysis in liver (Boden *et al.*, 2002). Moreover, raised FFA concentrations reduce PI3 kinase activation (Dresner *et al.*, 1999), possibly by interacting with the θ isoform of protein kinase C (PKC-θ) – an effect that has been implicated in muscle insulin resistance in rats fed a high-fat diet (Schmitz-Peiffer *et al.*, 1997). Prolonged elevation of FFA levels in normal subjects similarly induces insulin resistance, with activation of other membrane-associated PKC isoforms (βII and δ), apparently mediated by increased

diacylglycerol (DAG) formation (Itani *et al.*, 2002) (Figure 10.10).

Raised FFA levels associated with insulin resistance have also been implicated in endothelial dysfunction (Jiang *et al.*, 1999; Rask-Madsen and King, 2007) and polycystic ovarian syndrome (Holte, 1998; Glintborg *et al.*, 2005).

Ectopic triglyceride deposition

White adipocytes have evolved into the primary storage organ for surplus energy in the form of triglyceride (Chapter 4). In so doing, they also protect other tissues from accumulating excess triglyceride. There is now much evidence that ectopic triglyceride deposition in lean tissues (skeletal and heart muscle, liver, β cells and the arterial wall) can induce insulin resistance and impair other aspects of tissue function – so-called 'lipotoxicity' (Unger, 2003).

The deleterious effects of ectopic triglyceride deposition are evident in human diseases and experimental animal models in which white adipose tissue is greatly reduced. In humans, the rare lipoatrophic diabetes syndrome (Seip-Berardinelli) is characterized by the absence of subcutaneous and visceral abdominal fat from birth; triglyceride storage is markedly increased in liver and muscle, leading to severe insulin resistance, diabetes and recurrent ketosis (Robbins *et al.*, 1984; Joffe *et al.*, 2001) Leptin levels are very low, and appetite and food intake correspondingly increased. A similar phenotype is seen in the transgenic 'fatless' (A-ZIP/F-1) mouse, which lacks white adipose tissue and has greatly reduced leptin levels. Severe fatty infiltration of the liver is associated with raised FFA and triglyceride levels, and with insulin resistance, hyperinsulinaemia and diabetes (Moitra *et al.*, 1998; Reitman *et al.*, 2000). Surgical implantation of white adipose tissue from normal mice reverses all the metabolic derangements, suggesting that these are due to the lack of white fat (Gavrilova *et al.*, 2000).

Evidence that ectopic triglyceride deposition induces insulin resistance in the affected tissues in humans includes the finding that an increased intramyocellular triglyceride content is correlated closely with muscle insulin resistance (Figure 10.11); indeed, muscle lipid content was a better predictor of impaired insulin action than adiposity (Goodpaster *et al.*, 1997). Intracellular triglyceride accumulation could interfere with insulin signalling by increasing DAG content and thus inhibiting PKC (Figure 10.10).

Other clinical manifestations of ectopic lipid deposition in obesity may include non-alcoholic fatty liver and steatohepatitis (see Chapter 11), cardiac dysfunction and heart failure (Gavrilova *et al.*, 2000, Chapter 12), and β-cell dysfunction and apoptosis that may play a role in the development of type 2 diabetes (see below).

Leptin appears to play an important part in preventing triglyceride accumulation in non-adipose tissues, and in maintaining insulin sensitivity. In liver and muscle, leptin binding to its receptor (LEPB-R, or ObRb) activates a cascade of intracellular signals including the Janus kinase (JAK) and signal transduction and transcription (STAT) pathways and AMP-activated protein kinase (AMPK). These events culminate in increased glucose transport, β-oxidation of FFA, glycolysis and mitochondrial biogenesis (Frühbeck, 2006;). Moreover, activation of AMPK by leptin leads to inhibition of acetyl CoA carboxylase (ACC), and thus a decrease in acetyl CoA – the mediator that interferes with glucose metabolism in the glucose-fatty acid cycle (Figure 10.9). Thus, by promoting lipolysis and the oxidation of the resulting FFA, and by inhibiting lipogenic enzyme activity, leptin prevents triglyceride accumulation in lean tissues. Low leptin levels in human lipodystrophy and analogous animal models could therefore explain excess lipid

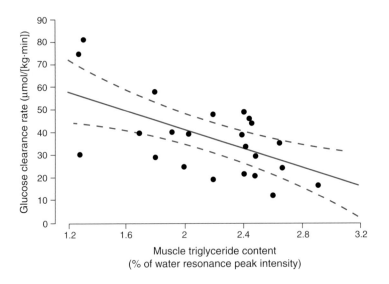

Figure 10.11 Ectopic triglyceride deposition in muscle is related to insulin resistance. Intramyocellular triglyceride content (measured using MR spectroscopy) was significantly inversely correlated with the metabolic clearance rate of glucose during a hyperinsulinaemic euglucaemic clamp. From Krssak *et al.*, 1999.

deposition in liver and muscle, contributing to insulin resistance. Consistent with this, leptin administration enhances the beneficial metabolic effects of adipose tissue transplantation in transgenic fatless mice; conversely, transplantation of leptin-deficient fat from *ob/ob* mice has no such effect – even though adiponectin levels were increased (Colombo *et al.*, 2002).

The fact that ectopic triglyceride accumulation tends to worsen with increasing obesity, even though circulating leptin levels increase in parallel with fat mass, is unexplained. It has been suggested that obese subjects become leptin-resistant, perhaps analogous to insulin resistance (Caro *et al.*, 1996), but direct evidence to support this hypothesis is lacking. Interestingly, some of leptin's actions could worsen insulin resistance. Leptin stimulates the release of tumour necrosis factor-α (TNF-α) from adipocytes, and this cytokine can interfere with insulin signalling (Hotamisligil *et al.*, 1996; see below). Chronically elevated leptin levels also stimulate the sympathetic nervous system, potentially aggravating insulin resistance as well as inducing hypertension (Beltowski, 2006; Wofford and Hall, 2004). Long-term hyperleptinaemia, with or without leptin resistance, could therefore become a maladaptive response that fails to prevent ectopic lipid accumulation and insulin resistance in obese subjects.

Adipokines

As already discussed, imbalances in the adipokines secreted by various fat depots could influence whole-body insulin sensitivity, and perhaps explain the association of visceral obesity with insulin resistance.

The metabolic actions of leptin and adiponectin have been described above. At a cellular level, adiponectin – like leptin – appears to activate AMPK, leading to reduced ACC activity and consequent increases in glucose utilization and uptake. FFA oxidation is also increased, while gluconeogenesis and lipogenesis are inhibited. These effects would result in improved insulin sensitivity (Yamauchi *et al.*, 2002; Yamauchi *et al.*, 2003). Production of uncoupling proteins is also enhanced, which would promote energy dissipation. Adiponectin may also inhibit atherogenesis – an effect revealed by cross-breeding transgenic mice that over-express adiponectin with apoE-knockout mice that usually develop atherosclerosis (Yamauchi *et al.*, 2003). The

metabolic effects of leptin and adiponectin are summarized in Figure 10.12.

Adipose tissue contains numerous macrophages and other inflammatory cells (Weisberg *et al.*, 2003; Chapter 4). When activated, for example by infections or hypoxia, these cells secrete numerous cytokines, notably TNF-α and IL-6 (Pickup, 2004). These acute-phase inflammatory mediators have various effects, including insulin resistance and activation of the sympathetic nervous system, hypothalamo-pituitary-adrenal (HPA) axis and the renin-angiotensin-aldosterone system (RAS) (Van Gaal, Mertens and De Block, 2006; Axelrod and Reisine, 1984; Chan, Tong and Critchley, 2002). This causes widespread pro-inflammatory, pro-thrombotic and haemodynamic changes as well as neuroendocrine disturbances and insulin resistance. Consistent with this notion, chronic low-grade infections such as hepatitis B and C have been implicated in the development of type 2 diabetes (Pradhan *et al.*, 2001; Mehta *et al.*, 2000) and cardiac and renal complications (Lo *et al.*, 2004; Cheng *et al.*, 2006; Soma *et al.*, 2000), especially in obese subjects and in non-Caucasian populations (Lao *et al.*, 2003; Ratziu, Trabut and Poynard, 2004).

Two important pro-inflammatory cytokines are TNF-α and IL-6. TNF-α has long been implicated in inflammatory conditions such as rheumatoid arthritis and also in the catabolic states associated with various malignancies (cancer cachexia) and severe heart failure (Aggarwal, 2000). TNF-α expression is increased in adipose tissue of obese humans and rodents (Hotamisligil, Shargill and Spiegelman, 1993; Hotamisligil *et al.*, 1995) and can contribute to insulin resistance, either at a paracrine level on adjacent adipocytes, or at distant sites. TNF-α has been shown to inhibit the phosphorylation of specific tyrosine residues on the insulin receptor and IRS-1 that normally follows insulin-receptor binding (Hotamisligil *et al.*, 1994).

IL-6 is secreted mainly by immune cells but also by adipose tissue, notably abdominal subcutaneous and visceral depots, which contribute up to one-third of the body's total IL-6 production (Mohamed-Ali *et al.*, 1997). Circulating IL-6 concentrations correlate with fat mass and BMI, and also with insulin resistance (Bastard *et al.*, 2000; Vozarova *et al.*, 2001; Kern *et al.*, 2001). In omental adipocytes, IL-6 (in the presence of dexamethasone) enhances leptin expression, while reducing expression of LPL; these effects,

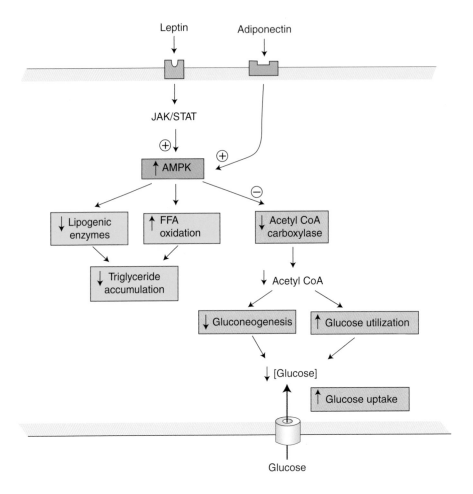

Figure 10.12 Metabolic actions of leptin and adiponectin. Both activate AMPK, which leads to enhanced utilization of both glucose and FFA, to decreased intracellular storage of triglycerides, and to a fall in intra-cellular glucose concentration, which steepens the transmembrane glucose gradient and promotes glucose uptake. These effects lead to enhanced insulin sensitivity.

which would promote lipolysis, are attenuated by insulin (Trujillo *et al.*, 2004). IL-6 apparently acts centrally to inhibit feeding, as intracerebroventricular injection of low doses causes hypophagia and reduced body fat, without causing peripheral effects such as the stimulation of acute-phase protein production by the liver (Wallenius *et al.*, 2002a; Wallenius *et al.*, 2002b). This central hypophagic effect may explain why IL-6 knockout mice become obese (Wallenius *et al.*, 2002b).

Chronic inflammation and insulin resistance

Obesity is associated with a low-grade chronic inflammatory state, probably mediated in part by cytokines produced by adipose tissue. Recent evidence strongly suggests that this contributes to insulin resistance.

The c-jun amino-terminal kinases (JNKs), I kappa kinase (IκK) and NF-κB are all important signalling molecules that can be activated by both inflammatory cytokines and FFA (Shoelson, Lee and Yuan, 2003), and may interfere with insulin action (Figure 10.13). In two mouse models of obesity, deletion of JNK was associated with improved insulin sensitivity, enhanced post-receptor signalling, and reduced adiposity (Hirosumi *et al.*, 2002). Similarly, deletion of IκK in hepatocytes protects against insulin resistance induced by high-fat feeding, obesity or ageing (Arkan *et al.*, 2005). Conversely, mice

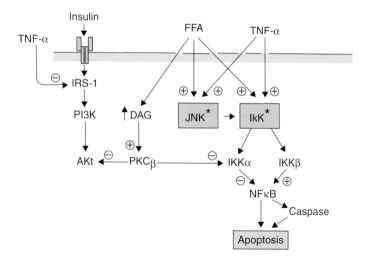

Figure 10.13 Intracellular pathways activated by inflammation, and which may contribute to insulin resistance. *: Deletion of JNK or IκK leads to improved insulin sensitivity; the precise mechanisms are as yet undetermined.

that selectively over-express IκK in hepatocytes developed marked hepatic lipid infiltration and inflammation as well as moderate muscle and systemic insulin resistance, leading to hyperglycaemia and a phenotype resembling type 2 diabetes (Cai *et al.*, 2005).

In human studies, intravenous triglyceride infusion increases DAG content in muscle, with activation of PKCβ (which inhibits PI3 kinase activity) this decreases levels of IκKα, which normally inhibits NF-κB activity (Itani *et al.*, 2002).

Role of other adipose tissue products

Adipose tissue secretes other factors that may contribute to insulin resistance, including monocyte chemoattractant protein-1 (MCP-1) (Kanda *et al.*, 2006), PAI-1 (Alessi and Juhan-Vague, 2006), acylation-stimulating protein (ASP) (Xia, Sniderman and Cianflone, 2002), and angiotensin and other components of the RAS (Engeli *et al.*, 2003). Also expressed in fat is the enzyme 11β-hydroxysteroid dehydrogenase type 1 (11β-HSD1), which catalyses the conversion of inactive cortisone to active cortisol in humans (Tomlinson and Stewart, 2005). Increased local availability of cortisol may promote differentiation of preadipocytes into mature adipocytes, further promoting fat accumulation. Resistin, an adipokine that was claimed to induce insulin resistance, is discussed in Chapter 4.

Obesity-induced ER stress

'Endoplasmic reticulum stress' (ER stress) describes the tendency of malformed proteins to be produced under conditions of high demand for protein synthesis – for example, failure to fold into the correct shape, due to underproduction of the 'chaperone' proteins that control the configuration of the newly-translated peptide (Hotamisligil, 2005; Kaufman *et al.*, 2002). Recent evidence suggests that ER stress can also cause insulin resistance, perhaps by producing malformed intracellular signalling proteins. ER stress may also contribute to cytokine-induced β-cell death. In particular, IL-1β and interferon-γ induce severe ER stress through nitric oxide (NO)-mediated depletion of ER calcium and inhibition of ER chaperones, respectively; these effects hamper β-cell defences and activate pro-apoptotic pathways. Mice deficient in a transcription factor X-box binding protein-1 (XBP-1), which normally attenuates the ER stress response, develop insulin resistance (Ozcan *et al.*, 2004). On the other hand, hepatic over-expression of a molecular chaperone, oxygen-regulated protein 150 (ORP150), which protects cells from ER stress, ameliorates insulin resistance and glucose tolerance in obese diabetic mice; enhanced insulin signalling and reduced expression of gluconeogenic enzymes have been implicated (Nakatani *et al.*, 2005).

Obesity and the development of type 2 diabetes

Even though obesity is a strong predictor for type 2 diabetes, most obese people (80%) remain normoglycaemic – albeit with insulin resistance and features of the metabolic syndrome, including cardiovascular disease in many cases (Colditz et al., 1995; Després and Lemieux, 2006). This indicates that the inability of the β cells to secrete enough insulin to overcome insulin resistance is a critical determinant for developing type 2 diabetes (Boden and Shulman, 2002).

Obesity predisposes to type 2 diabetes primarily by inducing insulin resistance, although the associated metabolic abnormalities may also contribute to the β-cell dysfunction, which ultimately causes blood glucose levels to rise into the diabetic range. Obesity is just one of many factors that can cause insulin resistance (see Table 10.4), and the contribution made by obesity varies widely among individuals.

Genetic determination of insulin resistance is apparently polygenic in most cases (Hattersley and Pearson, 2006; McCarthy and Zeggini, 2006). Candidate genes include:

- the β_3 adrenoceptor: a point mutation is associated with upper-body obesity and insulin resistance (Widen et al., 1995).
- the glycogen-associated regulatory subunit of protein phosphatase-1 that is expressed in skeletal muscle: a single nucleotide polymorphism

Table 10.4 Causes of insulin resistance.

Genetic	Acquired
Polygenic	Intrauterine malnutrition
	Obesity
	Physical inactivity and low physical fitness
	Increasing age
	Pregnancy
	Puberty
	Smoking
	Infections
	Drugs, e.g. glucocorticoids
	Endocrine disorders, e.g. Cushing syndrome

is associated with insulin resistance and hyper-insulinaemia (Hansen et al., 1995).

- the intestinal fatty-acid binding protein-2: a missense mutation of the FABP-2 is associated with insulin resistance (Baier et al., 1995).

Certain genetic variants of the mitochondrial genome, which encodes proteins that regulate oxidative phosphorylation and energy expenditure (Lane, 2006), are also associated with insulin resistance, especially in non-Caucasian populations (Fuku et al., 2007; Lee et al., 2005; Liou et al., 2007). Expression levels of OXPHOS, encoding oxidative phosphorylation enzymes, is reportedly decreased in insulin-resistant but normoglycaemic first-degree relatives of type 2 diabetic subjects, as well as in patients with type 2 diabetes (Patti et al., 2003). Overall, however, the contribution of each of these genes is probably small.

Malnutrition in utero and during the perinatal period is linked with insulin resistance, which is exacerbated by weight gain in infancy or later in life (Yajnik, 2002; Barker et al., 1993). In animal models, fetal protein malnutrition alters hepatic glucose metabolism and enhances 11β-HSD1 activity, but the relevance of this to humans is uncertain.

Pregnancy, drugs (e.g. glucocorticoids), infections (including hepatitis B and C), chronic inflammatory states and physical inactivity (see Chapter 8) all decrease insulin sensitivity. The latter also declining with age. Reductions in mitochondrial oxidative phosphorylation activity may contribute to age-related insulin resistance (Petersen et al., 2003), and also to inherited insulin resistance in subjects with a family history of type 2 diabetes (Petersen et al., 2004). Indeed, decreased mitochondrial density and function may be a common early defect in the pathogenesis of insulin resistance (Morino et al., 2005, 2006).

β-cell failure in type 2 diabetes

The ability of β cells to secrete enough insulin to overcome an individual's current level of insulin resistance ultimately determines whether normoglycaemia or hyperglycaemia will prevail.

β-cell failure was previously thought to be a late event in the development of type 2 diabetes, but it is now clear that it begins early and may be partly genetically determined. There is

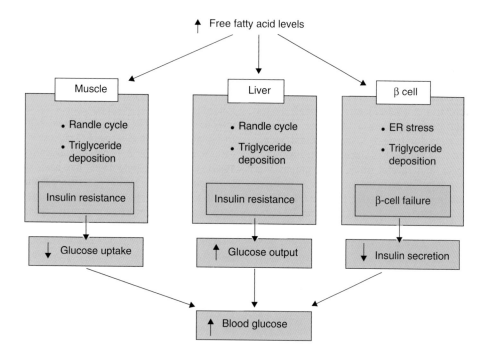

Figure 10.14 Obesity contributes to both insulin resistance and β-cell failure, the two defects that result in type 2 diabetes. The pathogenic roles of high FFA levels are highlighted here; other mechanisms also contribute (see text).

also evidence that the metabolic disturbances associated with obesity cause β-cell dysfunction and may hasten the failure of insulin secretion. Thus, obesity contributes to both the defects – insulin resistance and β-cell failure – that lead to type 2 diabetes (see Figure 10.14).

Causes of β-cell failure

These causes include genetic and acquired factors (Table 10.5). The role of obesity is discussed in detail below. As with insulin resistance, the

Table 10.5 Causes of β-cell dysfunction in type 2 diabetes.

Genetic	Acquired
Polygenic	Intrauterine malnutrition
	Obesity
	• High FFA levels (lipotoxicity)
	• Triglyceride deposition
	• ER stress
	Amyloid accumulation
	Hyperglycaemia (glucotoxicity)

relative importance of genetic and acquired factors, and the contribution of obesity, varies considerably between individuals.

A genetic predisposition to β-cell dysfunction is suggested by the finding that first-degree relatives of type 2 diabetic subjects show defects in insulin production that are characteristic of type 2 diabetes. These include a reduction in the first phase of insulin secretion (the acute 'spike' that immediately follows an intravenous glucose challenge) and disturbances of the normal pulsatile pattern of insulin secretion (Van Haeften *et al.*, 2000; O'Rahilly, Turner and Matthews, 1988). Strikingly, these defects are seen in lean, normoglycaemic subjects with normal insulin sensitivity, indicating that β-cell dysfunction predates insulin resistance in this population.

The genetic predisposition to β-cell failure in type 2 diabetes is likely to be both polygenic and multigenic; that is, numerous genes may potentially be involved, with different combinations operating in individual subjects (Hattersley and Pearson, 2006; McCarthy and Zeggini, 2006). Several genes have been identified of which mutations lead to maturity-onset diabetes of the young (MODY), which is characterized by inadequate insulin secretion. These include hepatic nuclear factor-4 (*HNF4A*; MODY 1), glucokinase (*GK*; MODY 2), *HNF1A* (MODY 3) and insulin promoter factor 1 (*IPF1*; MODY 4). However, specific genes underlying β-cell dysfunction in common type 2 diabetes have remained elusive until recently.

In 2006, the gene encoding transcription factor-7-like 2 (*TCF7L2*) was identified by the DECODE group in Iceland as a new susceptibility gene for type 2 diabetes (Grant *et al.*, 2006). This finding has since been replicated in European and several other racial groups that have a high prevalence of type 2 diabetes (Zeggini and McCarthy, 2007; Lehman *et al.*, 2007; Ng *et al.*, 2007). Studies suggest that *TCF7L2*, a transcription factor ubiquitously expressed and involved in the wnt signalling pathway, increases the risk of type 2 diabetes by reducing insulin secretion (Lyssenko *et al.*, 2007). In 2007, several other susceptibility gene loci for type 2 diabetes were identified through genome-wide association studies, including some such as *CDKAL1, SLC30A8* and *HHEX-KIF11-IDE,* which appear to impact on insulin secretion (Steinthorsdottir *et al.*, 2007; Frayling, 2007). Much interest is now focused on studying the mechanisms through which variants within these gene regions might affect insulin secretion.

Intrauterine malnutrition, and especially protein deficiency, can lead to lasting β-cell dysfunction in animal models and has also been implicated in humans (Hales and Barker, 1992). Certain drugs, such as thiazides and diazoxide, can also inhibit insulin secretion, but these effects are reversible.

Finally, insulin resistance at the level of the β cell itself and sustained hyperglycaemia may contribute to β-cell dysfunction and failure of insulin secretion. The β cell expresses insulin receptors, and selective knockout of these in transgenic mice leads to subnormal insulin secretion following a glucose challenge but a preserved response to another insulin secretagogue, arginine; this selective failure to respond to glucose is seen early in human type 2 diabetes (Kulkarni *et al.*, 1999). Chronic hyperglycaemia has been shown to impair β-cell function in experimental animals and is thought to play a role in the progressive decline of insulin secretion in human type 2 diabetes (Poitou and Robertson, 2002). Suggested mechanisms include down-regulation of glucose transporters (GLUT2) on the β cell, and altered gene transcription due to reactive oxygen species (free radicals) generated intracellularly under hyperglycaemic conditions. This aspect of glucotoxicity is potentially reversible, by glucose-lowering drugs or substantial weight loss.

Obesity and β-cell dysfunction

Defects of insulin secretion, including reductions in first-phase release and abnormal pulsatility, have also been described in obese subjects. Evidence suggests that high FFA levels and triglyceride deposition within the β cell can impair β-cell function and lead to damage and eventual cell death. Some of these effects may involve abnormal processing of the β-cell peptide, amylin (Figure 10.15).

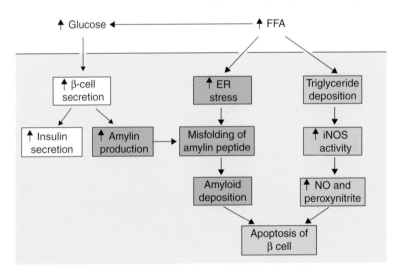

Figure 10.15 Possible mechanisms of β-cell dysfunction and death in obesity and type 2 diabetes.

In-vitro experiments show that sustained high FFA levels impair insulin secretion and eventually damage β cells. Isolated pancreatic islets exposed to high FFA concentrations for 24–48 hours show initially enhanced insulin release, followed by a progressive fall in insulin stores and secretion, even though proinsulin synthesis is increased. This suggests defective regulation of post-translation processing of proinsulin (Zhou and Grill, 1995; Bollheimer *et al.*, 1998) – a defect that is characteristic of type 2 diabetes (Kahn, 2004).

Chronically raised FFA levels are apparently toxic to β cells *in vivo* in animal models such as the Zucker Diabetic Fatty (ZDF) rat. This has a mutation of the leptin receptor (LEPR), leading to obesity with severe insulin resistance; this strain also develops β-cell apoptosis at 9 weeks of age, when hyperglycaemia develops. Longitudinal studies show that FFA levels rise progressively from 5 weeks, accompanied by marked increases in β-cell triglyceride content and disruption of islet morphology. The temporal relationship strongly suggests a pathogenic role of FFA in β-cell dysfunction (Lee *et al.*, 1994). Moreover, treatment of prediabetic ZDF rats with troglitazone (which lowers plasma FFA levels) prevents the progression to β-cell death and diabetes (Higa *et al.*, 1999). *In vitro*, troglitazone lowers triglyceride levels and improves insulin secretion in β cells from rats with insulin resistance induced by fructose feeding (Lee *et al.*, 1994).

There is some evidence that FFA are toxic to β cells in humans. After four days of intravenous lipid infusion to raise FFA concentrations, subjects with a family history of type 2 diabetes showed marked impairment of both the first- and second-phase insulin secretion (Kashyap *et al.*, 2003). Moreover, thiazolidinediones have been reported to preserve β-cell function in patients with impaired glucose tolerance (IGT) or type 2 diabetes (Leiter, 2005); however, the specificity of this effect is uncertain.

Ectopic triglyceride deposition has been documented in the β cells of the ZDF rat and other obese rodents, and has been implicated in β-cell damage and death. Measures that prevent islet triglyceride deposition (e.g. troglitazone treatment or under feeding) also prevent β-cell dysfunction and death (Ohneda, Inman and Unger, 1995). Possible mechanisms include up-regulation of inducible NOS (iNOS), increasing the production of NO which combines with reactive oxygen species to form peroxynitrite, a toxin that causes β-cell apoptosis (Shimabukuro *et al.*, 1997).

Amyloid deposition is another possible pathogenic mechanism. Deposits of amyloid within the β cell are common in type 2 diabetic subjects (up to 90% of cases) and also occur in about 10% of non-diabetic subjects (Hull *et al.*, 2004; Butler *et al.*, 2003; Zhao *et al.*, 2003). Amyloid deposition correlates with β-cell dysfunction in some models and is postulated to cause damage and death of the β cell, although the precise mechanisms remain uncertain.

β-cell amyloid consists largely of polymerized amylin (islet amyloid polypeptide (IAPP)), a β-cell peptide that is normally co-secreted with insulin. It is thought that increased production of amylin (in parallel with insulin hypersecretion) in the presence of ER stress, leads to misfolding of the peptide monomers, which aggregate to form amyloid (Hayden *et al.*, 2005). In transgenic mice that express human amylin in their β cells, high-fat feeding enhances amyloid deposition (Hull *et al.*, 2004), whereas this is reduced (with improved β-cell function) by treatment with rosiglitazone and metformin (Hull *et al.*, 2005).

Evolution of type 2 diabetes

Classical longitudinal studies followed blood glucose and insulin levels in obese subjects who progressed from normoglycaemia through IGT to type 2 diabetes (Mitrakou *et al.*, 1992; DeFronzo, 1992). The results are summarized in Figure 10.16. These were interpreted as showing that insulin resistance (manifested as raised insulin levels) was present in normoglycaemic obese subjects, and worsened as they developed IGT – which represented the peak of β-cell function. Beyond this stage, insulin production fell, attributed to the onset of β-cell failure, allowing glucose levels to rise into the diabetic range. The profile of insulin production, initially rising to a peak to compensate for insulin resistance and then declining, has been turned the 'Starling curve' of the pancreas (DeFronzo, 1992). Thus, insulin resistance was thought to precede β-cell failure by several years.

This scheme has now been superseded by evidence indicating that β-cell function is significantly impaired in normoglycaemic subjects before they develop IGT, and before severe

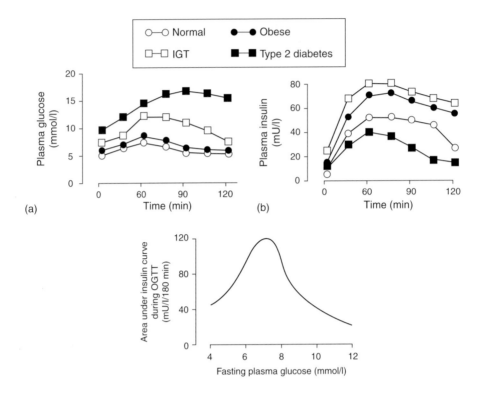

Figure 10.16 Upper panel: Changes in (a) plasma glucose and (b) plasma insulin concentrations, during the progression of obese subjects from normoglycaemia (with higher insulin levels than in lean subjects) to IGT (maximal insulin response) and finally type 2 diabetes (insulin levels fall, and glucose rises). Lower panel: The suggested sequence of insulin secretion – initial compensation followed by failure – was described by DeFronzo (1992) as the 'Starling curve' of the β cell.

insulin resistance supervenes (Mitrakou *et al.*, 1992; Kahn, 2001) (Figure 10.17). Impaired first-phase insulin release and reduced insulin sensitivity both predict the development of type 2 diabetes, even in notably insulin-resistant populations such as the Pima Indians (Lillioja *et al.*, 1993). In this population, transition from normoglycaemia to IGT is associated with increased body weight, reduced insulin-stimulated glucose disposal, and the progressive decline in first-phase insulin release; both the latter abnormalities worsen further with progression from IGT to type 2 diabetes (Weyer *et al.*, 1999).

Thus, both insulin resistance and β-cell dysfunction are essential defects in type 2 diabetes, but undoubtedly operate to different degrees among individuals (Kahn, 2004). Obesity appears to contribute to both.

As described in Chapter 18, successful bariatric surgery – which may cause loss of over 80% of excess weight – can improve glucose tolerance in hypoglycaemic individuals. Strikingly, established type 2 diabetes can be reversed, even in some long-standing cases. This suggests that β-cell failure is due more to functional impairment (perhaps from the effects of high FFA levels or β-cell triglyceride deposition) rather than to β-cell death.

Dyslipidaemia in obesity and the metabolic syndrome

In obesity, and especially in subjects with type 2 diabetes and the metabolic syndrome, a characteristic dyslipidaemia often occurs. Typical abnormalities are high triglyceride concentrations, low levels of high density lipoprotein cholesterol (HDL-cholesterol), which arise from abnormalities of lipoprotein metabolism, notably overproduction of very low density

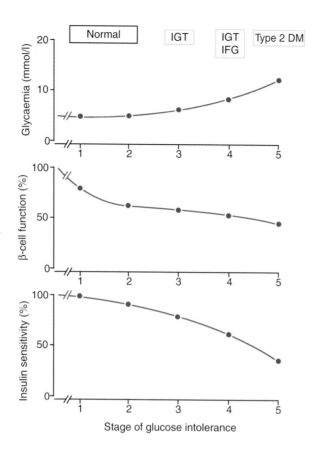

Figure 10.17 Current view of the progression of β-cell dysfunction and insulin resistance during the development of type 2 diabetes, from normoglycaemia (NGT) to impaired glucose tolerance (IGT) and impaired fasting glucose (IFG), and ultimately overt diabetes.

lipoprotein cholesterol (VLDL-cholesterol) and apolipoprotein B-100 (apo B), decreased catabolism of apo B-containing particles, and increased catabolism of HDL apoA-I particles.

In the postprandial phase, triglyceride-rich particles have both exogenous (chylomicrons) and endogenous (VLDL) origins, the former derived mainly from dietary fat and the latter secreted by the liver. Both chylomicrons and VLDL particles compete for the same removal pathways, that is lipolysis by lipoprotein lipase (LPL) and receptor-mediated uptake of remnant particles by the liver (Figure 10.18). As LPL has greater affinity for chylomicrons, VLDL particles secreted from the liver may accumulate postprandially because their clearance pathways become saturated. This process is exaggerated in the presence of increased production of VLDL, which is directly linked to enhanced FFA supply from visceral fat, and by impaired activity of

LPL (an insulin-sensitive enzyme) in insulin resistance.

Thus, a vicious cycle of overproduction and reduced clearance of VLDL leads to raised plasma triglyceride levels throughout the day in obesity and especially subjects with the metabolic syndrome and type 2 diabetes (Figure 10.19). In addition, recent evidence suggests that type 2 diabetes is accompanied by a relative deficiency of apolipoprotein C, which is critical for the hepatic clearance of VLDL. These abnormalities are compounded by the tendency of high FFA levels to impair the binding of lipid remnants to LPL and to endothelium-bound heparin sulphate in the liver, thus further reducing triglyceride clearance.

In the presence of overproduction and/or reduced clearance, the prolonged residence time of triglyceride in the circulation results in the excessive transfer of triglyceride to LDL and HDL

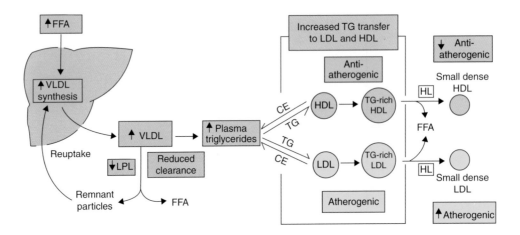

Figure 10.18 Disturbances of lipoprotein metabolism in obesity and the metabolic syndrome. CE: cholesteryl esters (transferred by CETP); HL: hepatic lipase; LPL: lipoprotein lipase; TG: triglyceride.

particles, and a concomitant transfer of cholesteryl esters to triglyceride under the influence of the enzyme, cholesterol ester transfer protein (CETP). Hepatic lipase (HL) mediates the hydrolysis of core triglyceride to produce small, dense LDL particles that are more readily taken up by subendothelial macrophages to form foam cells, the precursors of atherosclerotic plaques. Delayed clearance of triglyceride also promotes exchange of core lipids between HDL and triglyceride, resulting in enhanced formation of triglyceride-rich, small dense HDL particles. The latter are good substrates for hepatic lipase, resulting in enhanced catabolism of apoAI-rich HDL particles, and reduced reverse cholesterol transfer, thereby further reducing HDL levels and increasing atherogenic risk (Syvänne and Taskinen, 1997; Taskinen, 1992) (Figure 10.20).

Recent experiments point to complex abnormalities in the intracellular handling of lipoprotein in the liver that occur in the metabolic syndrome and type 2 diabetes. Various defects have been identified in the synthesis, folding and intracellular transport of apolipoproteins,

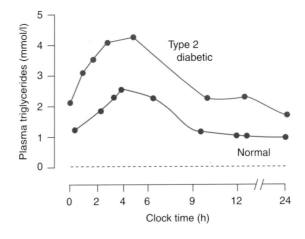

Figure 10.19 Plasma triglyceride concentrations are raised throughout the day in subjects with type 2 diabetes. This is due both to overproduction of VLDL by the liver, and to impaired clearance of triglyceride in insulin-resistant conditions. Adapted from Syvänne and Taskinen (1997), *Lancet* 350: SI20–3, with permission of the editor.

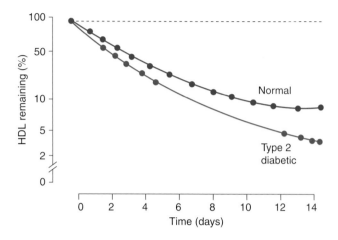

Figure 10.20 Catabolism of HDL cholesterol is accelerated in type 2 diabetic patients. From Golay *et al.* (1987).

and in their combination with lipid and trafficking of the resulting lipoproteins; these are suggested to contribute to dyslipidaemia (Adiels *et al.*, 2006; Chan, Barrett and Watts, 2006).

References

Adiels, M., Olofsson, S.O., Taskinen, M.R. and Boren, J. (2006) Diabetic dyslipidaemia. *Current Opinion in Lipidology*, **17**, 238–46.

Aggarwal, B.B. (2000) Tumour necrosis factors receptor associated signalling molecules and their role in activation of apoptosis, JNK and NF-kappaB. *Annals of the Rheumatic Diseases*, **59** (Suppl 1), i6–16.

Alberti, K., Zimmet, P., Shaw, J., IDF Epidemiology Task Force Consensus Group. (2005) The metabolic syndrome – a new worldwide definition. *Lancet*, **366**, 1059–62.

Alessi, M.C. and Juhan-Vague, I. (2006) PAI-1 and the metabolic syndrome: links, causes, and consequences. *Arteriosclerosis, Thrombosis, and Vascular Biology*, **26** (10), 2200–7.

Anderson, P.J., Chan, J.C.N., Chan, Y.L. *et al.* (1997) Visceral fat and cardiovascular risk factors in Chinese NIDDM patients. *Diabetes Care*, **20**, 1854–8.

Anderson, P.J., Critchley, J.A.J.H., Chan, J.C.N. *et al.* (2001) Factor analysis of the metabolic syndrome: obesity versus insulin resistance as the central abnormality. *International Journal of Obesity*, **25**, 1782–8.

Arkan, M.C., Hevener, A.L., Greten, F.R. *et al.* (2005) IKK-beta links inflammation to obesity-induced insulin resistance. *Nature Medicine*, **11** (2), 191–8.

Austin, M.A., Edwards, K.L., McNeely, M.J. *et al.* (2004) Heritability of multivariate factors of the metabolic syndrome in nondiabetic Japanese Americans. *Diabetes*, **53**, 1166–9.

Axelrod, J. and Reisine, T.D. (1984) Stress hormones: their interaction and regulation. *Science*, **224**, 452–9.

Baier, L.I., Sacchettini, J.C., Knowler, W.C. *et al.* (1995) An amino acid substitution in the human intestinal fatty acid binding protein is associated with increased fatty acid binding, increased fat oxidation, and insulin resistance. *The Journal of Clinical Investigation*, **95**, 1281–7.

Balkau, B. and Charles, M.A. (1999) Comment on the provisional report from the WHO consultation. European Group for the Study of Insulin Resistance (EGIR). *Diabetic Medicine: A Journal of the British Diabetic Association*, **16** (5), 442–3.

Banerji, M.A., Chaiken, R.L., Huey, H. *et al.* (1994) GAD antibody negative NIDDM in adult Black subjects with diabetic ketoacidosis and increased frequency of leukocyte antigen DR3 and DR4. Flatbush Diabetes. *Diabetes*, **43**, 741–5.

Barker, D.J.P., Hales, C.N., Fall, C.D. *et al.* (1993) Type 2 (non-insulin-dependent) diabetes mellitus, hypertension, and hyperlipidaemia (syndrome X): relation to reduced fetal growth. *Diabetologia*, **36**, 62–7.

Bastard, J.P., Jardel, C., Bruckert, E. *et al.* (2000) Elevated levels of interleukin 6 are reduced in serum and subcutaneous adipose tissue of obese women after weight loss. *The Journal of Clinical Endocrinology and Metabolism*, **85** (9), 3338–42.

Beltowski, J. (2006) Role of leptin in blood pressure regulation and arterial hypertension. *Journal of Hypertension*, **24** (5), 789–801.

Berg, A.H., Combs, T.P., Du, X. *et al.* (2001) The adipocyte-secreted protein Acrp30 enhances hepatic insulin action. *Nature Medicine*, **7** (8), 947–53.

Björntorp, P. (1991) Metabolic implications of body fat distribution. *Diabetes Care*, **14**, 1132–43.

Blouin, K., Després, J.P., Couillard, C. *et al.* (2005) Contribution of age and declining androgen levels to features of the metabolic syndrome in men. *Metabolism: Clinical and Experimental*, **54** (8), 1034–40.

Boden, G. (2002) Interaction between free fatty acids and glucose metabolism. *Current Opinion in Clinical Nutrition & Metabolic Care*, **5** (5), 545–9.

Boden, G. and Shulman, G.I. (2002) Free fatty acids in obesity and type 2 diabetes: defining their role in the development of insulin resistance and beta-cell dysfunction. *European Journal of Clinical Investigation*, **32** (Suppl 3), 14–23.

Boden, G., Cheung, P., Stein, T.P. *et al.* (2002) FFA cause hepatic insulin resistance by inhibiting insulin suppression of glycogenolysis. *American Journal of Physiology. Endocrinology and Metabolism*, **283** (1), E12–9.

Bollheimer, L.C., Skelly, R.H., Chester, M.W. *et al.* (1998) Chronic exposure to free fatty acid reduces pancreatic beta cell insulin content by increasing basal insulin secretion that is not compensated for by a corresponding increase in proinsulin biosynthesis translation. *The Journal of Clinical Investigation*, **101** (5), 1094–101.

Boyko, E.J., Fujimoto, W.Y., Leonetti, D.L. and Newell-Morris, L. (2000) Visceral adiposity and risk of type 2 diabetes: a prospective study among Japanese Americans. *Diabetes Care*, **23**, 465–71.

Butler, A.E., Janson, J., Bonner-Weir, S. *et al.* (2003) Beta-cell deficit and increased beta-cell apoptosis in humans with type 2 diabetes. *Diabetes*, **52** (1), 102–10.

Cai, D., Yuan, M., Frantz, D.F. *et al.* (2005) Local and systemic insulin resistance resulting from hepatic activation of IKK-beta and NF-kappaB. *Nature Medicine*, **11** (2), 183–90.

Carey, V.J., Walters, E.E., Colditz, G.A. *et al.* (1997) Body fat distribution and risk of non-insulin dependent diabetes mellitus in women. The Nurses' Health Study. *American Journal of Epidemiology*, **145**, 614–9.

Carnethon, M.R., Gidding, S.S., Nehgme, R. *et al.* (2003) Cardiorespiratory fitness in young adulthood and the development of cardiovascular disease risk factors. *Journal of American Medical Association*, **290**, 3092–100.

Caro, J.F., Kolaczynski, J.W., Nyce, M.R. *et al.* (1996) Decreased cerebrospinal-fluid/serum leptin ratio in obesity: a possible mechanism for leptin resistance. *Lancet*, **348** (9021), 159–61.

Chan, D.C., Barrett, P.H. and Watts, G.F. (2006) Recent studies of lipoprotein kinetics in the metabolic syndrome and related disorders. *Current Opinion in Lipidology*, **17**, 28–36.

Chan, J.C.N., Cheung, J.C.K., Lau, E.M.C. *et al.* (1996) The metabolic syndrome in Hong Kong Chinese – the inter-relationships amongst its components analysed by structural equation modelling. *Diabetes Care*, **19**, 953–9.

Chan, J.C.N., Tong, P.C.Y. and Critchley, J.A.J.H. (2002) The insulin resistance syndrome – mechanism of clustering of cardiovascular risk. *Seminars in Vascular Medicine*, **2**, 45–57.

Chan, J.M., Rimm, E.B., Colditz, G.A. *et al.* (1994) Obesity, fat distribution, and weight gain as risk factors for clinical diabetes in men. *Diabetes Care*, **17** (9), 961–9.

Chang, C.J., Wu, C.H., Yao, W.J. *et al.* (2000) Relationships of age, menopause and central obesity on cardiovascular disease risk factors in Chinese women. *International Journal of Obesity and Related Metabolic Disorders*, **24** (12), 1699–704.

Cheal, K.L., Abbasi, F., Lamendola, C. *et al.* (2004) Relationship to insulin resistance of the adult treatment panel III diagnostic criteria for identification of the metabolic syndrome. *Diabetes*, **53** (5), 1195–200.

Chen, J., Gu, D., Chen, C.S. *et al.* (2007) Association between the metabolic syndrome and chronic kidney disease in Chinese adults. *Nephrology, Dialysis, Transplantation*. **22**, 1100–6.

Chen, J., Muntner, P., Hamm, L. *et al.* (2004) The metabolic syndrome and chronic kidney disease in U.S. adults. *Annals of Internal Medicine*, **140**, 167–74.

Chen, L., Hwang, S., Tsai, S. *et al.* (2000) Glucose intolerance in Chinese patients with chronic hepatitis C. *World Journal of Gastroenterology*, **9**, 505–8.

Cheng, A.Y.S., Kong, A.P.S., Wong, V.W.S. *et al.* (2006) Chronic hepatitis B viral infection independently predicts renal outcome in type 2 diabetic patients. *Diabetologia*, **49**, 1777–84.

Cheung, N. and Byth, K. (2003) Population health significance of gestational diabetes. *Diabetes Care*, **26**, 2005–9.

Cho, Y.M., Park, K.S. and Lee, H.K. (2007) Genetic factors related to mitochondrial function and risk of diabetes mellitus. *Diabetes Research and Clinical Practice*, **77** (1), S172–7.

Colditz, G.A., Willett, W.C., Rotnitzky, A. and Manson, J.E. (1995) Weight gain as a risk factor for clinical diabetes mellitus in women. *Annals of Internal Medicine*, **122** (7), 481–6.

Colditz, G.A., Willett, W.C., Stampfer, M.J. *et al.* (1990) Weight as a risk factor for clinical diabetes in women. *American Journal of Epidemiology*, **132** (3), 501–13.

Colombo, C., Cutson, J.J., Yamauchi, T. *et al.* (2002) Transplantation of adipose tissue lacking leptin is unable to reverse the metabolic abnormalities associated with lipoatrophy. *Diabetes*, **51** (9), 2727–33.

Connolly, V., Unwin, N., Sherriff, P. *et al.* (2000) Diabetes prevalence and socioeconomic status: a population based study showing increased prevalence of type 2 diabetes mellitus in deprived areas. *Journal of Epidemiology and Community Health*, **54**, 173–7.

Corrao, M.A., Guindon, G.E., Cokkinides, V. and Sharma, N. (2000) Building the evidence base for global tobacco control. *Bulletin of the World Health Organization*, **78** (7), 884–90.

Couillard, C., Ruel, G., Archer, W.R. *et al.* (2005) Circulating levels of oxidative stress markers and endothelial adhesion molecules in men with abdominal obesity. *Journal of Clinical Endocrinology and Metabolism*, **90**, 6454–9.

DeFronzo, R.A. (1992) Pathogenesis of type 2 (non-insulin dependent) diabetes mellitus: a balanced overview. *Diabetologia*, **35**, 389–97.

DeFronzo, R.A. and Ferrannini, E. (1991) Insulin resistance. A multifaceted syndrome responsible for NIDDM, obesity, hypertension, dyslipidemia, and atherosclerotic cardiovascular disease. *Diabetes Care*, **14**, 173–94.

DeFronzo, R.A., Simonson, D. and Ferrannini, E. (1982) Hepatic and peripheral insulin resistance: a common feature of type 2 (non-insulin-dependent) and type 1 (insulin-dependent) diabetes mellitus. *Diabetologia*, **23** (4), 313–19.

Dekker, J.M., Girman, C., Rhodes, T. *et al.* (2005) Metabolic syndrome and 10-year cardiovascular disease risk in the Hoorn Study. *Circulation*, **112** (5), 666–73.

Després, J.P. and Lemieux, I. (2006) Abdominal obesity and metabolic syndrome. *Nature*, **444** (7121), 881–7.

Deurenberg, P., Deurenberg-Yap, M. and Guricci, S. (2002) Asians are different from Caucasians and from each other in their body mass index/body fat per cent relationship. *Obesity Reviews*, **3**, 141–6.

Dresner, A., Laurent, D., Marcucci, M. *et al.* (1999) Effects of free fatty acids on glucose transport and IRS-1-associated phosphatidylinositol 3-kinase activity. *The Journal of Clinical Investigation*, **103** (2), 253–9.

Dunaif, A. (1997) Insulin resistance and the polycystic ovary syndrome: mechanism and implications for pathogenesis. *Endocrine Reviews*, **18** (6), 774–800.

Engeli, S., Schling, P., Gorzelniak, K. *et al.* (2003) The adipose-tissue renin-angiotensin-aldosterone system: role in the metabolic syndrome? *The International Journal of Biochemistry & Cell Biology*, **35** (6), 807–25.

Everhart, J.E., Pettitt, D.J., Bennett, P.H. and Knowler, W.C. (1992) Duration of obesity increases the incidence of NIDDM. *Diabetes*, **41** (2), 235–40.

Executive Summary of the Third Report of The National Cholesterol Education Program (NCEP) (2001) Expert Panel on Detection Evaluation and Treatment of High Blood Cholesterol in Adults (Adult Treatment Panel III). *Journal of the American Medical Association*, **285** (19), 2486–97.

Ferrannini, E., Barrett, E.J., Bevilacqua, S. and DeFronzo, R.A. (1983) Effect of fatty acids on glucose production and utilization in man. *The Journal of Clinical Investigation*, **72** (5), 1737–47.

Ford, E.S. (2005) Risks for all-cause mortality, cardiovascular disease, and diabetes associated with the metabolic syndrome: a summary of the evidence. *Diabetes Care*, **28**, 1769–78.

Frayling, T.M. (2007) *Nature Reviews. Genetics*, **8** (9), 657–62.

Fraze, E., Donner, C.C., Swislocki, A.L. *et al.* (1985) Ambient plasma free fatty acid concentrations in noninsulin-dependent diabetes mellitus: evidence for insulin resistance. *The Journal of Clinical Endocrinology and Metabolism*, **61** (5), 807–11.

Frühbeck, G. (2006) Intracellular signalling pathways activated by leptin. *The Biochemical Journal.* **393** (Pt 1), 7–20.

Fuku, N., Park, K.S., Yamada, Y. *et al.* (2007) Mitochondrial haplogroup N9a confers resistance against type 2 diabetes in Asians. *American Journal of Human Genetics*, **80**, 407–15.

Gavrilova, O., Marcus-Samuels, B., Graham, D. *et al.* (2000) Surgical implantation of adipose tissue reverses diabetes in lipoatrophic mice. *The Journal of Clinical Investigation*, **105** (3), 271–8.

Glintborg, D., Stoving, R.K., Hagen, C. *et al.* (2005) Pioglitazone treatment increases spontaneous growth hormone (GH) secretion and stimulated GH levels in polycystic ovary syndrome. *The Journal of Clinical Endocrinology and Metabolism*, **90** (10), 5605–12.

Go, A., Chertow, G., Fan, D. *et al.* (2004) Chronic kidney disease and the risks of death, cardiovascular events, and hospitalization. *New England Journal of Medicine*, **351**, 1296–305.

Golay, A., Zech, L., Shi, M.Z., *et al.* (1987) High density lipoprotein (HDL) metabolism in noninsulin-dependent diabetes mellitus: measurement of HDL turnover using tritiated HDL. *Journal of Clinical Endocrinology and Metabolism*, **65** (3), 512–8.

Goodpaster, B.H., Thaete, F.L., Simoneau, J.A. and Kelley, D.E. (1997) Subcutaneous abdominal fat and thigh muscle composition predict insulin sensitivity independently of visceral fat. *Diabetes*, **46** (10), 1579–85.

Grant, S.F. *et al.* (2006) Variant of transcription factor 7-like 2 (TCF7L2) gene confers risk of type 2 diabetes. *Nature Genetics*, **48**, 320–3.

Griffin, M.E., Marcucci, M.J., Cline, G.W. *et al.* (1999) Free fatty acid-induced insulin resistance is associated with activation of protein kinase C theta and alterations in the insulin signalling cascade. *Diabetes*, **48** (6), 1270–4.

Grundy, S.M. (2007) Metabolic syndrome: a multiplex cardiovascular risk factor. *Journal of Clinical Endocrinology and Metabolism*, **92**, 399–404.

Guthrie, J.R., Taffe, J.R., Lehert, P. *et al.* (2004) Association between hormonal changes at menopause and the risk of a coronary event: a longitudinal study. *Menopause*, **11** (3), 315–22.

Haffner, S.M., Stern, M.P., Hazuda, H.P. *et al.* (1986) Upper body and centralized adiposity in Mexican Americans and non-Hispanic whites: relationship to body mass index and other behavioral and demographic variables. *International Journal of Obesity*, **10** (6), 493–502.

Hales, C.N. and Barker, D.J.P. (1992) Type 2 (non-insulin dependent) diabetes mellitus: The thrifty phenotype hypothesis. *Diabetologia*, **35**, 595–601.

Hamman, R.F., Wing, R.R., Edelstein, S.L. *et al.* (2006) Effect of weight loss with lifestyle intervention on risk of diabetes. *Diabetes Care*, **29** (9), 2102–7.

Hancox, R., Milne, B. and Poulton, R. (2004) Association between child and adolescent television viewing and adult health: a longitudinal birth cohort study. *Lancet*, **364**, 257–62.

Hansen, L., Hansen, T., Vestergaard, H. *et al.* (1995) A widespread amino acid polymorphism at codon 905 of the glycogen-associated regulatory subunit of protein phosphatase-1 is associated with insulin resistance and hypersecretion of insulin. *Human Molecular Genetics*, **4**, 1313–20.

Hattersley, A. and Pearson, E. (2006) Mini review: Pharmacogenetics and beyond: the interaction of therapeutic response, beta-cell physiology and genetics in diabetes. *Endocrinology* **147** (6), 2657–63.

Hayden, M.R., Tyagi, S.C., Kerklo, M.M. and Nicolls, M.R. (2005) Type 2 diabetes mellitus as a conformational disease. *Journal of Pancreas*, **6**, 287–302.

He, M., Tan, K.C., Li, E.T. and Kung, A.W. (2001) Body fat determination by dual energy X-ray absorptiometry and its relation to body mass index and waist circumference in Hong Kong Chinese. *International Journal of Obesity and Related Metabolic Disorder*, **25**, 748–52.

Higa, M., Zhou, Y.T., Ravazzola, M. *et al.* (1999) Troglitazone prevents mitochondrial alterations, beta cell destruction, and diabetes in obese prediabetic rats. *Proceedings of the National Academy of Sciences USA*, **96** (20), 11513–8.

Hirosumi, J., Tuncman, G., Chang, L. *et al.* (2002) A central role for JNK in obesity and insulin resistance. *Nature*, **420** (6913), 333–6.

Holte, J. (1998) Polycystic ovary syndrome and insulin resistance: thrifty genes struggling with over-feeding and sedentary life style? *Journal of Endocrinological Investigation*, **21** (9), 589–601.

Hong, Y., Pedersen, N., Brismar, K. and de Faire, U. (1997) Genetic and environmental architecture of the features of the insulin resistance syndrome. *American Journal of Human Genetics*, **60**, 143–52.

Hotamisligil, G.S. (2005) Role of endoplasmic reticulum stress and c-Jun NH2-terminal kinase pathways in inflammation and origin of obesity and diabetes. *Diabetes*, **54** (Suppl 2), S73–8.

Hotamisligil, G.S., Arner, P., Caro, J.F. *et al.* (1995) Increased adipose tissue expression of tumour necrosis factor-a in human obesity and insulin resistance. *The Journal of Clinical Investigation*, **95**, 2409–15.

Hotamisligil, G.S., Budavari, A., Murray, D. and Spiegelman, B.M. (1994) Reduced tyrosine kinase activity of the insulin receptor in obesity-diabetes. *The Journal of Clinical Investigation*, **94**, 1543–9.

Hotamisligil, G.S., Peraldi, P., Budavari, A. *et al.* (1996) IRS-1-mediated inhibition of insulin receptor tyrosine kinase activity in TNF-a and obesity-induced insulin resistance. *Science*, **271**, 665–8.

Hotamisligil, G.S., Shargill, N.S. and Spiegelman, B.M. (1993) Adipose expression of tumor necrosis factor-alpha: direct role in obesity-linked insulin resistance. *Science*, **259**, 87–91.

Hu, F.B., Willett, W.C., Li, T. *et al.* (2004) Adiposity as compared with physical activity in predicting mortality among women. *The New England Journal of Medicine*, **351** (26), 2694–703.

Hubert, H., Snider, J. and Winkleby, M. (2005) Health status, health behaviors, and acculturation factors associated with overweight and obesity in Latinos from a community and agricultural labor camp survey. *Preventive Medicine*, **40**, 642–51.

Hull, R.L., Andrikopoulos, S., Verchere, C.B. *et al.* (2003) Increased dietary fat promotes islet amyloid formation and beta-cell secretory dysfunction in a transgenic mouse model of islet amyloid. *Diabetes*, **52** (2), 372–9.

Hull, R.L., Shen, Z.P., Watts, M.R. *et al.* (2005) Long-term treatment with rosiglitazone and metformin reduces the extent of, but does not prevent, islet amyloid deposition in mice expressing the gene for human islet amyloid polypeptide. *Diabetes*, **54** (7), 2235–44.

Hull, R.L., Westermark, G.T., Westermark, P. and Kahn, S.E. (2004) Islet amyloid: a critical entity in the pathogenesis of type 2 diabetes. *Journal of Clinical Endocrinology and Metabolism*, **89**, 3629–43.

International Diabetes Federation. (2006) *Unite for diabetes 2006*, www.unitefordiabetes.org, last accessed 22 July 2008.

Inzucchi, S. and Sherwin, R. (2005) The prevention of type 2 diabetes mellitus. *Endocrinology and Metabolism Clinics of North America*, **34**, 199–219.

Isomaa, B., Almgren, P., Tuomi, T. *et al.* (2001) Cardiovascular morbidity and mortality associated with the metabolic syndrome. *Diabetes Care*, **24**, 683–9.

Itani, S.I., Ruderman, N.B., Schmieder, F. and Boden, G. (2002) Lipid-induced insulin resistance in human muscle is associated with changes in diacylglycerol, protein kinase C, and IkappaB-alpha. *Diabetes*, **51** (7), 2005–11.

Jia, W.P., Lu, J.X., Kiang, K.S. *et al.* (2003) Prediction of abdominal visceral obesity from body mass index, waist circumference and waist-hip ratio in Chinese adults: receiver operating characteristics curves analysis. *Biomedical Environmental Science*, **2003**, 206–11.

Jiang, Z.Y., Lin, Y.W., Clemont, A. *et al.* (1999) Characterization of selective resistance to insulin signalling in the vasculature of obese Zucker (fa/fa) rats. *The Journal of Clinical Investigation*, **104** (4), 447–57.

Johannsson, G., Marin, P., Lonn, L. *et al.* (1997) Growth hormone treatment of abdominally obese men reduces abdominal fat mass, improves glucose and lipoprotein metabolism and reduces diastolic blood pressure. *Journal of Clinical Endocrinology and Metabolism*, **82**, 727–34.

Kaaja, R.J. and Poyhonen-Alho, M.K. (2006) Insulin resistance and sympathetic overactivity in women. *Journal of Hypertension*, **24**, 131–41.

Kahn, S. (2001) The importance of β-cell failure in the development and progression of type 2 diabetes. *The Journal of Clinical Endocrinology and Metabolism*, **86**, 4047–58.

Kahn, S.E. (2004) The relative contributions of insulin resistance and beta-cell dysfunction to the pathophysiology of type 2 diabetes. *Diabetologia*, **46**, 3–19.

Kahn, R., Buse, J., Ferrannini, E., Stern, M., American Diabetes Association, European Association for the Study of Diabetes (2006) The metabolic syndrome: time for a critical appraisal: joint statement from the American Diabetes Association and the European Association for the Study of Diabetes. *Diabetes Care*, **28**, 2289–304.

Kanda, H., Tateya, S., Tamori, Y. *et al.* (2006) MCP-1 contributes to macrophage infiltration into adipose tissue, insulin resistance, and hepatic steatosis in obesity. *The Journal of Clinical Investigation*, **116** (6), 1494–1505.

Karter, A., Ferrara, A., Liu, J. *et al.* (2002) Ethnic disparities in diabetic complications in an insured population. *Journal of American Medical Association*, **287**, 2519–27.

Kashyap, S., Belfort, R., Gastaldelli, A. *et al.* (2003) A sustained increase in plasma free fatty acids impairs insulin secretion in nondiabetic subjects genetically predisposed to develop type 2 diabetes. *Diabetes*, **52** (10), 2461–74.

Kaufman, J.M. and Vermeulen, A. (2005) The decline of androgen levels in elderly men and its clinical and therapeutic implications. *Endocrine Reviews*, **26** (6), 833–76.

Kaufman, R.J., Scheuner, D., Schroder, M. *et al.* (2002) The unfolded protein response in nutrient sensing and differentiation. *Nature Reviews. Molecular Cell Biology*, **3** (6), 411–21.

Kern, P.A., Ranganathan, S., Li, C. *et al.* (2001) Adipose tissue tumor necrosis factor and interleukin-6 expression in human obesity and insulin resistance. *American Journal of Physiology. Endocrinology and Metabolism*, **280** (5), E745–51.

Kershaw, E.E. and Flier, J.S. (2004) Adipose tissue as an endocrine organ. *The Journal of Clinical Endocrinology and Metabolism*, **89** (6), 2548–56.

Knowler, W.C., Pettitt, D.J., Saad, M.F. *et al.* (1991) Obesity in the Pima Indians: its magnitude and relationship with diabetes. *The American Journal of Clinical Nutrition*, **53** (6 Suppl), 1543S–51S.

Ko, G.T.C., Chan, J.C.N. and Cockram, C.S. (2001) A low socioeconomic class is associated with diabetes and metabolic syndrome in Hong Kong Chinese. *European Journal of Epidemiology*, **17**, 289–95.

Ko, G.T.C., Chan, J.C.N., Tsang, L.W. *et al.* (2000) Smoking and diabetes in Chinese men. *Postgraduate Medical Journal*, **77**, 240–3.

Ko, G.T.C., Li, J.K.Y., Cheung, A.Y.K. *et al.* (1999) Two-hour post-glucose loading plasma glucose is the main determinant for the progression from impaired glucose tolerance to diabetes in Hong Kong Chinese. *Diabetes Care*, **22**, 2096–7.

Krssak, M., Petersen, K.F., Dresner, A. *et al.* (1999) Intramyocellular lipid concentrations are correlated with insulin sensitivity in humans: a 1H NMR spectroscopy study. *Diabetologia*, **42**, 113–6.

Kubaszek, A., Pihlajamaki, J., Komarovski, V. *et al.* (2003) Promoter polymorphisms of the TNF-alpha (G-308A) and IL-6 (C-174G) genes predict the conversion from impaired glucose tolerance to type 2 diabetes: the Finnish Diabetes Prevention Study. *Diabetes*, **52** (7), 1872–6.

Kulkarni, R.N., Bruning, J.C., Winnay, J.N. *et al.* (1999) Tissue-specific knockout of the insulin receptor in pancreatic beta cells creates an insulin secretory defect similar to that in type 2 diabetes. *Cell*, **96** (3), 329–39.

Kylin, E. (1923) Studien über das Hypertonie-Hyperglykämie-Hyperurikämie. *Zentralblatt für Innere Medizin*, **44**, 105–27.

Laaksonen, D.E., Niskanen, L., Punnonen, K. *et al.* (2004) Testosterone and sex hormone-binding globulin predict the metabolic syndrome and diabetes in middle-aged men. *Diabetes Care* **27**, 1036–41.

Lane, N. (2006) Mitochondrial disease: powerhouse of disease. *Nature*, **440**, 600–2.

Lao, T.T., Tse, K.Y., Chan, L.Y. *et al.* (2003) HBsAg carrier status and the association between gestational diabetes with increased serum ferritin concentration in Chinese women. *Diabetes Care*, **26**, 3011–6.

Lee, H.K., Park, K.S., Cho, Y.M. *et al.* (2005) Mitochondria-based model for fetal origin of adult disease and insulin resistance. *Annals of the New York Academy of Sciences*, **1042**, 1–18.

Lee, M.K., Miles, P.D., Khoursheed, M. *et al.* (1994) Metabolic effects of troglitazone on fructose-induced insulin resistance in the rat. *Diabetes*, **43** (12), 1435–9.

Lee, S.C., Hashim, Y., Li, J.K.Y. *et al.* (2001) The islet amyloid polypeptide (amylin) gene S20G mutation in Chinese subjects: Evidence for associations with type 2 diabetes and cholesterol levels. *Journal of Endocrinology*, **54**, 541–6.

Lee, Z.S., Critchley, J.A., Ko, G.T. *et al.* (2002) Obesity and cardiovascular risk factors in Hong Kong Chinese. *Obesity Reviews*, **3** (3), 173–82.

Lee, Z.S.K., Critchley, J.A.J.H., Tomlinson, B. *et al.* (2001) Urinary epinephrine and norepinephrine with obesity, insulin and the metabolic syndrome in Hong Kong Chinese. *Metabolism: Clinical and Experimental*, **50**, 135–43.

Lee, Y., Hirose, H., Ohneda, M. et al. (1994) Beta-cell lipotoxicity in the pathogenesis of non-insulin-dependent diabetes mellitus of obese rats: impairment in adipocyte-beta-cell relationships. *Proceedings of the National Academy of Sciences USA*, **91** (23), 10878–82.

Lehman, D.M. et al. (2007) *Diabetes*, **56**, 389–93.

Leiter, L.A. (2005) Beta-cell preservation: a potential role for thiazolidinediones to improve clinical care in type 2 diabetes. *Diabetic Medicine: A Journal of the British Diabetic Association*, **22** (8), 963–72.

Li, J.K.Y., Ng, M.C.Y., So, W.Y. et al. (2006) Phenotypic and genetic clustering of diabetes and metabolic syndrome in Chinese families with type 2 diabetes mellitus. *Diabetes/Metabolism Research and Reviews*, **22**, 46–52.

Li, T.Y., Rana, J.S., Manson, J.E. et al. (2006) Obesity as compared with physical activity in predicting risk of coronary heart disease in women. *Circulation*, **113** (4), 499–506.

Lillioja, S., Mott, D.M., Sprane, M. et al. (1993) Insulin resistance and insulin secretory dysfunction as precursors of non-insulin-dependent diabetes mellitus: prospective studies of Pima Indians. *New England Journal of Medicine*, **329**, 1988–92.

Liou, C.W., Lin, T.K., Huei, W.H. et al. (2007) A common mitochondrial DNA variant and increased body mass index as associated factors for development of type 2 diabetes: Additive effects of genetic and environmental factors. *Journal of Clinical Endocrinology and Metabolism*, **92**, 235–9.

Liu, K., Chan, Y., Chan, W. et al. (2003) Sonographic measurement of mesenteric fat thickness and its association with cardiovascular risk factors: comparison with subcutaneous and preperitoneal fat thickness, magnetic resonance imaging and anthropometric indexes. *International Journal of Obesity*, **27**, 1267–73.

Liu, K., Chan, Y., Chan, W. et al. (2006) Mesenteric fat thickness is an independent determinant of metabolic syndrome and defines subjects with increased carotid intima-media thickness. *Diabetes Care*, **29**, 379–84.

Liu, K., Chan, Y.L., Chan, J.C. et al. (2006) Mesenteric fat thickness as an independent determinant of fatty liver. *International Journal of Obesity*, **30** (5), 787–93.

Liu, Z., Zhang, Y.W., Chang, Y.S. and Fang, F.D. (2006) The role of cytoskeleton in glucose regulation. *Biochemistry* **71** (5), 476–80.

Lo, M.K.W., Lee, K.F., Chan, N. et al. (2004) Effects of gender, Helicobacter pylori (HP) and hepatitis B virus serology status on cardiovascular and renal complications in Chinese type 2 diabetic patients with overt nephropathy. *Diabetes, Obesity and Metabolism*, **6**, 223–30.

Lyssenko V., Lupi R., Marchetti P. et al. (2007) Mechanisms by which common variants in the TCF7L2 gene increase risk of type 2 diabetes. *The Journal of Clinical Investigation*, **117**, 2155–63.

Magnusson, I., Rothman, D.L., Katz, L.D. et al. (1992) Increased rate of gluconeogenesis in type II diabetes mellitus. A 13C nuclear magnetic resonance study. *The Journal of Clinical Investigation*, **90** (4), 1323–7.

Malik, S., Wong, N.D., Franklin, S.S. et al. (2004) Impact of the metabolic syndrome on mortality from coronary heart disease, cardiovascular disease, and all causes in United States adults. *Circulation*, **110**, 1245–50.

Martin, M.L. and Jensen, M.D. (1991) Effects of body fat distribution on regional lipolysis in obesity. *The Journal of Clinical Investigation*, **88**, 609–13.

Mathis, D., Vence, L. and Benoist, C. (2001) β-cell death during progression to diabetes. *Nature*, **414**, 792–8.

McCarthy, M. and Zeggini, E. (2006) Genetics of type 2 diabetes. *Current Report in Diabetes*, **6**, 147–54.

McNeely, M.J., Boyko, E.J., Shofer, J.B. et al. (2001) Standard definitions of overweight and central adiposity for determining diabetes risk in Japanese Americans. *The American Journal of Clinical Nutrition*, **74** (1), 101–7.

Medina, J., Fernandez-Salazar, L.I., Garcia-Buey, L. and Moreno-Otero, R. (2004) Approach to the pathogenesis and treatment of nonalcoholic steatohepatitis. *Diabetes Care*, **27** (8), 2057–66.

Mehta, S.H., Brancati, F.L., Sulkowski, M.S. et al. (2000) Prevalence of type 2 diabetes mellitus among persons with hepatitis C virus infection in the United States. *Annals of Internal Medicine*, **133** (8), 592–9.

Meigs, J.B., D'Agostino, R.B.S., Wilson, P.W. et al. (1997) Risk variable clustering in the insulin resistance syndrome. The Framingham Offspring Study. *Diabetes*, **46**, 1594–1600.

Meigs, J., Williams, K., Sullivan, L. et al. (2004) Using metabolic syndrome traits for efficient detection of impaired glucose tolerance. *Diabetes Care*, **27**, 1417–26.

Mi, J., Law, C., Zhang, K.L. et al. (2000) Effects of infant birth weight and maternal body mass index in pregnancy on components of the insulin resistance syndrome in China. *Annals of Internal Medicine*, **132**, 253–60.

Minokoshi, Y., Kim, Y.B., Peroni, O.D. et al. (2002) Leptin stimulates fatty-acid oxidation by activating AMP-activated protein kinase. *Nature*, **415** (6869), 339–43.

Mitrakou, A., Kelly, D., Mokan, M. et al. (1992) Role of reduced suppression of glucose production and diminished early insulin release in impaired glucose tolerance. *The New England Journal of Medicine*, **326**, 22–9.

Mohamed-Ali, V., Goodrick, S., Rawesh, A. et al. (1997) Subcutaneous adipose tissue releases interleukin-6, but not tumor necrosis factor-alpha, in vivo. *The Journal of Clinical Endocrinology and Metabolism*, **82** (12), 4196–200.

Moitra, J., Mason, M.M., Olive, M. et al. (1998) Life without white fat: a transgenic mouse. Genes and Development, 12 (20), 3168–81.

Molarius, A., Seidell, J.C., Sans, S. et al. (1999) Varying sensitivity of waist action levels to identify subjects with overweight or obesity in 19 populations of the WHO MONICA Project. Journal of Clinical Epidemiology, 52 (12), 1213–24.

Molarius, A., Seidell, J.C., Sans, S. et al. (1999) Waist and hip circumferences, and waist-hip ratio in 19 populations of the WHO MONICA Project. International Journal of Obesity and Related Metabolic Disorders, 23 (2), 116–25.

Morino, K., Petersen, K.F., Dufour, S. et al. (2005) Reduced mitochondrial density and increased IRS-1 serine phosphorylation in muscle of insulin-resistant offspring of type 2 diabetic parents. The Journal of Clinical Investigation, 115 (12), 3587–93.

Morino, K., Petersen, K.F. and Shulman, G.I. (2006) Molecular mechanisms of insulin resistance in humans and their potential links with mitochondrial dysfunction. Diabetes, 55 (Suppl 2), S9–15.

Morrish, N.J., Wang, S., Stevens, L.K. et al. (2001) Mortality and causes of death in the WHO Multinational Survey of Vascular Diseases in Diabetes. Diabetologia, 44 (Suppl 2), S14–21.

Muller, M., Grobbee, D.E., den Tonkelaar, I. et al. (2005) Endogenous sex hormones and metabolic syndrome in aging men. The Journal of Clinical Endocrinology and Metabolism, 90 (5), 2618–23.

Nakatani, Y., Kaneto, H., Kawamori, D. et al. (2005) Involvement of endoplasmic reticulum stress in insulin resistance and diabetes. The Journal of Biological Chemistry, 280 (1), 847–51.

Ng, M.C. et al. (2007) Replication and identification of novel variants at TCF7L2 associated with type 2 diabetes in Hong Kong Chinese. The Journal of Clinical Endocrinology and Metabolism, 92 (9), 3733–7.

Ng, M.C., So, W.Y., Cox, N.J. et al. (2004) Genome wide scan for metabolic syndrome and related quantitative traits in Hong Kong Chinese and confirmation of a susceptibility locus on chromosome 1q21–25. Diabetes, 53, 2676–83.

Ng, M.C.Y., Lee, S.C., Ko, G.T.C. et al. (2001) Familial early onset type 2 diabetes in Chinese: the more significant roles of obesity and genetics than autoimmunity. Diabetes Care, 24, 667–71.

Ng, M.C.Y., So, W.Y., Cox, N.J. et al. (2004) Genome wide scan for type 2 diabetes loci in Hong Kong Chinese and confirmation of a susceptibility locus on chromosome 1q21–q25. Diabetes, 53, 1609–13.

Ng, M.C.Y., Yeung, V.T.F., Chow, C.C. et al. (2000) Mitochondrial DNA A3243G mutation in patients with early or late onset type 2 diabetes mellitus in Hong Kong Chinese. Journal of Endocrinology, 52, 557–64.

Niswender, K.D. and Schwartz, M.W. (2003) Insulin and leptin revisited: adiposity signals with overlapping physiological and intracellular signalling capabilities. Frontiers in Neuroendocrinology, 24 (1), 1–10.

O'Rahilly, S., Turner, R. and Matthews, D. (1988) Impaired pulsatile secretion of insulin in relatives of patients with non-insulin-dependent diabetes. New England Journal of Medicine, 318, 1225–30.

Oh, J.Y., Hong, Y.S., Sung, Y.A. and Barrett-Connor, E. (2004) Prevalence and factor analysis of metabolic syndrome in an urban Korean population. Diabetes Care, 27, 2027–32.

Ohneda, M., Inman, L.R. and Unger, R.H. (1995) Caloric restriction in obese pre-diabetic rats prevents beta-cell depletion, loss of beta-cell GLUT 2 and glucose incompetence. Diabetologia, 38, 173–9.

Ozcan, U., Cao, Q., Yilmaz, E. et al. (2004) Endoplasmic reticulum stress links obesity, insulin action, and type 2 diabetes. Science, 306 (5695), 457–61.

Pan, X.R., Yang, W.Y., Li, G.W. and Liu, J. (1997) Prevalence of diabetes and its risk factors in China, 1994. National Diabetes Prevention and Control Cooperative Group. Diabetes Care, 20, 1664–9.

Park, Y.W., Zhu, S., Palaniappan, L. et al. (2003) The metabolic syndrome: prevalence and associated risk factor findings in the US population from the Third National Health and Nutrition Examination Survey, 1988–1994. Archives of Internal Medicine, 163 (4), 427–36.

Patti, M.E., Butte, A.J., Crunkhorn, S. et al. (2003) Coordinated reduction of genes of oxidative metabolism in humans with insulin resistance and diabetes: potential role of PGC1 and NRF1. Proceedings of the National Academy of Sciences USA, 100 (14), 8466–71.

Pecoits-Filho, R., Lindholm, B. and Stenvinkel, P. (2002) The malnutrition, inflammation, and atherosclerosis (MIA) syndrome – the heart of the matter. Nephrology, Dialysis, Transplantation, 17 (Suppl 11), 28–31.

Pereira, M., Kartashov, A., Ebbeling, C. et al. (2005) Fast-food habits, weight gain, and insulin resistance (the CARDIA study): 15-year prospective analysis. Lancet, 365, 36–42.

Petersen, K.F., Befroy, D., Dufour, S. et al. (2003) Mitochondrial dysfunction in the elderly: possible role in insulin resistance. Science, 300 (5622), 1140–2.

Petersen, K.F., Dufour, S., Befroy, D. et al. (2004) Impaired mitochondrial activity in the insulin-resistant offspring of patients with type 2 diabetes. New England Journal of Medicine, 350, 664–71.

Pickup, J. (2004) Inflammation and activated innate immunity in the pathogenesis of type 2 diabetes. Diabetes Care, 27 813–23.

Pitteloud, N., Mootha, V.K., Dwyer, A.A. et al. (2005) Relationship between testosterone levels, insulin sensitivity, and mitochondrial function in men. Diabetes Care, 28 (7), 1636–42.

Poitou, V. and Robertson, R. (2002) Minireview: secondary beta-cell failure in type 2 diabetes – a convergence of glucotoxicity and lipotoxicity. *Endocrinology*, **143**, 339–42.

Pradhan, A.D., Manson, J.E., Rifai, N. *et al.* (2001) C-reactive protein, interleukin 6 and risk of developing type 2 diabetes mellitus. *Journal of American Medical Association*, **286**, 327–34.

Rana, J.S., Li, T.Y., Manson, J.E. and Hu, F.B. (2007) Adiposity compared with physical inactivity and risk of type 2 diabetes in women. *Diabetes Care*, **30** (1), 53–8.

Randle, P.J., Hales, C.N., Garland, P.B. and Newsholme, E.A. (1963) The glucose fatty-acid cycle: its role in insulin sensitivity and the metabolic disturbances of diabetes mellitus. *Lancet*, **ii**, 785–9.

Rask-Madsen, C. and King, G.L. (2007) Mechanisms of disease: endothelial dysfunction in insulin resistance and diabetes. *Nature Clinical Practice Endocrinology & Metabolism*, **3** (1), 46–56.

Ratziu, V., Trabut, J.B. and Poynard, T. (2004) Fat, diabetes, and liver injury in chronic hepatitis C. *Current Gastroenterology Reports*, **6** (1), 22–9.

Reaven, G.M. (1988) Role of insulin resistance in human disease. Banting lecture 1988. *Diabetes*, **37**, 1595–607.

Reaven, G.M. (2006) The metabolic syndrome: is this diagnosis necessary? *American Journal of Clinical Nutrition*, **83**, 1237–47.

Reitman, M.L., Arioglu, E., Gavrilova, O. and Taylor, S.I. (2000) Lipoatrophy revisited. *Trends in Endocrinology and Metabolism*, **11** (10), 410–6.

Richelsen, B., Pedersen, S.B., Moller-Pedersen, T. and Bak, J.F. (1991) Regional differences in triglyceride breakdown in human adipose tissue: effects of catecholamines, insulin, and prostaglandin E2. *Metabolism: Clinical and Experimental*, **40** (9), 990–6.

Roglic, G., Unwin, N., Bennett, P. *et al.* (2005) The burden of mortality attributable to diabetes: realistic estimates for the year 2000. *Diabetes Care*, **28**, 2130–5.

Saad, M.F., Lillioja, S., Nyomba, B.L. *et al.* (1991) Racial differences in the relation between blood pressure and insulin resistance. *New England Journal of Medicine*, **324**, 733–9.

Sarafidis, P.A. and Ruilope, L.M. (2006) Insulin resistance, hyperinsulinemia, and renal injury: mechanisms and implications. *American Journal of Nephrology*, **26** (3), 232–44.

Sarnak, M., Levey, A.S., Schoolwerth, A. *et al.* (2003) Kidney disease as a risk factor for development of cardiovascular disease: a statement from the American Heart Association Councils on Kidney in Cardiovascular Disease, High Blood Pressure Research, Clinical Cardiology, and Epidemiology and Prevention. *Hypertension*, **42**, 1050–65.

Sawada, S., Lee, I., Muto, T. *et al.* (2003) Cardiorespiratory fitness and the incidence of type 2 diabetes: prospective study of Japanese men. *Diabetes Care*, **26**, 2918–22.

Schmitz-Peiffer, C., Browne, C.L., Oakes, N.D. *et al.* (1997) Alterations in the expression and cellular localization of protein kinase C isozymes epsilon and theta are associated with insulin resistance in skeletal muscle of the high-fat-fed rat. *Diabetes*, **46** (2), 169–78.

Shai, I., Jiang, R., Manson, J.E. *et al.* (2006) Ethnicity, obesity, and risk of type 2 diabetes in women: a 20-year follow-up study. *Diabetes Care*, **29**, 1585–90.

Shimabukuro, M., Ohneda, M., Lee, Y. and Unger, R.H. (1997) Role of nitric oxide in obesity-induced beta cell disease. *The Journal of Clinical Investigation*, **100**, 290–5.

Shoelson, S.E., Lee, J. and Yuan, M. (2003) Inflammation and the IKK beta/I kappa B/NF-kappa B axis in obesity- and diet-induced insulin resistance. *International Journal of Obesity and Related Metabolic Disorders*, **27** (Suppl 3), S49–52.

Shulman, G.I., Rothman, D.L., Jue, T. *et al.* (1990) Quantitation of muscle glycogen synthesis in normal subjects and subjects with non-insulin-dependent diabetes by 13C nuclear magnetic resonance spectroscopy. *The New England Journal of Medicine*, **322** (4), 223–8.

So, W.Y., Kong, A.P.S., Osaki, R. *et al.* (2006) Hong Kong Diabetes Registry 2: Glomerular filtration rate, cardiovascular endpoints and all-cause mortality in type 2 diabetic patients. *Diabetes Care*, **29**, 2046–52.

Soma, J., Saito, T., Taguma, Y. *et al.* (2000) High prevalence and adverse effect of hepatitis C virus infection in type II diabetic-related nephropathy. *Journal of the American Society of Nephrology*, **11** (4), 690–9.

Steinthorsdottir, V. *et al.* (2007) *Nature Genetics*, **39** (6), 770–5, 459.

Sundstrom, J., Riserus, U., Byberg, L. *et al.* (2006) Clinical value of the metabolic syndrome for long term prediction of total and cardiovascular mortality: prospective, population based cohort study. *British Medical Journal*, **332**, 878–82.

Suzuki, S., Oka, Y., Kadowaki, T. *et al.* (2003) Clinical features of diabetes mellitus with the mitochondrial DNA 3243 (A-G) mutation in Japanese: maternal inheritance and mitochondria-related complications. *Diabetes Research and Clinical Practice*, **59** (3), 207–17.

Swerdloff, R.S. and Wang, C. (1993) Androgens and aging in men. *Experimental Gerontology*, **28** (4–5), 435–46.

Swislocki, A.L., Chen, Y.D., Golay, A. *et al.* (1987) Insulin suppression of plasma-free fatty acid concentration in normal individuals and patients with type 2 (non-insulin-dependent) diabetes. *Diabetologia*, **30** (8), 622–6.

Syvänne, M. and Taskinen, M.R. (1997) Lipids and lipoproteins as coronary risk factors in non-insulin-dependent diabetes mellitus. *Lancet*, **350** (Suppl 1), SI20–3.

Tan, C.E., Ma, S., Wai, D. et al. (2004) Can we apply the National Cholesterol Education Program Adult Treatment Panel Definition of the Metabolic Syndrome to Asians? *Diabetes Care*, **27** (5), 1182–6.

Tan, K.C.B., Mackay, I.R., Zimmet, P.Z. et al. (2000) Metabolic and immunologic features of Chinese patients with atypical diabetes mellitus. *Diabetes Care*, **23**, 338–53.

Tan, K.C., Wat, N.M., Tam, S.C. et al. (2003) C-reactive protein predicts the deterioration of glycemia in Chinese subjects with impaired glucose tolerance. *Diabetes Care*, **26**, 2323–8.

Tanaka, S., Horimai, C. and Katsukawa, F. (2003) Ethnic differences in abdominal visceral fat accumulation between Japanese, African-Americans, and Caucasians: a meta-analysis. *Acta Diabetologia*, **40**, S302–4.

Tanaka, H., Shiohira, Y., Uezu, Y. et al. (2006) Metabolic syndrome and chronic kidney disease in Okinawa, Japan. *Kidney International*, **69**, 369–74.

Taskinen, M.R. (1992) Quantitative and qualitative lipoprotein abnormalities in diabetes mellitus. *Diabetes*, **41** (Suppl 2), 12–7.

The DECODA Study Group (2006) Prevalence of the metabolic syndrome in populations of Asian origin. Comparison of the IDF definition with the NCEP definition. *Diabetes Research and Clinical Practice*, **76**, 57–67.

Tomlinson, J.W. and Stewart, P.M. (2005) Mechanisms of disease: Selective inhibition of 11beta-hydroxysteroid dehydrogenase type 1 as a novel treatment for the metabolic syndrome. *Nature Clinical Practice Endocrinology & Metabolism*, **1** (2), 92–9.

Tong, P.C.Y., Ho, C.S., Yeung, V.T.F. et al. (2005) Low testosterone and insulin-like growth factor-I but high C-reactive protein are independent predictors for metabolic syndrome in Chinese middle-aged men with a family history of type 2 diabetes. *Journal of Clinical Endocrinology and Metabolism*, **90**, 6418–23.

Trujillo, M.E., Sullivan, S., Harten, I. et al. (2004) Interleukin-6 regulates human adipose tissue lipid metabolism and leptin production in vitro. *The Journal of Clinical Endocrinology and Metabolism*, **89** (11), 5577–82.

Tuomilehto, J., Lindstrom, J., Eriksson, J.G. et al. (2001) Prevention of type 2 diabetes mellitus by changes in lifestyle among subjects with impaired glucose tolerance. *New England Journal of Medicine*, **344**, 1343–50.

Unger, R.H. (2003) Mini review: weapons of lean body mass destruction: the role of ectopic lipids in the metabolic syndrome. *Endocrinology*, **144** (12), 5159–65.

Unwin, N., Harland, J., White, M. et al. (1997) Body mass index, waist circumference, waist-hip ratio and glucose intolerance in Chinese and Europid adults in Newcastle, UK. *Journal of Epidemiology and Community Health*, **51**, 160–6.

Van Gaal, L.F., Mertens, I.L. and De Block, C.E. (2006) Mechanisms linking obesity with cardiovascular disease. *Nature*, **444** (7121), 875–80.

Van Haeften, T., Pimento, W., Mitrakou, A. et al. (2000) Relative contributions of β-cell function and tissue insulin sensitivity to fasting and post-glucose-load glycemia. *Metabolism: Clinical and Experimental*, **49**, 1318–25.

Vaxillaire, M. and Froguel, P. (2008) Monogenic Diabetes of the Young, Pharacogenetics and relevance to multifactorial forms of type 2 diabetes. *Endocrine Reviews*, **29**(3), 254–64.

Vgontzas, A.N., Papanicolaou, D.A., Bixler, E.O. et al. (2000) Sleep apnea and daytime sleepiness and fatigue: relation to visceral obesity, insulin resistance, and hypercytokinemia. *The Journal of Clinical Endocrinology and Metabolism*, **85** (3), 1151–8.

Vozarova, B., Weyer, C., Hanson, K. et al. (2001) Circulating interleukin-6 in relation to adiposity, insulin action, and insulin secretion. *Obesity Research*, **9** (7), 414–7.

Wallenius, K., Wallenius, V., Sunter, D. et al. (2002a) Intracerebroventricular interleukin-6 treatment decreases body fat in rats. *Biochemical and Biophysical Research Communications*, **293** (1), 560–5.

Wallenius, V., Wallenius, K., Ahren, B. et al. (2002b) Interleukin-6-deficient mice develop mature-onset obesity. *Nature Medicine*, **8** (1), 75–9.

Wang, J., Qiao, Q., Miettinen, M. et al. (2004) The metabolic syndrome defined by factor analysis and incident type 2 diabetes in a Chinese population with high postprandial glucose. *Diabetes Care*, **27**, 2429–37.

Wang, Y., Rimm, E.B., Stampfer, M.J. et al. (2005) Comparison of abdominal adiposity and overall obesity in predicting risk of type 2 diabetes among men. *American Journal of Clinical Nutrition*, **81**, 555–63.

Wannamethee, S.G. and Shaper, A.G. (1999) Weight change and duration of overweight and obesity in the incidence of type 2 diabetes. *Diabetes Care*, **22** (8), 1266–72.

Wat, N.M., Lam, T.H., Janus, E.D. and Lam, K.S. (2001) Central obesity predicts the worsening of glycaemia in southern Chinese. *International Journal of Obesity and Related Metabolic Disorder*, **25**, 1789–93.

Wei, J., Sung, F., Li, C. et al. (2003) Low birth weight and high birth weight infants are both at an increased risk to have type 2 diabetes among schoolchildren in Taiwan. *Diabetes Care*, **26**, 343–8.

Weinstein, A.R., Sesso, H.D., Lee, I.M. et al. (2004) Relationship of physical activity vs body mass index with type 2 diabetes in women. *Journal of American Medical Association*, **292** (10), 1188–94.

Weisberg, S.P., McCann, D., Desai, M. et al. (2003) Obesity is associated with macrophage accumulation in adipose tissue. *The Journal of Clinical Investigation*, **112** (12), 1796–808.

Weyer, C., Bogardus, C., Mott, D.M. and Pratley, R.E. (1999) The natural history of insulin secretory dysfunction and insulin resistance in the pathogenesis of type 2 diabetes mellitus. *The Journal of Clinical Investigation*, **104** (6), 787–94.

Weyer, C., Funahashi, T., Tanaka, S. *et al.* (2001) Hypoadiponectinemia in obesity and type 2 diabetes: close association with insulin resistance and hyperinsulinemia. *The Journal of Clinical Endocrinology and Metabolism*, **86** (5), 1930–5.

WHO expert consultation. (2004) Appropriate body mass index for Asian populations and its implications for policy and intervention strategies. *Lancet*, **363**, 157–63.

Widen, E., Lehto, M., Kanninen, T. *et al.* (1995) Association of a polymorphism in the beta 3-adrenergic-receptor gene with features of the insulin resistance syndrome in Finns. *New England Journal of Medicine*, **333**, 348–51.

Wofford, M.R. and Hall, J.E. (2004) Pathophysiology and treatment of obesity hypertension. *Current Pharmaceutical Design*, **10** (29), 3621–37.

World Health Organization (1999) Department of Noncommunicable Disease Surveillance. Definition, diagnosis and classification of diabetes mellitus and its complications.

World Health Organization (2005) Preventing chronic diseases – a vital investment. http://www.who.int/chp/chronic_disease_report/en/index.html, (last accessed 1 June 2006).

Wu, A.Y., Kong, N.C., de Leon, F.A. *et al.* (2005) An alarmingly high prevalence of diabetic nephropathy in Asian type 2 diabetic patients: the MicroAlbuminuria Prevalence (MAP) Study. *Diabetologia*, **48**, 1674–5.

Xia, Z., Sniderman, A.D. and Cianflone, K. (2002) Acylation-stimulating protein (ASP) deficiency induces obesity resistance and increased energy expenditure in ob/ob mice. *The Journal of Biological Chemistry*, **277** (48), 45874–9.

Xiang, K., Wang, Y., Zheng, T. *et al.* (2004) Genome-wide search for type 2 diabetes/impaired glucose homeostasis susceptibility genes in the Chinese: significant linkage to chromosome 6q21–q23 and chromosome 1q21–q24. *Diabetes*, **53**, 228–34.

Xu, J.Y., Dan, Q.H., Chan, V. *et al.* (2005) Genetic and clinical characteristics of maturity-onset diabetes of the young in Chinese patients. *European Journal of Human Genetics*, **13**, 422–7.

Yajnik, C.S. (2002) The lifecycle effects of nutrition and body size on adult adiposity, diabetes and cardiovascular diseases. *Obesity Reviews*, **3**, 217–24.

Yajnik, C. and Yudkin, J. (2004) The Y-Y paradox. *Lancet*, **363**, 163.

Yamauchi, T., Kamon, J., Minokoshi, Y. *et al.* (2002) Adiponectin stimulates glucose utilization and fatty-acid oxidation by activating AMP-activated protein kinase. *Nature Medicine*, **8** (11), 1288–95.

Yamauchi, T., Kamon, J., Waki, H. *et al.* (2001) The fat-derived hormone adiponectin reverses insulin resistance associated with both lipoatrophy and obesity. *Nature Medicine*, **7** (8), 941–6.

Yamauchi, T., Kamon, J., Waki, H. *et al.* (2003) Globular adiponectin protected ob/ob mice from diabetes and ApoE-deficient mice from atherosclerosis. *The Journal of Biological Chemistry*, **278** (4), 2461–8.

Yokoi, N., Kanamori, M., Horikawa, Y. *et al.* (2006) Association studies of variants in the genes involved in pancreatic beta-cell function in type 2 diabetes in Japanese subjects. *Diabetes*, **55** (8), 2379–86.

Zeggini, E. and McCarthy, M.I. 2007. *Diabetologia*, **50**, 1–4.

Zhao, H.L., Lai, F.M.M., Tong, P.C.Y. *et al.* (2003) Prevalence and clinicopathological characteristics of islet amyloid in Chinese patients with type 2 diabetes. *Diabetes*, **52**, 2759–66.

Zhou, Y.P. and Grill, V. (1995) Long term exposure to fatty acids and ketones inhibits B-cell functions in human pancreatic islets of Langerhans. *The Journal of Clinical Endocrinology and Metabolism*, **80** (5), 1584–90.

Zhu, S., Heymsfield, S.B., Toyoshima, H. *et al.* (2005) Race-ethnicity-specific waist circumference cut-offs for identifying cardiovascular disease risk factors. *The American Journal of Clinical Nutrition*, **81** (2), 409–15.

Zhu, S., Wang, Z., Heshka, S. *et al.* (2002) Waist circumference and obesity-associated risk factors among whites in the third National Health and Nutrition Examination Survey: clinical action thresholds. *The American Journal of Clinical Nutrition*, **76** (4), 743–9.

Zimmet, P., Alberti, K.G. and Shaw, J. (2001) Global and societal implications of the diabetes epidemic. *Nature*, **414**, 782–7.

Liver Disease in Obesity

Key points

- Obesity is a major risk factor for non-alcoholic fatty liver disease (NAFLD). NAFLD is the cause of 70–90% of cases of liver disease in obese subjects and is the commonest liver disorder in Western countries.

- Obese subjects with NAFLD commonly have features of the metabolic syndrome, including insulin resistance, hyperglycaemia, dyslipidaemia and hypertension. NAFLD is widely regarded as the hepatic manifestation of the metabolic syndrome.

- Most cases have simple steatosis (fatty liver), which in itself is benign but can process in up to 40% of cases to non-alcoholic steatohepatitis (NASH) and in 10% to cirrhosis. Hepatocellular carcinoma is a recognized risk.

- Cardiovascular mortality is increased in obese subjects with NAFLD, with an excess risk that is not explicable by co-existent classical cardiovascular risk factors. The mechanism is unknown.

- Hepatocyte damage and inflammation are probably initiated by high FFA levels, release of cytokines via NF-κB and oxidative stress. Fibrosis may be enhanced by increased leptin (and perhaps insulin and glucose) levels and decreased adiponectin.

- Diagnosis of NAFLD requires exclusion of alcohol and other causes of liver dysfunction and may require liver biopsy to stage the disease. Liver imaging shows fatty change and may show the development of cirrhosis. Liver function tests are often normal and do not accurately predict the severity of liver damage. Older age and BMI, type 2 diabetes and an aspartate transaminase:alanine transaminase (AST:ALT) ratio >1.0 point to advanced fibrosis.

- Patients with simple steatosis should be reviewed frequently; advanced NAFLD requires specialist follow up with surveillance for oesophageal varices and hepatocellular carcinoma.

- Associated obesity, type 2 diabetes, dyslipidaemia and hypertension should be actively treated to decrease cardiovascular risk. Some therapies (e.g. metformin, thiazolidinediones and gastric banding) may improve liver histology and function.

Chapter 11   Liver Disease in Obesity

Nimantha de Alwis and Chris Day

Deposition of fat in the liver has long been recognized in obesity, but the range and potential gravity of obesity-associated liver disease have only recently been appreciated. Worldwide, obesity is becoming the major cause of non-alcoholic fatty liver disease (NAFLD), a disease spectrum ranging from simple fatty liver (steatosis), through non-alcoholic steatohepatitis (NASH) to hepatic fibrosis and ultimately cirrhosis (Figure 11.1). NAFLD was first described by Ludwig in 1980 and is now considered to be the most common liver disorder in the Western world. As the name suggests, it occurs in patients without a history of excessive alcohol consumption. Simple steatosis is benign, whereas NASH is characterized by hepatocyte injury, inflammation and fibrosis, which can lead to cirrhosis, liver failure and hepatocellular carcinoma (HCC).

NAFLD is strongly associated with obesity, insulin resistance, hypertension and dyslipidaemia and is widely regarded as the liver manifestation of the metabolic syndrome. The rapid spread of the obesity 'pandemic', coupled with the realization that the outcomes of obesity-related liver disease are not entirely benign, has led to rapid growth in clinical and basic studies of this hitherto neglected disorder. The resulting increase in our understanding of the natural history, clinical features and pathophysiology of NAFLD has now begun to inform the development of rational management strategies.

Epidemiology

The true prevalence of obesity-associated liver disease in unselected obese and overweight populations is largely unknown and the reported frequency varies widely, according to the population studied and the diagnostic methods used. The prevalence of hepatic steatosis appears to be 20–30% among Western adults – a consensus that has emerged from several recent well-conducted North American and European studies that used ultrasound or magnetic resonance imaging (Bedogni et al., 2005; Browning et al., 2004). In these populations, 30–50% of adults are overweight or obese (see Chapter 2). NASH is much rarer, affecting 2–3% of the general population of Western countries (Neuschwander-Tetri and Caldwell, 2003). Among severely obese patients (BMI $>35\,kg/m^2$) undergoing bariatric surgery, histological studies report prevalences of steatosis and NASH of 91% and 37%, respectively (Machado, Marques-Vidal and Cortez-Pinto, 2006). The prevalence of obesity-related liver disease in type 2 diabetes has not been systematically examined, but features of NAFLD were found in 70% of unselected Italian type 2 diabetic subjects (Targher et al., 2006a).

Pathogenesis of NAFLD in obesity

The process begins with deposition of triglyceride within hepatocytes, forming micro- or macrovesicular fat droplets (see Figure 11.3). This hepatic steatosis occurs in parallel with fat deposition in other tissues and is due to a combination of increased free fatty acid (FFA) supply to the liver from increased adipose tissue lipolysis, increased de novo lipogenesis and, to a lesser extent, reduced FFA oxidation and VLDL export (Browning and Horton, 2004). Simple hepatic steatosis is reversible: triglyceride deposits can be rapidly cleared from hepatocytes by restricting energy and fat intake (see above).

In some cases, steatosis progresses to inflammation and fibrosis, which can lead to irreversible liver damage. Possible genetic and environmental determinants of progression include polymorphisms in genes encoding the antioxidant enzymes superoxide dismutase 2 (SOD2), microsomal transfer protein (MTP), phosphatidyl e-methyl transferase (PEMT) and dietary intake of saturated fat and

Obesity: Science to Practice   Edited by Gareth Williams and Gema Frühbeck
© 2009 John Wiley & Sons, Ltd

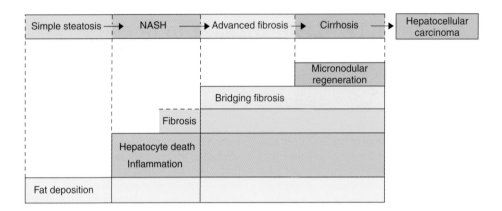

Figure 11.1 Spectrum of liver disease (NAFLD) associated with obesity.

antioxidant vitamins (De Alwis and Day, 2007). The pathogenesis of inflammation and fibrosis in NAFLD has been reviewed in detail (Day, 2006; Day, 2002) and current theories are summarized below and in Figure 11.2.

Inflammation

The key factor initiating inflammation appears to be an increased supply of FFA to the liver, due to obesity and the associated insulin resistance of adipose tissue. The latter may arise, at least in part, from infiltration of adipose tissue by macrophages, which release cytokines (TNFα, IL-6, IL-1β) that impair insulin signalling (Weisberg *et al.*, 2003). FFA taken up by the liver can be stored as triglyceride or oxidized, but also activate the transcription factor NFκB – the 'master regulator' controlling the transcription of genes encoding proinflammatory cytokines, chemokines and adhesion molecules. The subsequent release from hepatocytes of cytokines, in

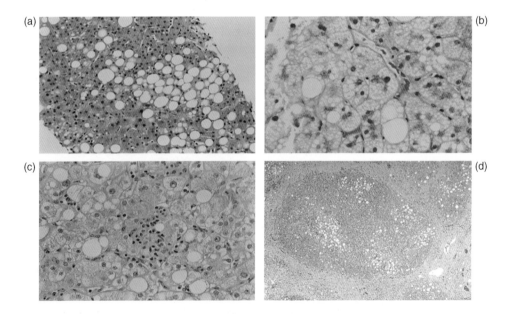

Figure 11.2 Histological features of NAFLD in obesity. (a,b) Simple steatosis, showing areas of (a) macrovesicular and (b) microvesicular fat deposition within hepatocytes. Haematoxylin and eosin stain, original magnification ×10 (2a) and ×20 (2b). (c) NASH, showing inflammatory cell infiltration around a focus of hepatocyte damage and death. (d) Cirrhosis, showing heavy fibrosis and micronodular regeneration. Haematoxylin and eosin stain, original magnification ×20. Courtesy Professor A.D. Burt (University of Newcastle, UK).

particular TNFα, activates classical inflammatory cells including Kupffer cells, and these produce more cytokines, in particular interleukin-12, capable of initiating hepatocyte injury, necrosis and apoptosis and of attracting other inflammatory cells. Hepatocyte damage is enhanced by oxidative stress free radical generation resulting from increased FFA oxidation. These cytokines also lead to hepatic insulin resistance, which contributes to increased hepatic FFA oxidation and may also aggravate extra-hepatic insulin resistance in muscle and adipose tissue.

Reduced production of the anti-inflammatory cytokine, adiponectin, by adipocytes in obesity may also contribute to the development of hepatic inflammation (Hui et al., 2004). Some evidence suggests that, as in alcoholic liver disease, gut-derived endotoxin may also play a role in activating Kupffer cells in NAFLD (Hui et al., 2004; Wigg et al., 2001). Obesity and type 2 diabetes mellitus have long been associated with small intestinal bacterial overgrowth.

Fibrosis

Hepatic fibrosis in NAFLD is due partly to the general response to inflammation and hepatocyte injury, which leads to the activation of collagen-producing hepatic stellate cells (HSC) and deposition of scar tissue. In addition, increasing evidence supports a role for other pro-fibrogenic mediators related to obesity and insulin resistance, which may activate HSC directly and without causing hepatic inflammation and necrosis. These putative mediators include leptin, angiotensin II and noradrenaline, all of which are secreted by adipose tissue and are raised in the serum of obese subjects (see Chapter 4). Furthermore, both hyperglycaemia and hyperinsulinaemia may have direct fibrogenic roles, as synthesis of fibrogenic growth factor and connective tissue growth factor by HSC is up-regulated by glucose and insulin (Paradis et al., 2001). The reduced circulating levels of adiponectin in obesity may also contribute directly to the development of liver fibrosis because it appears to exert potent anti-fibrotic as well as anti-inflammatory effects (Kamada et al., 2003).

Pathology of NAFLD

Hepatocellular steatosis is the hallmark of NAFLD. Triglyceride deposition is usually macrovesicular, with a single large fat droplet displacing the nucleus; a microvesicular pattern of several smaller well-defined intracytoplasmic droplets may also be seen (Figure 11.2a and b) (Brunt, 2004). Histological features of inflammation, hepatocyte damage and fibrosis are shown in Figure 11.3. Infiltrating inflammatory cells include macrophages and neutrophils, and hepatocyte apoptosis and necrosis may be seen. Collagen stains readily to show fibrosis; 'bridging' fibrosis that spans the hepatic lobules is a precursor of cirrhosis, which has a micronodular pattern (Figure 11.3).

Until recently, there was no consensus about what constitutes abnormal steatosis, or the histological features required to diagnose NASH. The National Institutes of Health (NIH) NAFLD Clinical Research Network have now published a validated histological scoring system that addresses the full spectrum of lesions of NAFLD, and have proposed a NAFLD activity score (NAS) for use in clinical trials (Kleiner et al., 2005). Importantly, in common with other liver diseases, the histological lesions of NASH are unevenly distributed throughout the liver; sampling error can potentially result in substantial inaccuracies in staging.

Natural history of NAFLD

In marked contrast to *alcoholic* steatohepatitis, the short-term prognosis of NAFLD is good. The largest prospective histological study of the natural history of NAFLD, with a mean follow-up of 13 years, has recently been published (Ekstadt et al., 2006). Data from this study and others suggest that the long-term prognosis of patients with NAFLD depends on the histological stage of disease at presentation (Day, 2005). These findings are summarized in Figure 11.4.

For patients with simple steatosis, 12–40% will develop NASH with early fibrosis after 8–13 years, without clinical or histological signs of cirrhosis. For patients presenting with NASH and early fibrosis, around 15% will develop cirrhosis and/or evidence of hepatic decompensation over the same time-period, increasing to 25% of patients with advanced pre-cirrhotic fibrosis at baseline. About 7% of subjects with compensated cirrhosis associated with NAFLD will develop a HCC within 10 years, and 50% will require a transplant or die from a liver–related cause (Sanyal, 2006). The risk of HCC in NAFLD-related cirrhosis is comparable to that in cirrhosis associated with alcohol or hepatitis C, and higher than in autoimmune diseases but lower than in chronic hepatitis B infection (Nair et al., 2002). This may partly explain the recently

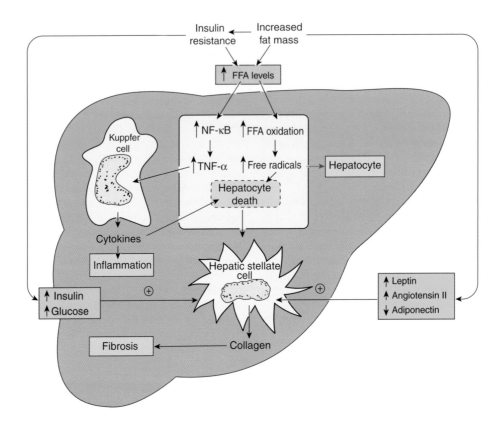

Figure 11.3 Pathogenesis of NAFLD in obesity. +: stimulation.

reported associations of HCC with high BMI and type 2 diabetes (Calle *et al.*, 2003).

Two recent studies have reported that the increased age-related mortality observed in patients with NAFLD is attributable to cardiovascular as well as liver-related deaths (Ekstadt *et al.*, 2006). This might be expected given the association between NAFLD and classical cardiovascular risk factors in the metabolic syndrome. However, recent data suggest that NAFLD may directly contribute to cardiovascular disease. Type 2 diabetic subjects with NAFLD showed higher prevalence and incidence of cardiovascular disease than those without NAFLD, independent of classical cardiovascular risk factors, glycaemic control, medication and features of the metabolic syndrome (Targher *et al.*, 2006b). NAFLD is also associated with increased carotid wall thickness (Targher *et al.*, 2006a) and endothelial dysfunction (Villanova *et al.*, 2005) – two powerful predictors of atheromatous disease – even when the confounding components of the metabolic syndrome are excluded. The mechanism of any direct effect of NAFLD on cardiovascular risk

remains unclear; possibilities include the release of atherogenic inflammatory cytokines and procoagulant factors from the steatotic liver (Targher and Arcaro, 2006).

Clinical presentation

NAFLD is a largely asymptomatic condition that may reach an advanced stage before it is suspected or diagnosed. Symptoms such as right upper quadrant discomfort, fatigue and lethargy have been reported but are inconsistent and uncommon presenting complaints.

Most patients are diagnosed following the incidental finding of abnormal liver enzyme tests performed during routine investigation or health-check. Several studies have demonstrated that NAFLD is the diagnosis in 70–90% of patients with abnormal liver enzymes who have negative viral hepatitis markers and no history of alcohol excess. Importantly, the vast majority (around 80%) of patients with NAFLD have *normal* liver enzyme levels, and there is no

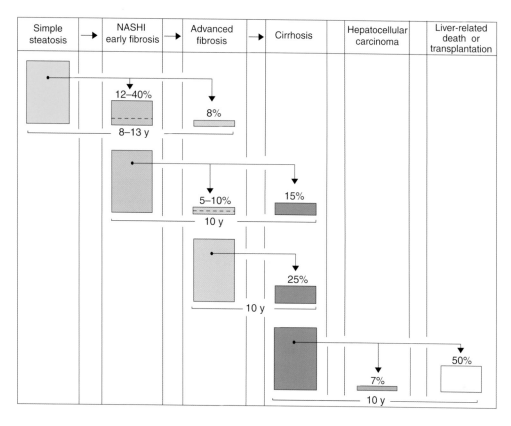

Figure 11.4 Natural history of NAFLD in obesity. Prognosis depends on the stage of liver damage when first ascertained. Duration of follow-up in each of the studies is indicated.

difference in histological severity between those with and without abnormal liver function tests (LFTs). Accordingly, NAFLD should be suspected and sought in all patients with established risk factors, whether or not LFTs are abnormal.

Investigation of suspected NAFLD

Most obese patients found to have liver disease will ultimately be diagnosed with NAFLD. Nevertheless, other diagnoses have to be considered and excluded: other causes of fatty liver and/or deranged liver function include alcohol, hepatotoxic drugs, viral hepatitis, pregnancy, autoimmune diseases including primary biliary cirrhosis and chronic active hepatitis, and rare hereditary diseases such as haemochromatosis, Wilson's disease and α-1 antitrypsin deficiency. Moreover, NAFLD associated with obesity can lead to cirrhosis and hepatocellular carcinoma, which have to be identified.

A flowchart for investigating patients with abnormal liver function or suspected NAFLD is shown in Figure 11.5. Initial assessment must include a careful history for alcohol intake and hepatotoxic drugs, and a standard 'liver screen' with serological markers for hepatitis B and C, autoantibodies (anti-mitochondrial and smooth muscle), serum ferritin, caeruloplasmin and α-1 antitrypsin phenotype. In the absence of evidence to the contrary, an alcohol intake at or below currently recommended 'sensible' limits (21 units per week for men, 14 for women) appears compatible with a diagnosis of NAFLD (Dixon, Bhathal and O'Brian, 2001), but the notorious unreliability of the alcohol consumption history must be remembered. The recently developed ALD/NAFLD Index (ANI), based on AST:ALT ratio, BMI, MCV and gender, has proved better at diagnosing alcohol-related fatty liver disease than individual conventional and newer biomarkers (Dunn et al., 2006).

Liver imaging, with ultrasound, CT or MRI scanning will be able to distinguish uniform

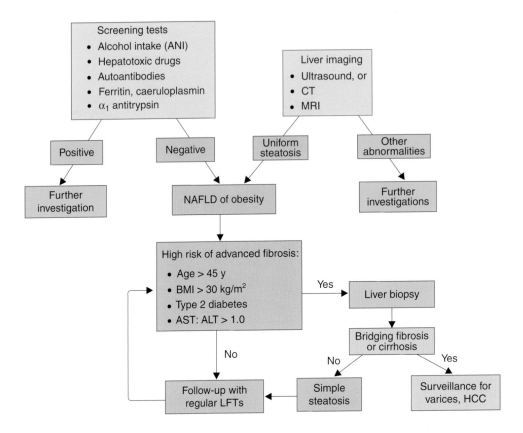

Figure 11.5 Algorithm for investigating suspected NAFLD or liver dysfunction in obese subjects.

fatty change consistent with NAFLD from cirrhosis or other hepatic pathologies. Currently available imaging modalities cannot differentiate patients with simple steatosis from those with NASH and fibrosis (Saadeh *et al.*, 2002), although newer imaging techniques (e.g. measurements of liver stiffness) may eventually prove effective.

A key issue in investigating patients with suspected NAFLD is to determine whether a liver biopsy is warranted. This can be justified either to establish the diagnosis of NAFLD or to stage the disease in order to inform prognosis and guide the management of patients with advanced or progressive liver damage. Cases should be carefully selected, because the large number of potential patients makes it impractical to perform liver biopsy in all.

In a patient with abnormal LFTs who has classical risk factors for NAFLD (obesity, especially with type 2 diabetes) and ultrasound liver scan steatosis, NAFLD can be diagnosed with relative confidence without a liver biopsy

after other common causes of abnormal LFTs have been excluded.

Non-invasive markers for staging NAFLD

Various clinical and laboratory markers have been shown to correlate with advanced fibrosis (bridging fibrosis or cirrhosis) in patients with NAFLD, notably age >45 years, BMI >30 kg/m^2, diagnosis of type 2 diabetes (or raised fasting blood glucose), and an aspartate transaminase: alanine transaminase (AST : ALT) ratio >1.0 (Guha *et al.*, 2006). At present, it would seem reasonable to restrict liver biopsy to patients with at least some, if not all, of these risk factors. These markers, together with platelet count and serum albumin concentration, have recently been combined into a NAFLD fibrosis score that accurately predicts the presence of advanced fibrosis in patients with NAFLD (Angulo *et al.* (2007)).

Other predictive algorithms, based on classical and emerging serum markers of fibrosis in NAFLD, are also in development. Non-invasive markers of steatohepatitis rather than fibrosis are also being sought: serum levels of a caspase cleavage product of the hepatocyte protein cytokeratin-18 (a putative marker of hepatocyte apoptosis) have recently been shown to predict NASH accurately (Wieckowska et al., 2006).

Management of patients with NAFLD

The management of patients with NAFLD is summarized in Figure 11.6.

The largely benign prognosis of patients with simple steatosis means that they can be managed conservatively, perhaps by a primary-care physician. By contrast, patients with NASH and fibrosis have increased propensity for disease progression and therefore require long-term specialist follow up. Advanced cases, with bridging fibrosis or cirrhosis, should be entered into appropriate surveillance programmes for oesophageal varices and hepatocellular carcinoma. It also seems likely that advanced cases will increasingly be candidates for novel 'second-line' therapies currently being evaluated in large randomized clinical trials (RCTs) – a further justification for accurate staging of the disease.

General measures

Definitive, evidence-based treatment recommendations for obesity-related liver disease have not yet been published, but should soon emerge from ongoing and planned RCTs. In the meantime, it is rational to direct treatment at associated features of the metabolic syndrome – obesity, insulin resistance, hypertension and dyslipidaemia – and at limiting alcohol and other hepatic toxins. Most patients with NAFLD will have some, if not all, features of the metabolic syndrome (Marchesini et al., 2003), and are therefore at increased risk of cardiovascular death. These cardiovascular risk factors require treatment regardless of the severity of any associated NAFLD; these measures will undoubtedly reduce mortality from cardiovascular disease and, as discussed below, may also improve the underlying liver disease.

Alcohol intake should not exceed the currently recommended sensible limits, because the only study to have examined this issue reported that light to moderate alcohol intake reduces the risk of steatosis and NASH in morbidly obese patients undergoing bariatric surgery, possibly by reducing insulin resistance and the risk of type 2 diabetes (Dixon, Bhathal and O'Brien, 2001).

Treatment of associated obesity

In theory, strategies aimed at achieving and maintaining weight loss in patients with NAFLD should improve hepatic histology, because reducing fat mass will decrease hepatic FFA supply and levels of pro-fibrotic adipocytokines, while increasing production of the anti-inflammatory and anti-fibrotic adiponectin.

Diet and exercise

Many uncontrolled studies show improvements in various parameters of NAFLD with diet-induced weight loss, but only two small (<20 patients) controlled trials have been published: one reported an improvement in ALT only, and

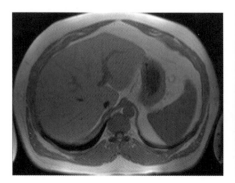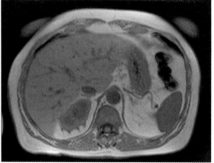

Figure 11.6 Fatty liver, imaged by MRI using two different scan conditions. Left panel: in-phase T1 weighted gradient echo (TR 105msec, TE 4.8msec at 1.5 Tesla). Right panel: Out of phase T1 weighted gradient echo (TR 105msec, TE 2.4msec at 1.5 Tesla).

the other a reduction in hepatic steatosis (Ueno et al., 1997).

To date, almost all studies of diet-induced weight loss have employed simple calorie restriction, whereas very few have manipulated specific dietary components. This area seems worthy of study, because intakes of both saturated fat and fibre are known to influence insulin resistance, while a diet high in saturated fat appears to be a risk factor for NASH in obese individuals (Musso et al., 2003). Dietary fat intake has also been shown to correlate with liver fat content and insulin resistance in short-term studies of obese, non-diabetic women – independently of changes in total-body, subcutaneous or abdominal fat (Westerbacka et al., 2005). The value of exercise in achieving and maintaining weight loss is well established; the only controlled study of weight loss that reported improvements in histology in treated patients combined calorie restriction with increased exercise (Ueno et al., 1997).

Pharmacological anti-obesity agents

Encouraging improvements in liver histology have been reported from pilot studies of the intestinal lipase inhibitor orlistat in patients with NASH (Harrison et al., 2004). Data from currently ongoing large RCTs of these drugs are awaited with interest. The cannabinoid receptor 1 (CB1) antagonist rimonabant has recently been shown to be effective in reducing weight and waist circumference, with improvements in several metabolic parameters including insulin resistance (Van Gaal et al., 2005). Its effects on the liver in NAFLD have not yet been reported, but as animal studies suggest that CB1 blockade may also inhibit liver fibrosis (Van Gaal et al., 2005), rimonabant seems ripe for study in this context.

Bariatric surgery

The various surgical procedures currently used for the treatment of obesity are described in Chapter 18. Biliopancreatic diversion appears to carry a significant risk of liver failure and worsening fibrosis, and should therefore be avoided in patients with NAFLD. Better results have been reported for gastric bypass and gastric banding surgery. Dixon et al. (2004) reported that adjustable gastric banding surgery in 36 patients with NASH decreased BMI from 47 to 34 kg/m² in 26 months, with significant improvements in histological features of steatosis, necroinflammation and fibrosis (Dixon et al., 2004).

Treatment of associated diabetes mellitus and insulin resistance

Evidence that insulin resistance may contribute to both inflammation and fibrosis in the liver has led to several pilot studies of metformin and other insulin-sensitizing agents in NAFLD patients with and without diabetes. There is as yet no direct evidence that hyperinsulinaemia per se adversely affects the liver, but the putative pathogenic role of insulin in causing fibrosis in NAFLD suggests that insulin or sulphonylureas might be best avoided if glycaemic control can be achieved with other agents that do not raise plasma insulin levels.

Pilot studies of metformin in diabetic and non-diabetic patients with NAFLD have shown inconsistent effects on LFTs and fat content, as determined by standard MRI or proton spectroscopy. However, the largest study to date, in non-diabetic NAFLD patients, has been more encouraging. In this 12-month, randomized open-label trial, metformin treatment (2 g/day) was associated with significantly higher rates of normalized aminotransferase levels and with significant decreases in liver fat, necroinflammation and fibrosis, compared with either vitamin E treatment or a weight-reducing diet (Bugianesi et al., 2005).

Thiazolidinediones

These anti-diabetic drugs act as agonists at the peroxisome proliferator activated receptor-γ (PPARγ). They improve insulin sensitivity, at least in part, via anti-steatotic effects in liver and muscle, which may in turn result from an increase in adiponectin secretion by adipocytes (see Chapter 5). Pilot studies of the second-generation thiazolidinediones, pioglitazone and rosiglitazone have reported encouraging improvements in insulin sensitivity, LFTs and liver histology; several large RCTs are currently in progress. A recent placebo-controlled RCT demonstrated that pioglitazone treatment in patients with NASH and impaired glucose tolerance (IGT) or type 2 diabetes had beneficial effects in reducing aminotransferase levels and insulin resistance and improving liver histology (Belfort et al., 2006).

Treatment of associated dyslipidaemia

Hypertriglyceridaemia affects 20–80% of patients with NAFLD. As with anti-obesity and insulin-sensitizing drugs, there are sound scientific reasons to support the use of fibrates – the conventional triglyceride-lowering agents – in patients with NAFLD. Fibrates are agonists at the PPARα receptor, a transcription factor that up-regulates the transcription of genes encoding various proteins that would be expected to reduce FFA delivery to the liver. However, the only controlled study with histological follow-up found that one year of clofibrate therapy had no effect on liver biochemistry or histology (Laurin et al., 1996).

There is no rationale for using HMG CoA reductase inhibitors (statins) to treat NAFLD, but they can be safely prescribed for 'conventional' indications, including type 2 diabetes regardless of cholesterol concentration. Importantly, there is no evidence that patients with pre-existing NAFLD are at increased risk of statin-induced idiosyncratic hepatotoxicity, or that statins are associated with a higher frequency of hepatic steatosis or serum ALT abnormalities in these subjects (Browning, 2006).

Treatment of associated hypertension

No studies have specifically examined the effect of different anti-hypertensive agents on the liver in hypertensive patients with NAFLD. Interestingly, however, evidence has recently emerged that angiotensin II receptor antagonists and ACE inhibitors are antifibrotic in animal models of hepatic fibrosis. This suggests that these agents are worth studying in clinical trials, especially as supportive pilot human data have recently been reported (Yokohama et al., 2004).

Liver-directed therapies for NAFLD

Increased understanding of the mechanisms of progressive liver damage in NAFLD has stimulated the search for specific therapies directed at the disease process itself, rather than at components of the metabolic syndrome.

Antioxidants

Several encouraging pilot studies of various agents indicate potential beneficial effects that may be related to their antioxidant effects. These include probucol (Merat et al., 2003), betaine (Abdelmalek et al., 2001) and vitamin E (α-tocopherol) (Lanvine, 2000). However, a recent RCT of vitamin E combined with vitamin C in patients with NASH found no overall improvement in hepatic fibrosis score compared with placebo.

Anti-cytokine agents

Beneficial effects of anti-TNFα therapies have been demonstrated in animal models of NASH, and the first human pilot study recently reported an improvement in aminotransferase levels. Given the emerging importance of pro-inflammatory cytokines in both liver pathology and insulin resistance in obesity, it seems likely that cytokines and their regulatory molecules, including NF-kB will become major therapeutic targets in both NAFLD and type 2 diabetes in the near future (Day, 2006).

Ursodeoxycholic acid (UDCA)

This agent is of theoretical interest because it has long been used as a hepatoprotectant. More recent evidence has suggested that bile acids may act as molecular chaperones capable of reducing endoplasmic reticulum (ER) stress (Ozcan et al., 2006). However, a large, placebo-controlled RCT in patients with NASH recently showed no benefit of UDCA (13–15 mg/kg/day) on liver histology after two years' treatment (Lindor et al., 2004).

Liver transplantation for patients with NAFLD

Patients with NAFLD who progress to decompensated cirrhosis or who develop HCC are candidates for liver transplantation. A favourable outcome depends on removing the factors that originally caused liver damage. Perhaps unsurprisingly, steatosis recurs in most patients within four years, with 50% developing NASH and fibrosis; cases of recurrent cirrhosis are also reported. Risk factors for recurrence are the presence of insulin resistance or type 2 diabetes pre- and post-transplantation, weight gain following transplantation, and a high cumulative steroid dose. These findings highlight the importance of ensuring weight and metabolic control in reducing the risk of disease recurrence, in a group of patients who will undoubtedly contribute increasing numbers to transplant programmes in the future.

References

Abdelmalek, M., Angulo, P., Jorgensen, R. *et al.* (2001) Betain, a promising new agent for patients with non-alcoholic steatohepatitis: results of a pilot study. *American Journal of Gastroenterology*, **96**, 2711–7.

Bedogni, G., Miglioli, L., Masutti, F. *et al.* (2005) Prevalence and risk factors for nonalcoholic fatty liver disease: The Dionysus nutrition and liver study. *Hepatology*, **42**, 44–52.

Belfort, R., Harrison, S.A., Brown, K. *et al.* (2006) A placebo controlled trial of pioglitazone in subjects with non-alcoholic steatohepatitis. *New England Journal of Medicine*, **355**, 2297–307.

Browning, J. (2006) Statins and hepatic steatosis: perspectives from the Dallas Heart Study. *Hepatology*, **44**, 466–71.

Browning, J.D. and Horton, J.D. (2004) Molecular mediators of hepatic steatosis and liver injury. *The Journal of Clinical Investigation*, **114**, 147–52.

Browning, J.D., Szczepaniak, L.S., Dobbins, R. *et al.* (2004) Prevalence of hepatic steatosis in an urban population in the United states: impact of ethnicity. *Hepatology*, **40**, 1387–95.

Brunt, E.M. (2004) Nonalcoholic steatohepatitis. *Seminars in Liver Disease*, **24**, 3–20.

Bugianesi, E., Gentilcore, E., Manini, R. *et al.* (2005) A randomised control trial of metformin versus vitamin E or prescriptive diet in nonalcoholic fatty liver disease. *American Journal of Gastroenterology*, **100**, 1082–90

Calle, E., Rodriguez, C., Walker-Thurmond, K. and Thun, M. (2003) Overweight, obesity and mortality from cancer in prospectively studied cohort of U.S. adults. *New England Journal of Medicine*, **348**, 1625–38.

Day, C.P. (2002) Pathogenesis of steatohepatitis. *Best Practice & Research in Clinical Gastroenterology*, **16**, 663–78

Day, C.P. (2005) Natural history of NAFLD: remarkably benign in the absence of cirrhosis. *Gastroenterology*, **129**, 375–8

Day, C.P. (2006) From fat to inflammation. *Gastroenterology*, **130**, 207–10

De Alwis, N.M.W. and Day, C.P. (2007) Genetics of alcoholic and non-alcoholic fatty liver disease. *Seminars in Liver Disease*, **27**, 44.

Dixon, J., Bhathal, P. and O'Brien, P. (2001) Non-alcoholic fatty liver disease: predictors of non-alcoholic steatohepatitis and liver fibrosis in the severely obese. *Gastroenterology*, **121**, 91–100.

Dixon, J., Bhathal, P., Hughes, N. and O'Brien, P. (2004) Improvement in liver histological analysis with weight loss. *Hepatology*, **39**, 1647–54

Dunn, W., Angulo, P., Sanderson, S. *et al.* (2006) Utility of a new model to diagnose an alcohol basis for steatohepatitis. *Gastroenterology*, **131**, 1057–63.

Ekstadt, M., Franzen, L.E., Mathiesen, U.L. *et al.* (2006) Long-term follow-up of patients with NAFLD and elevated liver enzymes. *Hepatology*, **44**, 865–73.

Guha, I.N., Parkes, J., Roderick, P.R. *et al.* (2006) Non-invasive markers associated with liver fibrosis in non-alcoholic fatty liver disease. *Gut*, **55**, 1650–60.

Harrison, S., Fincke, C., Helinski, D. *et al.* (2004) A pilot study of orlistat treatment in obese, nonalcoholic steatohepatitis patients. *Alimentary Pharmacology & Therapeutics*, **20**, 623–8

Hui, J., Hodge, A., Farrell, G. *et al.* (2004) Beyond insulin resistance in NASH: TNF-alpha or adiponectin? *Hepatology*, **40**, 46–54.

Kamada, Y., Tamura, S., Kiso, S. *et al.* (2003) Enhanced carbon tetrachloride-induced liver fibrosis in mice lacking adiponectin. *Gastroenterology*, **125**, 1796–807.

Kleiner, D., Brunt, E.M., Van Natta, M. *et al.* (2005) Design and validation of histologic scoring system for nonalcoholic fatty liver disease. *Hepatology*, **41**, 1313–21

Lanvine, J. (2000) Vitamin E treatment of nonalcoholic steatohepatitis in children: a pilot study. *The Journal of Pediatrics*, **136**, 734–8.

Laurin, J., Lindor, K., Crippin, J. *et al.* (1996) Ursodeoxycholic acid or clofibrate in the treatment of nonalcoholic induced steatohepatitis: a pilot study. *Hepatology*, **23**, 1464–7.

Lindor, K., Kowdley, K., Heathcote, E. *et al.* (2004) Ursodeoxycholic acid for treatment of non-alcoholic steatohepatitis: results of a randomized trial. *Hepatology*, **39**, 770–8

Machado, M., Marques-Vidal, P. and Cortez-Pinto, H. (2006) Hepatic histology in patients undergoing bariatric surgery. *Journal of Hepatology*, **45**, 600–6.

Marchesini, G., Bugianesi, E., Forlani, G. *et al.* (2003) Nonalcoholic fatty liver, steatohepatitis and the metabolic syndrome. *Hepatology*, **37**, 917–23.

Merat, S., Malekzadeh, R., Sohrabi, M. *et al.* (2003) Probucol in the treatment of nonalcoholic steatohepatitis: a double blind randomized controlled study. *Journal of Hepatology*, **38**, 414–8.

Musso, G., Gambino, R., De Michieli, F. *et al.* (2003) Dietary habits and their relations to insulin resistance and postprandial lipemia in nonalcoholic steatohepatitis. *Hepatology*, **37**, 909–16.

Nair, S., Mason, A., Eason, J. *et al.* (2002) Is obesity an independent risk factor for hepatocellular carcinoma in cirrhosis? *Hepatology*, **36**, 150–5.

Neuschwander-Tetri, B. and Caldwell, S. (2003) Non-alcoholic steatohepatitis: summary of an AASLD single topic conference. *Hepatology*, **37**, 1202–19.

Ozcan, U., Yilmaz, E., Ozcan, L. *et al.* (2006) Chemical chaperones reduce ER stress and restore glucose homeostasis in a mouse model of type 2 diabetes. *Science*, **313**, 1137–40.

Paradis, V., Perlemuter, G., Bonvosust, F. *et al.* (2001) High glucose and hyperinsulinaemia stimulate connective tissue growth factor expression: a potential mechanism involved in progression to fibrosis in non-alcoholic steatohepatitis. *Hepatology*, **34**, 738–44.

Saadeh, S., Younossi, Z.M., Remer, E.M. *et al.* (2002) The utility of radiological imaging in nonalcoholic fatty liver disease. *Gastroenterology*, **123**, 745–50

Targher, G. and Arcaro, G. (2007) Non-alcoholic fatty liver disease and increased risk of cardiovascular disease. *Atherosclerosis*, **191**, 235–50.

Targher, G., Bertolini, L., Padovani, R. *et al.* (2006a) Relation between carotid artery wall thickness and liver histology in subjects with nonalcoholic fatty liver disease. *Diabetes Care*, **29**, 1325–30.

Targher, G., Bertolini, L., Rodella, S. *et al.* (2006b) Associations between liver histology and cortisol secretion in subjects with nonalcoholic fatty liver disease. *Clinical Endocrinology*, **64**, 337–41.

Ueno, T., Sugawara, S., Sujaku, K. *et al.* (1997) Therapeutic effects of diet and exercise in obese patients with fatty liver. *Journal of Hepatology*, **27**, 103–10.

Van Gaal, L.F., Rissanen, A.M., Scheen, A.J. *et al.* (2005) Effects of the cannabinoid-1 receptor blocker rimonabant on weight reduction and cardiovascular risk factors in overweight patients: 1-year experience from the RIO-Europe study. *Lancet*, **365**, 1389–97.

Villanova, N., Moscatiello, S., Ramilli, S. *et al.* (2005) Endothelial dysfunction and cardiovascular risk profile in nonalcoholic fatty liver disease. *Hepatology*, **42**, 473–80.

Weisberg, S., McCann, D., Desai, M. *et al.* (2003) Obesity is associated with macrophage accumulation in adipose tissue. *The Journal of Clinical Investigation*, **112**, 1796–808.

Westerbacka, J., Lammi, K., Hakkinen, A.M. *et al.* (2005) Dietary fat content modifies liver fat in overweight nondiabetic subjects. *Journal of Clinical Endocrinology and Metabolism*, **90**, 2804–9.

Wieckowska, A., Zein, N.N., Yerian, L.M. *et al.* (2006) In vivo assessment of liver cell apoptosis as a novel biomarker of disease severity in nonalcoholic fatty liver disease. *Hepatology*, **44**, 27–33.

Wigg, A.J., Roberts-Thomson, I.C., Dymock, R.B. *et al.* (2001) The role of bacterial overgrowth, intestinal permeability, endotoxaemia, and tumour necrosis factor alpha in the pathogenesis of nonalcoholic steatohepatitis. *Gut*, **48**, 206–11.

Yokohama, S., Yoneda, M., Haneda, M. *et al.* (2004) Therapeutic efficacy of an angiotensinogen II receptor antagonist in patients with nonalcoholic steatohepatitis. *Hepatology*, **40**, 1222–5.

Cardiovascular Disease and Obesity

Key points

- Obesity is an independent risk factor for cardiovascular diseases, including hypertension, coronary-heart disease (CHD), cardiac failure, arrhythmias and cardiovascular death. The relationship is stronger with visceral obesity than with BMI. Epicardial fat and adipose tissue surrounding arteries may also influence cardiovascular outcomes, possibly through local effects of secreted products including adipokines and free fatty acids (FFA).

- Visceral obesity may increase cardiovascular risk by generating high FFA levels, which induce insulin resistance, stimulate very low density lipoprotein (VLDL) production by the liver, and promote triglyceride deposition in the myocardium. Compensatory hyperinsulinaemia may increase renal sodium retention, while raised leptin and insulin levels may activate the sympathetic nervous system (SNS), thus raising blood pressure. Atherogenic adipokines (e.g. PAI-1) are secreted by visceral fat, whereas levels of adiponectin, an anti-atherogenic and insulin-sensitizing adipokine, fall in obesity.

- Obesity, especially in the presence of hypertension and insulin resistance, causes important structural and functional changes in the heart. Increased volume and pressure loading of the left ventricle lead to left ventricular hypertrophy (LVH), which increases the risk of CHD, cardiac failure, arrhythmias and cardiac death. Right ventricular hypertrophy and left atrial enlargement may also occur.

- Obesity, especially visceral, strongly predicts hypertension, which affects 40% of obese subjects (six times more common than in lean people). Possible mechanisms include increased renin-angiotensin system (RAS) activity; raised levels of insulin and leptin, causing SNS activation; enhanced sodium retention due to hyperinsulinaemia; and loss of leptin's direct vasodilator action through 'leptin resistance'.

- Congestive heart failure is associated with obesity and can complicate LVH, especially in the presence of hypertension. Intracardiac triglyceride deposition may also impair contractile function. Paradoxically, low BMI may increase the risk of death in patients with severe heart failure, possibly because of the confounding effects of the associated hypercatabolic state ('cardiac cachexia').

- Obesity, especially visceral, is a major independent risk factor for CHD, its effects being amplified by coexistent risk factors such as hypertension, smoking, type 2 diabetes and dyslipidaemia. Peripheral arterial disease, including stroke and claudication, is also more common. Obesity causes endothelial dysfunction, an early marker of atherogenic risk; raised FFA levels and loss of leptin's vasodilator action may contribute.

- Obesity increases the risk of arrhythmias, especially chronic atrial fibrillation (associated with LVH and left atrial enlargement), QTc interval prolongation and sudden death.

- Some 'metabolically healthy obese' subjects are apparently spared cardiovascular complications, including hypertension, LVH and CHD, even in the presence of severe obesity. The reasons are unexplained.

- All obese patients require full cardiovascular assessment, including measurements of visceral obesity, blood pressure (measured with a wide cuff), and estimation of cardiovascular risk from smoking, blood glucose and lipids. ECG and echocardiography may require careful interpretation in the obese.

- Weight loss improves cardiovascular risk, lowering blood pressure, low density lipoprotein (LDL)-cholesterol and triglycerides, and raising high density lipoprotein (HDL)-cholesterol. Lifestyle modification can be supplemented in selected cases by anti-obesity drugs; bariatric surgery may be appropriate and can halve predicted cardiovascular risk.

- Hypertension should be managed by lifestyle improvement, aiming to reduce weight, increase exercise and limit sodium and alcohol intake. Antihypertensive drugs are indicated if lifestyle measures fail, and if blood pressure exceeds 140/90 mm Hg. ACE inhibitors (or angiotensin receptor blockers) are first-line therapy, supplemented if necessary by a thiazide diuretic, calcium-channel blocker or β-adrenoceptor blocker. Multiple drug therapy is usually required; drug choices should be informed by the patient's clinical condition, including complications such as angina.

Chapter 12 Cardiovascular Disease and Obesity

Gianluca Iacobellis and Arya M. Sharma

Obesity has long been considered an important cardiovascular risk factor – perhaps dating from Hippocrates' astute observation in 400 BC that 'sudden death was more common in those who are naturally fat than in the lean' (Chadwick and Mann, 1950). Obesity is often associated in the 'metabolic syndrome' with cardiovascular and metabolic abnormalities that predispose to hypertension and coronary-heart disease (CHD), and there is also evidence that obesity leads to other cardiovascular disorders, including congestive heart failure and cardiac arrhythmias (Poirier *et al.*, 2006; NIH, 1998; Sowers, 2003; Baik, Ascherio and Rimm, 2000; Widlansky *et al.*, 2004; Ajani, Lotufo and Gaziano, 2004) (see Table 12.1). The epidemiological evidence for these associations is reviewed in detail in Chapter 9.

The relationships between obesity and cardiovascular diseases are complex. The distribution of adiposity in the body seems to be more important than total fat mass, and visceral adiposity is a particularly powerful predictor of cardiovascular disease. Evidence is also emerging that adipose tissue adjacent to the heart and arteries may influence various cardiovascular functions and outcomes, while triglyceride deposited within the myocardium itself may adversely affect cardiac morphology and perhaps contribute to cardiac failure. The role of obesity per se is difficult to define, because it is often associated with comorbidities (insulin resistance, hypertension and dyslipidaemia) that themselves predispose to cardiovascular disease. Some studies suggest that 'uncomplicated' obesity in the absence of these comorbidities does not necessarily damage the cardiovascular system.

This chapter describes the cardiovascular disorders associated with obesity, together with their likely aetiology and clinical significance, and discusses recent findings that cast new light on the relationships between adiposity and the cardiovascular system.

General links between obesity and cardiovascular disease

As described in Chapter 9, the strength of the relationships between obesity and cardiovascular diseases depends on how obesity is measured. Many reports indicate that general increases in adiposity, reflected by a rising BMI, are associated with increasing risks of hypertension, coronary-heart disease (CHD) and death from cardiovascular causes. Paradoxically, however, a high BMI can apparently reduce the risk for certain cardiovascular end-points (see below). Moreover, measures of abdominal obesity such as waist circumference and waist:hip ratio (WHR) are much stronger predictors of cardiovascular disease, and this is the basis for the cut-off values for waist circumference used in clinical practice to define levels of risk associated with abdominal obesity (Figure 12.1).

The usefulness of BMI to predict cardiovascular outcomes has been challenged by numerous studies that demonstrated the greater importance of abdominal fat compared with total adiposity (Romero-Corral *et al.*, 2006; Després and Lemieux, 2006; Smith, 2006; Misra and Vikram, 2003; Janssen, Katzmarzyk and Ross, 2004; Kuk, Janiszewski and Ross, 2007; Rexrode *et al.*, 1998; Dagenais *et al.*, 2005; Yusuf *et al.*, 2005; Janssen, Katzmarzyk and Ross, 2005). For example, in a large prospective cohort study of women, Rexrode *et al.* (Janssen, Katzmarzyk and Ross, 2004) found that WHR and waist circumference were independently strongly associated with increasing risk for CAD, even among subjects whose BMI was $\leq 25 \, \text{kg/m}^2$. The Heart Outcomes Prevention Evaluation (HOPE) study confirmed that abdominal obesity specifically worsened the prognosis of patients with cardiovascular disease (Kuk, Janiszewski and

Obesity: Science to Practice   Edited by Gareth Williams and Gema Frühbeck

Table 12.1   Impact of obesity on the cardiovascular system.

Heart

- Hyperdynamic state
- Left ventricular hypertrophy, eccentric or concentric (with hypertension)
- Right ventricular hypertrophy
- Congestive cardiac failure
- Arrhythmias, especially atrial fibrillation
- Sudden death

Arterial disease

- Coronary-heart disease: angina, myocardial infarction
- Stroke
- Peripheral arterial disease
- Endothelial dysfunction and impaired vasorelaxation

Venous disease

- Deep venous thrombosis
- Pulmonary embolism

Hypertension

- Pulmonary hypertension

Side effects of anti-obesity drugs

- Fenfluramine (especially with phentermine): primary pulmonary hypertension and valvular heart disease
- Sibutramine: increase in heart rate, palpitation, occasional increase in blood pressure
- Orlistat: steatorrhea, interaction with Vit K (coumadin)
- Rimonabant: depression, suicidal ideation

Ross, 2007). The INTERHEART study has provided compelling evidence that measures of abdominal obesity, and not BMI, should be used to define cardiovascular risk (Yusuf et al., 2005). In this very large study (12 000 cases and 14 000 controls), WHR and waist circumference were strongly associated with the risk of myocardial infarction, across all ages and ethnic groups, and even after adjusting for other risk factors; by contrast, BMI showed a weaker and less consistent relationship. Using WHR rather than BMI increased by threefold the estimated risk of myocardial infarction attributed to obesity: the population-attributable risk (PAR) for the two highest quintiles of WHR was 24%, but only 8% for the two highest quintiles of BMI (see

Figure 12.2). Similarly, waist circumference and not BMI explained obesity-related health risks in adult Americans participating in the third National Health and Nutrition Examination Survey (NHANES III) (Dagenais et al., 2005).

Interestingly, a high BMI may be associated with better cardiovascular prognosis in some situations. For example, mortality was inversely related to BMI among Danish patients with acute myocardial infarction in the Trandalopril Cardiac Evaluation (TRACE) study; here, abdominal obesity was an independent predictor of all-cause mortality in men, but not in women (Køber et al., 2005). In older Chinese women, high BMI was also associated with lower mortality rates, after adjusting for waist circumference, although CAD risk among younger women did increase with BMI; across all ages, WHR was positively associated with CAD risk (Janssen, Katzmarzyk and Ross, 2005). As discussed below, a high BMI apparently protects against premature death in patients with severe heart failure (Fonarow et al., 2007; Horwich et al., 2001). The 'paradox' of high mortality at low BMI may be explained by smoking and other coexistent conditions that decrease body weight while shortening lifespan (see Chapter 9). Also, Kuk et al. (Kragelund et al., 2005) have reported that BMI is not correlated with visceral adiposity, after adjustment for age and waist circumference.

Taken together, all these data strongly support the proposal that visceral fat specifically confers cardiovascular and metabolic risk, and that BMI should be rejected in favour of measures of abdominal adiposity to stratify risk and perhaps to define obesity (Zhang et al., 2004).

Mechanisms of increased cardiovascular risk with visceral fat

The increased cardiovascular and metabolic risks conferred by intra-abdominal adipose tissue are probably due partly to its anatomical location – its secreted products are delivered directly to the liver via the portal system – and partly to its metabolic and secretory properties, which in turn are related to depot-specific patterns of expression of key receptors and adipokines (Figure 12.3).

Visceral fat shows more active lipolysis than subcutaneous fat, resulting from both enhanced sensitivity to catecholamine-induced lipolysis and relative insensitivity to the anti-lipolytic effect of insulin. The former is attributed to the relatively lower expression levels of the $\alpha2$-adrenoceptor (which inhibits lipolysis) compared with the β-adrenoceptors that stimulate

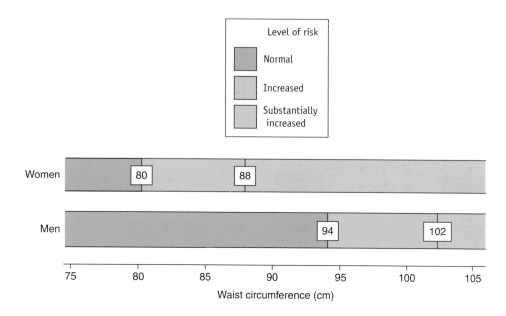

Figure 12.1 Thresholds of waist circumference in Caucasian men and women that define increased and substantially increased levels of cardiovascular and total risk.

it (see Chapter 4). The large amounts of free fatty acids (FFA) generated by lipolysis reach the liver, where they impair insulin's normal action to decrease hepatic glucose production by inhibiting gluconeogenesis and glycogen breakdown; unrestrained hepatic glucose production leads to hyperglycaemia and compensatory hyperinsulinaemia. High insulin levels may act

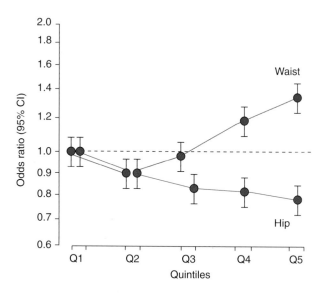

Figure 12.2 Waist circumference is a powerful predictor of myocardial infarction risk. In this study (INTER-HEART), the relationship between risk and the higher quintiles of waist circumference was much stronger than for equivalent quintiles of BMI. By contrast, hip circumference had an inverse relationship with infarction risk, with the higher quintiles apparently being protective. Data are adjusted for age, sex, BMI, smoking and other risk factors. From Yusuf *et al.* (2005) 'INTERHEART Study Investigators. Obesity and the risk of myocardial infarction in 27,000 participants from 52 countries: a case-control study'. *Lancet*, 366: 1640–9, with kind permission of *The Lancet*.

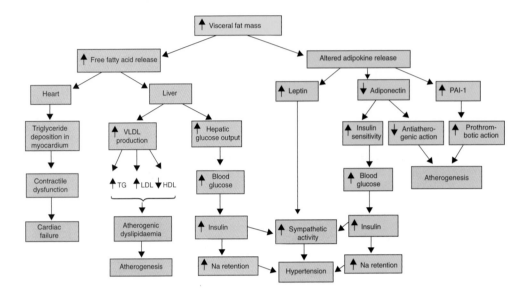

Figure 12.3 Properties of visceral adipose tissue and their cardiovascular consequences.

on the central nervous system (CNS) to stimulate the sympathetic nervous system (SNS), and on the kidney to increase sodium retention, both these effects tending to raise blood pressure.

Other hepatic consequences of high FFA uptake are excess triglyceride storage (causing steatosis, the first stage of non-alcoholic fatty liver disease, NAFLD) and increased VLDL secretion, leading eventually to the characteristic atherogenic dyslipidaemia of raised triglyceride and LDL levels, with reduced HDL-cholesterol (see Chapters 10 and 11). Raised systemic levels of FFA may also lead to enhanced triglyceride deposition in the myocardium, potentially impairing insulin signalling and contractile function (see below).

Visceral obesity also leads to disturbances in the relative proportions of circulating adipokines, and these may further increase cardiovascular risk (Fortuño et al., 2003). Visceral fat expresses and secretes high levels of leptin, which at least in experimental animals, acts centrally to stimulate the SNS, thus increasing pulse rate, peripheral resistance and blood pressure (Sader, Nian and Liu, 2003). This fat depot also secretes much PAI-1, which blocks the clearance of newly-formed thrombin and is thus prothrombotic and atherogenic. TNF-α, another adipokine secreted by visceral adipose tissue, interferes with signalling pathways

downstream of the insulin receptor; it may exert paracrine effects on adjacent cells (perhaps further reducing insulin sensitivity within the visceral fat depot) and possibly impair insulin action in the liver. By contrast, visceral adipose tissue secretes relatively little adiponectin, which – unlike other adipokines – shows a fall in its circulating levels in obesity and in insulin-resistant conditions. In experimental animals, adiponectin has anti-atherogenic and anti-inflammatory actions and enhances insulin sensitivity, and there is evidence that it may also exert such effects in humans (Fortuño et al., 2003; see Chapter 4).

Leptin and other adipokines have also been implicated in the adverse effects of obesity on left ventricular muscle (see below), and in sleep apnoea, which is also associated with hypertension and cardiovascular disease and death (see Chapter 13). Moreover, arteries have been shown to express receptors for several adipokines (Frühbeck, 2004), raising the possibility that these may have wider roles in cardiovascular regulation.

Impact of obesity on the heart

Various structural and functional changes in the heart – including left ventricular hypertrophy (LVH), heart failure and arrhythmias – have been linked with obesity. However, it is difficult to dissociate any effects of obesity per se from those of the comorbidities that commonly accompany it, notably hypertension (itself a cause of LVH, heart failure and arrhythmias) and the pro-atherogenic metabolic syndrome (see Table 12.2). Cardiac alterations in obese patients therefore reflect the collective impact of multiple haemodynamic, structural, functional, biochemical, metabolic and endocrine derangements. The outcomes differ according to the presence or absence of associated complications, notably hypertension and insulin resistance.

'Uncomplicated' obesity (i.e. without hypertension) results in an increase in blood volume, associated with the expanded tissue mass (Figure 12.4). Peripheral resistance is typically decreased in obesity (Iacobellis, 2004; Iacobellis et al., 2002; Iacobellis et al., 2004a), perhaps in part because of the increased

Table 12.2 Cardiovascular risk factors associated with a high BMI and/or waist circumference.

Metabolic

Dyslipidaemia

- Raised triglycerides
- Raised LDL (particularly small dense LDL particles) and VLDL-cholesterol
- Decreased HDL-cholesterol (especially HDL_2)

Insulin resistance

- Hyperinsulinaemia
- Glucose intolerance: impaired glucose tolerance (IGT), impaired fasting glucose (IFG)
- Type 2 diabetes

Hyperuricaemia

Haematological

- Procoagulant changes and decreased fibrinolysis
- Increased blood viscosity
- Low-grade chronic inflammation

Other

- Increased renin-angiotensin-aldosterone system (RAS) activity
- Increased sympathetic nervous system (SNS) activity
- Endothelial dysfunction
- Obstructive sleep apnoea

levels of leptin, which has a direct vasodilator action (see below); this is in contrast to the increased peripheral resistance seen in hypertension. Cardiac output rises in parallel with excess body weight, due mainly to increases in stroke volume, as pulse rate is only slightly elevated (Iacobellis et al., 2002). This hyperdynamic state increases the volume loading of the left ventricle in particular. Increased left ventricular (LV) wall stress tends to lead to LV dilatation and compensatory myocardial growth that results in LVH. In obesity, LVH is typically 'eccentric'; that is, the increase in LV wall thickness is in proportion to that of the LV cavity (see Figure 12.5). Increased left ventricular mass (LVM) is a significant abnormality, as it is an independent risk factor for coronary-heart disease (CHD), congestive heart failure, arrhythmias and cardiovascular and all-cause mortality (Gardin et al., 2001).

The reported relationship between obesity and LVM is variable. Many studies (e.g. Dorbala et al., 2006; Pascual, Pascual and Soria, 2003; Peterson et al., 2004; Crisostomo, Araujo and Camara, 1999) suggest that LVM is positively correlated with BMI, whereas others found no such relationship (Iacobellis, 2004; Iacobellis et al., 2002; Iacobellis et al., 2004b; Krishnan et al., 2005; Otto et al., 2004) (see Figure 12.6). The discrepancy may partly be explained by the weak links between BMI and cardiovascular disease, discussed above. Also, recent findings indicate that uncomplicated obesity (which was not considered separately in earlier studies) may not cause an inappropriate increase in LVM or alterations in LV morphology (Kuk, Janiszewski and Ross, 2007; Rexrode et al., 1998; Dagenais et al., 2005; Iacobellis, 2004; Iacobellis et al., 2002; Iacobellis et al., 2004a) – even when longstanding and in subjects with BMI $>50\,kg/m^2$ (Iacobellis et al., 2004b) (Figure 12.6). LV remodelling may not occur because of adaptive changes in the myocardium. These may involve the Wnt pathway, which is implicated in cardiac hypertrophy and which shows divergent regulation between obese and hypertensive hearts (Krishnan et al., 2005).

In obesity complicated by significant insulin resistance and hypertension – which commonly coexist in subjects with the metabolic syndrome – additional factors operate (Figure 12.7). High insulin levels related to insulin resistance are thought to increase the renal reabsorption of sodium (DeFronzo et al., 1975), further raising

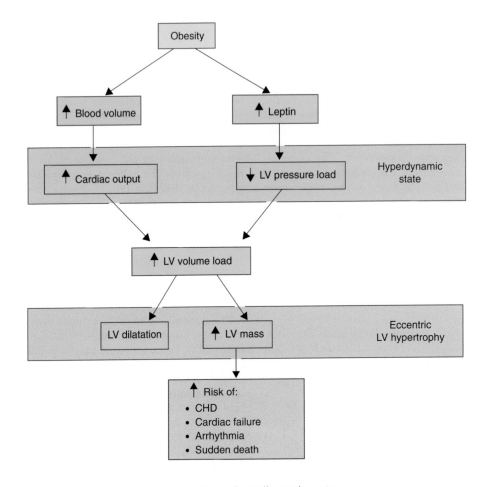

Figure 12.4 Impact of uncomplicated obesity on the cardiovascular system.

extracellular fluid and blood volumes and thus LV filling and volume loading. Increased blood viscosity, due to procoagulant changes triggered by inflammatory cytokines released from adipose tissue, worsens pressure loading. High insulin and leptin levels act on the central nervous system (CNS) to stimulate the sympathetic nervous system (SNS), causing arterial constriction and increased peripheral resistance and blood pressure, thus increasing LV pressure loading (Kamide, Rakugi and Higaki, 2002; Greenwood *et al.*, 2001). Moreover, leptin's direct vasodilator effect on arteries may be attenuated through 'leptin resistance' (Lembo *et al.*, 2000; Momin *et al.*, 2006), which would further elevate peripheral resistance – which is also raised in hypertension. The increases in LV volume and pressure loading, via LV wall stress, stimulate LV remodelling and LVH. In hypertension, LVH

progresses in a 'concentric' pattern, that is the LV wall thickness is increased disproportionately to the LV cavity (see Figure 12.5). With time, incremental rises in LV filling pressure and volume impair LV contractility, potentially leading to LV failure. As already mentioned, increased LVM is also an independent predictor of CHD, arrhythmias and death from both cardiovascular and other causes (Gardin *et al.*, 2001).

Certain metabolic and endocrine abnormalities of complicated obesity have been implicated in causing LVH in obesity. Hyperinsulinaemia may contribute (Iacobellis *et al.*, 2003a; Galvan, Galetta and Natali, 2000; Watanabe *et al.*, 1999; Malmqvist *et al.*, 2001; Sundström, Lind and Nyström, 2000), because LVM is identical to lean values in obese subjects with normal insulin sensitivity, but significantly raised in those who are insulin-resistant (Iacobellis *et al.*, 2003a). Insulin

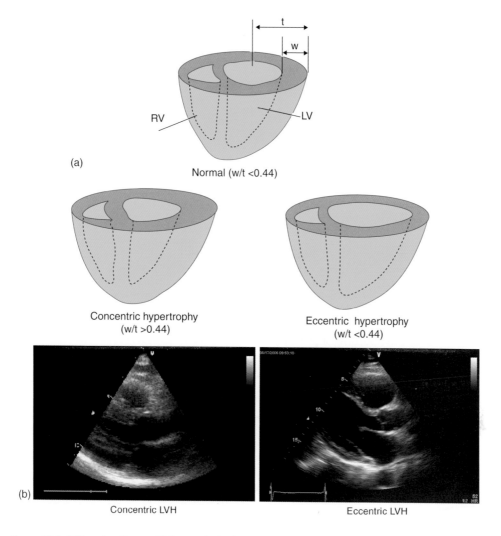

(a)

Normal (w/t <0.44)

Concentric hypertrophy
(w/t >0.44)

Eccentric hypertrophy
(w/t <0.44)

(b)

Concentric LVH

Eccentric LVH

Figure 12.5 Different patterns of left ventricular hypertrophy: (a) concentric hypertrophy, characteristic of hypertension – the left ventricular wall is disproportionately thickened, with the ratio of wall thickness/total left ventricular radius exceeding 0.44; (b) eccentric hypertrophy, typical of uncomplicated obesity – the left ventricular wall is thickened in proportion to the dilatation of the left ventricular cavity.

is known to stimulate myocardial growth and can induce pronounced LVH in the rat, acting either directly or via the IGF-1 receptor and/or by increasing IGF-1 bioavailability (Tanaka, Ryoke and Hongo, 1998; Delaughter *et al.*, 1999). As already mentioned, hyperinsulinaemia increases renal sodium retention and blood volume (DeFronzo *et al.*, 1975), and may act centrally to stimulate sympathetic outflow and peripheral vasoconstriction (Kamide, Rakugi and Higaki, 2002; Greenwood *et al.*, 2001); these effects would increase both volume and pressure loading on the left ventricle.

Certain adipokines may also modulate the left ventricle's response to obesity. Leptin has generated much interest but a clear picture is yet to emerge: some studies reported a positive correlation between leptin and LVM (Sader, Nian and Liu, 2003; Tritos, Manning and Danias, 2004; Paolisso *et al.*, 2000; Paolisso, Tagliamonte and Galderisi, 2001), whereas others found a negative correlation (Barouch, Berkowitz and Harrison, 2003) or no significant relationship (Pladevall, Williams and Guyer, 2003; Malmqvist *et al.*, 2002). Similarly, recent studies of the possible relationship between adiponectin

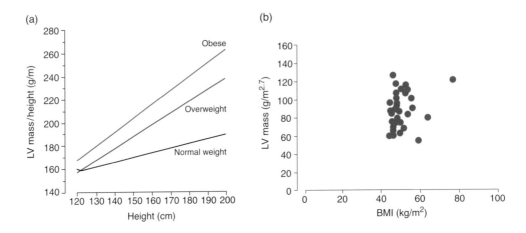

Figure 12.6 Different relationships reported between obesity and left ventricular mass (LVM). (a) The normal relationship between LVM/height has a steeper gradient in obese and overweight than in lean subjects, as reported by Gottdiener *et al.* (1994). (b) No significant relationship was found between indexed LVM and BMI in 'metabolically healthy obese' (MHO) subjects, even at BMI >50 kg/m² (Data adapted from Iacobellis *et al.* (2004)).

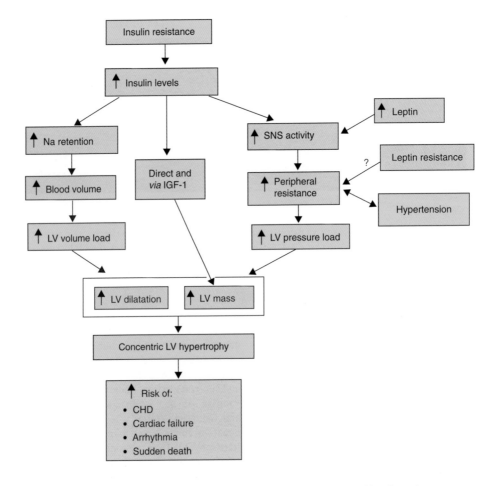

Figure 12.7 Cardiovascular impact of obesity in the presence of hypertension and insulin resistance.

levels and LVH have proved inconclusive (Hong *et al.*, 2004; Della Mea *et al.*, 2005; Mitsuhashi *et al.*, 2007; Iacobellis *et al.*, 2006a). Interestingly, uncomplicated obese subjects carrying a specific single nucleotide polymorphism (SNP) of the adiponectin gene (+276 G/G) show a relative increase in LVM (Iacobellis *et al.*, 2006a).

Impact on ventricular contractility

Obesity is associated with several abnormalities of ventricular contractility, affecting particularly the left ventricle, and apparent in both systole and diastole (Table 12.3).

Systolic dysfunction

The combination of increased stroke volume and cardiac output with decreased peripheral resistance results in hyperdynamic systolic function (Iacobellis, 2004; Iacobellis *et al.*, 2002; Iacobellis *et al.*, 2004a). Elevated LV end-diastolic pressure loading, together with LV hypertrophy, can predispose to LV systolic dysfunction. Usually, however, systolic function is not reduced at rest, and LV ejection fraction is often preserved even in severely obese subjects (Iacobellis, 2004; Iacobellis *et al.*, 2002; Iacobellis *et al.*, 2004a).

Novel, highly-sensitive imaging techniques have recently revealed subtle evidence of LV systolic dysfunction in obese subjects, even when LV ejection fraction remains normal (Peterson *et al.*, 2004; Wong *et al.*, 2004; Powell *et al.*, 2006). Tissue Doppler Imaging (TDI) and 'second harmonic imaging', which enhances

Table 12.3 Abnormalities of left ventricular function in obesity.

Systolic function

- Hyperdynamic state
- Reduced myocardial contractile velocity
- Increased long-axis strain

Diastolic function

- Prolonged relaxation
- Increased myocardial stiffness
- Delayed diastolic filling

Cardiac failure

the detection of the endocardial border of the LV cavity, have demonstrated abnormally low load-independent systolic myocardial velocity and increased long-axis strain in obese subjects. Significantly, these subclinical features of systolic dysfunction are accompanied by concentric LV remodelling (Peterson *et al.*, 2004). Obese subjects without cardiovascular disease may also have subtle changes of LV function even after adjustment for mean arterial pressure, age, gender and LVM (Peterson *et al.*, 2004; Wong *et al.*, 2004; Powell *et al.*, 2006).

Diastolic dysfunction

Obese patients commonly display features of diastolic dysfunction (Iacobellis, 2004; Iacobellis *et al.*, 2002; Iacobellis *et al.*, 2004a) (see Table 12.3). Diastolic dysfunction affects both morbid and uncomplicated obesity and is characterized either by early impairment of LV relaxation or increased myocardial stiffness (Figure 12.7).

The most common echocardiographic findings of diastolic dysfunction in obese subjects are a decreased early-to-late velocity ratio (E/A ratio), increased left atrial volume, prolongation of isovolumic relaxation time (IVRT) and abnormal TDI diastolic performance (Iacobellis, 2004; Iacobellis *et al.*, 2002; Iacobellis *et al.*, 2004a; Arias, Alonso-Fernandez, Garcia-Rio, 2006; Grandi, Zanzi and Fachinetti, 1999; Sasson *et al.*, 1996; Mureddu *et al.*, 1996). The delayed diastolic filling and prolonged LV relaxation may induce more forceful atrial contraction and progressive enlargement of the left atrium (Iacobellis, 2004; Iacobellis *et al.*, 2002; Iacobellis *et al.*, 2004a).

Abnormal LV relaxation occurs in both complicated and uncomplicated obesity, suggesting that diastolic function is impaired independently of the severity of obesity and the presence of comorbidities. It is still unclear whether this is an adaptive or pathological response. In uncomplicated obesity, diastolic dysfunction could be caused by the combined effect of haemodynamic and metabolic factors (Iacobellis, 2004), although these remain elusive. In complicated obesity, LV diastolic impairment may be related to insulin resistance and/or hyperinsulinaemia (Mureddu, Greco and Rosato, 1998), or to fasting hyperglycaemia (Jain, Avendano and Dharamsey, 1996). It has been suggested that insulin resistance can affect the biochemical mechanisms underlying diastolic relaxation, by impairing the inactivation of myocardial actin-myosin cross-links; this may be attributable to a lack of Ca^{2+} re-uptake from the sarcoplasmic reticulum (Mureddu, Greco and Rosato, 1998). High fasting insulin concentrations are significantly related to IVRT and less strongly to E/A, perhaps pointing to a greater effect of insulin on LV relaxation than on filling. However, abnormalities in insulin action do not seem sufficient to explain fully the diastolic impairment in obesity. Further studies are needed to clarify the underlying mechanisms, and whether impaired diastolic function can lead to systolic dysfunction in severely obese subjects.

Right ventricular changes

The right ventricle can also undergo remodelling and hypertrophy, especially in response to increased end-diastolic pressure and pulmonary hypertension (Valencia-Flores et al., 2004). Increased right ventricular mass is commonly observed in obese subjects; possible differences between complicated and uncomplicated obesity have not yet been systematically explored. Impaired relaxation and filling of the right ventricle have also been frequently observed in obese subjects.

Pulmonary hypertension may affect up to 70–90% of morbidly obese subjects (BMI $\geq 40 \, kg/m^2$), and its prevalence in patients with obstructive sleep apnoea is 15–20%. This was also a rare side effect of fenfluramine and dexfenfluramine, especially taken in combination with phentermine (see Chapter 17).

Atrial changes

Left atrial enlargement has been described in obese patients (Iacobellis et al., 2002) but has received little attention. This may partly reflect a physiological adaptation to the expanded blood volume, while impaired diastolic filling and abnormal LV relaxation may also contribute: delayed LV filling might induce more forceful atrial contraction and progressive enlargement of the left atrium. Left ventricular hypertrophy in long-standing obesity, especially

with hypertension, may also predispose to left atrial enlargement, but this can occur in normotensive obese individuals (Iacobellis et al., 2002).

Left atrial dilatation may explain the increased risk of atrial fibrillation associated with obesity (Iacobellis, 2005a). The coexistence of diastolic dysfunction and atrial fibrillation could be early features of the impaired systolic performance observed in morbidly obese subjects, as described above.

Obesity and hypertension

The importance of hypertension as a cardiovascular risk factor is indisputable, but the relationship between body weight and blood pressure is complex and incompletely understood.

Excess weight is one of the strongest predictors of the development of hypertension. Overall, hypertension is about six times more frequent in obese than in lean subjects (Poirier et al., 2006). The prevalence of hypertension (blood pressure $\geq 140/90 \, mm \, Hg$) rises progressively with increasing BMI among both men and women, from 15% among subjects with BMI $<25 \, kg/m^2$ to approximately 40% among those with BMI $\geq 30 \, kg/m^2$ (Drøyvold et al., 2005). Much clinical evidence suggests a causative link between increased adiposity and increased blood pressure, including the well-documented independent effect of decreases in BMI on lowering systolic and diastolic blood pressure in both women and men (Figure 12.8). A meta-analysis of randomized control trials (Drøyvold et al., 2005) concluded that diastolic pressure fell on average by 1 mm Hg per 1 kg of weight loss. In addition, some reports showed that weight loss enhances the response to antihypertensive treatment (Drøyvold et al., 2005).

All these observations confirm that obesity and hypertension are closely associated, and yet obesity as measured by BMI does not consistently predict hypertension-related cardiovascular risk. Indeed, a high BMI ($\geq 31 \, kg/m^2$) seems to mitigate cardiovascular changes in the systemic vascular bed caused by hypertension (Sharma and Chetty, 2005). Among older patients with hypertension, a wide range of BMI was associated with similar risks of death and stroke, whereas a low BMI ($<22 \, kg/m^2$) was associated with a higher risk of death than

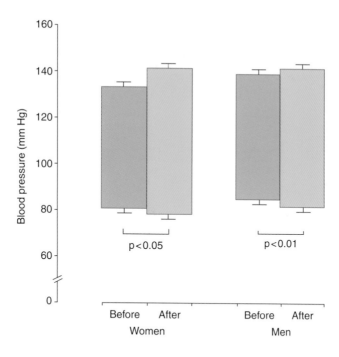

Figure 12.8 Diastolic blood pressure falls with weight loss in overweight men and women. In this study, average BMI fell by 2 kg/m² in both sexes. From W.B. Drøyvold, K. Midthjell, T.I. Nilsen and J. Holmen (2005) 'Change in body mass index and its impact on blood pressure: a prospective population study'. *International Journal of Obesity (London)*, 29: 650–5, with kind permission of the editor.

with a BMI in the median range of 26–29 kg/m² (Sharma *et al.*, 2001).

Measures of abdominal adiposity are better than BMI for stratifying cardiovascular risk related to high blood pressure, and visceral fat appears to play an important role in the development of hypertension. For example, greater abdominal visceral adiposity is associated with a significantly higher prevalence of hypertension, especially in non-obese men and women (Sharma, 2004a) and even in a lean Chinese population (Sharma *et al.*, 2002). Visceral adipose tissue masses outside the abdomen, such as mediastinal and epicardial fat, may also contribute (Schmieder and Messerli, 1993). Significantly larger volumes of mediastinal fat were found in hypertensive men than in normotensive men, matched for BMI and age (Wassertheil-Smoller *et al.*, 2000). Moreover, increased epicardial adipose tissue also correlates with increased diastolic blood pressure (Schmieder and Messerli, 1993). These observations raise the intriguing possibility that these previously neglected fat depots may be causally related to the development of

comorbidities such as hypertension and insulin resistance. Possible mechanisms, including the release of hormones and vasoactive cytokines, are discussed further below.

Mechanisms of hypertension in obesity

Many theories have been advanced to explain how an increase in fat mass might raise blood pressure (Figure 12.9). As yet, the role of visceral adipose tissue, including depots outside the abdomen, has not been fully clarified.

Hypertension has long been associated with various measures of insulin resistance in epidemiological studies, and a strong inverse relationship has been reported between insulin sensitivity and blood pressure (Figure 12.10). Possible explanations for the connection include the pressor effects of hyperinsulinaemia, namely to increase renal sodium reabsorption and thus blood volume, and central stimulation of the SNS to increase arterial vasoconstriction and renin release, thus activating

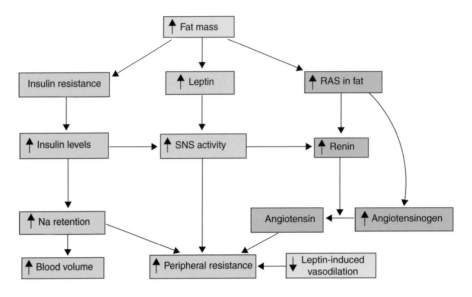

Figure 12.9 Possible mechanisms to explain the association of hypertension with obesity.

the systemic renin-angiotensin system (RAS) (Mikhail, Golub and Tuck, 1999; Pausova, 2006). These abnormalities probably underlie the increased peripheral resistance and volume expansion that are key to obesity-related hypertension.

The hormones and adipokines secreted by adipose tissue are also implicated. Both vascular smooth muscle cells and endothelial cells express functional leptin receptors (Gomez-Ambrosi *et al.*, 2006), and leptin at physiological concentrations is a direct,

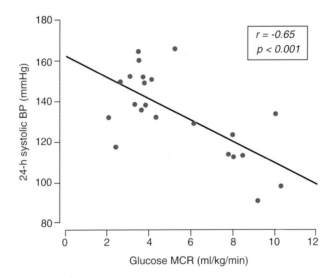

Figure 12.10 Hypertension is associated with insulin resistance. Average systolic blood pressure (measured over 24 hours using ambulatory monitoring) was inversely correlated with insulin sensitivity, assessed from the metabolic clearance rate of glucose during a hyperinsulinaemic euglycaemic clamp (see Chapter 3). From J.H. Pinkney *et al.* (1994) *Hypertension* 24, 362–4, with permission of the editor.

endothelium-dependent vasodilator (Lembo et al., 2000; Bełtowski, Wójcicka and Jamroz-Wiśniewska, 2006). It has been suggested that, in obese subjects, leptin resistance blunts this potential hypotensive action, and this would tend to raise peripheral resistance. Moreover, like insulin, leptin acting centrally activates the SNS in rodents (Correia et al., 2001) and may have similar effects in humans. Plasma leptin levels are commonly elevated in subjects with hypertension and are associated with increases in heart rate, plasma renin activity, and aldosterone and angiotensinogen levels (Mikhail, Golub and Tuck, 1999; Barton et al., 2003).

Activation of the systemic and adipose tissue RAS has also been implicated in obesity-related hypertension. Adipose tissue expresses all the components of the RAS, and upregulation of the genes encoding angiotensinogen, renin, angiotensin-converting enzyme (ACE) and the angiotensin II type 1 (AT_1) receptor has been observed in adipose tissue, in association with obesity-related hypertension (Lin et al., 2006; Iacobellis, 2005b; Sharma, 2004b). Expression of the AT_1 receptor gene is twofold greater in adipocytes from obese hypertensive than in obese normotensive persons. Animal studies indicate that adipocyte-derived angiotensinogen acts locally to stimulate adipocyte growth and differentiation, as well as lipid synthesis and storage in adipocytes (Kuk et al., 2006; Lin et al., 2006; Iacobellis, 2005b; Sharma, 2004b). Angiotensinogen produced in adipocytes may be released into the bloodstream, contributing to the circulating pool of angiotensinogen and angiotensin II. As well as potentially raising blood pressure, this might be expected to enhance the ectopic storage of triglyceride in tissues such as skeletal muscle and liver, thereby decreasing insulin sensitivity. Evidence from animal studies suggests that angiotensin-receptor blockers can promote redistribution of excess fat from these ectopic sites to mature adipocytes, resulting in improved insulin sensitivity (Lin et al., 2006; Iacobellis, 2005b; Sharma, 2004b).

Increased adiposity is also accompanied by downregulation of adiponectin, which enhances insulin sensitivity and inhibits atherosclerosis, and reduced adiponectin is associated with increased levels of inflammatory markers such as CRP and TNF-α. Endothelial abnormalities such as decreased nitric oxide responsiveness are common in obesity.

Impact of hypertension on cardiovascular risk in obesity

The presence of hypertension enhances the cardiovascular risk associated with obesity, notably for CHD, heart failure and arrhythmias. This is partly explained by the risks associated with LVH (Gardin et al., 2001).

Obesity and congestive heart failure

Congestive heart failure (CHF) is common, and increasing in its incidence and mortality rates are increasing. It has long been associated with obesity and with LVH, but as with other cardiovascular end-points, the relationship with obesity is not simple (Habbu, Lakkis and Dokainish, 2006).

Recent studies on patients with CHF point to an unexpected 'obesity paradox', in that increased BMI seems to protect against premature death in some circumstances. For example, in various cohorts of hospitalized patients with CHF, higher BMI was associated with lower in-hospital mortality risk (Fonarow et al., 2007; Curtis et al., 2005; Horwich et al., 2001; Lissin et al., 2002; Davos et al., 2003; Gustafsson et al., 2005). As discussed in Chapter 9, this may be partly explained by confounding factors, including smoking and the catabolic state termed 'cardiac cachexia', which reduce weight while increasing the risk of premature death. Consistent with this, Curtis et al. (2005) showed that overweight and obese patients were at lower risk of death than normal-weight patients, whereas underweight patients with stable CHF were at increased risk of death. Horwich et al. (2001) assessed patients with severe systolic CHF being evaluated for cardiac transplantation. During a 5-year follow up, unadjusted mortality was not statistically different among underweight, normal-weight, overweight and obese patients. However, after adjusting for age, gender, hypertension, diabetes and other haemodynamic variables, obese patients had a statistically significant survival benefit after 1 and 2 years, but not at 5 years. Lissin et al., (2002) found that obese patients had the best survival in unadjusted analysis among individuals with CHF, whereas Davos et al. (2003) found only a non-significant trend toward worse survival in obese subjects with chronic systolic CHF. The association between increasing BMI and lower mortality in CHF may depend on LV systolic function, in that systolic dysfunction confers an increased risk (Gustafsson *et al.*, 2005).

Obesity and coronary artery disease

In many studies, BMI has been strongly and independently associated with coronary-heart disease (CHD) and acute coronary syndrome, defined as unstable angina or acute myocardial infarction. In addition, the risk of developing CHD associated with obesity is substantially increased by other coexistent atherosclerotic risk factors, notably hypertension, smoking, type 2 diabetes and dyslipidaemia. Accordingly, the American Heart Association and American College of Cardiology guidelines for secondary prevention in CHD have identified obesity as a major modifiable cardiovascular risk factor (Smith *et al.*, 2001). This historic view is now being reappraised, with attention again focusing on the role of visceral adiposity.

One of the earliest epidemiological surveys to examine the influence of body weight on the development of cardiovascular disease was the Framingham Heart Study (Hubert, Feinleib, McNamara, 1983; Wilson *et al.*, 2002). Relationships between categories of BMI, cardiovascular disease risk factors and vascular disease end-points were examined in a population of American men aged 35 to 75 years, who were followed for up to 44 years. This, and other prospective studies with follow up data from over 20 years (such as the Manitoba Study, and the Harvard School of Public Health Nurses Study), found that obesity is an independent predictor of clinical CHD (Rabkin, Mathewson and Hsu, 1977; Kaplan *et al.*, 2002). In addition, excess adiposity, as measured by BMI, was associated with an increased risk of recurrent coronary events following acute myocardial infarction, in a large cohort of subjects who had survived a first infarct; risk was particularly high with BMI >30 kg/m² (Rea *et al.*, 2001). The Prevention of Events with Angiotensin Converting Enzyme-Inhibition (PEACE) Trial showed that in the presence of established CHD, obesity is associated with risk for major cardiovascular events in men, although not in women

(Domanski *et al.*, 2006). BMI has also been found to show a positive, graded relationship with death following acute myocardial infarction (Rana *et al.*, 2004; Hoit *et al.*, 1987).

Recent studies of the associations between obesity, cardiovascular events and total mortality in patients with coronary artery disease have highlighted the importance of visceral obesity and therefore the need to stratify cardiovascular risk according to measures of abdominal adiposity, rather than BMI. A recent meta-analysis of 40 studies comprising 250 152 patients (Romero-Corral *et al.*, 2006) showed that obese patients (BMI 30–35 kg/m²) had no increased risk for total mortality or cardiovascular mortality from CHD; those with BMI ≥35 kg/m² did not have increased total mortality but had the highest risk for cardiovascular mortality. By contrast, a low BMI (<20 kg/m²) was strongly associated with increased long-term risk of total mortality and cardiovascular events. Obesity was associated with higher all-cause mortality only in patients with history of cardiac by-pass (Romero-Corral *et al.*, 2006). Moreover, the recent literature suggests that obesity (BMI >30 kg/m²) is not associated with increased mortality and morbidity following coronary revascularization; indeed, a BMI of >30 kg/m² apparently conferred a short-term protective effect in patients undergoing percutaneous transluminal coronary angioplasty (Diercks *et al.*, 2006; Gurm *et al.*, 2002; Kim *et al.*, 2003; Reeves *et al.*, 2003; Brandt *et al.*, 2001; Minutello *et al.*, 2004).

Nevertheless, a high BMI must still be considered a major risk factor for developing CHD in young people (<40 years) (Imamura *et al.*, 2004) and underlines the need for aggressive management of obesity in this population.

Obesity and arrhythmias

Obese subjects of both sexes have been reported to be at higher risk of arrhythmias and sudden death as compared with non-obese individuals, even in the absence of clinical cardiac dysfunction (Poirier *et al.*, 2006).

Ventricular repolarization and QTc prolongation

Obesity has been associated with changes in ventricular repolarization, affecting the corrected QT (QTc) interval (Alpert *et al.*, 2000;

Lalani *et al.*, 2000; Kannel, Plehn and Cupples, 1988). Prolongation of the QTc interval is a well-known risk factor for potentially fatal ventricular arrhythmias, notably ventricular tachycardia and fibrillation. Positive correlations between BMI and QTc prolongation and QTc dispersion have been reported, whereas significant shortening of the QTc interval has been correlated with weight loss following bariatric surgery (el-Gamal *et al.*, 1995; Seyfeli *et al.*, 2006). Prolonged QTc interval was observed in 30% of subjects with impaired glucose tolerance (Papaioannou *et al.*, 2003) suggesting that obesity-related comorbidities, rather than adiposity alone, could impair ventricular repolarization; indeed, as described above for LV mass, no significant differences in baseline QTc interval and QTc dispersion parameters were found between lean and uncomplicated obese subjects (Pontiroli *et al.*, 2004; Brown *et al.*, 2001).

Atrial fibrillation

Many studies have indicated a relationship between obesity and atrial fibrillation, the most common arrhythmia. This was confirmed by a recent analysis by Wang *et al.* on a cohort of subjects from the Framingham Heart Study (Girola *et al.*, 2001). The risk of developing atrial fibrillation increased progressively with increasing BMI, independently of age, sex and hypertension. BMI seems to predispose especially to sustained atrial fibrillation rather than transitory or intermittent episodes. The association appears to be partially mediated by coexistent diabetes, with little apparent contribution from other cardiovascular risk factors (Iacobellis *et al.*, 2005c). Recent studies showed that obesity is an important determinant of new-onset atrial fibrillation after cardiac surgery (Wang *et al.*, 2004).

Various mechanisms have been suggested. Left atrial dilatation could be involved, perhaps due to impaired diastolic filling and abnormal LV relaxation; these abnormalities are frequently described in obese subjects (Iacobellis, 2005a). Delayed LV filling might induce more forceful atrial contractions and progressive enlargement of the left atrium. Recently, obesity-related obstructive sleep apnoea syndrome was suggested to induce cardiac changes such as increased left atrial

size and diastolic dysfunction, which could predispose to atrial fibrillation (Dublin *et al.*, 2006; Zacharias *et al.*, 2005).

In obese patients who develop atrial fibrillation, echocardiographic determination of left atrial structure and diastolic function are recommended, although this technique can be technically difficult in severely obese subjects. Since obesity is a potentially modifiable risk factor, its effective management should be considered in the treatment of atrial fibrillation.

Cardiac-associated adipose tissue

The mechanistic and functional links between increased adiposity and cardiac abnormalities remain controversial and incompletely understood. Recent research suggests that visceral adipose tissue lying outside the heart (epicardial fat), and triglyceride deposited within the myocardium, may both play important roles.

Epicardial adipose tissue

The presence of epicardial adipose tissue on the human myocardium and around the great vessels has been recognized since the mid-nineteenth century (Iacobellis *et al.*, 2005d; Reiner, Mazzoleni and Rodriguez, 1955). In the adult human heart, epicardial fat is commonly found in the atrioventricular and interventricular grooves, extending to the apex, with minor foci located subepicardically in the free walls of the atria and around the atrial appendages (Reiner *et al.*, 1959; Iacobellis *et al.*, 2003b; Iacobellis *et al.*, 2003c). In complicated obesity and hypertension, and especially in the presence of LVH, fat often fills the epicardial space and surrounds much of the surface of the heart (Figure 12.11). Epicardial fat usually amounts to only 0.02% of total adipose mass, but it appears largely unrelated to total adiposity body mass or BMI (Iacobellis and Leonetti, 2005; Iacobellis *et al.*, 2004b; Iacobellis *et al.*, 2007a; Iacobellis *et al.*, 2007b; Kankaanpaa *et al.*, 2006; Sacks and Fain, 2007).

Growing evidence suggests that this visceral fat depot could be an active tissue that locally modulates cardiac and vascular

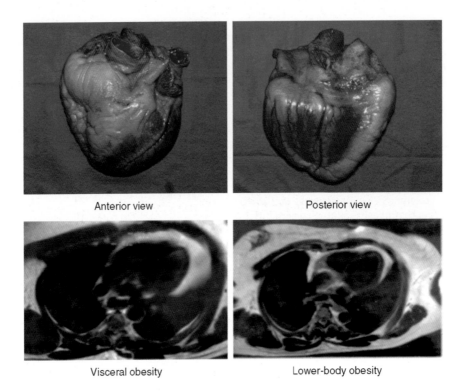

Anterior view   Posterior view

Visceral obesity   Lower-body obesity

Figure 12.11 Epicardial adipose tissue is increased in obesity, especially in association with left ventricular hypertrophy. (Upper panel) Macroscopic view of a hypertrophic heart weighing 900 g (normal weight is about 300 g), showing extensive epicardial fat deposits. G. Iacobellis, D. Corradi D and A.M. Sharma. (2005d) 'Epicardial adipose tissue: anatomic, biomolecular and clinical relation to the heart'. Courtesy of *Nature Clinical Practice Cardiovascular Medicine*, 2: 536–43. (Lower panel) MRI scan of the heart in a subject with visceral obesity (left), showing left ventricular hypertrophy and thicker epicardial fat than in a subject with lower-body obesity (right), who had normal visceral and epicardial fat masses. From G. Iacobellis, F. Assael, M.C. Ribaudo *et al.* (2003b) 'Epicardial fat from echocardiography: a new method for visceral adipose tissue prediction'. Courtesy of *Obesity Research*, 11: 304–10, with permission of the editor.

morphology and function in obesity (Jeong *et al.*, 2007). The close anatomical relationship between epicardial adipose tissue and the adjacent myocardium (they are not separated by fascia) could allow local paracrine interactions between these tissues (Figure 12.12). Nevertheless, its potential pathogenic role and use as marker of visceral adiposity and cardiovascular risk factor have only recently been considered (Iacobellis and Leonetti, 2005; Iacobellis *et al.*, 2004b; Iacobellis *et al.*, 2007a; Iacobellis *et al.*, 2007b; Kankaanpaa *et al.*, 2006; Sacks and Fain, 2007; Jeong *et al.*, 2007; Malavazos *et al.*, 2007; Willens *et al.*, 2007; Corradi *et al.*, 2004; Shirani, Berezowski and Roberts, 1995; Tansey, Aly and Sheppard, 2005).

Metabolic aspects of epicardial fat

The physiological role of epicardial adipose tissue in animals and humans is not completely clear. In neonatal animals, including humans, it contains both brown adipocytes and uncoupling protein-1; this suggests a role in thermogenesis that may be crucial in very early life, but it cannot explain the persistence of this fat depot into adult life, especially in non-hibernating species (Marchington, Mattacks and Pond, 1989; Pond, 2003; Pond, 2003; Marchington and Pond, 1990; Pond *et al.*, 1993; Pond and Mattacks, 1991). Epicardial adipose tissue has a higher turnover of FFA than in other fat depots; activities of lipogenic enzymes (e.g. acetyl CoA carboxylase) and of lipoprotein lipase are correspondingly low

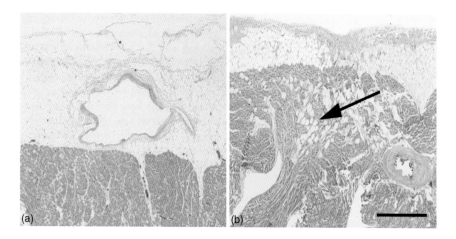

Figure 12.12 Microscopic appearance of the epicardial fat layer overlying (a) the left and (b) the right ventricles in a normal subject. Note the absence of any fascial layer separating the epicardial fat from the myocardium. The bar is 100 μm. From G. Iacobellis *et al.* (2005d) 'Is obesity a risk factor for atrial fibrillation?' *Nature Clinical Practice Cardiovascular Medicine*, 2, 134–5, with permission of the editor.

(Marchington, Mattacks and Pond, 1989; Pond, 2003; Pond, 2003; Marchington and Pond, 1990; Pond *et al.*, 1993; Pond and Mattacks, 1991). FFA are the main energy substrate for the myocardium, supplying 50–70% of its total needs under physiological conditions. However, high FFA levels are potentially dangerous because they can trigger arrhythmias. Epicardial fat could therefore serve two distinct functions – as a buffer, absorbing FFA and protecting the heart against high FFA levels, and perhaps as a local energy source at times of high demand, channelling FFA to the myocardium (Marchington, Mattacks and Pond, 1989; Pond, 2003; Marchington and Pond, 1990; Pond *et al.*, 1993; Pond and Mattacks, 1991). Epicardial fat may also influence general metabolism, because its volume is significantly related to insulin resistance and glucose intolerance in obese subjects (Iacobellis and Leonetti, 2005). However, the underlying mechanisms and the relationship with other depots of visceral fat remain to be determined.

Epicardial fat is also an important source of pro-inflammatory adipokines (TNF-α, IL-1, IL-6 and nerve growth factor) and of the anti-inflammatory adiponectin (Mazurek *et al.*, 2003; Iacobellis *et al.*, 2005e; Baker *et al.*, 2006; Chaldakov *et al.*, 2004; Date *et al.*, 2006; Kremen *et al.*, 2006). These products could affect the heart and coronary arteries through paracrine mechanisms and may also exert synergic effects.

Interestingly, macrophage infiltration into epicardial fat has been reported in subjects with CHD (Mazurek *et al.*, 2003), recalling the chronic inflammatory infiltration seen in the coronary artery wall and surrounding tissues adjacent to advanced atheromatous lessons. Inflammatory mediators such as TNF-α, released from epicardial fat in response to foci of inflammation around atheromatous plaques, may amplify the vascular inflammation and predispose to plaque rupture by inducing apoptosis and neovascularization in and around the plaque. Through its secretion of adiponectin, epicardial fat may also exert beneficial effects on the underlying coronary arteries; we recently found that adiponectin expression in epicardial fat is significantly higher in subjects with normal coronary arteries than in those with severe CHD (Iacobellis *et al.*, 2005e). Overall, the profile of adipokines secreted by epicardial fat could influence the evolution and outcome of CHD. Those adipokines may also act systemically: production of pro-inflammatory adipokines from epicardial fat has recently been implicated in the development of insulin resistance following cardiac surgery (Kremen *et al.*, 2006).

Iacobellis *et al.* (2004b) showed that epicardial adipose tissue may also affect the geometry and contractility of the heart. Echocardiographic studies found that epicardial fat volume correlates with LVM across a wide range of adiposity (Iacobellis *et al.*, 2004b), while its thickness is also related to right ventricular mass (Iacobellis *et al.*, 2007b).

Left ventricular hypertrophy is associated with a proportional increase in epicardial fat mass (Iacobellis *et al.*, 2005d; Iacobellis *et al.*, 2003b). In hypertrophic hearts, epicardial fat constitutes ~20% of total ventricular mass (see Figure 12.11) and will increase the work done by the heart (Corradi *et al.*, 2004), thus contributing to ventricular hypertrophy. Cardiac adiposity may also affect diastolic function, because increased epicardial fat thickness is significantly correlated with impairments of LV diastolic filling; this could lead to left atrial enlargement and the risk of atrial fibrillation (Iacobellis *et al.*, 2007b).

Overall, therefore, epicardial adipose tissue appears to be structurally and functionally important to the heart. Its suggested functions deserve further active exploration.

Intracardiac fat deposition

Ectopic triglyceride deposition in various tissues – notably liver and skeletal muscle – is a feature of obesity and may have pathological consequences such as insulin resistance. Excess triglyceride also accumulates within cardiomyocytes in obesity. Emerging evidence suggests that this may be directly toxic to the myocardium and that 'lipotoxicity' actively contributes to various cardiac disorders (McGavock *et al.*, 2006; Iacobellis and Sharma, 2006; Zhou *et al.*, 2000).

Intracellular lipid can be measured noninvasively using MR spectroscopy, and studies in lean and obese subjects show that myocardial triglyceride content rises progressively with BMI (Chiu *et al.*, 2001; Szczepaniak *et al.*, 2003; Reingold *et al.*, 2005). Suggested manifestations of cardiac lipotoxicity include LV hypertrophy and congestive heart failure. Experimental studies in isolated cardiomyocytes have shown alterations in substrate energy metabolism leading to impaired synthesis of ATP, which is pivotal for myocardial contraction and relaxation. Concomitant decreases in myocardial glucose uptake and oxidation, together with increased fatty acid oxidation, lead to reduced ATP availability and excessive triglyceride accumulation in cardiomyocytes (Wong and Marwick, 2007). Moreover, the switch from fat to glucose oxidation, which is initially adaptive, ultimately results in a decreased insulin sensitivity. Myocardial lipid concentrations are also elevated in obesity in relation with increased apoptosis, and the underexpression of fatty acid oxidative enzymes and the transcription factor, peroxisome proliferator-activated receptor-α, which regulates their activity; after age and BMI, the myocardial triglyceride level was the next most predictive variable of diastolic myocardial velocity, an index of LV relaxation (Zhou *et al.*, 2000; Chiu *et al.*, 2001; Szczepaniak *et al.*, 2003; Reingold *et al.*, 2005).

Overall, myocardial triglyceride deposition may account for at least part of the cardiomyopathy associated with obesity that cannot be explained by associated CAD or hypertension. In turn, this may contribute to the increasing incidence of congestive heart failure associated with obesity.

Peripheral vascular disease

Obesity is well known to be associated with peripheral vascular disease and with cardiovascular outcomes including stroke and intermittent claudication (Chadwick and Mann, 1950). The aetiology is multifactorial, and as with CAD, is often largely attributable to the combined insults of accompanying hypertension, dyslipidaemia and diabetes. However, certain aspects deserve specific mention.

Endothelial dysfunction

The endothelium is crucial to several important functions of arteries, including the regulation of coagulation, the prevention of thrombus formation and the control of vasomotor tone. The latter is particularly dependent on the production of powerful vasodilators, prostacyclin and nitric oxide (NO) by the endothelium; these diffuse to the underlying vascular smooth muscle and cause relaxation.

NO is particularly important. It is produced from arginine under the action of the specific endothelial isoform of the enzyme NO synthase, eNOS; expression of eNOS is upregulated, and NO production therefore enhanced, by various factors such as insulin, bradykinin and acetylcholine, acting through their respective receptors on the endothelium (Mombouli and Vanhoutte, 1999). Leptin has also been shown to induce

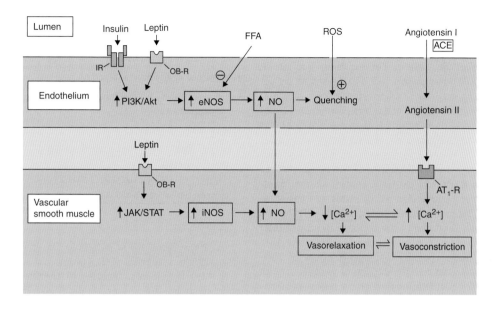

Figure 12.13 Role of the endothelium in causing arterial relaxation, showing the abnormalities in obesity that lead to endothelial dysfunction.

NO-dependent vasorelaxation (Lembo *et al.*, 2000). These 'endothelium-dependent' vaso-dilators are distinct from the 'endothelium-independent' vasodilators such as sodium nitro-prusside, which breaks down to yield NO directly. NO can be inactivated or 'quenched' by various compounds, including reactive oxygen species (ROS) generated, for example, by the advanced glycation end-products (AGE), which accumulate in diabetes and are taken up into cells via specific receptors (RAGE) (Figure 12.13).

Endothelium-dependent vasodilatation (usually in response to acetylcholine) can be measured using forearm blood-flow techniques. Impairment of this response – that is, endothelial motor dysfunction – is a striking feature of type 2 diabetes, insulin resistance, dyslipidaemia (especially hypertriglyceridaemia) and obesity (Steinberg *et al.*, 1996; Watts *et al.*, 1996; Shimokawa, 1999). Impaired vasorelaxation will raise peripheral resistance and therefore blood pressure. Moreover, this abnormality is particularly important because prospective studies have shown it to be a powerful predictor of atherogenesis, CAD and myocardial infarction (Schächinger, Britten and Zeiher, 2000). Loss of insulin action in inducing eNOS – a potential manifestation of insulin insensitivity – was previously held responsible for endothelial dysfunction in insulin-resistant states, but raised triglyceride and/or FFA levels now appear more likely (Lewis, Dart and Chin-Dusting, 1999; Steinberg *et al.*, 1997). The underlying mechanisms remain uncertain. Interestingly, endothelial dysfunction can be induced in humans and experimental animals by eating a high-fat meal that causes pronounced hyper-triglyceridaemia. This effect is surprisingly long-lasting – at least 24 hours in humans – indicating that an obesogenic diet, as well as adiposity per se, should be considered as a possible contributor to cardiovascular disease (Noronha *et al.*, 2005).

Perivascular adipose tissue

Perivascular fat, until recently dismissed as a structural support for arteries, is now thought to be involved in controlling vascular tone and it is possible that this effect may be disturbed in obesity.

An effect of perivascular fat on vascular tone was first described by Soltis, who found that noradrenaline-induced contraction of rat aorta was attenuated if the surrounding fat was not removed; he attributed this to uptake of nor-adrenaline by the fat (Soltis and Cassis, 1991). It is now clear that perivascular fat actively regulates arterial tone through various mechanisms

(Engeli, 2005; Henrichot *et al.*, 2005; Gollasch and Dubrovska, 2004; Löhn *et al.*, 2002; Dubrovska *et al.*, 2004; Verlohren *et al.*, 2004; Gao *et al.*, 2005). For example, Gao *et al.* (2005) have shown that it releases an as-yet uncharacterized adipocyte-derived vascular relaxation factor or factors. Gao *et al.* (2006) further demonstrated that perivascular fat produces superoxide, which enhances the arterial contractile response mediated by NAD(P)H oxidase and via activation of the tyrosine kinase and MAPK/ERK pathway. Leptin, another product of perivascular fat, operates as a vasodilator through a NO-mediated pathway (Frühbeck, 1999), and blunts the increase in intracellular Ca^{2+} induced by angiotensin-II (Figure 12.13).

Another possible pathogenic effect of perivascular fat is the induction of vascular smooth muscle proliferation through the release of adipocyte-derived growth factor(s) (Barandier, Montani and Yang, 2005). This could lead to thickening of the arterial media and the increased vascular stiffness seen in obesity (Montani *et al.*, 2004; Galvez *et al.*, 2006).

Thus, perivascular fat could potentially contribute to vasoconstriction and therefore hypertension, although direct evidence of dysfunction in obesity is yet to emerge.

Cardiovascular disease in 'metabolically healthy obesity'

Obesity is undoubtedly associated with cardiovascular disease (Poirier *et al.*, 2006; NIH, 1998; Sowers, 2003; Baik, Ascherio and Rimm, 2000; Widlansky *et al.*, 2004; Ajani, Lotufo and Gaziano, 2004; see Chapter 9). However, it is now apparent that generalized obesity does not inevitably lead to increased cardiovascular risk or adverse outcomes (Iacobellis and Sharma, 2007). Severely obese individuals have been described who lack cardiovascular risk factors such as hypertension, hyperglycaemia and dyslipidaemia, prompting the description of 'metabolically healthy obese' (MHO), proposed by Andres (Andres, 1980) and Simon (SIMS, 2001). This clinical entity appears relatively common, with prevalences of 8–37% reported in various European and North American populations (Brochu, Tchernof and Dionne, 2001; Karelis, Brochu, Rabasa-Lhoret, 2004a; Karelis *et al.*, 2004b; Karelis *et al.*, 2005; Shin *et al.*, 2006; Marini *et al.*, 2007; Marchesini *et al.*, 2004; Meigs

Table 12.4 Characteristics of 'metabolically healthy obese' (MHO) subjects.

- Relatively insulin-sensitive
- Normal or nearly normal blood glucose
- Normal or nearly normal lipid profile (oxidized LDL not elevated)
- Normal blood pressure
- Lower inflammatory markers than in typical obese subjects
- Carotid intima-media thickness intermediate between typical obese and lean subjects

et al., 2006; Iacobellis *et al.*, 2005a; Iacobellis *et al.*, 2005b; Iacobellis *et al.*, 2007c).

In MHO individuals, features of the metabolic syndrome are absent (Table 12.4). They are relatively insulin-sensitive, with normal glucose, lipid levels and blood pressure; levels of inflammatory markers (C-reactive protein, CRP) and oxidized LDL are close to lean values (Karelis, Brochu, Rabasa-Lhoret, 2004a; Karelis *et al.*, 2004b; Karelis *et al.*, 2005; Shin *et al.*, 2006; Marchesini *et al.*, 2004; Meigs *et al.*, 2006; Iacobellis *et al.*, 2005a; Iacobellis *et al.*, 2005b; Iacobellis *et al.*, 2007c). Estimated cardiovascular risk is low (Meigs *et al.*, 2006), and carotid intima-media thickness (a robust predictor of atheroma) is intermediate between lean and typical obese values (Marini *et al.*, 2007). Iacobellis *et al.* (2005a,b; 2006b) reported that 30% of an obese Italian population had 'uncomplicated' obesity with no cardiovascular or metabolic risk factors; their BMI ranged from 30.0–89.8 kg/m². Among the 'complicated' obese subjects, there was no relationship between BMI and any of the associated abnormalities – hyperglycaemia, raised total cholesterol, low HDL-cholesterol, hypertriglyceridaemia and increased liver enzymes – even at BMI >50 kg/m².

However, MHO subjects show some cardiovascular abnormalities associated with obesity, notably an expanded blood volume, decreased peripheral resistance and hyperdynamic systolic function (Iacobellis, 2004; Iacobellis *et al.*, 2002; Iacobellis *et al.*, 2004a; see Figure 12.4). This suggests that cardiac work must increase to supply the high oxygen consumption demanded by the increased body mass. This hyperkinetic state does not produce compensatory LVH, but is associated with dilatation of the aortic root, probably because of increased volume loading.

Overall, these observations indicate that obesity is not necessarily accompanied by cardiovascular and metabolic comorbidities. The reasons remain to be determined.

Investigation of cardiovascular disease in obesity

The wide range and potential gravity of cardiovascular disease in obese patients demand careful evaluation of risk and active management of weight and of other risk factors. The general assessment of the obese patient is covered in detail in Chapter 15.

All patients must have weight, height and an index of abdominal obesity (waist circumference or WHR) measured at presentation and whenever reviewed. Blood pressure must be checked, crucially with an appropriately-sized cuff, as a longer and wider cuff is needed for adequate compression of the brachial artery in the obese patient with a very large upper arm. The American Heart Association Council recommends that, for an arm circumference of 27–34 cm, the cuff should be 16×30 cm, increasing to 16×36 cm for a circumference of 35–44 cm, and to 16×42 cm (the 'adult thigh' cuff) for an arm circumference of 45–52 cm (Pickering et al., 2005).

Other risk factors – smoking, hyperglycaemia and dyslipidaemia – should be carefully evaluated from history and appropriate screening tests, and the cardiovascular risk predicted, for example using the Framingham risk calculator (Table 15.5).

An ECG should be performed, and other tests – for example echocardiography, 24-hour blood pressure monitoring, exercise tolerance testing and imaging of coronary or peripheral arteries – used as indicated from the history, examination and screening tests. It is important to note that certain investigations need to be interpreted with caution in obese subjects.

ECG in obesity

Several changes in the electrocardiogram (ECG) occur with obesity and are summarized in Table 12.5. As illustrated in Figure 12.14, the most common abnormalities are low QRS voltage and leftward deviation of the cardiac

Table 12.5 Electrocardiographic changes in obesity.

- Increased heart rate
- Prolonged PR interval
- Prolonged QRS interval
- Prolonged QTc interval
- Increased QT dispersion
- Increased late potentials
- Left axis deviation
- Decreased QRS voltage (may also be increased)
- Flattening of the T wave
- P wave changes of left atrial enlargement
- False-positive criteria for inferior myocardial infarction

axis, non-specific flattening of the T wave in the inferolateral leads (attributed to the horizontal displacement of the heart) and voltage criteria for left atrial enlargement (Otto et al., 2007). An increased incidence of false-positive criteria for inferior myocardial infarction has been described in obese individuals, probably due to diaphragmatic elevation (as also occurs in women in the final trimester of pregnancy) (Figure 12.14). Obesity is also associated with increased occurrence of abnormal small high-frequency ECG potentials (SAECG) (Gami et al., 2007) and with abnormal late potentials that outlast the normal QRS period during sinus rhythm.

All these abnormalities are found in obese patients with and without hypertension and/or diabetes. and often in the absence of clinical evidence of cardiac disease.

Echocardiography in obese subjects

Because of overlying fat, good images and measurements are often difficult to obtain. Echocardiographic measurements of LVM require careful interpretation in obese subjects. The absolute value of LVM is often high, but allowance must be made for the fact that all muscle mass is increased in obese people, although much less than fat mass. Accordingly, LVH should be 'indexed', that is, corrected against an appropriate characteristic of body habitus, in the same way that glomerular filtration rate is corrected for body surface area.

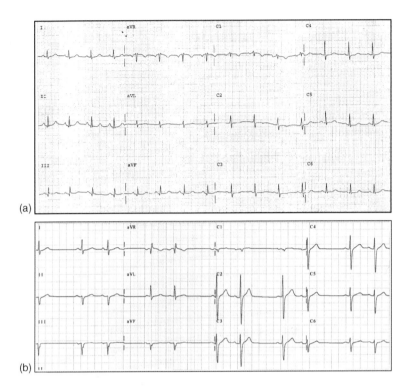

Figure 12.14 Typical ECG abnormalities in obesity: (a) subject with obesity complicated by hypertension (but without left ventricular hypertrophy), showing low-voltage QRS complexes, left axis deviation and T wave flattening in infero-lateral leads; (b) Q waves in the inferior leads, falsely suggesting a diagnosis of inferior myocardial infarction, together with Mobitz type I second-degree heart block. Courtesy of Dr. Alfonso Macías, Department of Cardiology, Clínica Universitaria de Navarra, Spain.

It has been suggested that LVM should be indexed according to height$^{2.7}$ ($h^{2.7}$) or to fat-free mass in kilograms of body weight (FMM_{kg}), when assessing LVM in obese populations (Iacobellis *et al.*, 2002; Daniels *et al.*, 1995). Interestingly, after indexing by lean body mass, there are no gender differences in LVM, and the relative effects of adiposity and blood pressure appear to be of similar magnitude.

Management of cardiovascular disease in obese subjects

The conventional management of obese patients begins with weight reduction through lifestyle changes, including dietary therapy and exercise. Many patients require a combined approach with lifestyle changes and pharmacological or even surgical interventions. The overall aim is to reduce cardiovascular risk by lowering cholesterol, glucose, insulin resistance and blood pressure, as well as proinflammatory and prothrombotic factors.

Even though obesity is recognized as a major cardiovascular risk factor and cardiovascular disease is an important cause of death in obese subjects, no specific guidelines have yet been proposed for the treatment of hypertension or coronary artery disease in the obese.

Effects of weight loss on cardiovascular disease

Weight loss is a primary intervention in obese patients, and if achieved, is frequently accompanied by significant improvements in cardiovascular risk as summarized in Table 12.6 (Aucott *et al.*, 2005). Net benefits include lowering of blood pressure, decreasing LDL-cholesterol and triglycerides and increasing HDL-cholesterol.

Table 12.6 Beneficial cardiovascular effects of weight reduction.

Haemodynamic

- Decreased blood volume
- Decreased stroke volume
- Decreased cardiac output
- Decreased pressure loading of left and right ventricles
- Improved left ventricular diastolic and systolic function

Cardiac structure

- Decreased left ventricular mass

Cardiac rhythm

- Decreased resting heart rate
- Decreased QT_c interval
- Increased heart rate variability

Blood pressure

- Decreased (or unchanged) peripheral resistance
- Decreased systolic and diastolic blood pressure
- Decreased pulmonary capillary wedge pressure

Arteries

- Improved endothelial function

Decreased resting oxygen consumption

Adapted from Poirier *et al.* (2006) *Circulation,* 113: 898–918

Weight management strategies involving lifestyle modification, drug therapy and bariatric surgery are covered in detail in Chapters 16–18. Here, we focus on the impact of these treatments on cardiovascular disease and risk.

Currently approved drugs for the long-term treatment of obesity include sibutramine, orlistat and rimonabant (Perrio *et al.*, 2007).

Sibutramine, a centrally-acting inhibitor of serotonin and noradrenaline reuptake, can reduce body weight and fat by enough to improve metabolic and cardiovascular risk factors. However, its sympathomimetic action (due to enhanced noradrenaline action) can lead in about 2% of cases to significant increases in blood pressure (Pickering *et al.*, 2005). This effect is idiosyncratic and unpredictable; careful monitoring of blood pressure is therefore necessary. Overall, however, a modest reduction (~5 mm Hg in systolic blood pressure and ~1 mm Hg in diastolic

pressure) can be expected in obese hypertensive patients whose blood pressure is well controlled at the outset with an ACE inhibitor, with or without concomitant thiazide diuretic therapy, and who lose weight with sibutramine (Sharma, 2001; James *et al.*, 2000; Shechter *et al.*, 2006; McMahon *et al.*, 2002; McMahon *et al.*, 2000). Short-term sibutramine therapy was recently found to be associated with weight loss and improved endothelial function in obese patients with CAD (Shechter *et al.*, 2006). Sibutramine has been also reported to decrease LVM in obese patients (Wirth *et al.*, 2006).

Orlistat, a gastrointestinal lipase inhibitor, has been associated with significant improvements in the general cardiovascular and metabolic risk profile (Douketis and Sharma, 2005), while obese patients with treated hypertension show a modest reduction in blood pressure (Derosa *et al.*, 2005).

Rimonabant, a selective CB1 cannabinoid receptor antagonist, reduces body weight and waist circumference and improves lipid profile and blood glucose in high-risk patients who are overweight or obese and/or have an atherogenic dyslipidaemia (Desprès *et al.*, 2005; Pi-Sunyer *et al.*, 2006). There does not seem to be an effect of rimonabant on blood pressure beyond that expected from weight loss alone.

Bariatric surgery, particularly laparoscopic adjustable gastric banding and the Roux-en-Y gastric bypass (RYGB), is increasingly used and achieves major weight loss, often of 25–30% of initial weight. General indications for bariatric surgery are discussed in Chapter 18.

The impact of bariatric surgery on the risk of CAD has been recently assessed (Sjöström *et al.*, 2004; Torquati *et al.*, 2007; Vogel *et al.*, 2007; Batsis *et al.*, 2007; Lubrano *et al.*, 2004; Ikonomidis *et al.*, 2007). Torquati *et al.* (2007) and Batsis *et al.* (2007) both found that bariatric surgery-induced weight loss significantly decreased the Framingham scores of 10-year predicted CAD risk (Torquati *et al.*, 2007); in the latter study, the risk score fell from 37% at baseline to 18% at follow up (Batsis *et al.*, 2007). Moreover, Willens *et al.* (2007) recently found that epicardial fat thickness, described above as index of visceral adiposity, decreased in severely obese patients who achieved substantial weight loss after bariatric surgery. The effect of bariatric surgery on different visceral and subcutaneous fat compartments needs to be fully characterized, but bariatric surgery would appear to be a powerful intervention to decrease cardiovascular risk and cardiovascular events in the morbidly obese.

Management of hypertension in obesity

Current guidelines do not provide specific recommendations for treating hypertension in obesity. Thus, therapeutic decisions have to be made from the potential benefits and risks of the available drugs, and the patient's own characteristics (Jordan et al., 2007). For example, β-adrenoceptor blockers reduce cardiac output and renin activity, both of which have been shown to be increased in obese patients; when used alone or in combination with an α-adrenoreceptor blocker, they decrease blood pressure more effectively in obese than in lean hypertensive individuals. However, β-blockers induce weight gain and insulin resistance, which may limit their use especially in young obese hypertensive patients without cardiac and renal complications.

Overall, it seems reasonable to follow evidence-based guidelines for managing hypertension in the general population (e.g. the Joint National Committee on Prevention, Detection, Evaluation and Treatment of High Blood Pressure (Anonymus, 2008)), and those formulated by the American Heart Association (AHA) and American Diabetes Association (ADA) for diabetic patients (Buse et al., 2007), who have a similar risk profile.

General approach

Patients with a systolic blood pressure of 130 to 139 mm Hg, or a diastolic blood pressure of 80 to 89 mm Hg, should start with lifestyle modification alone (with increased physical activity, reduction in dietary fat intake and increased consumption of fresh fruits and vegetables) with the aim of losing at least 5% of weight. Alcohol intake should be moderated, and sodium intake reduced. These measures should be continued alone for a maximum of three months, when if the blood pressure target level (130/80) is not achieved, treatment with one or more antihypertensive drugs should be started.

Patients with hypertension (systolic blood pressure >140 mm Hg or diastolic blood pressure >90 mm Hg) at presentation should receive drug therapy in addition to lifestyle improvement from the outset.

Most obese and diabetic patients will require two or more drugs to achieve blood pressure control. angiotensin-converting enzyme (ACE) inhibitors, angiotensin receptor blockers (ARBs), β-blockers, calcium channel inhibitors and thiazide diuretics have all been shown in clinical trials to reduce cardiovascular risk and so have particular potential benefits in these patients. Drugs should be added as needed to achieve blood pressure targets.

If ACE inhibitors, ARBs or diuretics are used, renal function and serum potassium levels should be monitored within the first three months. If stable, these should be followed up every six months thereafter.

In elderly hypertensive patients, blood pressure should be lowered gradually to avoid complications.

Antihypertensive drugs

ACE inhibitors may improve insulin sensitivity and have beneficial renal effects, preserving glomerular filtration rate and slowing the increase in urinary albumin losses (Remuzzi, Schieppati and Ruggenenti, 2002; American Diabetes Association, 2003). Some trials also suggest that ACE inhibitors may be associated with better cardiovascular outcomes compared to dihydropyridine calcium channel inhibitors (Turnbull et al., 2005; Varughese and Lip, 2005). Because of their broad spectrum of favourable effects, ACE inhibitors are currently regarded as the first-line antihypertensive drugs for obese patients, and for those with diabetes or renal disease; the ADA recommends them especially for type 2 diabetic patients over the age of 55 years and with high cardiovascular risk. ACE inhibitors may be used alone for lowering blood pressure, but are more effective when combined with a thiazide-type diuretic or other antihypertensive drugs.

Angiotensin receptor blockers (ARBs) are an alternative to ACE inhibitors and can be considered as first-line therapy for those who do not tolerate ACE inhibitors.

A low-dose *thiazide diuretic* generally should be one of the first two drugs used for managing hypertension in diabetic and obese patients. Previous concerns that these agents impair insulin secretion and worsen hyperglycaemia

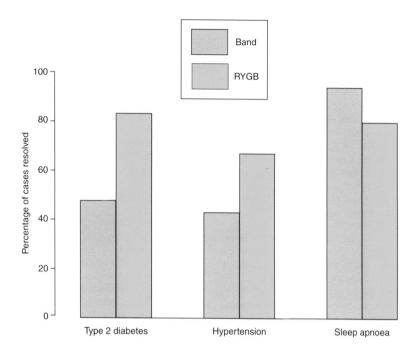

Figure 12.15 Effects of two bariatric surgical procedures – gastric banding and Roux-en-Y gastric bypass (RYGB) – on the prevalences of diabetes, hypertension and sleep apnoea in morbidly obese subjects. Both operations normalized blood pressure in a substantial proportion of cases, with nearly 70% following RYGB. From H. Buchwald, H. (2004) 'Barametric surgery': a systematic review and meta-analysis. *Journal of the American Medical Association*, 292, 1724–37, with permission of the editor.

were overstated, and thiazides do not cause more cardiovascular events than the other drug classes (Anonymus, 2008; Weinberger, 1985).

Calcium channel blockers are effective blood pressure-lowering agents and should be considered as additional therapy in patients who do not achieve adequate blood pressure control with ACE inhibitors or ARBs. They are also useful for patients with angina, and several trials have shown a reduction in cardiovascular events in diabetic subjects (Brown *et al.*, 2000; Black *et al.*, 2003).

β-blockers, especially β_1-selective agents, are useful as part of combination therapy, especially in subjects with ischaemic heart disease, but their value as monotherapy is less clear. They may also be less effective at preventing stroke than an ARB. β-blockers can cause weight gain and aggravate glucose tolerance; they can also mask the sympathetic symptoms of hypoglycaemia, which can pose problems particularly for insulin-treated diabetic subjects. However, these side effects are not absolute contraindications for their use.

Bariatric surgery

Successful bariatric surgery often lowers blood pressure, often to a substantial degree. For unknown reasons, the RYGB is particularly effective at restoring normotension, which is achieved in almost 70% of cases (Figure 12.15).

References

Ajani, U.A., Lotufo, P.A. and Gaziano, J.M. (2004) Body mass index and mortality among US male physicians. *Annals of Epidemiology*, **14**, 731–9.

Alpert, M.A., Terry, B.E., Cohen, M.V. *et al.* (2000) The electrocardiogram in morbid obesity. *The American Journal of Cardiology*, **85**, 908–10.

American Diabetes Association (2003) Treatment of hypertension in adults with diabetes. *Diabetes Care*, **26**, S80–2.

Andres, R. (1980) Effect of obesity on total mortality. *International Journal of Obesity and Related Metabolic Disorders*, **4**, 381–6.

Anonymous (2008) The Seventh Report of the Joint National Committee on Prevention, Detection, Evaluation, and Treatment of High Blood Pressure. National Heart, Lung, and Blood Institute, National High Blood Pressure. Education Program, NIH Publication No. 04-5230.

Arias, M.A., Alonso-Fernandez, A. and Garcia-Rio, F. (2006) Left ventricular diastolic abnormalities in obese subjects. *Chest*, **130**, 1282–3.

Aucott, L., Poobalan, A., Smith, W.C. *et al.* (2005) Effects of weight loss in overweight/obese individuals and long-term hypertension outcomes: a systematic review. *Hypertension*, **45**, 1035–41.

Baik, I., Ascherio, A. and Rimm, E.B. (2000) Adiposity and mortality in men. *American Journal of Epidemiology*, **152**, 264–71.

Baker, A.R., Silva, N.F., Quinn, D.W. *et al.* (2006) Human epicardial adipose tissue expresses a pathogenic profile of adipocytokines in patients with cardiovascular disease. *Cardiovascular Diabetology*, **5**, 1.

Barandier, C., Montani, J.P. and Yang, Z. (2005) Mature adipocytes and perivascular adipose tissue stimulate vascular smooth muscle cell proliferation: effects of aging and obesity. *American Journal of Physiology. Heart and Circulatory Physiology*, **289**, H1807–13.

Barouch, L.A., Berkowitz, D.E. and, Harrison, R.Wl. (2003) Disruption of leptin signaling contributes to cardiac hypertrophy independently of body weight in mice. *Circulation*, **108**, 754–9.

Barton, M., Carmona, R., Ortmann, J. *et al.* (2003) Obesity-associated activation of angiotensin and endothelin in the cardiovascular system. *The International Journal of Biochemistry & Cell Biology*, **35**, 826–37.

Batsis, J.A., Romero-Corral, A., Collazo-Clavell, M.L. *et al.* (2007) Effect of weight loss on predicted cardiovascular risk: change in cardiac risk after bariatric surgery. *Obesity (Silver Spring)*, **15**, 772–84.

Bełtowski, J., Wójcicka, G. and Jamroz-Wiśniewska, A. (2006) Role of nitric oxide and endothelium-derived hyperpolarizing factor (EDHF) in the regulation of blood pressure by leptin in lean and obese rats. *Life Sciences*, **79**, 63–71.

Black, H.R., Elliott, W.J., Grandits, G. *et al.* and CONVINCE Research Group (2003) Principal results of the Controlled Onset Verapamil Investigation of Cardiovascular End Points (CONVINCE) trial. *The Journal of the American Medical Association*, **289**, 2073–82.

Brandt, M., Harder, K., Walluscheck, K.P. *et al.* (2001) Severe obesity does not adversely affect perioperative mortality and morbidity in coronary artery bypass surgery. *European Journal of Cardio-Thoracic Surgery*, **19**, 662–6.

Brochu, M., Tchernof, A. and Dionne, I.J. (2001) What are the physical characteristics associated with a normal metabolic profile despite a high level of obesity in postmenopausal women? *The Journal of Clinical Endocrinology and Metabolism*, **86**, 1020–5.

Brown, D.W., Giles, W.H., Greenlund, K.J. *et al.* (2001) Impaired fasting glucose, diabetes mellitus, and cardiovascular disease risk factors are associated with prolonged QTc duration: results from the Third National Health and Nutrition Examination Survey. *Journal of Cardiovascular Risk*, **8**, 227–33.

Brown, M.J., Palmer, C.R., Castaigne, A. *et al.* (2000) Morbidity and mortality in patients randomised to double-blind treatment with a long-acting calcium-channel blocker or diuretic in the International Nifedipine GITS study: Intervention as a Goal in Hypertension Treatment (INSIGHT). *Lancet*, **356**, 366–72.

Buchwald, H. *et al.* (2004) Barametric surgery: a systematic review and meta-analysis. *Journal of the American Medical Association*, **292**, 1724–37

Buse, J.B., Ginsberg, H.N., Bakris, G.L. *et al.* and American Heart Association, American Diabetes Association (2007) Primary prevention of cardiovascular diseases in people with diabetes mellitus: a scientific statement from the American Heart Association and the American Diabetes Association. *Diabetes Care*, **30**, 162–72 (simultaneously published in *Circulation* **115**, 114–26).

Chadwick, J. and Mann, W.N. (1950) *The Medical Works of Hippocrates. Aphorisms, sect. II 44*, Charles C Thomas Co, Springfield, IL, 154.

Chaldakov, G.N., Fiore, M., Stankulov, I.S. *et al.* (2004) Neurotrophin presence in human coronary atherosclerosis and metabolic syndrome: a role for NGF and BDNF in cardiovascular disease? *Progress in Brain Research*, **146**, 279–89.

Chiu, H.C., Kovacs, A., Ford, D.A. *et al.* (2001) A novel mouse model of lipotoxic cardiomyopathy. *The Journal of Clinical Investigation*, **107**, 813–22.

Corradi, D., Maestri, R., Callegari, S. *et al.* (2004) The ventricular epicardial fat is related to the myocardial mass in normal, ischemic and hypertrophic hearts. *Cardiovascular Pathology*, **13**, 313–6.

Correia, M.L., Morgan, D.A., Sivitz, W.I. *et al.* (2001) Leptin acts in the central nervous system to produce dose-dependent changes in arterial pressure. *Hypertension*, **37**, 936–42.

Crisostomo, L.L., Araujo, L.M. and Camara, E. (1999) Comparison of left ventricular mass and function in obese versus nonobese women <40 years of age. *The American Journal of Cardiology*, **84**, 1127–9.

Curtis, J.P., Selter, J.G., Wang, Y. *et al.* (2005) The obesity paradox: body mass index and outcomes in patients with heart failure. *Archives of Internal Medicine*, **165**, 55–61.

Dagenais, G.R., Yi, Q., Mann, J.F. *et al.* (2005) Prognostic impact of body weight and abdominal obesity in women and men with cardiovascular disease. *American Heart Journal*, **159**, 54–60.

Daniels, S.R., Kimball, T.R., Morrison, J.A. *et al.* (1995) Effect of lean body mass, fat mass, blood pressure, and sexual maturation on left ventricular mass in children and adolescents: statistical, biological, and clinical significance. *Circulation*, **92**, 3249–54.

Date, H., Imamura, T., Ideguchi, T. *et al.* (2006) Adiponectin produced in coronary circulation regulates coronary flow reserve in nondiabetic patients with angiographically normal coronary arteries. *Clinical Cardiology*, **29**, 211–4.

Davos, H., Doehner, W., Rauchhaus, M. *et al.* (2003) Body mass and survival in patients with chronic heart failure without cachexia: the importance of obesity. *Journal of Cardiac Failure*, **9**, 29–35.

DeFronzo, R.A., Cooke, C.R., Andres, R. *et al.* (1975) The effect of insulin on renal handling of sodium, potassium, calcium, and phosphate in man. *The Journal of Clinical Investigation*, **55**, 845–55.

Delaughter, M.C., Taffet, G.E., Fiorotto, M.L. *et al.* (1999) Local insulin-like growth factor I expression induces physiologic, then pathologic, cardiac hypertrophy in transgenic mice. *The FASEB Journal*, **13**, 1923–9.

Della Mea, P., Lupia, M., Bandolin, V. *et al.* (2005) Adiponectin, insulin resistance, and left ventricular structure in dipper and nondipper essential hypertensive patients. *American Journal of Hypertension*, **18**, 30–5.

Derosa, G., Cicero, A.F., Murdolo, G. *et al.* (2005) Efficacy and safety comparative evaluation of orlistat and sibutramine treatment in hypertensive obese patients. *Diabetes, Obesity & Metabolism*, **7**, 47–55.

Després, J.P., Golay, A., Sjöström, L. and Rimonabant in Obesity-Lipids Study Group (2005) Effects of rimonabant on metabolic risk factors in overweight patients with dyslipidemia. *The New England Journal of Medicine*, **353**, 2121–34.

Després, J.P. and Lemieux, I. (2006) Abdominal obesity and metabolic syndrome. *Nature*, **444**, 881–7.

Diercks, D.B., Roe, M.T., Mulgund, J. *et al.* (2006) The obesity paradox in non-ST-segment elevation acute coronary syndromes: results from the Can Rapid Risk Stratification of Unstable Angina Patients Suppress Adverse Outcomes with Early Implementation of the American College of Cardiology/American Heart Association Guidelines Quality Improvement Initiative. *American Heart Journal*, **152**, 140–8.

Domanski, M.J., Jablonski, K.A., Rice, M.M. *et al.* and PEACE Investigators (2006) Obesity and cardiovascular events in patients with established coronary disease. *European Heart Journal*, **27**, 1416–22.

Dorbala, S., Crugnale, S., Yang, D. and Di Carli, M.F. (2006) Effect of body mass index on left ventricular cavity size and ejection fraction. *The American Journal of Cardiology*, **97**, 725–9.

Douketis, J.D. and Sharma, A.M. (2005) Obesity and cardiovascular disease: pathogenic mechanisms and potential benefits of weight reduction. *Seminars in Veterinary Medicine*, **5**, 25–33.

Drøyvold, W.B., Midthjell, K., Nilsen, T.I. and Holmen, J. (2005) Change in body mass index and its impact on blood pressure: a prospective population study. *International Journal of Obesity (London)*, **29**, 650–5.

Dublin, S., French, B., Glazer, N.L. *et al.* (2006) Risk of new-onset atrial fibrillation in relation to body mass index. *Archives of Internal Medicine*, **166**, 2322–8.

Dubrovska, G., Verlohren, S., Luft, F.C. and Gollasch, M. (2004) Mechanisms of ADRF release from rat aortic adventitial adipose tissue. *The American Journal of Physiology*, **286**, H1107–13.

el-Gamal, A., Gallagher, D., Nawras, A. *et al.* (1995) Effects of obesity on QT, RR, and QTc intervals. *The American Journal of Cardiology*, **75**, 956–9.

Engeli, S. (2005) Is there a pathophysiological role for perivascular adipocytes? *American Journal of Physiology. Heart and Circulatory Physiology*, **289**, H1794–5.

Fonarow, G.C., Srikanthan, P., Costanzo, M.R. *et al.* (2007) ADHERE Scientific Advisory Committee and Investigators. An obesity paradox in acute heart failure: analysis of body mass index and in-hospital mortality for 108,927 patients in the Acute Decompensated Heart Failure National Registry. *American Heart Journal*, **153**, 74–81.

Fortuño, A., Rodriguez, A., Gomez-Ambrosi, J. *et al.* (2003) Adipose tissue as an endocrine organ: role of leptin and adiponectin in the pathogenesis of cardiovascular diseases. *Journal of Physiology and Biochemistry*, **59**, 51–60.

Frühbeck, G. (1999) Pivotal role of nitric oxide in the control of blood pressure after leptin administration. *Diabetes*, **48**, 903–8.

Frühbeck, G. (2004) The adipose tissue as a source of vasoactive factors. *Current Medicinal Chemistry – Cardiovascular & Hematological Agents*, **2**, 197–208.

Galvan, A.Q., Galetta, F. and Natali, A. (2000) Insulin resistance and hyperinsulinemia: no independent relation to left ventricular mass in humans. *Circulation*, **102**, 2233–8.

Galvez, B., de Castro, J., Herold, D. *et al.* (2006) Perivascular adipose tissue and mesenteric vascular function in spontaneously hypertensive rats. *Arteriosclerosis, Thrombosis, and Vascular Biology*, **26**, 1297–302.

Gami, A.S., Hodge, D.O., Herges, R.M. *et al.* (2007) Obstructive sleep apnea, obesity, and the risk of incident atrial fibrillation. *Journal of the American College of Cardiology*, **49**, 565–71.

Gao, Y.J., Takemori, K., Su, L.Y. *et al.* (2006) Perivascular adipose tissue promotes vasoconstriction: the role of superoxide anion. *Cardiovascular Research*, **71**, 363–73.

Gao, Y.J., Zeng, Z.H., Teoh, K. *et al.* (2005) Perivascular adipose tissue modulates vascular function in the human internal thoracic artery. *The Journal of Thoracic and Cardiovascular Surgery*, **130**, 1130–6.

Gardin, J.M., McClelland, R., Kitzman, D. *et al.* (2001) M-mode echocardiographic predictors of six- to seven-year incidence of coronary heart disease, stroke, congestive heart failure, and mortality in an elderly cohort (the Cardiovascular Health Study). *The American Journal of Cardiology*, **87**, 1051–7.

Girola, A., Enrini, R., Garbetta, F. *et al.* (2001) QT dispersion in uncomplicated human obesity. *Obesity Research*, **9**, 71–7.

Gollasch, M. and Dubrovska, G. (2004) Paracrine role for periadventitial adipose tissue in the regulation of arterial tone. *Trends in Pharmacological Sciences*, **25**, 647–53.

Gomez-Ambrosi, J., Salvador, J., Silva, C. *et al.* (2006) Increased cardiovascular risk markers in obesity are associated with body adiposity: role of leptin. *Thrombosis and Haemostasis*, **95**, 991–6.

Gottdiener, J.S., Reda, D.J., Materson, B.J., Massie, B.M., Notargiacomo, A., Hamburger R.J., Williams, D.W. and Henderson, W.G. (1994) Importance of obesity, race and age to the cardiac structural and functional effects of hypertension. The Department of Veterans Affairs Cooperative Study Group on Antihypertensive Agents. *Journal of the American College of Cardiology* **24**, 1492–8.

Grandi, A.M., Zanzi, P. and Fachinetti, A. (1999) Insulin and diastolic dysfunction in lean and obese hypertensives. *Hypertension*, **34**, 1208–14.

Greenwood, J.P., Scott, E.M., Stoker, J.B. and Mary, D.A. (2001) Hypertensive left ventricular hypertrophy: relation to peripheral sympathetic drive. *Journal of the American College of Cardiology*, **15**, 1711–7.

Gurm, H.S., Whitlow, P.L., Kip, K.E. and BARI Investigators (2002) The impact of body mass index on short- and long-term outcomes inpatients undergoing coronary revascularization. Insights from the bypass angioplasty revascularization investigation (BARI). *Journal of the American College of Cardiology*, **39**, 834–40.

Gustafsson, F., Kragelund, C.B., Torp-Pedersen, C. *et al.* and DIAMOND study group (2005) Effect of obesity and being overweight on long-term mortality in congestive heart failure: influence of left ventricular systolic function. *European Heart Journal*, **26**, 58–64.

Habbu, A., Lakkis, N.M. and Dokainish, H. (2006) The obesity paradox: fact or fiction? *The American Journal of Cardiology*, **98**, 944–8.

Henrichot, E., Juge-Aubry, C.E., Pernin, A. *et al.* (2005) Production of chemokines by perivascular adipose tissue: a role in the pathogenesis of atherosclerosis? *Arteriosclerosis, Thrombosis, and Vascular Biology*, **25**, 2594–9.

Hoit, B.D., Gilpin, E.A., Maisel, A.A. *et al.* (1987) Influence of obesity on morbidity and mortality after acute myocardial infarction. *American Heart Journal*, **114**, 1334–41.

Hong, S.J., Park, C.G., Seo, H.S. *et al.* (2004) Associations among plasma adiponectin, hypertension, left ventricular diastolic function and left ventricular mass index. *Blood Pressure*, **13**, 236–42.

Horwich, T.B., Fonarow, G.C., Hamilton, M.A. *et al.* (2001) The relationship between obesity and mortality in patients with heart failure. *Journal of the American College of Cardiology*, **38**, 789–95.

Hubert, H.B., Feinleib, M. and McNamara, P.M. (1983) Obesity as independent risk factor for cardiovascular disease: a 26-year follow-up of the participants in the Framingham Heart Study. *Circulation*, **67**, 968–77.

Iacobellis, G. (2004) True uncomplicated obesity is not related to increased left ventricular mass and systolic dysfunction. *Journal of the American College of Cardiology*, **44**, 2257.

Iacobellis, G. (2005a) Is obesity a risk factor for atrial fibrillation? *Nature Clinical Practice Cardiovascular Medicine*, **2**, 134–5.

Iacobellis, G. (2005b) Imaging of visceral adipose tissue: an emerging diagnostic tool and therapeutic target. *Current Drug Targets – Cardiovascular & Haematological Disorders*, **5**, 345–53.

Iacobellis, G. and Leonetti, F. (2005) Epicardial adipose tissue and insulin resistance in obese subjects. *The Journal of Clinical Endocrinology and Metabolism*, **90**, 6300–2.

Iacobellis, G. and Sharma, A.M. (2006) Adiposity of the heart. *Annals of Internal Medicine*, **145**, 554–5.

Iacobellis, G. and Sharma, A.M. (2007) Obesity and the heart: redefinition of the relationship. *Obesity Reviews*, **8**, 35–9.

Iacobellis, G., Assael, F., Ribaudo, M.C. *et al.* (2003b) Epicardial fat from echocardiography: a new method for visceral adipose tissue prediction. *Obesity Research*, **11**, 304–10.

Iacobellis, G., Corradi, D. and Sharma, A.M. (2005d) Epicardial adipose tissue: anatomical, biomolecular and clinical relation to the heart. *Nature Clinical Practice Cardiovascular Medicine*, **2**, 536–43.

Iacobellis, G., Curione, M., Di Bona, S. *et al.* (2005c) Effect of acute hyperinsulinemia on ventricular repolarization in uncomplicated obesity. *International Journal of Cardiology*, **99**, 161–3.

Iacobellis, G., Leonetti, F., Singh, N. and Sharma, A.M. (2007b) Relationship of epicardial adipose tissue with atrial dimensions and diastolic function in morbidly obese subjects. *International Journal of Cardiology*, **115**, 272–3.

Iacobellis, G., Moschetta, A., Buzzetti, R. *et al.* (2007c) Aminotransferase activity in morbid and uncomplicated obesity: predictive role of fasting insulin. *Nutrition, Metabolism, and Cardiovascular Diseases* **17**, 442–7.

Iacobellis, G., Moschetta, A., Ribaudo, M.C. *et al.* (2005b) Normal serum alanine aminotransferase activity in uncomplicated obesity. *World Journal of Gastroenterology*, **11**, 6018–21.

Iacobellis, G., Pellicelli, A.M., Grisorio, B. *et al.* (2007a) Relation of subepicardial adipose tissue with carotid intima media thickness in HIV-infected subjects. *The American Journal of Cardiology*, **99**, 1470–2.

Iacobellis, G., Petrone, A., Leonetti, F. and Buzzetti, R. (2006a) Left ventricular mass and +276 G/G single nucleotide polymorphism of the adiponectin gene in uncomplicated obesity. *Obesity (Silver Spring)*, **14**, 368–72.

Iacobellis, G., Pistilli, D., Gucciardo, M. et al. (2005e) Adiponectin expression in human epicardial adipose tissue in vivo is lower in patients with coronary artery disease. *Cytokine*, **29**, 251–5.

Iacobellis, G., Ribaudo, M.C., Assael, F. et al. (2003c) Echocardiographic epicardial adipose tissue is related to anthropometric and clinical parameters of metabolic syndrome: a new indicator of cardiovascular risk. *The Journal of Clinical Endocrinology and Metabolism*, **88**, 5163–8.

Iacobellis, G., Ribaudo, M.C., Leto, G. et al. (2002) Influence of excess fat on cardiac morphology and function: study in uncomplicated obesity. *Obesity Research*, **10**, 767–73.

Iacobellis, G., Ribaudo, M.C., Zappaterreno, A. et al. (2003a) Relationship of insulin sensitivity and left ventricular mass in uncomplicated obesity. *Obesity Research*, **11**, 518–24.

Iacobellis, G., Ribaudo, M.C., Zappaterreno, A. et al. (2004a) Adapted changes in left ventricular structure and function in severe uncomplicated obesity. *Obesity Research*, **12**, 1616–21.

Iacobellis, G., Ribaudo, M.C., Zappaterreno, A. et al. (2004b) Relation between epicardial adipose tissue and left ventricular mass. *The American Journal of Cardiology*, **94**, 1084–7.

Iacobellis, G., Ribaudo, M.C., Zappaterreno, A. and Leonetti, F. (2005a) Prevalence of uncomplicated obesity in a Italian obese population. *Obesity Research*, **13**, 1116–22.

Ikonomidis, I., Mazarakis, A., Papadopoulos, C. et al. (2007) Weight loss after bariatric surgery improves aortic elastic properties and left ventricular function in individuals with morbid obesity: a 3-year follow-up study. *Journal of Hypertension*, **25**, 439–47.

Imamura, H., Izawa, A., Kai, R. et al. (2004) Trends over the last 20 years in the clinical background of young Japanese patients with coronary artery disease. *Circulation Journal*, **68**, 186–91.

Jain, A., Avendano, G. and Dharamsey, S. (1996) Left ventricular diastolic function in hypertension and role of plasma glucose and insulin: comparison with diabetic heart. *Circulation*, **93**, 1396–402.

James, W.P., Astrup, A., Finer, N. et al. (2000) Effect of sibutramine on weight maintenance after weight loss: a randomised trial. STORM Study Group. Sibutramine Trial of Obesity Reduction and Maintenance. *Lancet*, **356** (9248), 2119–25.

Janssen, I., Katzmarzyk, P.T. and Ross, R. (2004) Waist circumference and not body mass index explains obesity-related health risk. *The American Journal of Clinical Nutrition*, **79**, 379–84.

Janssen, I., Katzmarzyk, P.T. and Ross, R. (2005) Body mass index is inversely related to mortality in older people after adjustment for waist circumference. *Journal of the American Geriatrics Society*, **53**, 2112–8.

Jeong, J.W., Jeong, M.H., Yun, K.H. et al. (2007) Echocardiographic epicardial fat thickness and coronary artery disease. *Circulation Journal*, **71**, 536–9.

Jordan, J., Engeli, S., Redon, J. et al. and European Society of Hypertension Working Group on Obesity (2007) European Society of Hypertension Working Group on Obesity: background, aims and perspectives. *Journal of Hypertension*, **25**, 897–900.

Kamide, K., Rakugi, H. and Higaki, J. (2002) The renin-angiotensin and adrenergic nervous system in cardiac hypertrophy in fructose-fed rats. *American Journal of Hypertension*, **15**, 66–71.

Kankaanpaa, M., Lehto, H.R., Parkka, J.P. et al. (2006) Myocardial triglyceride content and epicardial fat mass in human obesity: relationship to left ventricular function and serum free fatty acid levels. *The Journal of Clinical Endocrinology and Metabolism*, **91**, 4689–95.

Kannel, W.B., Plehn, J.F. and Cupples, L.A. (1988) Cardiac failure and sudden death in the Framingham Study. *American Heart Journal*, **115**, 869–75.

Kaplan, R.C., Heckbert, S.R., Furberg, C.D. and Psaty, B.M. (2002) Predictors of subsequent coronary events, stroke, and death among survivors of first hospitalized myocardial infarction. *Journal of Clinical Epidemiology*, **55**, 654–64.

Karelis, A.D., Brochu, M. and Rabasa-Lhoret, R. (2004) Can we identify metabolically healthy but obese individuals (MHO)? *Diabetes & Metabolism*, **30**, 569–72.

Karelis, A.D., St-Pierre, D.H., Conus, F. et al. (2004) Metabolic and body composition factors in subgroups of obesity: what do we know? *The Journal of Clinical Endocrinology and Metabolism*, **89**, 2569–75.

Karelis, A.D., Faraj, M., Bastard, J.P. et al. (2005) The metabolically healthy, but obese individual presents a favorable inflammation profile. *The Journal of Clinical Endocrinology and Metabolism* **90**, 4145–50.

Kim, J., Hammar, N., Jakobsson, K. et al. (2003) Obesity and the risk of early and late mortality after coronary artery bypass graft surgery. *American Heart Journal*, **146**, 555–60.

Køber L., Torp-Pedersen C., Carlsen JE et al. (1995) A clinical trial of the angiotensin-converting–enzyme inhibitor trandolapril in patients with left ventricular dysfunction after myocardial infarction. *The New England Journal of Medicine*, **333**, 1670–76.

Kragelund, C., Hassager, C., Hildebrandt, P. et al. and Trace study group (2005) Impact of obesity on long-term prognosis following acute myocardial infarction. *International Journal of Cardiology*, **98**, 123–31.

Kremen, J., Dolinkova, M., Krajickova, J. et al. (2006) Increased subcutaneous and epicardial adipose tissue production of proinflammatory cytokines in cardiac surgery patients: possible role in postoperative insulin resistance. *The Journal of Clinical Endocrinology and Metabolism*, **91**, 4620–7.

Krishnan, R., Becker, R.J., Beighley, L.M. and Lopez-Candales, A. (2005) Impact of body mass index on markers of left ventricular thickness and mass calculation: results of a pilot analysis. *Echocardiography*, **22**, 203–10.

Kuk, J.L., Janiszewski, P.M. and Ross, R. (2007) Body mass index and hip and thigh circumferences are negatively associated with visceral adipose tissue after control for waist circumference. *The American Journal of Clinical Nutrition*, **85**, 1540–4.

Kuk, J.L., Katzmarzyk, P.T., Nichaman, M.Z. *et al.* (2006) Visceral fat is an independent predictor of all-cause mortality in men. *Obesity Research*, **14**, 336–41.

Lalani, A.P., Kanna, B., John, J. *et al.* (2000) Abnormal signal-averaged electrocardiogram (SAECG) in obesity. *Obesity Research*, **8**, 20–8.

Lembo, G., Vecchione, C., Fratta, L. *et al.* (2000) Leptin induces direct vasodilation through distinct endothelial mechanisms. *Diabetes*, **49**, 293–7.

Lewis, T.V., Dart, A.M. and Chin-Dusting, J.P. (1999) Endothelium-dependent relaxation by acetylcholine is impaired in hypertriglyceridemic humans with normal levels of plasma LDL cholesterol. *Journal of the American College of Cardiology*, **33**, 805–12.

Lin, S., Cheng, T.O., Liu, X. *et al.* (2006) Impact of dysglycemia, body mass index, and waist-to-hip ratio on the prevalence of systemic hypertension in a lean Chinese population. *The American Journal of Cardiology*, **97**, 839–42.

Lissin, W., Gauri, A.J., Froelicher, V.F. *et al.* (2002) The prognostic value of body mass index and standard exercise testing in male veterans with congestive heart failure. *Journal of Cardiac Failure*, **8**, 206–15.

Löhn, M., Dubrovska, G., Lauterbach, B. *et al.* (2002) Periadventitial fat releases a vascular relaxing factor. *The FASEB Journal*, **16**, 1057–63.

Lubrano, C., Cornoldi, A., Pili, M. *et al.* (2004) Reduction of risk factors for cardiovascular diseases in morbid-obese patients following biliary-intestinal bypass: 3 years' follow-up. *International Journal of Obesity and Related Metabolic Disorders*, **28**, 1600–6.

Malavazos, A.E., Ermetici, F., Coman, C. *et al.* (2007) Influence of epicardial adipose tissue and adipocytokine levels on cardiac abnormalities in visceral obesity. *International Journal of Cardiology* **121**, 132–4.

Malmqvist, K., Isaksson, H., Ostergren, J. and Kahan, T. (2001) Left ventricular mass is not related to insulin sensitivity in never-treated primary hypertension. *Journal of Hypertension*, **19**, 311–7.

Malmqvist, K., Ohman, K.P., Lind, L. *et al.* (2002) Relationships between left ventricular mass and the renin-angiotensin system, catecholamines, insulin and leptin. *Journal of Internal Medicine*, **252**, 430–9.

Marchesini, G., Melchionda, N., Apolone, G. and QUOVADIS. Study Group (2004) The metabolic syndrome in treatment-seeking obese persons. *Metabolism: Clinical and Experimental*, **53**, 435–40.

Marchington, J.M., Mattacks, C.A. and Pond, C.M. (1989) Adipose tissue in the mammalian heart and pericardium: structure, foetal development and biochemical properties. *Comparative Biochemistry and Physiology B*, **94**, 225–32.

Marchington, J.M. and Pond, C.M. (1990) Site specific properties of pericardial and epicardial adipose tissue: the effects of insulin and high-fat feeding on lipogenesis and the incorporation of fatty acids in vivo. *International Journal of Obesity*, **14**, 1013–22.

Marini, M.A., Succurro, E., Frontoni, S. *et al.* (2007) Metabolically healthy but obese women have an intermediate cardiovascular risk profile between healthy non-obese women and obese insulin resistant women. *Diabetes Care,* **30**, 2145–7.

Mazurek, T., Zhang, L., Zalewski, A. *et al.* (2003) Human epicardial adipose tissue is a source of inflammatory mediators. *Circulation*, **108**, 2460–6.

McGavock, J.M., Victor, R.G., Unger, R.H. and Szczepaniak, L.S. (2006) Adiposity of the heart, revisited. *Annals of Internal Medicine*, **144**, 517–24.

McMahon, F.G., Fujioka, K., Singh, B.N. *et al.* (2000) Efficacy and safety of sibutramine in obese white and African American patients with hypertension: a 1-year, double-blind, placebo-controlled, multicenter trial. *Archives of Internal Medicine*, **160**, 2185–91.

McMahon, F.G., Weinstein, S.P., Rowe, E. *et al.* and Sibutramine in Hypertensives Clinical Study Group (2002) Sibutramine is safe and effective for weight loss in obese patients whose hypertension is well controlled with angiotensin-converting enzyme inhibitors. *Journal of Human Hypertension*, **16**, 5–11.

Meigs, J.B., Wilson, P.W., Fox, C.S. *et al.* (2006) Body mass index, metabolic syndrome, and risk of type 2 diabetes or cardiovascular disease. *The Journal of Clinical Endocrinology and Metabolism*, **91**, 2906–12.

Mikhail, N., Golub, M.S. and Tuck, M.L. (1999) Obesity and hypertension. *Progress in Cardiovascular Diseases*, **42**, 39–58.

Minutello, R.M., Chou, E.T., Hong, M.K. *et al.* (2004) Impact of body mass index on in-hospital outcomes following percutaneous coronary intervention (report from the New York State Angioplasty Registry). *The American Journal of Cardiology*, **93**, 1229–32.

Misra, A. and Vikram, N.K. (2003) Clinical and pathophysiological consequences of abdominal adiposity and abdominal adipose tissue depots. *Nutrition*, **19**, 457–66.

Mitsuhashi, H., Yatsuya, H., Tamakoshi, K. *et al.* (2007) Adiponectin level and left ventricular hypertrophy in Japanese men. *Hypertension*, **49**, 1448–54.

Mombouli, J.V. and Vanhoutte, P.M. (1999) Endothelial dysfunction: from physiology to therapy. *Journal of Molecular and Cellular Cardiology*, **31**, 61–74.

Momin, A.U., Melikian, N., Shah, A.M. *et al.* (2006) Leptin is an endothelial-independent vasodilator in humans with coronary artery disease: evidence for tissue specificity of leptin resistance. *European Heart Journal*, **27**, 2294–9.

Montani, J.P., Carroll, J.F., Dwyer, T.M. *et al.* (2004) Ectopic fat storage in heart, blood vessels and kidneys in the pathogenesis of cardiovascular diseases. *International Journal of Obesity and Related Metabolic Disorders*, **28** (Suppl 4), S58–65.

Mureddu, G.F., de Simone, G., Greco, R., Rosato, G.F. and Contaldo, F. (1996) Left ventricular filling pattern in uncomplicated obesity. *The American Journal of Cardiology*, **77**, 509–14.

Mureddu, G.F., Greco, R. and Rosato, G.F. (1998) Relation of insulin resistance to left ventricular hypertrophy and diastolic dysfunction in obesity. *International Journal of Obesity and Related Metabolic Disorders*, **22**, 363–8.

NIH (1998) Clinical Guidelines on the Identification, Evaluation, and Treatment of Overweight and Obesity in Adults: the evidence report. *Obesity Research*, **6**, (Suppl 2), 51S–209S.

Noronha, B.T., Li, J.M., Wheatcroft, S.B. *et al.* (2005) Inducible nitric oxide synthase has divergent effects on vascular and metabolic function in obesity. *Diabetes*, **54**, 1082–9.

Otto, M.E., Belohlavek, M., Khandheria, B. *et al.* (2004) Comparison of right and left ventricular function in obese and nonobese men. *The American Journal of Cardiology*, **93**, 1569–72.

Otto, M.E., Belohlavek, M., Romero-Corral, A. *et al.* (2007) Comparison of cardiac structural and functional changes in obese otherwise healthy adults with versus without obstructive sleep apnea. *The American Journal of Cardiology*, **99**, 1298–302.

Paolisso, G., Manzella, D., Montano, N. *et al.* (2000) Plasma leptin concentrations and cardiac autonomic nervous system in healthy subjects with different body weights. *The Journal of Clinical Endocrinology and Metabolism*, **85**, 1810–4.

Paolisso, G., Tagliamonte, M.R. and Galderisi, M. (2001) Plasma leptin concentration, insulin sensitivity, and 24-hour ambulatory blood pressure and left ventricular geometry. *American Journal of Hypertension*, **14**, 114–20.

Papaioannou, A., Michaloudis, D., Fraidakis, O. *et al.* (2003) Effects of weight loss on QT interval in morbidly obese patients. *Obesity Surgery*, **13**, 869–73.

Pascual, M., Pascual, D.A. and Soria, F. (2003) Effects of isolated obesity on systolic and diastolic left ventricular function. *Heart (British Cardiac Society)*, **89**, 1152–6.

Pausova, Z. (2006) From big fat cells to high blood pressure: a pathway to obesity-associated hypertension. *Current Opinion in Nephrology and Hypertension*, **15**, 173–8.

Perrio, M.J., Wilton, L.V. and Shakir, S.A. (2007) The safety profiles of orlistat and sibutramine: results of prescription-event monitoring studies in England. *Obesity (Silver Spring)*, **15**, 2712–22.

Peterson, L.R., Waggoner, A.D., Schechtman, K.B. *et al.* (2004) Alterations in left ventricular structure and function in young healthy obese women: assessment by echocardiography and tissue Doppler imaging. *Journal of the American College of Cardiology*, **43**, 1399–404.

Pickering, T.G., Hall, J.E., Appel, L.J. *et al.* (2005) Recommendations for blood pressure measurement in humans and experimental animals: part 1: blood pressure measurement in humans: a statement for professionals from the Subcommittee of Professional and Public Education of the American Heart Association Council on High Blood Pressure Research. *Circulation*, **111**, 697–716.

Pinkney, J.H. *et al.* (1994) *Hypertension*, **24**, 362–4.

Pi-Sunyer, F.X., Aronne, L.J., Heshmati, H.M. *et al.* and RIO-North America Study Group (2006) Effect of rimonabant, a cannabinoid-1 receptor blocker, on weight and cardiometabolic risk factors in overweight or obese patients: RIO-North America: a randomized controlled trial. *The Journal of the American Medical Association*, **295**, 761–75.

Pladevall, M., Williams, K. and Guyer, H. (2003) The association between leptin and left ventricular hypertrophy: a population-based cross-sectional study. *Journal of Hypertension*, **21**, 1467–73.

Poirier, P., Giles, T.D., Bray, G.A. *et al.* and American Heart Association, Obesity Committee of the Council on Nutrition, Physical Activity, Metabolism (2006) Obesity and cardiovascular disease: pathophysiology, evaluation, and effect of weight loss: an update of the 1997 American Heart Association Scientific Statement on Obesity and Heart Disease from the Obesity Committee of the Council on Nutrition, Physical Activity, and Metabolism. *Circulation*, **113**, 898–918.

Pond, C.M. (2003) The contribution of wild animal biology to human physiology and medicine: adipose tissue associated with lymphoid and cardiac tissues. *Ecoscience*, **10**, 1–9.

Pond, C.M. and Mattacks, C.A. (1991) The effect of noradrenalin and insulin on lipolysis in adipocytes isolated from nine different adipose depots of guinea-pigs. *International Journal of Obesity*, **15**, 609–18.

Pond, C.M., Mattacks, C.A., Colby, R.H. and Tyler, N.J.C. (1993) The anatomy, chemical composition and maximum glycolytic capacity of adipose tissue in wild Svalbard reindeer in winter. *Journal of Zoology*, **229**, 17–40.

Pontiroli, A.E., Pizzocri, P., Saibene, A. *et al.* (2004) Left ventricular hypertrophy and QT interval in obesity and in hypertension: effects of weight loss and of normalisation of blood pressure. *International Journal of Obesity and Related Metabolic Disorders*, **28**, 1118–23.

Powell, B.D., Redfield, M.M., Bybee, K.A. *et al.* (2006) Association of obesity with left ventricular remodeling and diastolic dysfunction in patients without coronary artery disease. *The American Journal of Cardiology*, **98**, 116–20.

Rabkin, S.W., Mathewson, F.A. and Hsu, P.H. (1977) Relation of body weight to development of ischemic heart disease in a cohort of young North American men after a 26 year observation period: the Manitoba Study. *The American Journal of Cardiology*, **39**, 452–8.

Rana, J.S., Mukamal, K.J., Morgan, J.P. *et al.* (2004) Obesity and the risk of death after acute myocardial infarction. *American Heart Journal*, **147**, 841–6.

Rea, T.D., Heckbert, S.R., Kaplan, R.C. *et al.* (2001) Body mass index and the risk of recurrent coronary events following acute myocardial infarction. *The American Journal of Cardiology*, **88**, 467–72.

Reeves, B.C., Ascione, R., Chamberlain, M.H. and Angelini, G.D. (2003) Effect of body mass index on early outcomes in patients undergoing coronary artery bypass surgery. *Journal of the American College of Cardiology*, **42**, 668–76.

Reiner, L., Mazzoleni, A. and Rodriguez, F.L. (1955) Statistical analysis of the epicardial fat weight in human hearts. *AMA Archives of Pathology*, **60**, 369–73.

Reiner, L., Mazzoleni, A., Rodriguez, F.L. and Freudenthal, R.R. (1959) The weight of the human heart. I. Normal cases. *AMA Archives of Pathology*, **68**, 58–73.

Reingold, J.S., McGavock, J.M., Kaka, S. *et al.* (2005) Determination of triglyceride in the human myocardium using magnetic resonance spectroscopy: reproducibility and sensitivity of the method. *American Journal of Physiology. Endocrinology and Metabolism*, **289**, E935–9.

Remuzzi, G., Schieppati, A. and Ruggenenti, P. (2002) Clinical practice. Nephropathy in patients with type 2 diabetes. *The New England Journal of Medicine*, **346**, 1145–51.

Rexrode, K.M., Carey, V.J., Hennekens, C.H. *et al.* (1998) Abdominal adiposity and coronary heart disease in women. *The Journal of the American Medical Association*, **280**, 1843–8.

Romero-Corral, A., Montori, V.M., Somers, V.K. *et al.* (2006) Association of bodyweight with total mortality and with cardiovascular events in coronary artery disease: a systematic review of cohort studies. *Lancet*, **368**, 666–78.

Sacks, H.S. and Fain, J.N. (2007) Human epicardial adipose tissue: a review. *American Heart Journal*, **153**, 907–17.

Sader, S., Nian, M. and Liu, P. (2003) Leptin: a novel link between obesity, diabetes, cardiovascular risk, and ventricular hypertrophy. *Circulation*, **108**, 644–6.

Sasson, Z., Rasooly, Y., Gupta, R. and Rasooly, I. (1996) Left atrial enlargement in healthy obese: prevalence and relation to left ventricular mass and diastolic function. *The Canadian Journal of Cardiology*, **12**, 257–63.

Schächinger, V., Britten, M.B. and Zeiher, A.M. (2000) Prognostic impact of coronary vasodilator dysfunction on adverse long-term outcome of coronary heart disease. *Circulation*, **101**, 1899–906.

Schmieder, R.E. and Messerli, F.H. (1993) Does obesity influence early target organ damage in hypertensive patients? *Circulation*, **87**, 1482–8.

Seyfeli, E., Duru, M., Kuvandik, G. *et al.* (2006) Effect of obesity on P-wave dispersion and QT dispersion in women. *International Journal of Obesity (London)*, **30**, 957–61.

Sharma, A.M. (2001) Sibutramine in overweight/obese hypertensive patients. *International Journal of Obesity and Related Metabolic Disorders*, **25** (Suppl 4), S20–3.

Sharma, A.M. (2004a) Mediastinal fat, insulin resistance, and hypertension. *Hypertension*, **44**, 117–8.

Sharma, A.M. (2004b) Is there a rationale for angiotensin blockade in the management of obesity hypertension? *Hypertension*, **44**, 12–9.

Sharma, A.M. and Chetty, V.T. (2005) Obesity, hypertension and insulin resistance. *Acta Diabetologica*, **42** (suppl 1), S3–8.

Sharma, A.M., Pischon, T., Engeli, S. and Scholze, J. (2001) Choice of drug treatment for obesity-related hypertension: where is the evidence? *Journal of Hypertension*, **19**, 667–74.

Sharma, A.M., Janke, J., Gorzelniak, K. *et al.* (2002) Angiotensin blockade prevents type 2 diabetes by formation of fat cells. *Hypertension*, **40**, 609–11.

Shechter, M., Beigel, R., Freimark, D. *et al.* (2006) Short-term sibutramine therapy is associated with weight loss and improved endothelial function in obese patients with coronary artery disease. *The American Journal of Cardiology*, **97**, 1650–3.

Shimokawa, H. (1999) Primary endothelial dysfunction: atherosclerosis. *Journal of Molecular and Cellular Cardiology*, **31**, 23–37.

Shin, M.J., Hyun, Y.J., Kim, O.Y. *et al.* (2006) Weight loss effect on inflammation and LDL oxidation in metabolically healthy but obese (MHO) individuals: low inflammation and LDL oxidation in MHO women. *International Journal of Obesity (London)*, **30**, 1529–34.

Shirani, J., Berezowski, K. and Roberts, W.C. (1995) Quantitative measurement of normal and excessive (cor adiposum) subepicardial adipose tissue, its clinical significance, and its effect on electrocardiographic QRS voltage. *The American Journal of Cardiology*, **76**, 414–8.

Sims, A. (2001) Are there persons who are obese, but metabolically healthy? *Metabolism: Clinical and Experimental*, **50**, 1499–504.

Sjöström, L., Lindroos, A.K., Peltonen, M. *et al.* (2004) Swedish Obese Subjects Study Scientific Group. Lifestyle, diabetes, and cardiovascular risk factors 10 years after bariatric surgery. *The New England Journal of Medicine*, **351**, 2683–93.

Smith, S.C., Jr, Blair, S.N., Bonow, R.O. *et al.* (2001) AHA/ACC Guidelines for Preventing Heart Attack and Death in Patients With Atherosclerotic Cardiovascular Disease: 2001 update. A statement for healthcare professionals from the American Heart Association and the American College of Cardiology. *Journal of the American College of Cardiology*, **38**, 1581–3.

Smith, S.R. (2006) Importance of diagnosing and treating the metabolic syndrome in reducing cardiovascular risk. *Obesity (Silver Spring)*, **14** (Suppl 3), 128S–34S.

Soltis, E.E. and Cassis, L.A. (1991) Influence of perivascular adipose tissue on rat aortic smooth muscle responsiveness. *Clinical and Experimental Hypertension*, **275**, 681–92.

Sowers, J.R. (2003) Obesity as a cardiovascular risk factor. *The American Journal of Medicine*, **8** (Suppl 8A), 37S–41S.

Steinberg, H.O., Chaker, H., Leaming, R. *et al.* (1996) Obesity/insulin resistance is associated with endothelial dysfunction. Implications for the syndrome of insulin resistance. *The Journal of Clinical Investigation*, **97**, 2601–2610.

Steinberg, H.O., Tarshoby, M., Monestel, R. *et al.* (1997) Elevated circulating free fatty acid levels impair endothelium-dependent vasodilation. *The Journal of Clinical Investigation*, **100**, 1230–9.

Sundström, J., Lind, L. and Nyström, N. (2000) Left ventricular concentric remodeling rather than left ventricular hypertrophy is related to the insulin resistance syndrome in elderly men. *Circulation*, **101**, 2595–600.

Szczepaniak, L.S., Dobbins, R.L., Metzger, G.J. *et al.* (2003) Myocardial triglycerides and systolic function in humans: in vivo evaluation by localized proton spectroscopy and cardiac imaging. *Magnetic Resonance in Medicine*, **49**, 417–23.

Tanaka, N., Ryoke, T. and Hongo, M. (1998) Effects of growth hormone and IGF-I on cardiac hypertrophy and gene expression in mice. *The American Journal of Physiology*, **275**, H393–9.

Tansey, D.K., Aly, Z. and Sheppard, M.N. (2005) Fat in the right ventricle of the normal heart. *Histopathology*, **46**, 98–104.

Torquati, A., Wright, K., Melvin, W. and Richards, W. (2007) Effect of gastric bypass operation on Framingham and actual risk of cardiovascular events in class II to III obesity. *Journal of the American College of Surgeons*, **204**, 776–82.

Tritos, N.A., Manning, W.J. and Danias, P.G. (2004) Role of leptin in the development of cardiac hypertrophy in experimental animals and humans. *Circulation*, **109**, 67.

Turnbull, F., Neal, B., Algert, C. *et al.* and Blood Pressure Lowering Trialists' Collaboration (2005) Effects of different blood pressure-lowering regimens on major cardiovascular events in individuals with and without diabetes mellitus: results of prospectively designed overviews of randomized trials. *Archives of Internal Medicine*, **165**, 1410–9.

Valencia-Flores, M., Rebollar, V., Santiago, V. *et al.* (2004) Prevalence of pulmonary hypertension and its association with respiratory disturbances in obese patients living at moderately high altitude. *International Journal of Obesity and Related Metabolic Disorders*, **28**, 1174–80.

Varughese, G.I. and Lip, G.Y. (2005) Antihypertensive therapy in diabetes mellitus: insights from ALLHAT and the Blood Pressure-Lowering Treatment Trialists'

Collaboration meta-analysis. *Journal of Human Hypertension*, **19**, 851–3.

Verlohren, S., Dubrovska, G., Tsang, S.-Y. *et al.* (2004) Visceral periadventitial adipose tissue regulates arterial tone of mesenteric arteries. *Hypertension*, **44**, 271–6.

Vogel, J.A., Franklin, B.A., Zalesin, K.C. *et al.* (2007) Reduction in predicted coronary heart disease risk after substantial weight reduction after bariatric surgery. *The American Journal of Cardiology*, **99**, 222–6.

Wang, T.J., Parise, H., Levy, D. *et al.* (2004) Obesity and the risk of new-onset atrial fibrillation. *The Journal of the American Medical Association*, **292**, 2471–7.

Wassertheil-Smoller, S., Fann, C., Allman, R.M. *et al.* (2000) Relation of low body mass to death and stroke in the systolic hypertension in the elderly program. The SHEP Cooperative Research Group. *Archives of Internal Medicine*, **160**, 494–500.

Watanabe, K., Sekiya, M., Tsuruoka, T. *et al.* (1999) Effect of insulin resistance on left ventricular hypertrophy and dysfunction in essential hypertension. *Journal of Hypertension*, **17**, 1153–60.

Watts, G.F., O'Brien, S.F., Silvester, W. and Millar, J.A. (1996) Impaired endothelium-dependent and independent dilatation of forearm resistance arteries in men with diet-treated non-insulin-dependent diabetes: role of dyslipidaemia. *Clinical Science*, **91**, 567–73.

Weinberger, M.H. (1985) Blood pressure and metabolic responses to hydrochlorothiazide, captopril, and the combination in black and white mild-to-moderate hypertensive patients. *Journal of Cardiovascular Pharmacology*, **7** (Suppl 1), S52–5.

Widlansky, M.E., Sesso, H.D., Rexrode, K.M. *et al.* (2004) Body Mass Index and total and cardiovascular mortality in men with a history of cardiovascular disease. *Archives of Internal Medicine*, **164**, 2326–32.

Willens, H.J., Byers, P., Chirinos, J.A. *et al.* (2007) Effects of weight loss after bariatric surgery on epicardial fat measured using echocardiography. *The American Journal of Cardiology*, **99**, 1242–5.

Wilson, P.W., D'Agostino, R.B., Sullivan, L. *et al.* (2002) Overweight and obesity as determinants of cardiovascular risk: the Framingham experience. *Archives of Internal Medicine*, **162**, 1867–72.

Wirth, A., Scholze, J., Sharma, A.M. *et al.* (2006) Reduced left ventricular mass after treatment of obese patients with sibutramine: an echocardiographic multicentre study. *Diabetes, Obesity & Metabolism*, **8**, 674–81.

Wong, C.H. and Marwick, T.H. (2007) Alterations in myocardial characteristics associated with obesity: detection, mechanisms, and implication. *Trends in Cardiovascular Medicine*, **17**, 1–5.

Wong, C.Y., O'Moore-Sullivan, T., Leano, R. *et al.* (2004) Alterations of left ventricular myocardial characteristics associated with obesity. *Circulation*, **110**, 3081–7.

Yusuf, S., Hawken, S., Ounpuu, S. *et al.* and Interheart Study Investigators (2005) Obesity and the risk of myocardial infarction in 27,000 participants from 52 countries: a case-control study. *Lancet*, **5**, 1640–9.

Zacharias, A., Schwann, T.A., Riordan, C.J. *et al.* (2005) Obesity and risk of new-onset atrial fibrillation after cardiac surgery. *Circulation*, **112**, 3247–55.

Zhang, X., Shu, X.O., Gao, Y.T. *et al.* (2004) Anthropometric predictors of coronary heart disease in Chinese women. *International Journal of Obesity and Related Metabolic Disorders*, **28**, 734–40.

Zhou, Y.T., Grayburn, P., Karim, A. *et al.* (2000) Lipotoxic heart disease in obese rats: implications for human obesity. *Proceedings of the National Academy of Sciences of the United States of America*, **97**, 1784–89.

Obesity and Other Diseases

Chapter 13

Key points

- Obesity increases the risk of osteoarthritis of the knees, hips and hands; excessive pressure loading and changes in adipokines that damage cartilage and bone may contribute. Shoulder tendinitis and plantar fasciitis are also more common, and fracture risk in children is increased.

- Lung volumes are decreased due to mechanical restriction. Obstructive sleep apnoea (OSA), with intermittent occlusion of the upper airway and oxygen desaturation during sleep, is due to compression by surrounding fat and perhaps inflammatory and central actions of adipokines. Complications of OSA include hypertension, heart failure and premature death. Snoring and daytime sleepiness are characteristic, and polysomnography demonstrates episodic awakening and desaturation. Continuous positive airway pressure (CPAP) ventilation at night greatly improves symptoms and prognosis. Obesity/hyperventilation syndrome (OHS) results from inadequate ventilatory drive and causes pulmonary hypertension and premature death. CPAP and weight loss can be helpful.

- Polycystic ovarian syndrome (PCOS) is characterised by failure of ovulation, causing multiple ovarian cysts and infertility. Obesity affects 40% of cases, while a family history of PCOS increases by 4–10 fold the risk of developing the disorder. Insulin resistance is present, and 10% of subjects have type 2 diabetes. Increased androgen levels (possibly stimulated by hyperinsulinaemia) lead to hirsutism; acanthosis nigricans may occur. A high luteinizing hormone (LH): follicle stimulating hormone (FSH) ratio and ovarian cysts on ultrasound scanning suggest the diagnosis. Metformin or thiazolidinediones can restore ovulation and fertility.

- Obese men show falls in testosterone, although levels of the active metabolite (dihydrotestosterone) remain normal. Sperm count and motility are reduced, sometimes causing infertility.

- Growth hormone (GH) levels are reduced, due to both reduced secretion and enhanced clearance, but growth is not impaired. Sympathetic activity may be enhanced, perhaps to central stimulation by raised insulin and/or leptin levels. Vitamin D3 is sequestered in fat and its bioavailability reduced; subclinical secondary hyperparathyroidism may affect 25–40% of obese subjects.

- Gastrointestinal complications of obesity include hiatus hernia and gastro-oesophageal reflux; the latter is implicated in the premalignant Barrett's oesophagus. Gallstones are sevenfold more common in obese women.

- Obesity and overweight predispose to many malignancies. Prevalence and deaths are increased for cancers of the oesophagus, colon and rectum, liver, gall-bladder, pancreas and kidney. Postmenopausal obese women are at increased risk of breast, uterine, cervical and ovarian cancers, while obese men have a higher prevalence of poorly-differentiated prostate cancer. Aetiological factors may include raised insulin and IGF-1 levels. Haematological malignancies (especially lymphomas) are more common; pro-inflammatory cytokines generated by adipose tissue, and perhaps physical inactivity and overconsumption of dairy products, may also contribute.

Chapter 13   Obesity and Other Diseases

Mimi Chen and Robert Andrews

In addition to its metabolic and cardiovascular consequences, obesity can contribute to the development and progression of many other diseases (Table 13.1). These range from osteoarthritis of weight-bearing joints to endocrine disorders such as polycystic ovarian disease and various cancers. Obesity also has a considerable psychological and psychiatric impact, discussed in detail in Chapter 14.

Musculoskeletal disorders

Musculoskeletal disorders are an important cause of impaired quality of life, disability and lost productivity, and collectively are the most expensive disease category for European healthcare (Lindgren, 1998). Obesity has long been associated with osteoarthritis and soft-tissue disorders, but no convincing links have been identified with rheumatoid arthritis or other inflammatory joint diseases.

Osteoarthritis

Osteoarthritis is the most common musculoskeletal disorder. Obesity is a well-known risk factor for both the development and progression of osteoarthritis in weight-bearing joints, notably the knees (Felson *et al.*, 1988) and to a lesser extent the hips (Reijman *et al.*, 2007) (Figure 13.1). The relative risk of developing osteoarthritis of the knees rises by over 100-fold (from 0.1 to 13.6) as BMI increases from $\leq 20\,\text{kg/m}^2$ to $\geq 36\,\text{kg/m}^2$, as compared with the risk at a 'normal' BMI of $24–24.9\,\text{kg/m}^2$ (Coggon *et al.*, 2001). Population-based case-control studies indicate that, in men, even a modest rise in BMI within the normal range significantly increases the risk of developing osteoarthritis of the knees (Holmberg, Thelin and Thelin, 2005). Osteoarthritis of the knees and hips progresses more rapidly in obese subjects, who are more likely to need joint replacement; perhaps surprisingly, however, obesity does not increase the risk of these operations failing and requiring revision (Amin *et al.*, 2006). Interestingly, osteoarthritis of the hands is also more common in obese people (Figure 13.1), whereas the foot and ankle joints are relatively spared.

The association between obesity and osteoarthritis is poorly understood. The classical explanation – excessive mechanical loading of the joints during locomotion – appears valid for the hips and knees, which suffer additional strain because the varus (bow-legged) deformity of obese legs disturbs the normal vertical alignment of these weight-bearing joints (Figure 13.2). However, this cannot explain the sparing of weight-bearing joints below the knee, or osteoarthritis of the hands. Recent research points to altered metabolism of cartilage and bone, leading to loss of cartilage and remodelling of damaged bone, with increased density and overgrowth to form the characteristic osteophytes. These changes may be induced by increased local concentrations of adipokines (leptin and resistin) released by the expanded fat mass, and the concomitant fall in adiponectin (see Chapter 4). An increased ratio of leptin to adiponectin in synovial fluid may trigger cartilage destruction and thus contribute to the initiation and/or progression of osteoarthritis (Pottie *et al.*, 2006; Alexander, 2004). These circulating factors may help to explain the involvement of non-weight-bearing joints, and also how weight loss can protect against both the development and progression of osteoarthritis.

Other disorders

Obesity increases the risk of developing tendinitis of the shoulder, causing a 'painful arc syndrome' and plantar fasciitis (Wearing *et al.*, 2006; Wendelboe *et al.*, 2004). Shoulder tendinitis may

Obesity: Science to Practice   Edited by Gareth Williams and Gema Frühbeck
© 2009 John Wiley & Sons, Ltd

Table 13.1 Impact of obesity on other systems of the body.

Musculoskeletal system

- Osteoarthritis of hips, knees and hands
- Tendinitis of shoulders, plantar fasciitis
- Increased fracture risk in children

Respiratory system

- Mechanical restriction of ventilation
- Obstructive sleep apnoea (OSA)
- Obesity/hypoventilation syndrome (OHS)

Endocrine system

- Polycystic ovarian syndrome (PCOS)
- Female infertility, complications of pregnancy
- Male infertility, erectile dysfunction
- Reduced growth hormone secretion and levels (growth not impaired)
- Secondary hyperparathyroidism (subclinical)

Gastrointestinal tract

- Hiatus hernia
- Gastro-oesophageal reflux and Barrett's oesophagus
- Gallstones (especially in women)
- Non-alcoholic fatty liver disease (Chapter 11)

Malignancies (see Table 13.6)

Skin

- Acanthosis nigricans

Psychological and psychiatric disorders (Chapters 14 and 20)

be due to excessive pressure loading of the rotator cuff muscles and tendons, while plantar fasciitis is thought to result from reduced flexibility of the ankle joint and increased tensile loading of the sole. Heel pain may also arise from reduced elasticity of the underlying fat pad, increasing the force transmitted to the heel. Overall, subjects with a BMI >30 kg/m^2 have a fourfold increased risk of developing musculoskeletal pain involving the back, hip, knee, ankle and foot (Wearing *et al.*, 2006).

The risk of bone fracture following trauma is altered by obesity, with opposite effects in children and adults. Obese children are at increased risk of fractures, possibly because bone mineral density is lower as a result of reduced physical activity and poor nutrition. By contrast, obesity may protect against fractures in older adults. A recent meta-analysis found a 17% reduction in the risk of hip fractures in men and women with a mean age of 63 years whose BMI was >30 kg/m^2, as compared with subjects with a BMI of 25 kg/m^2 (De Laet *et al.*, 2005). Suggested mechanisms include the enhanced bone density of the femoral head and neck, which has been demonstrated in White women (Castro *et al.*, 2005), as well as greater cushioning by the overlying fat layer.

Respiratory system

Obesity adversely affects several aspects of respiratory function, partly through mechanical restriction of respiration, as well as poorly

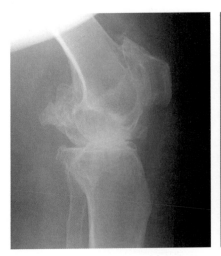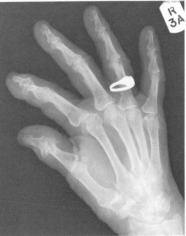

Figure 13.1 Osteoarthritis of the knee and hand in an obese subject. Images reproduced by courtesy of Ros Andrews, Bristol from own x-ray collection.

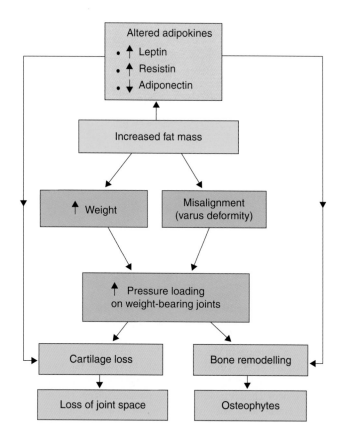

Figure 13.2 Possible mechanisms to explain the role of obesity in the development and progression of osteoarthritis.

explained indirect effects. Apart from a suggestion that it may predispose to childhood asthma (see Chapter 21), there is no evidence that obesity causes or worsens intrinsic lung disease.

Lung volumes

Obesity restricts expansion of the chest wall and downward movement of the diaphragm. As weight increases, all lung volumes decline, the greatest impact being on the functional residual capacity (FRC) and expiratory reserve volume (ERV), as shown in Figure 13.3. In one study, subjects with a BMI of 30 kg/m^2 showed reductions in FRC and ERV of 25 and 53%, respectively, compared with the values at a BMI of 20 kg/m^2 (Jones and Nzekwu, 2006). Cohort studies have demonstrated that vital capacity (VC) falls by ~25 ml for each 1 kg of excess weight (Chen, Horne and Dosman, 1993). With increasing weight, airway resistance increases, and forced expiratory volume in 1 second (FEV1) falls, possibly because small airways tend to close as lung volumes decline (Jones and

Nzekwu, 2006). Reduced static lung volumes, together with enhanced respiratory drive, possibly in response to the increased mechanical loading of the chest wall and abdomen, can cause otherwise healthy obese people to feel breathless, especially when respiratory demand is increased through physical activity (Chen, Horne and Dosman, 1993; El-Gamal et al., 2005).

Obstructive sleep apnoea (OSA)

OSA is characterized by episodes of partial and/or complete occlusion of the pharynx during sleep, leading to cessation of breathing for at least 10 seconds and sometimes for over a minute. Sleep is disturbed by restlessness, snoring (often very loud), the typical prolonged apnoeic episodes, and recurrent awakening; morning headache and daytime sleepiness and impaired concentration are also typical (Table 13.2).

Obesity is the most important risk factor for OSA. The general prevalence of OSA in middle-aged men and women is respectively

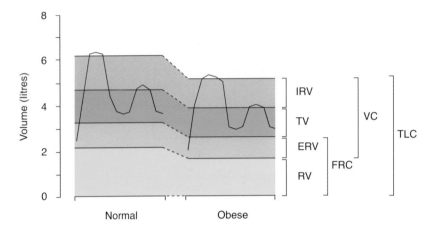

Figure 13.3 Impact of obesity on lung volumes. ERV: expiratory reserve volume; FRC: functional residual capacity; IRV: inspiratory reserve volume; RV: residual volume; TLC: total lung capacity; TV: tidal volume; VC: vital capacity.

4–9% and 1–2%, but this rises over 10-fold to 40–70% in morbidly obese subjects whose BMI is >35 kg/m². Furthermore, weight gain of 10% is associated with a 6-fold increase in the risk of developing OSA (Svatikova *et al.*, 2005).

Until recently, the association was attributed to excess fat in the neck compressing the upper airway. Morbidly obese men with OSA show a reduction in pharyngeal cross-sectional area that is proportional to surrounding fat deposition (Figure 13.4). Conversely, weight loss in obese subjects results in an increased pharyngeal area and a corresponding reduction

Table 13.2 Symptoms of obstructive sleep apnoea (OSA).

Daytime symptoms

- Excessive daytime sleepiness
- Morning headaches
- Impaired concentration
- Depression
- Irritability

Nocturnal symptoms

- Snoring
- Recurrent awakening
- Restlessness, particularly affecting the legs
- Nocturnal choking, gasping and snorting
- Breathing cessation for over 10 seconds

Other symptoms

- Decreased libido
- Impotence

in the severity of the OSA (Busetto *et al.*, 2005). Interestingly, recent evidence implicates raised levels of pro-inflammatory adipokines, notably TNF-α and interleukin-6 (IL-6), released especially by visceral fat, in the development of OSA. Consistent with this suggestion, pilot studies using metanercept (a fusion protein that mimics the TNF-deactivating action of the soluble TNF-α receptor) have shown significant reductions in the frequency of apnoeic episodes and in daytime sleepiness in obese subjects with OSA (Vgontzas, Bixler and Chrousos, 2005). Suggested pathogenic mechanisms include decreased respiratory drive (especially at night), inflammation of the upper airways and soft-tissue oedema (Vgontzas, Bixler and Chrousos, 2005).

OSA is a serious condition that damages quality of life for the sufferers (and often their partner) and also increases morbidity and risk of premature death, especially from cardiovascular diseases (Marin *et al.*, 2005). Cardiovascular complications include hypertension, myocardial infarction and heart failure, for which OSA doubles the 5-year mortality rate from 12% to 24% (Marin *et al.*, 2005; Wang *et al.*, 2007). Deleterious effects of periodic deoxygenation and excessive cardiac loading from exaggerated inspiratory effort may contribute (Stradling, 2007).

Awareness of OSA among physicians is poor, and the diagnosis is often missed and treatment delayed. The diagnosis is based on the characteristic symptoms (Table 13.2); the sleep history is often graphically provided by the patient's partner. The Epworth Sleepiness Scale (Table 13.3) is useful for quantifying daytime symptoms (Johns, 1991). A neck circumference of >42 cm

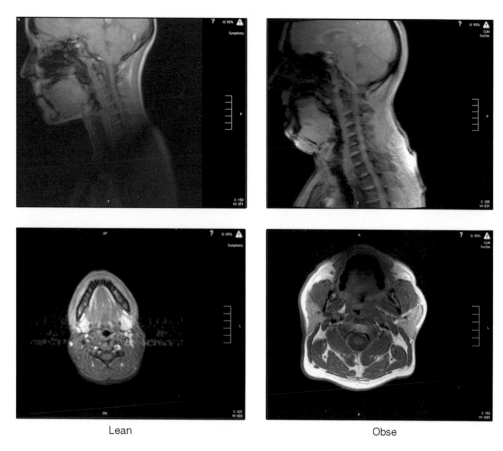

Lean   Obse

Figure 13.4 MRI scans of the head and neck in a lean subject (left) and an obese subject with OSA (right). The obese subject shows encroachment of the upper airway by surrounding adipose tissue. Images courtesy of Dr. Secundino Fernández, Department of Othorrhinolaringology, Clínica Universitaria de Navarra, Spain.

in men and >38 cm in women is strongly predictive of clinically significant OSA. Sleep studies (polysomnography) are diagnostic, demonstrating both the apnoeic episodes (with increased inspiratory effort against a closed pharynx), and the resulting fall in transcutaneous oxygen tension (Figure 13.5). Once the diagnosis is established, the Apnoea/Hypopnoea Index (AHI), which quantifies sleep disruption and oxygen desaturation, is useful to determine the severity of the OSA (American Academy of Sleep Medicine Task Force, 1991).

Treatment of OSA requires specialist intervention. Continuous positive airway pressure (CPAP) ventilation during the night, delivered using a tightly-fitting mask over the mouth and nose, keeps the upper airway open; this dramatically reduces the frequency of apnoea and oxygen desaturation, with a striking improvement in symptoms and quality of life (Stradling, 2007). Blood pressure and cardiac function also

improve, and life expectancy may be extended (Stradling, 2007). Weight loss also improves symptoms, but may require a long time to be effective. Some patients with structural abnormalities of the lower face or neck may be helped by surgical reconstruction, but operations to remove the uvula and redundant soft palate have now fallen out of favour.

Obesity/hypoventilation syndrome (OHS)

This rare condition, strongly associated with obesity, can occur alone or may develop secondarily to OSA. It has also been called the 'Pickwickian Syndrome' after Joe, the obese and hypersomnolent boy in Dickens' *The Pickwick Papers*.

OHS is due to inadequate ventilatory drive, presumably at the level of the respiratory centre, leading to severe hypoxaemia and ultimately hypercapnic respiratory failure. Associated features are pulmonary hypertension and right-sided heart

Table 13.3 The Epworth sleepiness scale.

The scale is used to quantify the level of daytime sleepiness. Each of the eight situations listed below is scored from 0 to 3 for the likelihood of dozing, using the following scale:

0 = No chance of dozing

1 = Slight chance of dozing

2 = Moderate chance of dozing

3 = High chance of dozing

Situations:

- Sitting and reading
- Watching television
- Sitting inactive in a public place (e.g. a meeting or in the theatre)
- As a passenger in a car for an hour, without a break
- Lying down to rest in the afternoon, when circumstances permit
- Sitting and talking to someone
- Sitting quietly after lunch without alcohol
- In a car, while stopped for a few minutes in traffic

Interpretation of results:

0−9 = Average daytime sleepiness

10−15 = Excessive daytime sleepiness

16−24 = Moderate to severe daytime sleepiness, requiring investigation

failure (cor pulmonale), which are unexplained. Life expectancy is severely reduced: in one study, the 18-month mortality rate was 23%, compared with 9% among obese subjects without OHS (Nowbar *et al.*, 2004). The causes of ventilatory failure and the unresponsiveness to hypoxaemia and hypercapnia are not known. Postulated factors include respiratory muscle dysfunction, reduced respiratory drive and blunted chemosensitivity to low oxygen and high carbon dioxide levels; 'resistance' to central actions of leptin has been implicated (Piper and Grunstern, 2007).

As with OSA, the diagnosis and treatment are often neglected. A high index of suspicion, coupled with a careful history, is required and the measurement of arterial oxygen and carbon dioxide tensions is diagnostic. Treatment is by CPAP, to prevent apnoea and hypopnoea; non-invasive mechanical intervention, to alleviate daytime hypercapnia; and weight loss, which improves both pulmonary function and central ventilatory drive.

Endocrine system

Endocrine disorders are well-recognized but overall rare causes of human obesity, classical examples being Cushing's syndrome and hypothyroidism (see Chapter 8). Conversely, obesity influences the secretion and/or actions of several hormones, although most of the effects are relatively subtle and have no obvious clinical consequences. An important exception is polycystic ovarian syndrome (PCOS), in which obesity is a major aetiological factor. In addition, the presence of obesity may influence the interpretation of various endocrine investigations.

Polycystic ovarian syndrome (PCOS)

This disorder is named for the characteristic multiple ovarian cysts (Figure 13.6), which are persisting immature Graafian follicles that have failed to discharge their ova. Fertility is therefore impaired. Failure of ovulation also means that the corpus luteum does not form, so that levels of progesterone, its main secretory product, do not show the normal rise in the second (luteal) phase of the menstrual cycle. This in turns prevents the normal progesterone-driven hyperplasia of the endometrium, resulting in long or irregular cycles or amenorrhoea.

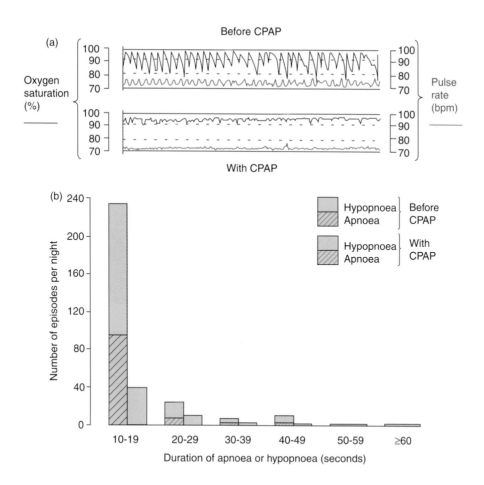

Figure 13.5 Sleep studies in subjects with OSA. (a) Representative 30-min tracings, showing hypopnoeic and apnoeic episodes, with resulting falls in oxygen saturation (black tracing) and increases in pulse rate (blue tracing). The improvement with CPAP is shown in the lower panel. (b) Effect of CPAP on the frequency of episodes of hypopnoea and apnoea. The histogram shows the frequency of episodes per night, sorted according to their duration, in a subject with moderately severe OSA, before and during CPAP.

Other clinical features include variable manifestations of increased androgen levels, notably hirsutism and acne, and occasionally acanthosis nigricans, a dark, velvety thickening of the skin – particularly in the axilla, groin and nape of the neck – which is associated with insulin resistance (see Table 13.4 and Figure 13.7). Insulin resistance and glucose intolerance are common, the overall prevalence of type 2 diabetes and IGT being about 10 and 35%, respectively (Norman et al., 2007).

Aetiology of PCOS

Obesity is a powerful risk factor for the development of PCOS, affecting up to 40% of cases. The time-course and distribution of obesity are important factors in the development of PCOS, and its influence apparently begins *in utero*. The daughters of women who were obese during pregnancy are at increased risk of developing hyperandrogenism and PCOS, possibly because exposing the fetus to the obese mother's increased androgen levels may programme the future deposition of excess fat, especially in visceral sites (Abbott, Dumesic and Franks, 2002). Subsequently, obesity in early childhood (~7 years) and in the early 20s confers the greatest risk of developing menstrual problems and PCOS by the age of 33 years (Lake, Power and Cole, 1997). Women with central and visceral obesity are most likely to develop PCOS, probably because their circulating levels of free testosterone and insulin are higher than

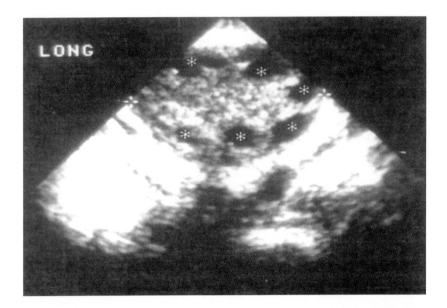

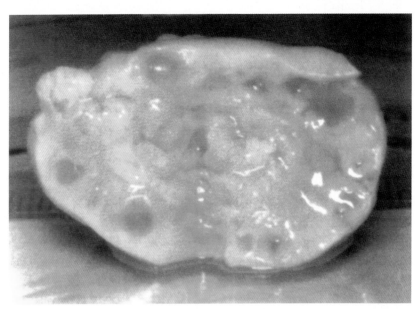

Figure 13.6 Polycystic ovarian syndrome (PCOS). The characteristic cysts (below) are readily visible on ultrasound scanning (above). Images reproduced courtesy of Dr D. Kiddy and Professor Steven Franks, Imperial College School of Medicine, London.

in women with lower-body adiposity (Kirschner *et al.*, 1990).

Genetic susceptibility is also important, and women with a family history of PCOS are 4–10 times more likely to develop the condition (Urbanek, 2007). Twin studies suggest that several genes, each with significant impact, are responsible; over 70 candidate genes have been studied, but none has yet been convincingly implicated (Urbanek, 2007).

The endocrine abnormalities of PCOS are not fully explained. Characteristic features include a raised LH:FSH ratio and absence of the LH surge that normally triggers ovulation. Progesterone levels are persistently low, while androgen concentrations (free testosterone

Table 13.4 Clinical features of the polycystic ovarian syndrome (PCOS), and their pathophysiological basis. The major endocrine abnormalities are also shown.

Clinical features

- Obesity (40% of cases)
- Long irregular cycles
- Amenorrhoea
- Infertility
- Hirsutism
- Acanthosis nigricans

- Arrested folliculogenesis
- Absence of corpus luteum
- Anovulation
- Increased androgen levels
- Insulin resistance

Endocrine abnormalities

- Oestradiol: persistently follicular-phase levels
- Progesterone: persistently low (no luteal-phase rise)
- LH: sustained high levels, but no preovulatory surge
- LH:FSH ratio: raised
- Testosterone and androstenedione: levels raised
- Sex hormone binding globulin (SHBG): levels decreased
- Insulin: levels raised, with insulin resistance

and androstenedione) are raised. Elevated insulin concentrations and/or decreased sensitivity of the hypothalamo-pituitary-ovarian axis to insulin probably play a role, because weight loss and insulin-sensitizing drugs that lower insulin levels can correct the endocrine abnormalities and restore ovulation. High circulating insulin levels apparently stimulate thecal cells in the ovarian follicles to produce androgens.

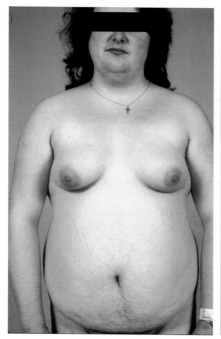 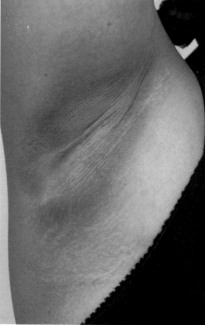

Figure 13.7 Clinical features of PCOS, showing hirsutism (left) and acanthosis nigricans (right). Images reproduced by courtesy of Dr. Cameron Kennedy, University Hospitals Bristol, UK.

Diagnosis and treatment

The history of irregular or absent periods and/or infertility, especially in an obese woman, should lead to the endocrine investigations described above. Ovarian ultrasound scanning will typically show multiple cysts (Figure 13.6).

Treatment centres on improving insulin sensitivity, through weight loss or drugs such as metformin and thiazolidinediones (Norman *et al.*, 2007). Weight loss of 2–5%, especially if combined with exercise, can lower androgen levels and improve hirsutism (although this may take many months), and can ultimately restore ovulation and regularize the cycles. Metformin and thiazolidinediones may induce ovulation without substantial weight loss; women need to be warned of this possible effect, and contraceptive advice offered if appropriate.

Other effects on female reproductive function

Obesity can also interfere with reproductive function in women who do not have PCOS, with a tendency to reduced LH and FSH concentrations and decreased oestradiol production, even though menstruation may be normal (De Pergola *et al.*, 2006). Fertility can also be reduced. Compared with normal-weight women, those with a BMI of >30 kg/m² have a 2.7-fold higher risk of infertility, and those who succeed in becoming pregnant have a 25–37% increased risk of miscarrying (Linne, 2004). Obese women are less likely to respond to treatment for infertility, and

have a greater risk of early pregnancy loss following *in-vitro* fertilization treatment (Pasquali, Patton and Gambineri, 2007).

Pregnancy can be hazardous for the obese woman and her child (Table 13.5). The mother has higher risks of developing hypertension, gestational diabetes and complications of delivery such as prolonged labour; rates of Caesarean section are higher than in normal-weight women. The children of obese mothers are more likely to die *in utero* and to suffer congenital abnormalities, head trauma, shoulder dystocia and death within the first year (Linne, 2004). Weight loss can considerably improve an obese woman's chances of becoming pregnant and the outcomes of pregnancy, and this should be strongly encouraged before any attempt to conceive (Clark *et al.*, 1998).

Prolactin secretion shows subtle disturbances in obese women, and in obese men (Kok *et al.*, 2004). Basal levels and pulses both show increases that are proportional to BMI and visceral fat mass, and the normal mid-sleep peak is delayed (Figure 13.8). There is also blunting of the increases in prolactin secretion normally evoked by various stimuli, such as hypoglycaemia, thyrotrophin releasing hormone (TRH) and metoclopramide. These abnormalities are reversed by weight loss, suggesting that they are secondary to obesity (Kok *et al.*, 2006). Any impact on female reproduction is uncertain, and lactation is not obviously affected.

Male reproductive function

Obese men have relatively low testosterone and high oestrogen levels compared with lean men,

Table 13.5   Hazards of obesity in pregnancy.

For the mother	For the baby
Increased risk of:	*Increased risk of:*
• Gestational diabetes	• Spina bifida and other congenital abnormalities
• Hypertension	• Death *in utero*
• Pre-eclampsia	• Birth trauma: head injury, shoulder dystocia, brachial plexus lesions, fracture of clavicle
• Preterm delivery	• Increased perinatal mortality
• Increased risk of induced delivery	
• Prolonged delivery	
• Increased risk of caesarean sections	
• Thromboembolism	
• Vulval or perineal tears	

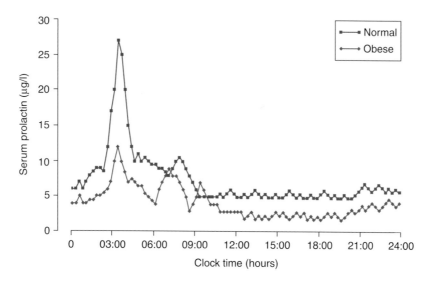

Figure 13.8 Effects of obesity on the 24-h profile of circulating prolactin levels. From Kok *et al.* (2004).

other androgens being unaffected. Fertility may be impaired, but there are no overt signs of male hypogonadism or feminization (Kokkoris and PiSunyer, 2003); the presence of these features should prompt a search for other genetic or endocrine conditions.

Total and free testosterone levels decline as BMI rises (Vermeulen, 1996). This may be due to increased activity of the aromatase in adipose tissue, which converts testosterone to oestradiol and so also raises oestrogen concentrations. Concomitantly, sex hormone binding globulin (SHBG) falls. Concentrations of the testosterone precursor, androstenedione, remain essentially normal, suggesting that testosterone production is not blocked. Levels of dihydrotestosterone (DHT) the most active form of the hormone, remain normal, as do the adrenal-derived androgens, DHEA and DHEAS (Kley, Edelmann and Kruskemper, 1980; Vermeulen *et al.*, 1993). LH does not rise as would normally be expected with low testosterone levels, possibly indicating altered sensitivity to negative feedback at the hypothalamus and/or pituitary. FSH levels are reduced, possibly because of the increased oestrogens produced by the aromatization of testosterone in adipose tissue (Kokkoris and PiSunyer, 2003).

The impact of obesity on male fertility has been neglected until recently. Erectile dysfunction becomes more common with increasing BMI, with the prevalence rising from 17% in lean men to 45% in those with a BMI of $>30\,kg/m^2$

(Kratzik *et al.*, 2005; Cheng and Ng, 2007). Furthermore, the concentration, total sperm count and the number of motile sperm all fall as weight increases; overall, obese men have a 10% greater chance of being infertile than those of normal weight (Nguyen *et al.*, 2007).

With weight loss, testosterone and SHGB levels return to normal and erectile function improves (Esposito *et al.*, 2004). The effect on semen quality is unknown.

Growth hormone and IGF-1

The growth hormone/IGF-1 axis is influenced by nutritional state at several levels (Figure 13.9). For example, growth hormone (GH) secretion is stimulated by the orexigenic gut peptide ghrelin, and inhibited by IGF-1, whose free levels are indirectly regulated by insulin. The pattern of GH secretion affects the sensitivity of its target tissues to its actions, and therefore the hormone's effects. It has been suggested that the greater pulsatility of GH release in men, compared with the relatively continuous profile in women, may determine the different patterns of linear growth between the sexes.

In obese subjects, plasma GH levels are decreased due to a combination of reduced basal and diurnal secretion and enhanced metabolic clearance. The normal circadian rhythm is maintained, but GH pulses are sparser and smaller, and the nocturnal peak is diminished

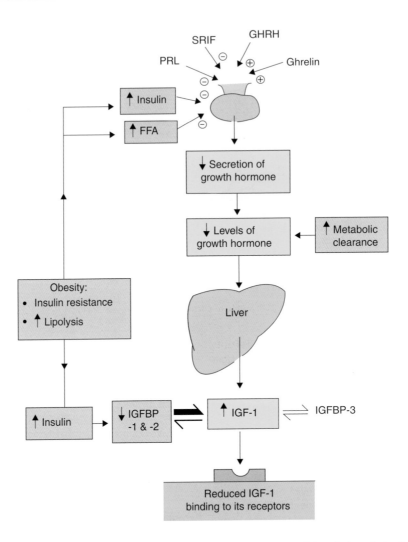

Figure 13.9 Effects of obesity on the growth hormone/IGF-1 axis. Abnormalities of the axis in obesity are highlighted in yellow, and possible causative factors in blue. FFA: free fatty acids; GHRH: growth hormone releasing hormone; IGFBP: IGF-1 binding proteins; PRL: prolactin; SRIF: somatostatin.

(Scacchi, Pincelli and Cavagnini, 1999; Kokkoris and PiSunyer, 2003). Plasma GH levels are reduced in proportion to BMI, typically by 75% (Veldhuis et al., 1991). Moreover, GH responses to stimuli such as exercise, hypoglycaemia, arginine, clonidine and growth hormone-releasing hormone (GHRH), are attenuated (Scacchi, Pincelli and Cavagnini, 1999; Kokkoris and PiSunyer, 2003; Kanaley et al., 1999). In some cases, GH responses are so blunted that GH deficiency may be suspected; however, in contrast to GH-deficient subjects, obese individuals do not show delayed growth. True growth hormone deficiency can be distinguished using a combined arginine and GHRH stimulation test, applying

BMI-specific cut-off values (Ghigo, Aimaretti and Corneli, 2008). Basal and stimulated GH secretion return to normal following weight loss (Edén Engström et al., 2006).

The causes of impaired GH secretion in obesity are uncertain, but may include the inhibitory effects of chronically raised insulin and free fatty acid (FFA) levels (Alvarez-Castro et al., 2004), and abnormalities in the hypothalamic systems that regulate growth hormone release, such as ghrelin and neuropeptide Y (Alvarez-Castro et al., 2004).

The growth-promoting and metabolic effects of GH are mediated by IGF-1, which is secreted mainly by the liver in response to GH (Figure 13.9). Some IGF-1 is also produced locally in GH target tissues.

Circulating IGF-1 is mostly bound to its binding proteins, notably IGFBP-1, -2 and -3, with only 1% of the total being free to act on IGF-1 receptors on target tissues. The abundant IGFBP-3 binds the most GH, but IGFBP-1 and -2 have short half-lives and their production is regulated (inhibited) by insulin; these therefore largely determine the availability of free IGF-1. In obese subjects, levels of IGFBP-1 and -2 are decreased (presumably by hyperinsulinaemia), while IGFBP-3 is increased. Overall, free IGF-1 is usually elevated, but this is offset by reduced binding of IGF-1 to its tissue receptors (Hochberg et al., 1992).

Adrenocortical function

Many obese subjects show increased cortisol secretion, but clearance is also enhanced, so that 24-hour plasma cortisol levels remain unchanged. Cortisol hypersecretion is probably driven by increased activity of the hypothalamo-pituitary-adrenocortical (HPA) axis, possibly due to increased responsiveness to stress and eating, which normally causes a slight rise in plasma cortisol (Ljung et al., 1996; Björntorp, 2001).

Cortisol action on its target tissues may also be influenced by obesity, as obese subjects apparently have organ-specific alterations in the activity of 11-β hydroxysteroid dehydrogenase type 1 (11β-HSD 1) the enzyme that converts the inactive cortisone to cortisol. 11β-HSD 1 activity is decreased in the liver, but increased in fat, which would therefore be exposed to higher local cortisol concentrations. In theory, this might promote the differentiation of adipose tissue stromal cells to mature adipocytes (see Chapter 4), thus encouraging fat deposition. Specific inhibitors of 11β-HSD 1 are currently undergoing clinical evaluation as potential anti-obesity agents.

Changes in HPA activity are presumed to be secondary to obesity. The effects of weight loss have not been comprehensively examined; one small study found no effect on the responses to corticotrophin-releasing factor (CRF) (Yanovski et al., 1997).

Thyroid function

Minor disturbances in Thyroid stimulating hormone (TSH) and thyroid hormone levels are seen in obesity, although values remain within the normal reference range. TSH and free and total triiodothyronine (T_3) concentrations may be relatively higher than in lean subjects (Iacobellis et al., 2005; Manji et al., 2006), whereas TRH and thyroxine levels (free and total) show no differences (Kokkoris and PiSunyer, 2003). One study reported that TSH levels were positively correlated with BMI, possibly because leptin stimulates TRH and TSH release (Kokkoris and PiSunyer, 2003).

Overfeeding lean subjects increases plasma T_3, while decreasing levels of reverse T_3, (rT_3), the inactive metabolite of thyroxine (Davidson and Chopra, 1979). Conversely T_3 falls, and rT_3 increases, in obese subjects who lose weight through diet or bariatric surgery (Alagna et al., 2003).

Adrenal medulla and sympathetic function

Adrenaline and noradrenaline secreted by the adrenal medulla, and noradrenaline released from sympathetic nerve endings, have major catabolic effects including lipolysis and enhanced liver glucose production; they also promote thermogenesis in brown fat and other tissues (see Chapters 4 and 5).

Some studies suggest that obesity is associated with a general increase in sympathetic tone, which may be partly due to stimulation of central sympathetic centres by raised circulating levels of insulin (Rocchini, 1991) or leptin (Grassi et al., 2005). In humans, increased firing of sympathetic nerves supplying muscle and fat has been demonstrated, while circulating noradrenaline and adrenaline levels remain normal.

One consequence of increased sympathetic activity may be hypertension, through vasoconstriction and enhanced renin release by the juxtaglomerular apparatus, leading to relatively increased angiotensin II and perhaps aldosterone production (Ruano et al., 2005; Hiramatsu et al., 1981; see Chapter 12). Renin and aldosterone concentrations in obese subjects are higher than in lean individuals but remain within the normal range. With weight loss, renin and aldosterone levels fall and are accompanied by a decrease in blood pressure (Hiramatsu et al., 1981; Engeli et al., 2005).

Some prospective studies have reported that plasma noradrenaline concentrations are relatively low in subjects who subsequently become obese (van Baak, 2001; Lee et al., 2001). It has been suggested that this may reflect low sympathetic drive to the thermogenic tissues and that reduced energy expenditure might explain the susceptibility to obesity; the importance of this effect remains uncertain. Obese adults may show reduced adrenaline levels following stimulation by a glucose load or exercise (Vettor *et al.*, 1997). As this defect is not seen in obese children, it appears to be an acquired abnormality rather than a causative factor in obesity (Del Rio, 2000; Vettor *et al.*, 1997).

Calcium metabolism

Recent work suggests that many obese patients – perhaps 25–40% – have evidence of subclinical secondary hyperparathyroidism, with raised parathyroid hormone (PTH) levels and decreased ionized calcium (Carlin *et al.*, 2006). Total serum calcium remains normal, while urinary calcium excretion is increased, possibly encouraged by shifts in calcium binding in the circulation that may explain the fall in ionized calcium and the secondary rise in PTH (Andersen *et al.*, 1986). vitamin D levels are also reduced, possibly because of decreased bioavailability of vitamin D3, which is sequestered in fat (Worstmann *et al.*, 2000).

These abnormalities are reversed by weight loss (Sanchez-Hernandez *et al.*, 2005), but not when this is achieved by bariatric surgery (Andersen *et al.*, 1988); this is presumably because malabsorptive procedures impair the uptake of dietary calcium (see Chapter 18). There is a theoretical risk of vitamin D deficiency during chronic treatment with the lipase inhibitor, orlistat, because fat-soluble vitamins are normally absorbed together with digested lipid products, whose uptake across the gut mucosa is blocked by the drug (see Chapter 17).

Gastrointestinal tract

Hiatus hernia and associated gastro-oesophageal reflux are well-recognized as complications of obesity (Stene-Larsen *et al.*, 1988), although Lundell *et al.* (1995) did not find significant relationships between the severity of reflux and various measures of adiposity. The associations are attributed to raised intra-abdominal pressure due to visceral fat accumulation.

Gastro-oesophageal reflux is potentially important, because it predisposes to Barrett's oesophagus, that is, transformation of the normal squamous epithelium of the oesophagus into a gastric-type mucosa. This is a

pre-malignant condition and probably accounts for the association of obesity with carcinoma of the oesophagus (see below and Figure 13.10).

Gallstones are another classical comorbidity of obesity, especially in women. In the North American Nurses' Health Study, the risk of developing clinically significant gallstones increased progressively as BMI rose, reaching a 7-fold higher risk for women whose BMI was $>45\,\text{kg/m}^2$ (Stampfer *et al.*, 1992). In men, the association is weaker and more clearly related to visceral obesity (Heaton *et al.*, 1991). Gallstone formation is apparently enhanced in obesity because the bile becomes supersaturated with cholesterol, rather than through impaired contraction of the gall bladder (Busch and Matern, 1991). Some studies suggest that weight loss – especially if rapid, as with bariatric surgery or a very low calorie diet (VLCD) – may increase the risk of cholelithiasis (Stampfer *et al.*, 1992; see Chapter 18).

Obesity and cancer

Large-scale studies have demonstrated that obesity (and even overweight) increases the risk of developing several forms of cancer, including several that are not classically viewed as hormone-dependent (Table 13.6). In both men and women, increasing BMI is significantly associated with higher death rates from cancers of the oesophagus, colon and rectum, liver, gall bladder, pancreas and kidney, as well as non-Hodgkin lymphoma and multiple myeloma. In addition, men are at increased risk of dying from stomach and prostate cancer, and women from cancers of the breast, uterus, cervix and ovary (Calle *et al.*, 2003). The associations between obesity and particular malignancies may be affected by body fat distribution, and may result from diverse factors including diet and abnormal levels of hormones and inflammatory cytokines (Calle and Kaaks, 2004).

Gastrointestinal cancers

The relative risk of most gastrointestinal cancers increases with rising BMI. One study in men found that, compared with normal-weight subjects, those with a BMI of $35–39\,\text{kg/m}^2$ had a 1.5-fold increased risk of pancreatic cancer and a 4.5-fold higher risk of hepatocellular cancer (Calle *et al.*, 2003). The association with hepatocellular cancer is probably explained by non-alcoholic fatty

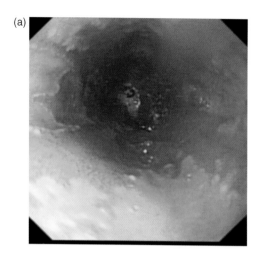 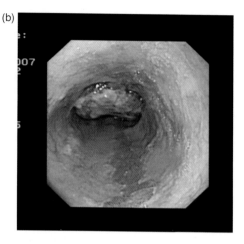

Figure 13.10 Oesophageal complications of obesity: (a) Barrett's oesophagus, with ascending gastric-type mucosa (appearing darker); (b) carcinoma of the oesophagus with Barrett's oesophagus. Images reproduced by courtesy of Dr. N Sarwar, Royal Liverpool University Hospital.

liver disease, which develops in conjunction with the metabolic syndrome and can lead to cirrhosis (Chapter 11).

Other gastrointestinal cancers have been associated with the hyperinsulinaemia of obesity, and insulin may promote the development and

Table 13.6 Obesity predisposes to malignancies.

Type of cancer	Male	Female
Oesphageal	1.63	1.39
Stomach	1.94	1.08
Colorectal	1.84	1.36
Hepatocellular	4.52	1.68
Pancreatic	1.49	1.41
Lung	0.67	0.66
Breast (post-menopausal)		1.70
Uterine		2.77
Cervical		3.20
Ovarian		1.51
Prostate (poorly-differentiated)	1.34	
Kidney	1.70	1.70
Non-Hodgkin lymphomas	1.49	1.95
Multiple myeloma	1.71	1.44
Leukaemia (all types)	1.70	0.93

The table shows the relative risk of various cancers, in men and women with BMI 35–40 kg/m², as compared with the normal-weight population with BMI 18.4–24.9 kg/m². Adapted from Calle *et al.* (2003).

growth of these tumours. Hyperglycaemia has also been implicated, particularly in pancreatic cancer, perhaps through generating excess superoxides that trigger cell damage and proliferation (Giovannucci and Michaud, 2007). This suggestion is supported by the findings that diabetic subjects have an increased risk of gastrointestinal cancers, which can be nullified by treatment with insulin-sensitizing drugs such as metformin (Johnson *et al.*, 2002).

Obesity-related changes in the growth hormone/IGF-1 axis, resulting in increased levels of free IGF-1, have been implicated in the development of colorectal carcinoma (Giovannucci and Michaud, 2007). Consistent with this is the enhanced risk of colonic cancer in people with acromegaly who have very high IGF-1 levels. IGF-1, like insulin and epidermal growth factor (EGF), can promote the growth of gastrointestinal and other tumours under experimental conditions.

The prevalence of oesophageal cancer has increased in recent years, especially among young men (Holmes and Vaughan, 2007); as already mentioned, this association is probably due to gastro-oesophageal reflux, which predisposes to Barrett's oesophagus and ultimately neoplasia (Figure 13.10).

Haematological malignancies

Obesity is associated with an increased risk of non-Hodgkin lymphoma, diffuse large B-cell lymphoma, follicular lymphoma, chronic lymphocytic leukaemia and multiple myeloma. Possible causes include the low-grade chronic inflammation that accompanies obesity, with increased production of pro-inflammatory cytokines such as interleukin-6, TNF-α and leptin. These cytokines regulate T- and B-cell responses and enhance B-cell proliferation and survival, thus providing an environment that favours the development of these disorders (Skibola, 2007).

The reduced physical activity levels and poor diet that are commonly associated with obesity may also play a role. Physical inactivity and high consumption of dairy and saturated fats is suggested to increase the risk of non-Hodgkin lymphoma, whereas a diet rich in fish, fruit and vegetables is apparently protective (Skibola, 2007). One possible mechanism for the increased risk associated with dairy products relates to the high calcium content of these foods, which may inhibit the formation of 1,25 dihydroxy vitamin D, the active form of the vitamin. Vitamin D has potentially potent anti-carcinogenic properties, because it inhibits growth and triggers apoptosis in pre-neoplastic cells (Skibola, 2007).

Prostate cancer

Some studies have demonstrated an overall increased risk of prostate cancer with increasing BMI or body weight, whereas others have failed to confirm any such association (Giovannucci and Michaud, 2007). This discrepancy may be explained by the differing effects of key hormones on the development of specific types of prostate cancer. Androgens are thought to promote the initiation and progression of well-differentiated prostate cancer, while protecting against poorly-differentiated tumours. By contrast, hyperinsulinaemia has been associated with an increased risk of poorly-differentiated prostate cancer, while leptin may also play a role in these tumours (Giovannucci and Michaud, 2007). Recent cohort studies (Schatzl et al., 2001) indicate that obese subjects have an increased risk of poorly-differentiated, androgen independent prostate cancers – which would be expected from the low testosterone and raised insulin and leptin levels characteristic of obesity. Unfortunately, these tumours are more aggressive and less likely to respond to conventional therapy.

Breast cancer

Obesity is strongly associated with an increased risk of developing breast cancer after the menopause, with a 3% increase in risk for each 1 kg/m² gain in BMI. There is no evidence that the risk of pre-menopausal breast cancer is enhanced (Carmichael, 2006). The association between obesity and post-menopausal breast cancer may be partly explained by elevated circulating oestrogen concentrations, resulting from enhanced conversion of androgens to oestrogen by aromatase in adipose tissue. The mitogenic effects of increased circulating insulin and IGF-1 levels may also contribute. A recent suggestion is that adipokines (particularly leptin, TNF-α and IL-6), secreted by local adipocytes in the breast and by remote adipose tissue, may promote breast neoplasia (Modesitt and van Nagell, 2005; Schäffler, Schölmerich and Buechler, 2007).

Gynaecological cancers

Endometrial cancer

Obesity is estimated to account for 39% of all cases of endometrial cancer, with a 10-fold increased risk in women who are 20 kg or more above their ideal body weight (Kaaks, Lukanova and Kurzer, 2002). The 'unopposed oestrogen' hypothesis has been advanced to explain this association. Obesity increases adrenal and ovarian secretion of androgens (see above), which inhibits ovulation and therefore decreases progesterone production. Concomitantly, oestrogen levels are increased through aromatization of androgens in peripheral fat. In the absence of progesterone, oestrogen increases mitotic activity and DNA replication errors in endometrial cells, resulting in endometrial hypoplasia, somatic mutations, and eventually endometrial cancer (Modesitt and van Nagell, 2005).

Cervical cancer

Some studies have reported a modestly increased risk of cervical adenocarcinoma in obese women (Modesitt and van Nagell, 2005). These tumours comprise only 15% of all cervical cancers and there is no evidence of any association between obesity and the more common squamous-cell cervical cancers. Obese women appear to be less compliant with general screening recommendations for cervical cancer, and this may explain the increased mortality from all cervical cancers in this group.

Ovarian cancer

The significance of obesity appears complex. There may be an association between adolescent obesity and pre-menopausal ovarian cancer, but there appears to be no link between ovarian cancer and obesity later in life (Modesitt and van Nagell, 2005). Nonetheless, the risk of dying from ovarian cancer appears to be increased in obese women.

Psychological and psychiatric disorders

The enormous psychological burdens that obesity can inflict have only been fully recognized in the last 20 years or so. These include stigmatization, victimization at school, prejudice and discrimination; the effects are evident in adulthood and extend into adult life, and can damage education, employment and personal relationships. Health-care workers, notably doctors, need to be aware of this, not least because they (together with family members) have been identified by obese people as the most common sources of bias against them (Puhl and Brownell, 2006).

Psychiatric diseases associated with obesity include anxiety, depression and two distinct eating disorders, binge-eating disorder (BED) and night-eating syndrome (NES) (Spitzer *et al.*, 1993; Rand, Macgregor and Stunkard, 1997). As well as potentially reducing quality of life, these conditions can damage the patient's adherence to treatment and its eventual outcome. In women, obesity is associated with a higher risk of major depression; by contrast, the risk is decreased in men. Bipolar disorder appears to be more common among the morbidly obese (Alciati *et al.*, 2007). Interestingly, the risk of substance abuse is apparently reduced among obese people (Simon *et al.*, 2006).

Psychological and psychiatric disorders, and their interplay with social factors, are discussed in detail in Chapters 14 and 20.

References

Abbott, D.H., Dumesic, D.A. and Franks, S. (2002) Developmental origin of polycystic ovary syndrome – a hypothesis. *Journal of Endocrinology*, **174** (1), 1–5.

Alagna, S., Cossu, M.L., Masala, A. *et al.* (2003) Evaluation of serum leptin levels and thyroid function in morbidly obese patients treated with bariatric surgery. *Eating and Weight Disorders*, **8** (2), 95–9.

Alciati, A., D'Ambrosio, A., Foschi, D., Corsi, F., Mellado, C. and Angst, J. (2007) Bipolar spectrum disorders in severely obese patients seeking surgical treatment. *Journal of Affective Disorders*, **101**, (1–3), 131–8.

Alexander, C.J. (2004) Idiopathic osteoarthritis: time to change paradigms? *Skeletal Radiology*, **33** (6), 321–4. Epub 2004 Jan 9.

Allison, D.B., Mentore, J.L., Heo, M. *et al.* (1999) Antipsychotic-induced weight gain: a comprehensive research synthesis. *The American Journal of Psychiatry*, **156** (11), 1686–96.

Alvarez-Castro, P., Isidro, M.L., Garcia-Buela, J. *et al.* (2004) Marked GH secretion after ghrelin alone or combined with GH-releasing hormone (GHRH) in obese patients. *Clinical Endocrinology*, **61**, 250–5.

American Academy of Sleep Medicine Task Force (1999). Sleep-related breathing disorders in adults: recommendations for syndrome definition and measurement techniques in clinical research. The Report of an American Academy of Sleep Medicine Task Force. *Sleep.* **22**(5), 667–89.

Amin, A.K., Patton, J.T., Cook, R.E. and Brenkel, I.J. (2006) Does obesity influence the outcome at five years following total knee replacement for osteoarthritis? *Journal of Bone and Joint Surgery*, **88**, 335–40.

Andersen, T., McNair, P., Fogh-Andersen, N. *et al.* (1986) Increased parathyroid hormone as a consequence of changed complex binding of plasma calcium in morbid obesity. *Metabolism: Clinical and Experimental*, **35** (2), 147–51.

Andersen, T., McNair, P., Hyldstrup, L. *et al.* (1988) Secondary hyperparathyroidism of morbid obesity regresses during weight reduction. *Metabolism: Clinical and Experimental*, **37** (5), 425–8.

Andrews, R.C. and Walker, B.R. (1999) Glucocorticoids and insulin resistance: old hormones, new targets. *Clinical Science*, **96** (5), 513–23.

Björntorp, P. (2001) Do stress reactions cause abdominal obesity and comorbidities? *Obesity Reviews*, **2** (2), 73–86.

Bole-Feysot, C., Goffin, V., Edery, M. *et al.* (1998) Prolactin (PRL) and its receptor: actions, signal transduction pathways and phenotypes observed in PRL receptor knockout mice. *Endocrine Reviews*, **19** (3), 225–68.

Busch, N. and Matern, S. (1991) Current concepts in cholesterol gallstone pathogenesis. *European Journal of Clinical Investigation*, **21**, 453–60.

Busetto, L., Enzi, G., Inelmen, E.M. *et al.* (2005) Obstructive sleep apnea syndrome in morbid obesity: effects of intragastric balloon. *Chest*, **128** (2), 618–23.

Calle, E.C. and Kaaks, R. (2004) Overweight, obesity and cancer: epidemiological evidence and proposed mechanisms. *Nature Reviews. Cancer*, **4**, 579–91.

Calle, E.E., Rodriguez, C., Walker-Thurmond, K. and Thun, M.J. (2003) Overweight, obesity, and mortality from cancer in a prospectively studied cohort of U.S. adults. *The New England Journal of Medicine*, **348** (17), 1625–38.

Carlin, A.M., Rao, D.S., Meslemani, A.M. *et al.* (2006) Prevalence of vitamin D depletion among morbidly obese patients seeking gastric bypass surgery. *Surgery for Obesity and Related Disorders*, **2** (2), 98–103.

Carmichael, A.R. (2006) Obesity as a risk factor for development and poor prognosis of breast cancer. *British Journal of Obstetrics and Gynaecology*, **113** (10), 1160–6.

Castro, J.P. *et al.* (2005) Differential effect of obesity on bone mineral density in White, Hispanic and African American women: a cross sectional study. *Nutrition & Metabolism*, **2**, 9.

Chen, Y., Horne, S.L. and Dosman, J.A. (1993) Body weight and weight gain related to pulmonary function decline in adults: a six year follow up study. *Thorax*, **48**, 375–80.

Cheng, J.Y. and Ng, E.M. (2007) Body mass index, physical activity and erectile dysfunction: a U-shaped relationship from population-based study. *International Journal of Obesity*, **31**(10), 1571–78.

Clark, A.M., Thornley, B., Tomlinson, L. *et al.* (1998) Weight loss in obese infertile women results in improvement in reproductive outcome for all forms of fertility treatment. *Human Reproduction (Oxford, England)*, **13** (6), 1502–5.

Coggon, D., Reading, I., Croft, P. *et al.* (2001) Knee osteoarthritis and obesity. *International Journal of Obesity*, **25**, 622–7.

Cordido, F., Fernandez, T., Martinez, T. *et al.* (1998) Effect of acute pharmacological reduction of plasma free fatty acids on growth hormone (GH) releasing hormone-induced GH secretion in obese adults with and without hypopituitarism. *Journal of Clinical Endocrinology and Metabolism*, **83**, 4350–4.

Davidson, M.B. and Chopra, I.J. (1979) Effect of carbohydrate and noncarbohydrate sources of calories on plasma 3,5,3′-triiodothyronine concentrations in man. *Journal of Clinical Endocrinology and Metabolism*, **48** (4), 577–81.

De Laet, C. *et al.* (2005) Body mass index as a predictor of fracture risk: a meta-analysis. *Osteoporosis International*, **16**, 1330–8.

De Pergola, G., Maldera, S., Tartagni, M. *et al.* (2006) Inhibitory effect of obesity on gonadotropin, estradiol, and inhibin B levels in fertile women. *Obesity*, **14** (11), 1954–60.

Del Rio, G. (2000) Adrenomedullary function and its regulation in obesity. *International Journal of Obesity and Related Metabolic Disorders*, **24** (Suppl 2), S89–91.

Dieguez, C. and Casanueva, F.F. (1995) Influence of metabolic substrates and obesity on growth hormone secretion. *Trends in Endocrinology and Metabolism*, **6**, 55–9.

Edén Engström, B., Burman, P., Holdstock, C. *et al.* (2006) Effects of bypass on the GH/IGF-1 axis in severe obesity and a comparison with GH deficiency. *European Journal of Endocrinology/European Federation of Endocrine Societies*, **154** (1), 53–9.

El-Gamal, H., Khayat, A., Shikora, S. and Unterborn, J.N. (2005) Relationship of dyspnea to respiratory drive and pulmonary function tests in obese patients before and after weight loss. *Chest*, **128**, 3870–4.

Engeli, S., Bohnke, J., Gorzelniak, K. *et al.* (2005) Weight loss and the renin-angiotensin-aldosterone system. *Hypertension*, **45** (3), 356–62.

Esposito, K., Giugliano, F., Di Paolo, C. *et al.* (2004) Effect of lifestyle changes on erectile dysfunction in obese men: a randomized controlled trial. *Journal of the American Medical Association*, **23**; **291**, (24), 2978–84.

Felson, D.T., Anderson, J.J., Naimark, A. *et al.* (1988) Obesity and knee osteoarthritis. The Framingham Study. *Annals of Internal Medicine*, **109** (1), 18–24.

Freemark, M., Fleenor, D., Driscoll, P. *et al.* (2001) Body weight and fat deposition in prolactin receptor-deficient mice. *Endocrinology*, **142** (2), 532–7.

Ghigo, E., Aimaretti, G. and Corneli, G. (2008) Diagnosis of adult GH deficiency. Growth Hormone and IGF Research, **18**(1), 1–16.

Giovannucci, E. and Michaud, D. (2007) The role of obesity and related metabolic disturbances in cancers of the colon, prostate, and pancreas. *Gastroenterology*, **132** (6), 2208–25.

Grassi, G., Facchini, A., Trevano, F.Q. *et al.* (2005) Obstructive sleep apnea-dependent and -independent adrenergic activation in obesity. *Hypertension*, **46**, 321–50.

Heaton, K., Braddon, F., Emmett, P. *et al.* (1991) Why do men get gallstones? Roles of abdominal fat and hyperinsulinemia. *European Journal of Gastroenterology & Hepatology*, **3**, 745–51.

Hiramatsu, K., Yamada, T., Ichikawa, K. *et al.* (1981) Changes in endocrine activities relative to obesity in patients with essential hypertension. *Journal of the American Geriatrics Society*, **29** (1), 25–30.

Hochberg Z. Hertz, P., Colin, V. *et al.* (1992) The distal axis of growth hormone (GH) in nutritional disorders: GH-binding protein, insulin-like growth factor-I (IGF-I), and IGF-I receptors in obesity and anorexia nervosa. *Metabolism: Clinical and Experimental*, **41** (1), 106–12.

Holmberg, S., Thelin, A. and Thelin, N. (2005) Knee osteoarthritis and body mass index: a population-based case-control study. *Scandinavian Journal of Rheumatology*, **34** (1), 59–64.

Holmes, R.S. and Vaughan, T.L. (2007) Epidemiology and pathogenesis of esophageal cancer. *Seminars in Radiation Oncology*, **17**, 2–9.

Iacobellis, G., Ribaudo, M.C., Zappaterreno, A. *et al.* (2005) Relationship of thyroid function with body mass index, leptin, insulin sensitivity and adiponectin in euthyroid obese women. *Clinical Endocrinology*, **62** (4), 487–91.

Jensen, T.K., Andersson, A.M., Jorgensen, N. *et al.* (2004) Body mass index in relation to semen quality and reproductive hormones among 1,558 Danish men. *Fertility and Sterility*, **82** (4), 863–70.

Johns, M.P. (1991) A new method for measuring daytime sleepiness: The Epworth Sleepiness Scale. *Sleep*, **14**, 540–5.

Johnson, J.A., Majumdar, S.R., Simpson, S.H. and Toth, E.L. (2002) Decreased mortality associated with the use of metformin compared with sulfonylurea monotherapy in type 2 diabetes. *Diabetes Care*, **25** (12), 2244–8.

Jones, R.L. and Nzekwu, M.U. (2006) The effects of body mass index on lung volumes. *Chest*, **130**, 827–33.

Kaaks, R., Lukanova, A. and Kurzer, M.S. (2002) Obesity, endogenous hormones, and endometrial cancer risk: a synthetic review. *Cancer Epidemiology, Biomarkers & Prevention: A publication of the American Association for Cancer Research, cosponsored by the American Society of Preventive Oncology*, **11** (12), 1531–43.

Kanaley, J.A., Weatherup-Dentes, M.M., Jaynes, E.B. and Hartman, M.L. (1999) Obesity attenuates the growth hormone response to exercise. *Journal of Clinical Endocrinology and Metabolism*, **84**, 3156–61.

Kirschner, M.A., Samojlik, E., Drejka, M. *et al.* (1990) Androgen-estrogen metabolism in women with upper body versus lower body obesity. *Journal of Clinical Endocrinology and Metabolism*, **70** (2), 473–9.

Kley, H.K., Edelmann, P. and Kruskemper, H.L. (1980) Relationship of plasma sex hormones to different parameters of obesity in male subjects. *Metabolism: Clinical and Experimental*, **29** (11), 1041–5.

Kok, P., Roelfsema, F., Frolich, M. *et al.* (2004) Prolactin release is enhanced in proportion to excess visceral fat in obese women. *Journal of Clinical Endocrinology and Metabolism*, **89** (9), 4445–9.

Kok, P., Roelfsema, F., Langendonk, J.G. *et al.* (2006) Increased circadian prolactin release is blunted after body weight loss in obese premenopausal women. *American Journal of Physiology. Endocrinology and Metabolism*, **290** (2), E218–24.

Kokkoris, P. and PiSunyer, F.X. (2003) Obesity and endocrine disease. *Endocrinology and Metabolism Clinics of North America*, **32**, 895–914.

Kratzik, C.W., Schatzl, G., Lunglmayr, G. *et al.* (2005) The impact of age, body mass index and testosterone on erectile dysfunction. *Journal of Urology*, **174** (1), 240–3.

Lake, J.K., Power, C. and Cole, T.J. (1997) Women's reproductive health: the role of body mass index in early and adult life. *International Journal of Obesity and Related Metabolic Disorders*, **21** (6), 432–8.

Lee, Z.S., Critchley, J.A., Tomlinson, B. *et al.* (2001) Urinary epinephrine and norepinephrine interrelations with obesity, insulin, and the metabolic syndrome in Hong Kong Chinese. *Metabolism: Clinical and Experimental*, **50** (2), 135–43.

Lindgren, B. (1998) The economic impact of musculoskeletal disorders. *Acta Orthopaedica Scandinavica Suppl*, **281**, 58–60.

Linne, Y. (2004) Effects of obesity on women's reproduction and complications during pregnancy. *Obesity Reviews*, **5** (3), 137–43.

Ljung, T., Andersson, B., Bengtsson, B.A. *et al.* (1996) Inhibition of cortisol secretion by dexamethasone in relation to body fat distribution: a dose-response study. *Obesity Research*, **4** (3), 277–82.

Lundell, L., Ruth, M., Sandberg, N. and Bove-Nielsen, M. (1995) Does massive obesity promote abnormal gastroesophageal reflux? *Digestive Diseases and Sciences*, **40**, 4632–5.

Manji, N., Boelaert, K., Sheppard, M.C. *et al.* (2006) Lack of association between serum TSH or free T4 and body mass index in euthyroid subjects. *Clinical Endocrinology*, **64** (2), 125–8.

Marin, J.M., Carrizo, S.J., Vicente, E. and Agusti, A.G. (2005) Long-term cardiovascular outcomes in men with obstructive sleep apnoea-hypopnoea with or without treatment with continuous positive airway pressure: an observational study. *Lancet*, **365**, 1046–53.

Modesitt S.C. van Nagell, J.R., Jr. (2005) The impact of obesity on the incidence and treatment of gynecologic cancers: a review. *Obstetrical & Gynecological Survey*, **60** (10), 683–92.

Nguyen, R.H., Wilcox, A.J., Skjaerven, R. and Baird, D.D. (2007) Men's body mass index and infertility. *Human Reproduction (Oxford, England)*, **22**, 2488–930.

Norman, R.J., Dewailly, D., Legro, R.S. and Hickey, T.E. (2007) Polycystic ovarian syndrome. *Lancet*, **370**, 685–97.

Nowbar, S. Burkart, K.M. Gonzales, R., Fedorowicz A, Gozansky W.S., Gaudio J.C., Taylor M.R., and Zwillich C.W. (2004) Obesity-associated hypoventilation in hospitalized patients: prevalence, effects, and outcome, *The American Journal of Medicine*, **116**(1), 1–7.

Pasquali, R., (2006) Obesity, fat distribution and infertility *Maturitas*, **54** (4), 363–71.

Pasquali, R., S Patton, L. and Gambineri, A., (2007) Obesity and infertility. *Current Opinion in Endocrinology, Diabetes and Obesity*, **14**, 482–7.

Piper, A.J. and Grunstern, R.R. (2007) Current perspectives on the obesity hypoventilation syndrome. *Current Opinion in Pulmonary Medicine*, **13**, 490–6.

Pottie, P., Presle, N., Terlain, B. *et al.* (2006) Obesity and osteoarthritis: more complex than predicted. *Annals of the Rheumatic Diseases*, **65**, 1403–5.

Puhl, R.M. and Brownell, K.D. (2006) Confronting and coping with weight stigma: an investigation of overweight and obese adults. *Obesity*, **14**, 1802–15.

Rand C.S. Macgregor, A.M. and Stunkard, A.J. (1997) The night eating syndrome in the general population and among postoperative obesity surgery patients. *International Journal of Eating Disorders*, **22** (1), 65–9.

Reijman, M., Pols, H.A.P., Bergink, A.P. *et al.* (2007) Body mass index associated with onset and progression of osteoarthritis of the knee but not of the hip: The Rotterdam Study. *Annals of the Rheumatic Diseases*, **66**, 158–62.

Reynolds, R.M. and Walker, B.R. (2003) Human insulin resistance: the role of glucocorticoids. *Diabetes, Obesity & Metabolism*, **5** (1), 5–12.

Rocchini, A.P. (1991) Insulin resistance and blood pressure regulation in obese and nonobese subjects. Special lecture. *Hypertension*, **17**(6 Pt2), 837–42.

Ruano, M., Silvestre, V., Castro, R. *et al.* (2005) Morbid obesity, hypertensive disease and the renin-angiotensin-aldosterone axis. *Obesity Surgery*, **15** (5), 670–6.

Sanchez-Hernandez, J., Ybarra J., Gich, I. *et al.* (2005) Effects of bariatric surgery on vitamin D status and secondary hyperparathyroidism: a prospective study. *Obesity Surgery* **15** (10) 1389–95.

Scacchi, M., Pincelli, A.I. and Cavagnini, F. (1999) Growth hormone in obesity. *International Journal of Obesity and Related Metabolic Disorders*, **23** (3), 260–71.

Schäffler, A., Schölmerich, J. and Buechler, C. (2007) Mechanisms of disease: adipokines and breast cancer – endocrine and paracrine mechanisms that connect adiposity and breast cancer. *National Clinical Practice, Endocrinology and Metabolism*, **3**, 345–54.

Schatzl, G., Madersbacher, S., Thurridl, T. *et al.* (2001) High-grade prostate cancer is associated with low serum testosterone levels. *Prostate*, **47** (1), 52–8.

Schmid, C., Goede, D.L., Hauser, R.S. and Brandle, M. (2006) Increased prevalence of high body mass Index in patients presenting with pituitary tumours: severe obesity in patients with macroprolactinoma. *Swiss Medical Weekly*, **15** (15–16), 254–8.

Simon G.E. Von Korff, M., Saunders, K. *et al.* (2006) Association between obesity and psychiatric disorders in the US adult population. *Archives of General Psychiatry*, **63**, 824–30.

Skibola, C.F. (2007) Obesity, diet and risk of non-Hodgkin lymphoma. *Cancer Epidemiology, Biomarkers & Prevention*: A publication of the American Association for Cancer Research, cosponsored by the American Society of Preventive Oncology, **16** (3), 392–5.

Spitzer, R.L., Yanovski, S., Wadden, B.T. *et al.* (1993) Binge eating disorder: its further validation in a multisite study. *International Journal of Eating Disorders*, **13**, 137–53.

Stampfer, M., Maclure, K., Colditz, G. *et al.* (1992) Risk of symptomatic gallstones in women with severe obesity. *The American Journal of Clinical Nutrition*, **55**, 652–8.

Stene-Larsen, G., Weberg, R., Larsen, I. *et al.* (1988) Relationship of overweight to hiatus hernia and reflux oesophagitis. *Scandinavian Journal of Gastroenterology*, **23**, 427–32.

Stradling, J. (2007) Obstructive sleep apnoea. *British Medical Journal*, **335**, 314–5.

Svatikova, A., Wolk, R., Gami, A.S. *et al.* (2005) Interaction between obstructive sleep apnoea and the metabolic syndrome. *Current Diabetes Reports*, **5**, 53–8.

Urbanek, M. (2007) The genetics of the polycystic ovary syndrome. *National Clinical Practice, Endocrinology and Metabolism*, **3** (2), 103–11.

van Baak, M.A. (2001) The peripheral sympathetic nervous system in human obesity. *Obesity Reviews*, **2** (1), 3–14.

Vaswani, A.N. (1985) Effect of weight reduction on the renin-aldosterone axis. *Journal of the American College of Nutrition*, **4** (2), 225–31.

Veldhuis, A., Iranmesh, K.K., Ho, M.J. *et al.* (1991) Dual defects in pulsatile growth hormone secretion and clearance subserve the hyposomatotropism of obesity in man. *Journal of Clinical Endocrinology and Metabolism*, **72**, 51–9.

Vermeulen, A. (1996) Decreased androgen levels and obesity in men. *Annals of Medicine*, **28** (1), 13–5.

Vermeulen, A., Kaufman, J.M., Deslypere, J.P. and Thomas, G. (1993) Attenuated luteinizing hormone (LH) pulse amplitude but normal LH pulse frequency, and its relation to plasma androgens in hypogonadism of obese men. *Journal of Clinical Endocrinology and Metabolism*, **76** (5), 1140–6.

Vettor, R., Macor, C., Rossi, E. *et al.* (1997) Impaired counterregulatory hormonal and metabolic response to exhaustive exercise in obese subjects. *Acta Diabetologica*, **34** (2), 61–6.

Vgontzas, A.N., Bixler, E.O. and Chrousos, G.P. (2005) Sleep apnoea is a manifestation of the metabolic syndrome. *Theoretical Review. Sleep Medicine Reviews*, **9**, 211–24.

Wake, D.J. and Walker, B.R. (2006) Inhibition of 11beta-hydroxysteroid dehydrogenase type 1 in obesity. *Endocrine*, **29** (1), 101–8.

Wang, G.J., Volkow, N.D., Logan, J. *et al.* (2001) Brain dopamine and obesity. *Lancet*, **357**, (9253) 354–7.

Wang, H., Parker, J.D., Newton, G.E. *et al.* (2007) Influence of obstructive sleep apnea on mortality in patients with heart failure. *Journal of the American College of Cardiology*, **49**, 1625–31.

Wearing, S.C. *et al.* (2006) Musculoskeletal disorders associated with obesity: a biomechanical perspective. The International Association for the Study of Obesity. *Obesity Reviews*, **7**, 239–50.

Wendelboe A.M., Hegmann, K.T., Gren, L.H. *et al.* (2004) Associations between body-mass index and surgery for rotator cuff tendinitis. *Journal of Bone and Joint Surgery. American Volume*, **86-A** (4), 743–7.

Worstmann, J., Matsuoka, L.Y., Chen, T.C. *et al.* (2000) Decreased bioavailability of vitamin D in obesity. *The American Journal of Clinical Nutrition*, **72**, 690–3.

Yanovski, J.A., Yanovski, S.Z., Gold, P.W., and Chrousos G.P. (1997) Differences in corticotropin-releasing hormone-stimulated adrenocorticotropin and cortisol before and after weight loss. *Journal of Clinical Endocrinology and Metabolism*, **82** (6), 1874–8.

Zemel, M.B., Shi, H., Greer, B. *et al.* (2000) Regulation of adiposity by dietary calcium. *The FASEB Journal*, **14** (9), 1132–8.

Social and Psychological Factors in Obesity

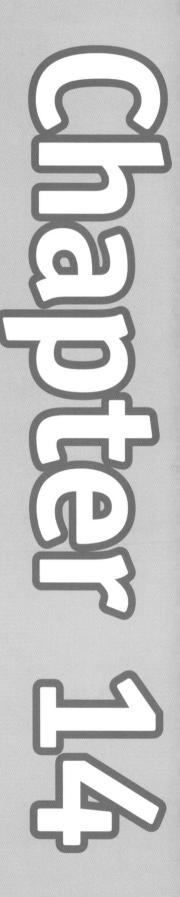

Key points

- Obese people are prone to social disadvantage and psychological problems, which can derive partly from their obesity and also serve to initiate and perpetuate the obese state. Individual 'resilience' is important in mitigating the impact of adverse psychosocial factors.

- Adverse stereotyping of obese people – typically as undisciplined, inactive, unappealing and responsible for their weight problem – is widespread in westernized countries and becomes established early in childhood.

- Prejudice and discrimination against obese people are common. Obese people, especially women, are systematically disadvantaged in school and higher education, employment and earning potential, and in health care and medical insurance.

- Stigmatization and victimization can damage obese people's social interactions throughout adolescence and adulthood, and ultimately impede significant relationships including marriage.

- Depression is associated with obesity, especially if severe (risk is increased fivefold at BMI $\geqslant 40\,kg/m^2$) and in women, who have an increased risk of major depression and suicide. Depression is more common in those undergoing obesity treatment than in the general population and often emerges during adolescence; it often improves with weight loss, but recurs with weight regain.

- Body-image distress and low self-esteem are common in obese people from the teens onwards, especially in females. Quality of life is also impaired, particularly in those with multiple concurrent chronic illnesses.

- Better public and professional understanding of the importance of psychosocial factors in obesity should help to improve the medical management of the condition as well as relieving distress.

Chapter 14   Social and Psychological Factors in Obesity

Andrew J. Hill

Body weight has a major influence on people's perception of themselves and others. In many cultures, the prevailing attitude is 'anti-fat'; stigmatization and discrimination because of obesity are widespread and become established early in childhood. Obesity adversely affects key areas of life including education, employment, healthcare and social interaction, especially for women. Psychological well-being can also be damaged, with increased risks of depression, poor self-esteem and impaired quality of life. In some cases, psychological factors interfere with adherence to treatment and so reduce the effectiveness of weight-management strategies.

This chapter reviews the numerous interactions between obesity and social and psychological functions, and highlights the importance of the latter in both theoretical and practical aspects of managing obesity.

Stereotyping of obesity

The idea that body shape is somehow related to personality and behavioural style has long been held. Sheldon's 'somatotypes', popularized in the 1940s, distinguished the endomorph, ectomorph and mesomorph, corresponding respectively to fat, thin and medium body shapes; endomorphs were described as having strong needs for food, people and affection. Nowadays, these generalizations are overshadowed by morally-laden assertions that obese people lack physical attractiveness and self-control. This negative stereotyping of obesity is clear in the judgments made by children and adults and is determined surprisingly early in life.

A child's eye view

Children's attitudes to obesity emerged from research into perceptions of disability. In one

of the earliest studies (Richardson *et al.*, 1961), 10–11 year olds were asked to rank their liking for six line-drawings showing a child as physically normal, in a leg brace, in a wheelchair, with facial disfigurement, without a hand, or overweight. The child with no obvious disability was most preferred, whereas the fat child was ranked lowest. Similar research up to the mid-1980s confirmed the consistency of this finding, with the fat child almost always placed last or next to last. Girls and children in Western societies showed the least tolerant attitudes to their obese peers (DeJong and Kleck, 1986). A recent follow up study, over 40 years after the original, shows that dislike of obese stereotypes has strengthened, especially among girls: the fat child was placed bottom by an even greater proportion of children than in the original study, whereas the healthy non-disabled child was more consistently chosen first (Latner and Stunkard, 2003) (Figure 14.1). Strikingly, this polarization of views has occurred against a backdrop of increasing obesity, suggesting that stigmatization has increased despite its greater familiarity to children.

Children also have adverse perceptions of obese people's personalities. In an early study (Staffieri, 1967), 6–10 year old boys were asked to assign each of 39 adjectives to drawings of thin and fat body figures. The fat body shape was more frequently labelled 'lazy', 'stupid', 'sloppy', 'dirty', 'naughty', mean', 'ugly', and 'gets teased', whereas least frequent descriptions included 'best friend' and 'has lots of friends'. Subsequent research, using drawings or photographs with written descriptions or rating scales rather than the artificial forced allocation of attributes, has confirmed children's negative views of the obese (Figure 14.2). Thin figures also tend to receive fewer positive endorsements for some traits – indicating that some children reject any deviation from normal body

Obesity: Science to Practice   Edited by Gareth Williams and Gema Frühbeck
© 2009 John Wiley & Sons, Ltd

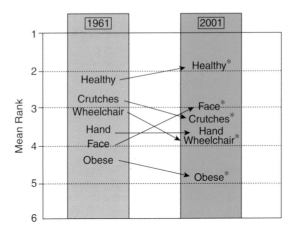

Figure 14.1 Ranked preferences by 10–11 year old children of line drawings representing a healthy child, or a child with a physical abnormality, including obesity. Data are shown from surveys in 1961 (Richardson *et al.*, 1961) and 2001 (Latner and Stunkard, 2001). Scores that changed significantly in 2001 are asterisked.

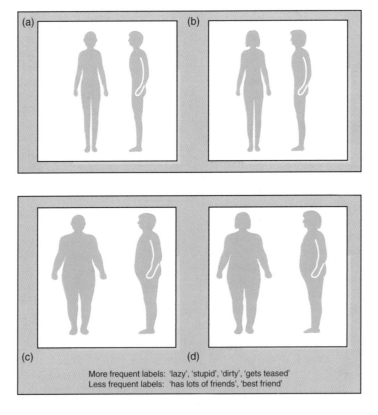

Figure 14.2 Examples of body figure drawings used to investigate children's stereotyping of thin (a and b) and fat (c and d) body shapes. Some commonly-attributed perceptions of the fat shapes are also shown. From A.J Hill and E. Silver (1995) 'Fat, friendless and unhealthy: 9-year old children's perception of body shape stereotypes'. *International Journal of Obesity*, **19**, 423–30, with kind permission.

shape – but there is consistently greater negativity towards fatness.

This stereotyping is apparently established by the age of 5 and possibly earlier. The 4–6 year old American children studied by Musher-Eizenman *et al.* (2004) rated a fat body shape the most negatively, with only 16% choosing it as a friend and 7% as best friend (compared with 46 and 38%, respectively, for an average body shape). Cramer and Steinwert (1998) found that 3–5 year old children, especially girls, were significantly more likely to choose a drawing of a fat figure to identify the 'mean' child in a story line, compared with a thin or average-shaped figure. Interestingly, low- and average-weight children preferred an average-shaped playmate, whereas overweight children were more likely to choose a thin figure.

Overall, it is evident that some very young children have absorbed the prevalent 'fat-is-bad' stereotype, but the degree to which this is internalized, comprehended and acted upon is still unclear.

Adult attitudes

Adults perpetuate the 'anti-fat' stereotyping, with obese people generally seen as undisciplined, inactive, unappealing and having emotional or psychological problems. The only positive perception in the obesity stereotype is that obese people are more humorous and warm. Even this can be demeaning: overweight and obese characters in TV fictional roles are more likely to be the targets rather than the deliverers of humour (Greenberg *et al.*, 2003). They are also more likely to be shown eating than thin characters. Moreover, overweight females appear less often in the media than the frequency of overweight and obese women in the general population; perhaps the social unacceptability of obesity is confirmed by its invisibility.

Determining people's genuine attitudes to obesity can be difficult because many prefer to disguise their true feelings, perhaps to avoid causing offence or appearing badly to the researcher. Accordingly, some studies may have underestimated the strength of anti-obesity prejudice. Alternative approaches such as the Implicit Association Test, developed to investigate stigma based on age, race and gender, are now being investigated.

'Implicit attitudes', that is associations beyond conscious evaluation, can be assessed as the strength of association between obesity and negative attributes during a timed response task. Such studies have shown that strong negative associations with obesity are held by the general public (Schwartz *et al.*, 2006), by physical education students (O'Brien, Hunter and Banks, 2007), and even by health professionals who treat obesity (Teachman and Brownell, 2001). Intriguingly, obese subjects also displayed implicit anti-fat attitudes (albeit weaker), indicating that weight bias is both commonplace and potent.

Social disadvantage

Negative stereotyping leads to prejudice and ultimately to discrimination. There is now convincing evidence that social disadvantage and discrimination due to obesity occur in almost every important area of life, including education, the workplace, health care and social relationships (Puhl and Brownell, 2001).

Education

Obesity can impact on educational experience and achievement throughout school and higher education, as well as peer interactions at school.

School

An emerging literature shows obese children to have lower IQ scores, to score lower in school tests, or more likely to be placed in remedial classes (Tara and Potts-Datema, 2005). Poor learning outcomes can be seen in children as young as 6 years old (Datar and Sturm, 2006). Poor parental education and family income may contribute, but do not explain all these associations; substantial evidence is lacking, but other suggested factors include the increased risk of mental health problems in obese children, poor peer relationships and increased absenteeism.

The relationship between childhood IQ and adult BMI is complex. Analysis of a Scottish cohort showed that lower childhood IQ was associated with higher adult BMI (Lawlor *et al.*, 2006). Allowing for the person's highest educational qualification removed this association, but educational attainment was itself negatively associated with adult BMI. Moreover, extrinsic factors such as parental intelligence and education, school and neighbourhood characteristics, accounted for much of the association between educational attainment and adult BMI. This implies that poor academic performance in obese children may be attributable to their social, familial and physical circumstances rather than to any intrinsic limitation of intellectual ability.

Higher education

The first report of obesity-related educational disadvantage was published in the mid-1960s and concerned university acceptance. US high school students were less likely than their lean peers to be accepted by universities, despite making similar numbers of applications and having comparable academic qualifications (Canning and Mayer, 1966). This bias was most clear in obese females. Subsequently, obese female students were found to receive less financial support from their families than normal-weight students (Crandall, 1991). Thus, university selection procedures and parental attitudes both acted as barriers to higher educational achievement.

Consequences of barriers to education were evident in a well-known longitudinal study of young Americans. Young women overweight at 16 years old had completed fewer years of school than their lean peers when followed up 7 years later, although overweight had no adverse educational consequence for young men (Gortmaker *et al.*, 1993). In a very large cohort of young Swedish men, those obese at age 18 had poorer school marks and less chance of getting into higher education than their lean peers, even after accounting for intelligence and parental socio-economic status (Karnehed *et al.*, 2006). Obese men may be less affected than women but are not immune to the disadvantages that can constrain academic achievement.

The workplace

Two recent surveys highlight the current bias against obese employees in the UK, which may reflect the situation in many westernized countries. One reported that 80% of 300 senior managers and directors of major UK companies believed there was prejudice in business against obese people, who were perceived as lacking the personal qualities to succeed, notably self-control, energy and drive (Personnel Today, 2007). In the second, nearly 50% of 2000 personnel professionals surveyed felt that obesity negatively affected the employee's output, while 30% regarded obesity as a valid medical reason for not employing a person (Personnel Today, 2005). Moreover, given the choice of two identically-qualified applicants, one normal-weight and one obese, 93% would employ the normal-weight candidate.

Research over the last 25 years, often using simulated employment situations, has confirmed that management and personnel biases are translated into workplace discrimination. In one study, public health administrators were sent a letter asking for information about career prospects in the health professions. A simulated overweight applicant (e.g. wearing padded clothes in a photograph) received fewer responses than a normal-weight control, and those who received a reply were told they were less likely to enter a graduate programme or get a good job after training (Benson *et al.*, 1980). In another study that controlled for facial appearance, college students were less likely to hire an overweight applicant for a position involving sales (and therefore interaction with the public) but were equally likely to hire for a business post (Rothblum, Miller and Garbutt, 1998). Klesges *et al.* (1990) asked adults with employment experience to make recruitment decisions and personal judgments on the basis of job descriptions, CVs and short videotaped interviews. Obese and diabetic applicants were both less likely to be hired, but for different reasons, the obese person being viewed as having poor work habits and more likely to have emotional and interpersonal problems. Finally, even being seated next to an overweight person while waiting for a job interview led to candidates being rated more negatively by people role-playing hiring decisions (Hebl and Mannix, 2003) – perhaps providing evidence of 'stigma by association'.

Economic penalties

There is strong evidence that being obese decreases earnings, especially in women. Gortmaker *et al.*

(1993) found that young American women who had been obese adolescents had lower household incomes and higher rates of household poverty; strikingly, adolescent obesity had no discernible financial penalty for men. Two studies that revisited this cohort up to 12 years later both confirmed that obese women continued to have lower wages. Various socio-economic factors and family confounders could not explain this, suggesting that employer discrimination was responsible (Baum and Ford, 2004). The financial penalty for white women who weighed two standard deviations above the cohort mean represented a reduction in wages equivalent to 1.5 years of education or 3 years' work experience (Cawley, 2004). An economic penalty specific to obese women has also been observed in a UK birth cohort (Sargent and Blanchflower, 1994). Cawley and Danziger (2005) have also shown that obesity in White women is a barrier to gaining employment after having been on state benefit, something not apparent in African–Americans. Overall, obese women are both less likely to gain employment and to receive equitable wages.

Health care

Obese people are at increased medical risk from the disorder and its complications (see Chapter 9), and yet many are disadvantaged by bias and inequality in the provision of health care. Factors include adverse attitudes by health professionals and the failure by them and insurance systems to recognize obesity as a medical disease.

As mentioned above, health professionals share similar anti-obesity biases with the general population. These negative stereotypes have also been observed in doctors, medical students, nurses and dieticians (Puhl and Brownell, 2001). The absence of self-control and will-power are again common perceptions and linked to beliefs about personal responsibility controlling food intake. Professional health training and practice have yet to overcome these strong cultural associations; significantly, obesity has until recently been conspicuously absent from many medical curricula (Banasiak and Murr, 2001).

Many doctors remain ambivalent about their involvement in obesity management (Puhl and Brownell, 2001). One factor may be their pessimism about the outcome, because doctors perceive obesity treatment as less effective than that of other chronic conditions, such as smoking or depression (Foster et al., 2003). Doctors' negativity may, in turn, discourage obese people from seeking advice. For example, obese women working in a large US community hospital were four times more likely than normal-weight workers to delay or cancel doctors' appointments, citing embarrassment about their weight as the most common reason (Olson, Schumaker and Yawn, 1994). White, but not Black, obese women are also less likely to use preventative services, even though they use medical services more because of obesity-related diseases (e.g. Meisinger, Heier and Loewel, 2004; Østbye et al., 2005). Disincentives included the prospect of being weighed or the health practitioner making comments about the person being overweight.

Closer inspection suggests that this blanket portrayal is over-simplistic. Many studies have examined small samples and not measured the extent of negativity or included positive attitudes. The literature on nurses' attitudes confirms that some respondents hold negative views, while others show a more complex mix (Brown, 2006). General medical practitioner's attitudes to overweight people ranged from neutral to negative rather than entirely negative, and were generally better than their attitudes to smokers (Harvey and Hill, 2001). Moreover, negative attitudes are not necessarily reflected in how health professionals behave towards their patients, and some recent studies indicate that patients' perceptions of their doctors are more positive. Only 13% of bariatric surgery patients (mean BMI, 55 kg/m^2) reported being 'usually' or 'always' treated disrespectfully by doctors (Anderson and Wadden, 2004) – substantially fewer than in previous studies. Also, a study of obese women revealed general satisfaction with their overall health care, with very few reports of negative interactions with doctors apart from dissatisfaction with their doctor's poor weight management skills (Wadden et al., 2000).

The impact of obesity on medical insurance is well documented in North America (Puhl and Brownell, 2001) and may become increasingly relevant elsewhere. Obesity treatment is excluded from US health insurance plans, while the Internal Revenue Service does not allow the costs of obesity treatment to be claimed against tax. This situation reflects the perceptions that obesity is not a disease but is self-inflicted, and that treatment is expensive and unsuccessful. Employer-sponsored health insurance in the US is also distorted by obesity. Obese people receiving this insurance have lower wages than those who do not (Bhattacharya and Bundorf, 2005), implying that employers compensate for the higher healthcare costs of the obese by reducing their wages. The wage reduction was consistent with estimated healthcare costs for men, but greater than those calculated for obese women. Once again, women appear to bear the brunt of obesity discrimination.

Social consequences

Many obese people face teasing, victimization and social rejection. The hurt experienced extends beyond the events themselves, and everyday social situations may become anxiety-laden and ultimately avoided. The most frequently encountered stigmatizing situations reported by a sample of obese Americans (Table 14.1) include comments from doctors, family, children and strangers. Being fat would seem to give others the licence to pass judgment on appearance, the cause of obesity and the necessary remedy.

Indeed, 40% of US obese adults report having been mistreated over their weight, over half of them by their spouse and two-thirds by strangers (Falkner et al., 1999). Between 50–70% of obese teenagers are teased about their weight, with little difference between boys and girls (e.g. Haines et al., 2006; Hayden-Wade et al., 2005; Hill and Waterston, 2002). Most perpetrators are peers rather than family members.

Table 14.1   The most common stigmatizing situations reported by US adults, in descending order of frequency.

- Comments from children

  'As an adult, having a child make fun of you.'

  'A child coming up to you and saying something like, "You're fat!"'

- Others making negative assumptions about you

  'Other people having low expectations of you because of your weight.'

  'Having people assume you have emotional problems because you are overweight.'

- Physical barriers

  'Not being able to fit into seats at restaurants, theatres and other public places.'

  'Not being able to find clothes that fit.'

- Being stared at

  'Being stared at in public.'

  'Groups of people pointing and laughing at you in public.'

- Inappropriate comments from doctors

  'Having a doctor make cruel remarks, ridicule you, or call you names.'

  'A doctor blaming unrelated physical problems on your weight.'

- Nasty comments from family

  'A spouse/partner calling you names because of your weight.'

  'A parent or other relative nagging you to lose weight.'

- Nasty comments from others

  'Having strangers suggest diets to you.'

  'Being offered fashion advice from strangers.'

- Being avoided, excluded, ignored

  'Being unable to get a date because of your size.'

  'Being singled out as a child by a teacher, school nurse, etc. because of your size.'

From A. Myers and J.C. Rosen (1999) 'Obesity stigmatization and coping: relation to mental health symptoms, body image, and self-esteem'. *International Journal of Obesity*, **23**, 221–30.

Stigmatization can have behavioural consequences. For example, a high proportion of subjects in the Swedish Obese Study (SOS) that evaluated bariatric surgery reported significant concerns about social activities, especially in public (Sullivan *et al.*, 1993). Women were particularly affected: nearly two-thirds were troubled by (and generally avoided) going out to a restaurant, while holidaying away from home worried over 50%, and buying clothes or public bathing nearly 90%.

Social relationships

Obesity can affect social relationships, especially from the teens onwards. Interestingly, despite early stereotyping mentioned above, obesity has little impact on children's popularity among their own peers – at least in community samples of primary school-aged children and as measured by peer friendship nominations and choice of companions in and outside school (Phillips and Hill, 1998). However, different rules apply to teenagers. Data from the US National Longitudinal Survey of Adolescent Health (Strauss and Pollack, 2003) showed that overweight and obese adolescents were significantly more likely to have three or fewer friendship nominations from their peers, as compared with normal-weight controls – who were more likely to have six or more nominations. Obese teenagers also received fewer reciprocal nominations from those whom they had nominated themselves (Figure 14.3), suggesting that friendship ties involving obese adolescents are weaker as well as less plentiful.

These distorted friendship patterns do not necessarily affect the development of the close relationships associated with adolescent and adult well-being. General social interaction among adults may not suffer, possibly because of extra effort invested to compensate for anticipated problems (Miller *et al.*, 1995a, 1995b). However, sexual relationships and marriage prospects may be damaged. Obese teenage girls are less likely to have romantic relationships than their normal-weight peers (Pearce, Boergers and Prinstein, 2002), while normal-weight young adults tended to reject overweight individuals as potential sexual partners (Chen and Brown, 2005).

US and UK cohort studies confirm the costs to marriage. Gortmaker *et al.* (1993) found that girls obese at 16 years of age were 20% less likely to be married 7 years later than their lean peers, while overweight men were 11% less

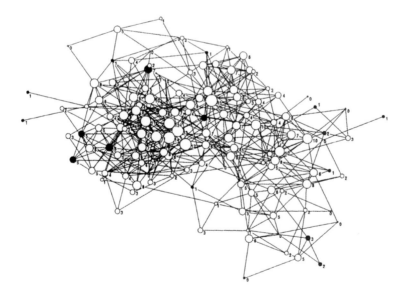

Figure 14.3 The social network map of adolescents in school. Each dot represents an adolescent; black dots are overweight or obese subjects. The size of the dot represents the number of peer nominations received, and those closer to the centre received more reciprocated nominations. From R.S. Strauss, and H.A. Pollack (2003) 'Social marginalization of overweight children'. *Archives of Pediatric & Adolescent Medicine*, **157**, 746–52, © American Medical Association, 2003. All rights reserved.

likely to be married. The National Longitudinal Survey of Youth confirmed that obese young adults – like those with short stature or high alcohol consumption – had lower marriage rates than their lean counterparts (Fu and Goldman, 1996), but once married were no more likely to get divorced (Fu and Goldman, 2000). Obesity that persists from childhood to adulthood reduces the likelihood of women (but not men) having a current sexual partner (Viner and Cole, 2005). When obese people do marry, they are more likely to choose an overweight partner (Jacobson *et al.*, 2006).

Psychological well-being

The psychological consequences of growing up and being fat in an antagonistic climate have generally received less attention than the physical sequelae. This situation is changing as psychosocial outcomes become valued in their own right, and with the recognition that psychological state affects the success of obesity treatment uptake and adherence. Psychological distress is variable within most groups of people and obesity is no exception: some obese individuals have serious psychological problems, whereas others have mild or few difficulties. An important challenge is to identify who suffers psychologically from their obesity, how they display their distress, and how to reduce this in the overall context of weight management.

Mood disorders

The older literature on the relationship between obesity and depression or anxiety is inconclusive, probably due to inconsistencies in assessing psychopathology and in study populations. Greater clarity is now emerging from prospective studies using improved methodologies.

Current views on the association between obesity and depression are summarized in Table 14.2. Numerous studies have highlighted the disproportionate burden on women. The US National Longitudinal Alcohol Epidemiologic Survey collected data from more than 40000 adults in 1992, including interview-based assessments of past-year depression and suicide attempts, and self-reported height and weight. Obesity (BMI >30 kg/m^2) was associated with a statistically significant 37% increased risk of major depression in women, but a 37% *decreased* risk of depression

Table 14.2   Current views on the association between obesity and depression.

The relationship between obesity and depression:

- Is weak overall, but stronger with severe obesity (BMI ⩾ 40 kg/m^2)
- Is stronger in females
- Is stronger in obese people undergoing treatment than in the general population
- Emerges during adolescence
- Is observed throughout the developed world

in men (Figure 14.4); similarly, women were at increased risk and men at reduced risk of suicide attempts (Carpenter *et al.*, 2000). The latter finding was confirmed by the lowering of suicide risk with increasing BMI observed in a study of over 1 million Swedish men (Magnusson *et al.*, 2005), and the US Survey NHANES III showed obese women (but not obese men) to be at increased risk of depression within the previous month (Onyike *et al.*, 2003). The latter study showed a near-doubling of obesity-associated depression risk in women, which was overshadowed by the fivefold higher risk in those with a BMI of ⩾40 kg/m^2. Wadden *et al.* (2006) have confirmed the high risk faced by those with severe obesity: 25% of a sample of patients with BMI of >40 kg/m^2 were assessed as having a mood disorder that would benefit from treatment.

These points were emphasized by the SOS surgical intervention study (perhaps the largest clinical sample yet to investigate mood disorders), which also examined the effects of successful treatment. At baseline, the first 1700 patients showed much higher levels of emotional disorder than healthy lean controls (Sullivan *et al.*, 1993). Obese men (mean BMI, 34 kg/m^2) and women (mean BMI, 38 kg/m^2) were over four times more likely to have clinical anxiety and seven times more likely to be clinically depressed. Two years after surgery, and following a marked reduction in BMI, both anxiety and depression were reduced; the proportion who were depressed fell from 9% to 4% and the decrease in depression scores was correlated with weight loss. By contrast, levels of anxiety and depression in obese subjects not receiving surgery did not change over this period (Karlsson, Sjöström and Sullivan, 1998) (Figure 14.5).

Studies of obese adolescents mirror many of the findings reported above – notably that depression is most apparent in obese girls and in those

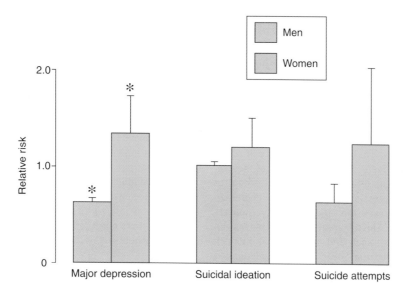

Figure 14.4 The relative risk of major depression is significantly increased in obese women but decreased in obese men, compared with normal-weight controls (relative risk = 1.0). Risk of suicidal behaviour was also higher in obese women, but not significantly so. From K.M. Carpenter *et al.* (2000) 'Relationship between obesity and DSM-IV major depressive disorder, suicide ideation, and suicide attempts: results from a general population study'. *American Journal of Public Health*, **90**, 251–7, with kind permission.

undergoing treatment – and may also cast light on factors that link obesity with depression. In this younger age group, depression can be at least partially accounted for by the individual's weight concerns (Daniels, 2005), their perceived isolation from peers (Xie *et al.*, 2005), or a combination of social isolation and experiences of shame (Sjöberg, Nilsson and Leppert, 2005). In adults, physical ill-health appears to be the most potent mediator, as it is for quality of life (e.g. Jorm *et al.*, 2003); influences of age and ethnicity have also been observed (Heo *et al.*, 2006).

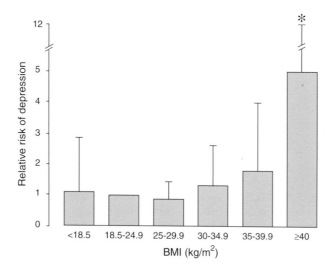

Figure 14.5 The relationship of risk of depression with BMI, relative to normal-weight subjects (BMI 18.5–24.0 kg(m²). From C.U. Onyike *et al.* (2003) 'Is obesity associated with major depression? Results from the third National Health and Nutrition Examination Survey'. *American Journal of Epidemiology*, **158**, 1139–47, with kind permission.

Possible causal relationships have also been explored by longitudinal studies. Several reports show that depression in adolescence is associated with later weight gain and a two-fold greater increase in the risk of subsequent obesity (e.g. Goodman and Whitaker, 2002; Richardson *et al.*, 2003; Franko *et al.*, 2005). At this age, and over a relatively short period, obesity appears to pose little risk for the onset of depression. By contrast, obesity in adults aged ⩾50 years doubled the risk of depression five years later, even after controlling for baseline depression, whereas being depressed did not increase the risk of obesity (Roberts *et al.*, 2003). This apparent contradiction may be explained by age- and time-critical interactions between the two conditions. Supporting this view are observations from a Finnish birth cohort, in which persistent obesity (at both ages 14 and 31 years) was most clearly associated with depression, and only in females (Herva *et al.*, 2006). Thus, obesity that develops early and persists into adulthood has the greatest social and psychological consequences, especially for women.

Body image and weight self-perception

Many, but not all, obese people are dissatisfied and preoccupied with their physical appearance – so-called 'body-image distress'. Risks for body-image distress include binge eating and previous stigmatizing experiences (Rosen, 2002). The relationship with binge eating and other eating disorders is discussed further in Chapter 20.

Body-image distress is expressed in many ways, including the wish to be considerably thinner and dislike of specific aspects of physical appearance, particularly the size and shape of the waist, stomach, thighs and buttocks – feelings that are shared by many non-obese women. Interestingly, body dissatisfaction is not consistently correlated with obesity except at the highest levels of BMI (e.g. Sarwer, Wadden and Foster, 1998; Hill and Williams, 1998); other factors such as depression may be more strongly related to body-image problems (see Chapter 20).

Individuals' perception of their weight is imperfect. For example, the ONS Omnibus Survey in the UK found that 75% of overweight but only 44% of obese respondents correctly assigned themselves to those categories (Wardle and Johnson, 2002). Characteristically, overweight or obese men fail to recognize their weight problem while normal-weight women tend to classify themselves as overweight (Chang and Christakis, 2003). Interestingly, many parents have distorted views of their children's weight, with overweight in boys especially passing undetected. In one UK study, parents correctly rated only 25% of overweight children and 43% of those obese (Jeffery *et al.*, 2005). This misperception is important given that recognizing overweight is a necessary first step to taking action. Misjudgments of body size are not apparently due to sensory errors; instead, body-image perception is influenced by various personal attitudes, beliefs and thoughts that must modify the widely-held negative view of obesity.

Self-esteem

Obesity is associated with a decrease in global self-esteem, although the effect is relatively modest; a meta-analysis reveals a significant 40% reduction in scores of self-esteem (Miller and Downey, 1999).

The association is relatively weak during childhood but strengthens through adolescence and into adulthood, and again is more apparent in females (Miller and Downey, 1999). As with depression, the causal interactions are likely to be complex. Low self-esteem can impair an obese person's ability to make necessary changes in behaviour, and thus could initiate and perpetuate obesity. Overall, low self-esteem is probably a minor contributor, albeit one that can interact with other risk factors for weight gain. Conversely, obesity can damage an individual's self-worth. Perhaps surprisingly, self-esteem – like obesity itself – is highly resistant to change. Self-esteem is a higher-order, internalized schema that is based on deep knowledge that is acquired early and often derives from emotionally significant experiences to which an individual has little conscious access; any threat to stability tends to produce anxiety and is therefore avoided.

Multi-domain approaches have helped to characterize self-esteem, especially in children and adolescents (Harter, 1993). Harter regards self-esteem as the personal evaluation of competence in various 'domains' that the individual deems important. People with low self-esteem perceive themselves as falling short of their ideals in particular domains of skills or valued personal attributes. Children's domains of

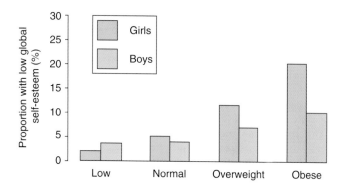

Figure 14.6 The relationship between global self-worth and weight. The graph shows the proportion of 9–13 year old girls and boys in each weight category who gave themselves a low score for global self-worth. From J. Franklin *et al.* (2006) 'Obesity and risk of low self-esteem: a state-wide survey of Australian children'. *Pediatrics*, **118**, 2481–7, with kind permission.

competence are largely set by their parents (e.g. scholastic competence, behaviour) and peers (physical appearance, social and athletic competences). The range of domains expands through adolescence into adulthood, taking in attributes such as job competence, romantic appeal and sense of humour.

Low self-esteem is established early in obese girls, who at the age of 9–10 years score themselves significantly lower on physical appearance and athletic competence than their normal-weight peers; obese boys are largely spared at this age (Phillips and Hill, 1998). By age 11, obese girls in a large Australian cohort included social rejection in their negative attributes, while boys associated their obesity with reduced physical appearance and athletic competence, although not as profoundly as the girls (Franklin *et al.*, 2006). In this study, obese adolescents were 2–4 times more likely than their normal-weight peers to give themselves low scores in one or more competence domains, especially their physical appearance: 63% of obese girls and 33% of obese boys depicted themselves as clearly unattractive. Overweight and obese children – especially girls – give themselves low scores for a global measure of self-worth (see Figure 14.6). Nonetheless, only 20% of the obese girls scored in this low range. This emphasizes the fact that low self-esteem should not be assumed in every obese child, adolescent or adult. Indeed, obesity coupled with high self-esteem may provide lessons for understanding 'resilience' (see below) and ultimately how to improve psychological well-being.

Quality of life

Many studies have shown that obesity diminishes health-related quality of life in children and adults, sometimes very profoundly. For example, one group of obese children referred to hospital found that 49% had impaired quality of life – comparable with children receiving chemotherapy for cancer (Schwimmer, Burwinkle and Varni, 2003). Less dramatic decreases in quality of life have been observed in community-based samples of overweight and obese children (Williams *et al.*, 2005); the discrepancy may be attributable to differences in obesity severity or the experience of treatment. For obese adolescents, impaired quality of life is predicted by the degree of overweight, presence of depressive symptoms, poor perceived peer support and low socioeconomic status (Zeller and Modi, 2006).

Quality of life research in obese adults has employed either generic measures (e.g. the widely-used SF-36) or obesity-specific instruments. The SF-36, which comprises standardized scores across a range of physical, social and psychological health 'dimensions', was used to examine the relationships between BMI, health and well-being within the Australian Longitudinal Study on Women's Health (Brown *et al.*, 2000). Among 14 000 women aged 18–23 years, overweight and obese subjects scored significantly lower in physical functioning, vitality and general health but did not differ from normal-weight controls in any of the main psychological health measures. However, overweight and obese middle-aged women (45–49 years) showed a different pattern

(Brown, Dobson and Mishra, 1998): they scored significantly lower than those of average weight on all the physical and psychological health scales, with the greatest deficits in the heaviest.

A UK study using the SF-36 showed that obese men and women (combined) scored lower than their normal-weight counterparts on every scale, with the most severely obese (BMI >40 kg/m²) being the lowest (Doll, Petersen and Stewart-Brown, 2000). This study also examined the impact of concurrent chronic illnesses, which affected about half of this cohort. People with obesity and other chronic illnesses reported particularly poor physical and psychological health, while the coexistence of obesity among people with comparably severe chronic illness was associated with a significant deterioration in physical but not emotional well-being (Figure 14.7). The conclusion that obese individuals with multiple co-occurring chronic illnesses are most at risk of psychological distress is supported by other studies (e.g. Heo *et al.*, 2003); these findings also imply that previous assessments of psychological well-being in obese people may have been confounded by coexisting physical health problems.

Several obesity-specific measures of quality of life, focusing on the most relevant areas of function, have been developed to complement the generic approaches. One of the most widely used and reliable is the IWQOL-Lite (short version of the Impact of Weight on Quality of Life questionnaire), which has five scales that address physical function, self-esteem, sexual life, public distress and work (Kolotkin *et al.*, 2001; Duval *et al.*, 2006). Most of the questions start with the phrase 'Because of my weight ...'. These assessments confirm the lack of enjoyment of sexual activity and avoidance of sexual encounters described earlier, especially in women and the most obese (Kolotkin *et al.*, 2006). In general, obesity-specific quality of life scores mirror changes in weight during and after weight-reduction programmes, showing improvement with weight loss and deterioration with weight regain (Engel *et al.*, 2003).

Resilience

The psychological impact of obesity is broadly related to features such as the severity of obesity, its duration and persistence and gender; however, there is also great individual variation. Many obese people have high self-esteem, do not suffer major depression, are in well-paid employment and have good social relationships. This implies individual resistance to the negative effects of obesity – so called resilience. Resilience

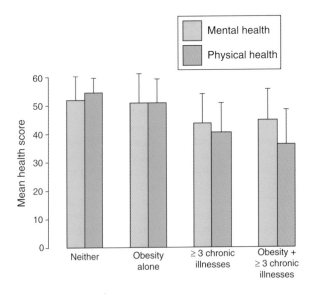

Figure 14.7 The impact of obesity and coexistent chronic diseases on quality of life. The graph shows the mean mental health and physical health component scores from the SF-36 in adults with and without obesity and chronic illnesses. Error bars indicate standard deviation. From H.A. Doll *et al.* (2000) 'Obesity and physical and emotional well-being: Associations between body mass index, chronic illness, and the physical and mental components of the SF-36 questionnaire'. *Obesity Research*, **8**, 160–70, with kind permission.

is an acquired process rather than a personality trait and is a function of individual, family and community factors; it offers a different perspective to the more traditional risk factor approach, focusing on strengths rather than deficits (Fergus and Zimmerman, 2005). Resilience has been considered mainly in children in the contexts of violence and deprivation and seems likely to provide valuable insights in obesity research.

Underpinning resilience is good social support, such as close family relationships or supportive peers. Unfortunately, experiences of social rejection and victimization are relatively common for obese people. The frequency of these experiences has been linked to poor mental health, body dissatisfaction and low self-esteem (Myers and Rosen, 1999). Scrutiny by others in public situations erodes confidence and, by limiting social activities, reduces the individual's social networks. There is a substantial literature outside obesity showing how social support underpins a person's ability to cope with life stress. There is certainly evidence that having a close supportive relationship or confidant delays the reduction in physical functional capacity experienced by older obese adults (Surtees, Wainwright and Khaw, 2004). As already noted, perceived isolation is partly responsible for depression in obese teenagers; conversely, it is possible that the support of close friends may protect against depression. The social experience afforded by weight-loss groups and other user-led support organizations for obese people may provide similar benefits.

The way forward

This chapter has highlighted the numerous, complex and variable interactions between obesity and psychosocial factors. In order to understand these better, and to exploit that knowledge to improve the health and well-being of obese people, new ways of thinking are needed.

First, it is necessary to move beyond simple cause–effect explanations in order to understand how social disadvantage and the psychological problems develop in obese people and how they initiate and perpetuate obesity. Obese people face psychosocial challenges that are repeated and may have occurred since childhood. Current low self-esteem, perceived isolation and all their consequences may therefore be the products of a long history of experiences of rejection and achievement failures; they also

direct future experiences, both behaviourally by discouraging social interactions and cognitively through confirmatory biases. The cumulative impact of multiple life-events and circumstances can be unravelled using the life-course epidemiological approach, which has been used to explore health and social inequality (Davey Smith, 2003). This methodology is now being applied to obesity. Analysing data from a Swedish cohort followed for 14 years from the age of 16, Novak, Ahlgren and Hammarström (2006) concluded that the social disadvantage of overweight reflected the accumulation of multiple adversities from adolescence into young adulthood; importantly, the pathways differed for men and women. This approach may help describe the complexity of the processes, and to identify key times in childhood and adolescence when interventions to reduce stigma and negativity might be effective.

Second, the crucial importance of psychosocial factors in determining the success or failure of weight-management strategies needs to be fully appreciated. Significant and maintained weight loss seems likely to improve psychosocial status: body image, quality of life and social competence all improve with weight loss, and all deteriorate as weight is regained. Conversely, psychological problems such as depression and low self-esteem are known to reduce the uptake, completion and success of treatment (e.g. Zeller et al., 2004). Effective seeking, identification and management of psychosocial problems are essential to enable disempowered patients to break out of the vicious cycle of overweight and negative effect.

Finally, the nature of obesity itself has to be considered in a fresh light. The pervasive ideology of blame – based on ill-conceived notions of will-power and which holds obese people responsible for their weight problem and their failure to solve it – needs to be replaced with a better understanding of the complex biological and environmental causes of obesity. Governmentally-set targets such as those in the UK and the portrayal of obesity as a lifestyle disorder have done little to help people lose weight. Indeed, shifting the onus of responsibility on to the individual identifies obesity as a personal failing. Friedman (2003) has called for 'A war on obesity, not the obese'. There can be no doubt that better public and professional knowledge about obesity will help to relieve the psychological and social burdens of obesity, and to improve the medical management of the condition.

References

Anderson, D.A. and Wadden, T.A. (2004) Bariatric surgery patients' views of their physicians' weight-related attitudes and practices. *Obesity Research*, **12**, 1587–95.

Banasiak, M. and Murr, M.M. (2001) Medical school curricula do not address obesity as a disease. *Obesity Surgery*, **11**, 671–9.

Baum, C.L. and Ford, W.F. (2004) The wage effects of obesity: a longitudinal study. *Health Economics*, **13**, 885–99.

Benson, P.L., Severs, D., Tatgenhorst, J. and Loddengaard, N. (1980) The social costs of obesity: a non-reactive field study. *Social Behaviour and Personality*, **8**, 91–6.

Bhattacharya, J. and Bundorf, M.K. (2005) *The Incidence of the Healthcare Costs of Obesity*. Working Paper 11303, National Bureau of Economic Research, Cambridge, MA.

Brown, I. (2006) Nurses' attitudes towards adult patients who are obese: literature review. *Journal of Advanced Nursing*, **53**, 221–32.

Brown, W.J., Dobson, A.J. and Mishra, G. (1998) What is a healthy weight for middle aged women? *International Journal of Obesity*, **22**, 520–8.

Brown, W.J., Mishra, G., Kenardy, J. and Dobson, A. (2000) Relationships between body mass index and well-being in young Australian women. *International Journal of Obesity*, **24**, 1360–8.

Canning, H. and Mayer, J. (1966) Obesity – its possible effects on college acceptance. *New England Journal of Medicine*, **275**, 1172–4.

Carpenter, K.M., Hasin, D.S., Allison, D.B. and Faith, M.S. (2000) Relationship between obesity and DSM-IV major depressive disorder, suicide ideation, and suicide attempts: results from a general population study. *American Journal of Public Health*, **90**, 251–7.

Cawley, J. (2004) The impact of obesity on wages. *The Journal of Human Resources*, **39**, 451–74.

Cawley, J. and Danziger, S. (2005) Morbid obesity and the transition from welfare to work. *Journal of Policy Analysis and Management*, **24**, 727–43.

Chang, V.W. and Christakis, N.A. (2003) Self-perception of weight appropriateness in the United States. *American Journal of Preventive Medicine*, **24**, 332–9.

Chen, E.Y. and Brown, M. (2005) Obesity stigma in sexual relationships. *Obesity Research*, **13**, 1393–7.

Cramer, P. and Steinwert, T. (1998) Thin is good, fat is bad: how early does it begin? *Journal of Applied Developmental Psychology*, **19**, 429–51.

Crandall, C.S. (1991) Do heavy-weight students have more difficulty paying for college? *Personality and Social Psychology Bulletin*, **17**, 606–11.

Daniels, J. (2005) Weight and weight concerns: Are they associated with reported depressive symptoms in adolescents? *Journal of Pediatric Health Care*, **19**, 33–41.

Datar, A. and Sturm, R. (2006) Childhood overweight and elementary school outcomes. *International Journal of Obesity*, **30**, 1449–60.

Davey Smith, F.G. (ed.) (2003) *Health Inequalities: Lifecourse Approaches*, The Policy Press, Bristol.

DeJong, W. and Kleck, R.E. (1986) The social psychological effects of overweight, in *Physical Appearance, Stigma, and Social Behaviour: The Ontario Symposium* (eds C.P. Herman, M.P. Zanna and E.T. Higgins), Lawrence Erlbaum, Hillsdale.

Doll, H.A., Petersen, S.E.K. and Stewart-Brown, S.L. (2000) Obesity and physical and emotional well-being: Associations between body mass index, chronic illness, and the physical and mental components of the SF-36 questionnaire. *Obesity Research*, **8**, 160–70.

Duval, K., Marceau, P., Pérusse, L. and Lacasse, Y. (2006) An overview of obesity-specific quality of life questionnaires. *Obesity Reviews*, **7**, 347–60.

Engel, S.G., Crosby, R.D., Kolotkin, R.L. *et al.* (2003) Impact of weight loss and regain on quality of life: mirror image or differential effect? *Obesity Research*, **11**, 1207–13.

Falkner, N.H., French, S.A., Jeffery, R.W. *et al.* (1999) Mistreatment due to weight: prevalence and sources of perceived mistreatment in women and men. *Obesity Research*, **7**, 572–6.

Fergus, S. and Zimmerman, M.A. (2005) Adolescent resilience: a framework for understanding healthy development in the face of risk. *Annual Review of Public Health*, **26**, 399–419.

Foster, G.D., Wadden, T.A., Makris, A.P. *et al.* (2003) Primary care physicians' attitudes about obesity and its treatment. *Obesity Research*, **10**, 1168–77.

Franklin, J., Denyer, G., Steinbeck, K.S. *et al.* (2006) Obesity and risk of low self-esteem: a state-wide survey of Australian children. *Pediatrics*, **118**, 2481–7.

Franko, D.L., Striegel-Moore, R.H., Thompson, D. *et al.* (2005) Does adolescent depression predict obesity in black and white young adult women? *Psychological Medicine*, **35**, 1505–13.

Friedman, J.M. (2003) A war on obesity, not the obese. *Science*, **299**, 856–8.

Fu, H. and Goldman, N. (1996) Incorporating health into models of marriage choice: demographic and sociological perspectives. *Journal of Marriage & the Family*, **58**, 740–58.

Fu, H. and Goldman, N. (2000) The association between health-related behaviours and the risk of divorce in the USA. *Journal of Biological Science*, **32**, 63–88.

Goodman, E. and Whitaker, R.C. (2002) A prospective study of the role of depression in the development and persistence of adolescent obesity. *Pediatrics*, **109**, 497–504.

Gortmaker, S.L., Must, A., Perrin, J.M. *et al.* (1993) Social and economic consequences of overweight in adolescence and young adulthood. *New England Journal of Medicine*, **329**, 1008–12.

Greenberg, B.S., Eastin, M., Hofschire, L. *et al.* (2003) Portrayals of overweight and obese individuals on commercial television. *American Journal of Public Health*, **93**, 1342–8.

Haines, J., Neumark-Sztainer, D., Eisenberg, M.E. and Hannan, P.J. (2006) Weight teasing and disordered eating behaviours in adolescents: longitudinal findings from Project EAT (Eating Among Teens). *Pediatrics*, **117**, e209–15.

Harter, S. (1993) Causes and consequences of low self-esteem in children and adolescents, in *Self-esteem: The Puzzle of Low Self-regard* (eds R.F. Baumeister), Plenum, New York, pp. 87–116.

Harvey, E.L. and Hill, A.J. (2001) Health professionals' views of overweight people and smokers. *International Journal of Obesity*, **25**, 1253–61.

Hayden-Wade, H.A., Stein, R.I., Ghaderi, A. *et al.* (2005) Prevalence, characteristics, and correlates of teasing experiences among overweight children vs. non-overweight peers. *Obesity Research*, **13**, 1381–92.

Hebl, M.R. and Mannix, L.M. (2003) The weight of obesity in evaluating others: a mere proximity effect. *Personality and Social Psychology Bulletin*, **29**, 28–38.

Heo, M., Allison, D.B., Faith, M.S. *et al.* (2003) Obesity and quality of life: mediating effects of pain and comorbidities. *Obesity Research*, **11**, 209–16.

Heo, M., Pietrobelli, A., Fontaine, K.R. *et al.* (2006) Depressive mood and obesity in US adults: comparison and moderation by sex, age, and race. *International Journal of Obesity*, **30**, 513–9.

Herva, A., Laitinen, J., Miettunen, J. *et al.* (2006) Obesity and depression: Results from the longitudinal Northern Finland 1966 Birth Cohort Study. *International Journal of Obesity*, **30**, 520–7.

Hill, A.J. and Silver, E. (1995) Fat, friendless and unhealthy: 9-year old children's perception of body shape stereotypes. *International Journal of Obesity*, **19**, 423–30.

Hill, A.J. and Waterston, C.L. (2002) Fat-teasing in pre-adolescent children: the bullied and the bullies. *International Journal of Obesity*, **26** (Suppl 1), 20.

Hill, A.J. and Williams, J. (1998) Psychological health in a non-clinical sample of obese women. *International Journal of Obesity*, **22**, 578–83.

Jacobson, P., Torgerson, J.S., Sjöström, L. and Bouchard, C. (2006) Spouse resemblance in body mass index: Effects on adult obesity prevalence in the offspring generation. *American Journal of Epidemiology*, **165**, 101–8.

Jeffery, A.N., Voss, L.D., Metcalf, B.S. *et al.* (2005) Parents' awareness of overweight in themselves and their children: cross sectional study within a cohort (EarlyBird 21). *British Medical Journal*, **330**, 23–4.

Jorm, A.F., Korten, A.E., Christensen, H. *et al.* (2003) Association of obesity with anxiety, depression and emotional well-being: a community survey.

Australian and New Zealand Journal of Public Health, **27**, 434–40.

Karlsson, J., Sjöström, L. and Sullivan, M. (1998) Swedish obese subjects (SOS) – an intervention study of obesity. Two year follow-up of health-related quality of life (HRQL) and eating behaviour after gastric surgery for severe obesity. *International Journal of Obesity*, **22**, 113–26.

Karnehed, N., Rasmussen, F., Hemmingsson, T. and Tynelius, P. (2006) Obesity and attained education: cohort study of more than 700000 Swedish men. *Obesity*, **14**, 1421–8.

Klesges, R.C., Klem, M.L., Hanson, C.L. *et al.* (1990) The effects of applicant's health status and qualifications on simulated hiring decisions. *International Journal of Obesity*, **14**, 527–35.

Kolotkin, R.L., Binks, M., Crosby, R.D. *et al.* (2006) Obesity and sexual quality of life. *Obesity*, **14**, 472–9.

Kolotkin, R.L., Crosby, R.D., Kosloski, K.D. and Williams, G.R. (2001) Development of a brief measure to assess quality of life in obesity. *Obesity Research*, **9**, 102–11.

Latner, J.D. and Stunkard, A.J. (2003) Getting worse: the stigmatisation of obese children. *Obesity Research*, **11**, 452–6.

Lawlor, D.A., Clark, H., Davey Smith, G. and Leon, D.A. (2006) *International Journal of Obesity*, **30**, 1758–65.

Magnusson, P.K.E., Rasmussen, F., Lawlor, D.A. *et al.* (2005) Association of body mass index with suicide mortality: a prospective cohort study of more than one million men. *American Journal of Epidemiology*, **163**, 1–8.

Meisinger, C., Heier, M. and Loewel, H. (2004) The relationship between body weight and health care among German women. *Obesity Research*, **12**, 1473–80.

Miller, C.T. and Downey, K.T. (1999) A meta-analysis of heavyweight and self-esteem. *Personality and Social Psychology Revue*, **3**, 68–84.

Miller, C.T., Rothblum, E.D., Brand, P.A. and Felicio, D.M. (1995a) Do obese women have poorer social relationships than nonobese women? Reports by self, friends, and coworkers. *Journal of Personality*, **63**, 65–85.

Miller, C.T., Rothblum, E.D., Felicio, D.M. and Brand, P.A. (1995b) Compensating for stigma: Obese and non-obese women's reactions to being visible. *Personality & Social Psychology Bulletin*, **21**, 1093–106.

Musher-Eizenman, D.R., Holub, S.C., Miller, A.B. *et al.* (2004) Body size stigmatization in preschool children: the role of control attributions. *Journal of Pediatric Psychology*, **29**, 613–20.

Myers, A. and Rosen, J.C. (1999) Obesity stigmatization and coping: relation to mental health symptoms, body image, and self-esteem. *International Journal of Obesity*, **23**, 221–30.

Novak, M., Ahlgren, C. and Hammarström, A. (2006) A life-course approach in explaining social inequity in obesity among young adult men and women. *International Journal of Obesity*, **30**, 191–200.

O'Brien, K.S., Hunter, J.A. and Banks, M. (2007) Implicit anti-fat bias in physical educators: physical attributes, ideology and socialization. *International Journal of Obesity*, **31**, 308–14.

Olson, C.L., Schumaker, H.D. and Yawn, B.P. (1994) Overweight women delay medical care. *Archives of Family Medicine*, **3**, 888–92.

Onyike, C.U., Crum, R.M., Lee, H.B. *et al.* (2003) Is obesity associated with major depression? Results from the third National Health and Nutrition Examination Survey. *American Journal of Epidemiology*, **158**, 1139–47.

Østbye, T., Taylor, D.H., Yancy, W.S. and Krause, K.M. (2005) Associations between obesity and receipt of screening mammography, papanicolaou tests, and influenza vaccination: results from the Health and Retirement Study (HRS) and the Asset and Health Dynamics Among Oldest old (AHEAD) Study. *American Journal of Public Health*, **95**, 1623–30.

Pearce, M.J., Boergers, J. and Prinstein, M.J. (2002) Adolescent obesity, overt and relational peer victimization, and romantic relationships. *Obesity Research*, **10**, 386–93.

Personnel Today (2005) Fattism is the last bastion of employee discrimination. http://www.personneltoday.com/Articles/2005/10/25/32213/obesity-research-fattism-is-the-last-bastion-of-employee.html (last accessed 12 July 20080.

Personnel Today (2007) Overweight employees are disadvantaged in the workplace. http://www.personneltoday.com/Articles/2007/01/02/38721/overweight-employees-are-disadvantaged-in-the-workplace.html (last accessed 12 July 2008).

Phillips, R.G. and Hill, A.J. (1998) Fat, plain, but not friendless: Self-esteem and peer acceptance of obese pre-adolescent girls. *International Journal of Obesity*, **22**, 287–93.

Puhl, R. and Brownell, K.D. (2001) Bias, discrimination and obesity. *Obesity Research*, **9**, 788–805.

Richardson, L.P., Davis, R., Poulton, R. *et al.* (2003) A longitudinal evaluation of adolescent depression and adult obesity. *Archives of Pediatric & Adolescent Medicine*, **157**, 739–45.

Richardson, S.A., Hastorf, A.H., Goodman, N. and Dornbusch, S.M. (1961) Cultural uniformity in reaction to physical disabilities. *American Sociological Review*, **26**, 241–7.

Roberts, R.E., Deleger, S., Strawbridge, W.J. and Kaplan, G.A. (2003) Prospective association between obesity and depression: evidence from the Alameda County Study. *International Journal of Obesity*, **27**, 514–21.

Rosen, J.C. (2002) Obesity and body image, in *Eating Disorders and Obesity*, 2nd edn (eds C.G. Fairburn and K.D. Brownell), Guilford Press, New York, pp. 399–402.

Rothblum, E.D., Miller, C.T. and Garbutt, B. (1988) Stereotypes of obese job applicants. *International Journal of Eating Disorders*, **7**, 277–83.

Sargent, J.D. and Blanchflower, D.G. (1994) Obesity and stature in adolescence and earnings in young adulthood. *Analysis of a British Birth Cohort. Archives of Pediatric & Adolescent Medicine*, **148**, 681–7.

Sarwer, D.B., Wadden, T.A. and Foster, G.D. (1998) Assessment of body image dissatisfaction in obese women: specificity, severity, and clinical significance. *Journal of Consulting and Clinical Psychology*, **66**, 651–4.

Schwartz, M.B., Vartanian, L.R., Nosek, B.A. and Brownell, K.D. (2006) The influence of one's own body weight on implicit and explicit anti-fat bias. *Obesity*, **14**, 440–7.

Schwimmer, J.B., Burwinkle, T.M. and Varni, J.W. (2003) Health-related quality of life of severely obese children and adolescents. *Journal of the American Medical Association*, **289**, 1813–9.

Sjöberg, R.L., Nilsson, K.W. and Leppert, J. (2005) Obesity, shame, and depression in school-aged children: a population-based study. *Pediatrics*, **116**, e389–92.

Staffieri, J.R. (1967) A study of social stereotype of body image in children. *Journal of Personality and Social Psychology*, **7**, 101–4.

Strauss, R.S. and Pollack, H.A. (2003) Social marginalization of overweight children. *Archives of Pediatric & Adolescent Medicine*, **157**, 746–52.

Sullivan, M., Karlsson, J., Sjöström, L. *et al.* (1993) Swedish obese subjects (SOS) – an intervention study of obesity. Baseline evaluation of health and psychosocial functioning in the first 1743 subjects examined. *International Journal of Obesity*, **17**, 503–12.

Surtees, P.G., Wainwright, N.W.J. and Khaw, K-T. (2004) Obesity, confidant support and functional health: cross-sectional evidence from the EPIC-Norfolk cohort. *International Journal of obesity*, **28**, 748–58.

Tara, H. and Potts-Datema, W. (2005) Obesity and student performance at school. *Journal of School Health*, **75**, 291–5.

Teachman, B.A. and Brownell, K.D. (2001) Implicit anti-fat bias among health professionals: Is anyone immune? *International Journal of Obesity*, **25**, 1525–31.

Viner, R.M. and Cole, T.J. (2005) Adult socioeconomic, educational, social, and psychological outcomes of childhood obesity: a national birth cohort study. *British Medical Journal*, **330**, 1354–8.

Wadden, T.A., Anderson, D.A., Foster, G.D. *et al.* (2000) Obese women's perceptions of their physicians' weight management attitudes and practices. *Archives of Family Medicine*, **9**, 854–60.

Wadden, T.A., Butryn, M.L., Sarwer, D.B. *et al.* (2006) Comparison of psychosocial status in treatment-seeking women with class III vs. class I-II obesity. *Obesity*, **14** Suppl (2), 90S–8S.

Wardle, J. and Johnson, F. (2002) Weight and dieting: examining levels of weight concern in British adults. *International Journal of Obesity*, **26**, 1144–9.

Williams, J., Wake, M., Hesketh, K. *et al.* (2005) Health-related quality of life of overweight and obese children. *Journal of the American Medical Association*, **293**, 70–6.

Xie, B., Chou, C.P., Spruijt-Metz, D. *et al.* (2005) Effects of peer isolation and social support availability on the relationship between body mass index and depressive symptoms. *International Journal of Obesity*, **29**, 1137–43.

Zeller, M., Kirk, S., Claytor, R. *et al.* (2004) Predictors of attrition from a pediatric weight management program. *Journal of Pediatrics*, **144**, 466–70.

Zeller, M.H. and Modi, A.C. (2006) Predictors of health-related quality of life in obese youth. *Obesity*, **14**, 122–30.

Assessment and Investigation of Obesity

Key points

- Full evaluation of the obese patient is essential to identify the causes of obesity, assess associated health risks and determine the patient's suitability for treatment.

- Almost all obesity is related to an obesogenic lifestyle, but other causes should be actively sought and treated. Numerous drugs increase weight, notably glucocorticoids, antidiabetic agents, antipsychotics and anti-epileptic medications. Endocrine diseases that induce obesity include hypothyroidism and Cushing syndrome. Rare genetic causes include inherited conditions such as Prader-Willi syndrome and mutations affecting leptin and the proopiomelanocortin neurones, which mediate its appetite-suppressing effect.

- The severity of obesity and associated health risks can be determined from BMI and waist circumference (or waist:hip ratio). Many risks increase when BMI exceeds $25 \, \text{kg/m}^2$ (overweight), while cardiovascular and diabetes risk increases markedly when waist circumference exceeds 102 cm (men) or 88 cm (women). Precise measurements of body or visceral fat mass are occasionally useful for defining risk more precisely.

- The development of obesity should be documented with its relationship to life events, pregnancy, family history of obesity and diabetes, and drug therapy. Previous attempts to lose weight and their outcomes, and possible reasons for failure, should be explored.

- Intake of food, sweetened drinks and alcohol, and physical and sedentary activities should be documented. Obese people tend to under-report their energy intake and overestimate physical activity.

- Smoking exacerbates obesity-related cardiovascular and health risks while decreasing body weight. Smoking cessation often causes significant weight gain, which may deter smokers from stopping the habit.

- Psychological state should be assessed, including depression, possible eating disorders and the patient's motivation and readiness for lifestyle change.

- Obesity (especially central) is a major risk factor for type 2 diabetes. Fasting glucose should be checked, proceeding to an oral glucose tolerance test in high-risk cases. Impaired fasting glucose (IFG) and impaired glucose tolerance (IGT) also increase health risks.

- Central obesity increases cardiovascular risk, with coronary-heart and peripheral arterial disease, myocardial infarction, heart failure and hypertension. Clinical features may be unimpressive; high-risk patients need further investigation to diagnose complications such as heart failure and arterial disease.

- Dyslipidaemia associated with obesity and the metabolic syndrome comprises moderately raised triglyceride levels and low HDL cholesterol. Triglyceride levels exceeding 2.0 mmol/l, together with a waist circumference above 102 cm (men) or 88 cm (women), denote high cardiovascular risk.

- Other conditions associated with obesity include obstructive sleep apnoea, gastro-oesophageal reflux (which predisposes to oesophageal carcinoma), polycystic ovarian syndrome, fatty liver disease (which can progress to cirrhosis) and several malignancies. All these conditions must be considered when reviewing an obese patient, and appropriate screening tests conducted.

Chapter 15 Assessment and Investigation of Obesity

Luc Van Gaal and Ilse Mertens

Comprehensive assessment of the obese patient is an essential precursor to the effective management of the condition. There are several complementary aims. The severity of obesity must be assessed in terms of the amount and distribution of body fat. Potential causes of obesity must be considered; although the vast majority of cases are primarily related to lifestyle, certain drugs and genetic or endocrine conditions can be responsible, and these may require specific treatment. The presence or risk of the many comorbidities of obesity must be determined, together with the overall likely impact on the subject's health and prognosis. The patient's lifestyle should be evaluated, not only as a potential contributor to obesity, but also to gauge his or her motivation for change and thus the likelihood of success of any treatment. Finally, the patient's suitability for various forms of obesity management (lifestyle modification, pharmacotherapy or bariatric surgery) must be assessed.

This chapter covers the clinical assessment of obesity, highlighting the key points that should be sought from the personal and family history and a thorough physical examination. Routine screening tests are described, together with additional specific investigations that can be used to evaluate adiposity and the complications of obesity. Areas of active research in this area are also highlighted as appropriate.

As background, relevant aspects of the causes of obesity (described in Chapters 7 and 8) and the comorbidities of obesity (Chapters 9–13) will first be summarized.

Causes of obesity

In routine clinical practice, all but a small percentage of cases of obesity are ultimately attributable to lifestyle factors, superimposed on a background of genetically determined susceptibility that overall accounts for 40–70% of the variation in body weight (Farooqi and O'Rahilly, 2006). An obesogenic lifestyle comprises variable combinations of an excessive energy intake and/or decreased energy expenditure, particularly through physical inactivity. The interplay of these factors is discussed in detail in Chapters 7 and 8.

The crucial role of lifestyle highlights the importance of a detailed history of food intake and physical activity patterns – remembering that obese people frequently underestimate their food intake and over-report their physical activity levels (see Chapter 3).

Other causes of obesity (Table 15.1) must be borne in mind throughout a consultation with an obese patient. Although unlikely, identifying a primary cause for obesity will often require specific investigations and treatment that may be curative.

Drug-induced obesity

Numerous drugs can cause an increase in fat mass and weight gain (World Health Organization, 1997), including several in common clinical practice, and some (e.g. antidiabetic and antihypertensive agents) that are frequently used in obese patients. The main obesogenic drugs are shown in Table 15.2, and the mechanisms through which they cause obesity are discussed further in Chapter 8.

The main offenders are antipsychotic drugs (particularly the newer 'atypical' agents), antidepressants, antiepileptics, progestational contraceptives, and especially glucocorticoids and – with the exception of metformin – antidiabetic agents (Bray, 2004). Weight gain is often 2–4 kg with glucocorticoids or insulin,

Obesity: Science to Practice   Edited by Gareth Williams and Gema Frühbeck
© 2009 John Wiley & Sons, Ltd

Table 15.1 Causes of obesity.

Lifestyle-related ('simple') obesity: >95% of all cases

- genetic susceptibility
- obesogenic lifestyle

Obesogenic drugs (see Table 15.2)

Endocrine disorders

- Hypothyroidism
- Polycystic ovarian syndrome (PCOS)
- Cushing syndrome
- Pituitary disease: panhypopituitarism, growth hormone deficiency
- Hypothalamic lesions

Inherited syndromes

- Prader-Willi syndrome
- Bardet-Biedl syndrome
- Alström syndrome

Monogenic disorders

Due to mutations affecting:

- Leptin (*LEP*)
- Leptin receptor (*LEPR*)
- Proopiomelanocortin (*POMC*)
- Prohormone convertase 1 (*PHC-1*)
- Neurotrophic tyrosine kinase receptor type 2 (*NTRK2*)

Table 15.2 Obesogenic drugs.

Glucocorticoids

Antidiabetic drugs

- Insulin
- Sulphonylureas and glitinides
- Thiazolidinediones

Psychoactive drugs

- Antipsychotics
  - Classical (chlorpromazine, haloperidol)
  - Atypical (olanzepine, clozapine)
- Antidepressants (tricyclics)

Antiepileptic drugs

- Valproate
- Carbamazepine
- Gabapentin

Endocrine agents

- Progestagen-based contraceptives
- Hormone replacement therapy
- Tamoxifen

β-adrenoceptor blockers

- Propranolol

Miscellaneous

- Cyproheptadine
- Pizotifen
- Flunarizine
- Antihistamines
- Cyclophosphamide
- Fluorouracil

and may reach 15 kg with antipsychotic and antiepileptic drugs.

Continuing treatment with drugs that promote weight gain can greatly reduce the chances of success in managing obesity through lifestyle modification or pharmacotherapy. A comprehensive drug history must be taken to identify possible iatrogenic causes of obesity and determine whether these could be withdrawn or reduced, or whether other medications that do not cause weight gain could be substituted. Some possible alternatives to the more common obesogenic drugs are discussed in Chapter 17.

Endocrine disorders

Several endocrine conditions are associated with obesity, although most are very rare (Table 15.1).

Hypothyroidism leads in two-thirds of cases to weight gain, which is usually modest; marked obesity is rare (Knudsen *et al.*, 2005). This is mainly due to falls in basal metabolic rate and in physical activity. As hypothyroidism is relatively common (its prevalence is approximately 4% in most adult populations), the condition should be actively sought. Classical clinical features such as cold intolerance, hoarse voice, constipation and myxoedematous facies (Figure 15.1) may or may not be evident.

Polycystic ovarian syndrome (PCOS) is commonly (40–50% of cases) associated with obesity

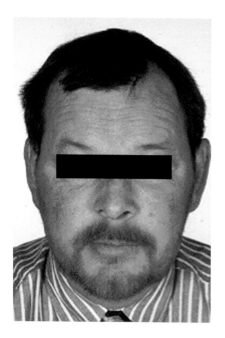

Figure 15.1 Hypothyroidism, showing the puffy myxo-edematous facies, sallow complexion and thinning of the lateral part of the eyebrows. The patient's weight gain was reversed by thyroxine replacement. Image reproduced by courtesy of Professor Gareth Williams, University of Bristol, UK.

and insulin resistance, and carries a relatively high prevalence of glucose intolerance and type 2 diabetes (see Chapter 13). Clinical features include menstrual irregularity, anovulation and infertility, with hirsutism and acanthosis nigricans – the latter being a marker of severe insulin resistance.

Cushing syndrome is rare, but classically includes truncal obesity with a 'buffalo hump' (a fat pad overlying the lower cervical spine) and a plethoric, rounded 'moon face' (Figure 15.2). Other typical features are a thin skin with easy bruising, purple striae (which owe their colour to the subdermal vascular plexus being visible through the thinned skin), hypertension, and wasting of the limbs with proximal myopathy.

Obesity is a feature of panhypopituitarism, growth hormone deficiency and hypogonadism. Hypothalamic lesions are a rare but striking cause of obesity, usually with hyperphagia and other autonomic disturbances such as temperature and thirst dysregulation. Usual causes are tumours, notably craniopharyngioma or a pituitary macroadenoma extending above the sella (see Figure 21.8 on page 517). Other causes include trauma, or iatrogenic damage from surgery or radiotherapy. Hyperphagia and

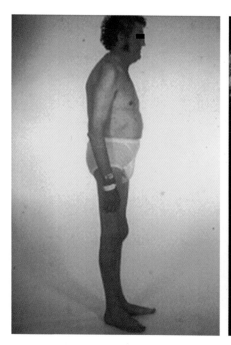
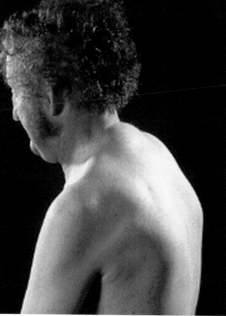

Figure 15.2 Cushing syndrome, showing (left) truncal obesity with proximal limb wasting, a rounded and plethoric 'moon' face and (right) a 'buffalo hump'. Image reproduced by courtesy of Professor Gareth Williams, University of Bristol, UK.

obesity are probably due to destruction of the POMC neurones of the arcuate (tuberoinfundibular) nucleus that mediate the appetite-suppressing action of leptin (see Chapter 6).

Insulinomas are extremely rare, but are often associated with hyperphagia and weight gain, induced by recurrent hypoglycaemia.

'Syndromic' and monogenic causes of obesity

Obesity is part of the phenotype of many genetic syndromes, notably over 20 Mendelian disorders (Chung and Leibel, 2005; Farooqi, 2005) (Table 15.1). Most of these are characterized by morbid obesity that begins in childhood, together with specific dysmorphic or developmental features. These disorders, and their diagnosis and management, are discussed in detail in Chapter 21.

The most common inherited syndrome is Prader-Willi syndrome (PWS), with early-onset hyperphagia and obesity, short stature, hypogonadism, poor muscle tone and learning difficulties (see Figure 21.9 on page 517). Many of the other syndromes are also characterized by neurodevelopmental delay, organ-specific abnormalities and dysmorphic features (Table 21.2 on page 523).

Several monogenic obesity syndromes, due to mutations affecting the peripheral and central pathways that regulate body fat mass, have now been recognized (Mutch and Clément, 2006). These include mutations affecting the genes encoding leptin, the leptin receptor, and the melanocortin-4 receptor (MC4-R) (see Figures 21.10 and 21.11 on page 519). These typically present with childhood-onset hyperphagia and severe obesity. Overall, they are very rare, although MC4-R mutations may account for 4–6% of cases of morbid obesity that begin in childhood.

Comorbidities and health risks of obesity

Obesity predisposes to and is associated with many diseases that can adversely affect health and life expectancy (Table 15.3). These are covered in detail in Chapters 9–13, and the key points relevant to the routine assessment of the obese patient, and of the associated risk to health, are summarized here.

Table 15.3 Comorbidities of obesity.

Type 2 diabetes and glucose-intolerant states

Cardiovascular disease

- Coronary-heart disease
- Myocardial infarction
- Heart failure
- Hypertension
- Peripheral vascular disease

Dyslipidaemia

- Raised LDL, low HDL
- Raised triglycerides

Obesity-related liver disease

- Steatosis and steatohepatitis
- Cirrhosis and hepatocellular carcinoma
- Obstructive sleep apnoea

Gastrointestinal tract

- Gastro-oesophageal reflux and Barrett's oesophagus
- Oesophageal carcinoma
- Gallstones

Reproductive system

- Female: PCOS and infertility
- Male: subfertility and erectile dysfunction

Musculoskeletal

- Osteoarthritis (especially hips, knees and hands)
- Gout

Skin

- Acanthosis nigricans
- Infections (bacterial and fungal)

Malignancies (see Table 15.7)

Disorders highlighted in green are features of the metabolic syndrome.

Type 2 diabetes

Central and particularly visceral obesity is a major risk factor for the development of insulin resistance, glucose intolerance and ultimately type 2 diabetes (Wang *et al.*, 2005; Boyko *et al.*, 2000; Chapter 10). In turn, both obesity and type 2 diabetes increase cardiovascular risk (Haffner *et al.*, 1998; Tominaga *et al.*, 1999). The presence of type 2 diabetes therefore confers high risk on the obese patient, making it important to ascertain the glycaemic status in all cases.

Diabetes can be diagnosed from a raised fasting plasma glucose concentration (>7.0 mmol/l) and/or from an elevated plasma glucose (>11.1 mmol/l) 2 hours after a 75-g oral glucose tolerance test (OGTT) (Table 15.4). A fasting plasma glucose in the range 6.1–6.9 mmol/l identifies the condition of 'impaired fasting glucose' (IFG), which although in the sub-diabetic range, confers increased risk. In addition, a 2-hour post-OGTT plasma glucose of 7.8–11.0 mmol/l indicates impaired glucose tolerance, which carries increased cardiovascular risk as well as a 30–50% chance of progressing to type 2 diabetes within a few years (Tominaga *et al.*, 1999; Unwin *et al.*, 2002; Nathan *et al.*, 2006). Thus, both tests may be needed to define an individual's glycaemic status. Fasting glucose, the preferred test to detect diabetes, should be measured first, with non-diabetic subjects then proceeding on another day to an OGTT (American Diabetes Association, 2007).

Cardiovascular disease

Obesity is an independent risk factor for cardiovascular disease (coronary-heart disease, heart failure, stroke and peripheral arterial disease), and this risk is enhanced by associated comorbidities such as type 2 diabetes, hypertension and dyslipidaemia as well as by smoking and a positive family history (Haffner *et al.*, 1998; Tominaga *et al.*, 1999; see Chapter 11).

It is important to evaluate cardiovascular risk in obese subjects who do not have previous or clinically obvious cardiovascular disease. This is needed for prognostic reasons and to determine the scope and intensity of eventual therapy for obesity itself and for associated risk factors. Various guidelines have been proposed to assess global cardiovascular risk, including the Framingham risk score (Grundy, 2006) (Table 15.5) and the Prospective Cardiovascular Münster Study risk calculator (Assmann, Cullen and Schulte, 2002). These are appropriate for obese patients, and appear better than estimating cardiovascular risk from the presence of features of the metabolic syndrome (Stern *et al.*, 2004; McNeill *et al.*, 2005; Wilson *et al.*, 1998). Both Framingham and Münster scores take account of well-established and potent risk factors such as age, sex, family history, total cholesterol and smoking. Also, there is continuing disagreement over the

Table 15.4 States of glucose tolerance defined by criteria set by the American Diabetes Association (1997) and World Health Organization (1999).

		2-h plasma glucose, mmol/l (mg/dl)		
		< 7.8 (140)	7.8–11.0 (140–199)	≥ 11.1 (200)
Fasting plasma glucose, mmol/l (mg/dl)	< 6.1 (110)	Normal	IGT	Diabetes on an isolated 2-h hyperglycaemia IPH (isolated postchallenge hyperglycaemia)
	6.1–6.9 (110–125)	IFG	IFG and IGT	
	≥ 7.0 (126)	Diabetes on an isolated fasting hyperglycaemia		Diabetes on both fasting and 2-h hyperglycaemia

IFG, impaired fasting glucose; IGT, impaired glucose tolerance; IPH, isolated postchallenge hyperglycaemia.

criteria that define the metabolic syndrome (Table 15.6), and even uncertainty that this entity actually exists (Kahn *et al.*, 2005). A meta-analysis by Ford (2005) has shown that the presence of features of the metabolic syndrome is a strong predictor for the development of type 2 diabetes, but has a weaker relationship with cardiovascular disease and all-cause mortality.

Obstructive Sleep Apnoea (OSA)

Obesity is the most powerful risk factor for OSA, the association being attributed to central actions of leptin and other adipokines as well as compression by fat of the pharynx (Gami, Caples and Somers, 2003; see Chapter 13). OSA impairs the sufferer's quality of life and is implicated in the initiation and progression of hypertension and cardiovascular disease, notably heart failure (Shamsuzzaman, Gersh and Somers, 2003). Ultimately, OSA shortens life expectancy. Symptoms may be vague and pass unnoticed by the patient and physician alike, but timely diagnosis and treatment with continuous positive airway pressure (CPAP) can markedly improve quality of life and prognosis.

A high index of suspicion is therefore required, and the characteristic history sought routinely (see below).

Obesity-related liver disease

'Non-alcoholic fatty liver disease' (NAFLD) associated with obesity and the metabolic syndrome affects over 70% of obese subjects (including those with type 2 diabetes) and is now the most common cause of hospital referral for disturbed liver function (Taylor, 2007; see Chapter 12). Fatty infiltration of the liver (steatosis) in obesity may contribute to insulin resistance (Frayn, Arner and Yki-Jarvinen, 2006; Van Gaal, Mertens and De Block, 2006). The previous assumption that steatosis is benign is now known to be fallacious: inflammation ('steatohepatitis') can develop, leading ultimately to hepatic fibrosis, cirrhosis and an increased risk of hepatocellular carcinoma (Grant and Lisker-Melman, 2004). The presence and severity of liver disease therefore needs to be determined. All but the final stages are essentially asymptomatic, which complicates screening and investigation.

Table 15.5 Framingham risk score. From Grundy *et al.* (2006) *American Journal of Clinical Nutrition*, **83**(6), 1248–51, with kind permission.

Risk Assessment Tool for Estimating 10-year Risk of Developing Hard Coronary Heart Disease (CHD) (Myocardial Infarction and Coronary Death) The *risk assessment tool* below uses recent data from the Framingham Heart Study to estimate 10-year risk for 'hard' coronary heart disease outcomes (myocardial infarction and coronary death). This tool is designed to estimate risk in adults aged 20 and older who do not have heart disease or diabetes. The tool is accessed at www.nhlbihin.net/atpiii/calculator and the subject's data are entered as in the fields below.

Age: ☐ years

Gender: Female / Male

Total Cholesterol: ☐ mg/dL

HDL Cholesterol: ☐ mg/dL

Smoker: No / Yes

Systolic Blood Pressure: ☐ mm/Hg

Currently on medication for high blood pressure? No / Yes

Calculate 10-Year Risk

- *Total and HDL cholesterol*: values should be the average of at least two measurements.
- *Smoker*: The designation 'smoker' means any cigarette smoking in the past month.
- *Systolic blood pressure*: The value obtained at the time of assessment, regardless of whether the person is taking antihypertensive therapy (treated hypertension carries residual risk).

Table 15.6 Varying definitions of the metabolic syndrome.

Clinical measure	IDF	AHA/NHLBI
		Any 3 of the 5 following features:
Body weight/fat distribution	Waist circumference increased:	Waist circumference increased:
	• Men: ≥94 cm	Men: ≥102 cm
	• Women: ≥80 cm	Women: ≥88 cm
	Plus any 2 of the following:	
Fasting plasma lipid levels	Raised triglycerides (TG):	Raised triglycerides (TG):
	TG ≥1.70 mmol/l (150 mg/dl), or taking TG-lowering drugs	TG ≥1.70 mmol/l (150 mg/dl), or taking TG-lowering drugs
	Low HDL-cholesterol:	Low HDL-cholesterol:
	• Men: <1.03 mmol/l (40 mg/dl)	• Men: <1.03 mmol/l (40 mg/dl)
	• Women: <1.30 mmol/l (50 mg/dl), or taking cholesterol-lowering drugs	• Women: <1.30 mmol/l (50 mg/dl), or taking cholesterol-lowering drugs
Blood pressure	Hypertension:	Hypertension:
	• Systolic ≥130 mm Hg and/or	• Systolic ≥130 mm Hg and/or
	• Diastolic ≥85 mm Hg, and/or taking hypotensive drugs	• Diastolic ≥85 mm Hg, and/or taking hypotensive drugs
Fasting plasma glucose (FPG) concentration	Hyperglycaemia:	Hyperglycaemia:
	• FPG ≥5.6 mmol/l (100 mg/dl), or diagnosed type 2 diabetes	• FPG ≥5.6 mmol/l (100 mg/dl), or diagnosed type 2 diabetes

From the International Diabetes Federation (IDF) (Alberti *et al.*, 2006) and the American Heart Association (ADA)/ American National Heart, Lungs and Blood Institute (NHLBI) (2005), with kind permission. See also Reaven (1988), World Health Organization (1999), Balkau and Charles (1999), Einhorn *et al.* (2003), NCEP (2002) and Grundy *et al.* (2005).

Gastrointestinal tract

Gastroesophageal reflux, with or without hiatus hernia, is probably the most common gastro-intestinal complication of obesity and is especially significant because it predisposes to the premalignant Barrett's oesophagus and thus to oesophageal carcinoma, which is commoner among obese subjects (see Chapter 13 and Figure 13.10 on page 337).

Cholesterol gallstone formation is a well-recognized complication of obesity – especially in middle-aged women – and may also be precipitated by rapid weight loss (Bray, 2004; Erlinger, 2000).

Reproductive system

Obese women may show menstrual disturbances and infertility. PCOS is accompanied by obesity in about 50% of cases; insulin resistance is common (and sometimes accompanied by acanthosis nigricans) and type 2 diabetes affects about 40% (Rotterdam Conference, 2004; Gambineri *et al.*, 2002). Insulin resistance and hyperinsulinaemia may underlie the endocrine changes (sustained high oestrogen levels, raised androgen concentrations) that cause menstrual irregularity, anovulation and infertility. Weight loss or insulin-sensitising drugs often restore ovulation and improve androgenic features – highlighting the importance of making the diagnosis.

Obese men are at increased risk of infertility (with reduced numbers and quality of spermatozoa) and erectile dysfunction (see Chapter 13).

Musculoskeletal disorders

Osteoarthritis affecting the hips, knees and also hands is more common among obese subjects; adverse effects of adipokines on cartilage and bone may contribute, as well as excessive mechanical loading on the joints (Wearing *et al.*, 2006; Gelber *et al.*, 1999; Bliddal and Christansen, 2006; see Chapter 13). Obesity is reportedly the single most important causative factor for severe disabling knee pain (Jinks, Jordan and Croft, 2006) and osteoarthritis of this joint (Coggon *et al.*, 2001). Gout is also associated with the metabolic syndrome. Bone density tends to be increased in obese adults, but osteopenia and osteoporosis can occur.

Skin disorders

Acanthosis nigricans – overgrowth of the dermis thought to be due to high insulin levels acting through the epidermal growth factor (EGF) receptor – is a marker of severe insulin resistance. The characteristic dark velvety appearance is usually seen in the axillae, groin or on the nape of the neck (see Figure 13.7 on page 331).

Other skin lesions in obesity include pale stretch marks around the abdomen, trunk or upper arms (which are distinct from the purplish-red striae of Cushing syndrome). Various infections of the skin and subcutaneous tissues appear to be more common in obese subjects, notably candidiasis, intertrigo, erythrasma, tinea cruris and folliculitis. Rarer infections include cellulitis and necrotising fasciitis, sometimes with gas-forming organisms ('gas gangrene') (Scheinfeld, 2004; Garcia Hidalgo, 2002).

Malignancies

Obesity has emerged as a significant risk factor for numerous cancers and haematological malignancies, and not just those with a 'hormonal' basis. Importantly, the risks of certain malignancies are now known to become signifi-cant for patients who are overweight rather than obese. Overall, over 70 000 of the 3.5 million new cases of cancer each year in the European Union are estimated to be attributed to overweight or obesity (McMillan, Sattar and McArdle, 2006). Physical inactivity may also be an independent risk factor for example for breast and colon cancers (Verrijken *et al.*, 2006; Friedenreich and Orenstein, 2002).

The malignancies most convincingly associated with obesity are listed in Table 15.7. Possible mechanisms are discussed in Chapter 13.

Colonic and rectal cancers are independently associated with obesity, especially in men; physical inactivity and a high fat intake may also contribute (Murphy *et al.*, 2000). The association with Barrett's oesophagus and oesophageal cancer has been mentioned above.

Breast cancer risk appears to be increased, but only in postmenopausal women (Van Gaal and Mertens, 1998; IARC, 2002). Weight gain during adult life may be an important risk factor (McTiernan, 2000). Diagnosis may also be delayed because of the reluctance of obese women to consult doctors, and the difficulty

Table 15.7 Malignancies associated with obesity with relative risk to each sex.

Type of cancer	Male	Female
Oesphageal	1.63	1.39
Stomach	1.94	1.08
Colorectal	1.84	1.36
Hepatocellular	4.52	1.68
Pancreatic	1.49	1.41
Lung	0.67	0.66
Breast (post-menopausal)		1.70
Uterine		2.77
Cervical		3.20
Ovarian		1.51
Prostate (poorly-differentiated)	1.34	
Kidney	1.70	1.70
Non-Hodgkin lymphoma	1.49	1.95
Multiple myeloma	1.71	1.44
Leukaemia (all types)	1.70	0.93

of detecting small tumours in obese breasts (Verrijken *et al.*, 2006). Endometrial cancer, which usually occurs in postmenopausal women, is consistently associated with obesity (Bray, 2002; Rose, 1996).

In men, obesity (and perhaps high fat intake) increases the risk of poorly-differentiated prostate cancer (Verrijken *et al.*, 2006; Barnard *et al.*, 2002).

In both sexes, haematological malignancies associated with overweight and obesity include non-Hodgkin lymphoma, myeloma and chronic lymphocytic leukaemia (see Chapter 13).

Practical assessment of obesity

Practical assessment requires a comprehensive history, physical examination and appropriate further investigations. The aims are to assess the severity and degree of health risk associated with obesity, to identify possible underlying causes of obesity, and the presence of any comorbidities or complications of obesity. Diagnostic features and tests for other causes of obesity are given in Table 15.8, and for comorbidities of obesity in Table 15.9.

Personal history

History and evolution of obesity

The time-course of obesity may provide important clues about its causes, risks and eventual management. Onset in childhood, especially if marked and before 5 years of age, should raise the suspicion of an inherited syndrome or a monogenic cause, although an obesogenic lifestyle alone is now causing morbid obesity among children (see Figure 21.3). Gradual and progressive weight gain from early adult life is typical of lifestyle-related obesity, while a cyclical 'yo-yo' pattern of repeated unsuccessful attempts to lose weight is often seen (Kushner and Roth, 2003).

Possible relationships of weight gain to life-events, pregnancies and drug treatment should be determined. The nature and duration of any previous attempts to lose weight (including unconventional or alternative medicine) should also be documented, together with how successful these were and what the reasons for failure might have been (Bray, 2004).

Weight gain during early adulthood is also important because it appears to confer additional

Table 15.8 Diagnostic features and further investigations for underlying causes of obesity.

Cause	History	Examination	Further investigation
Drug-induced obesity	Exposure to obesogenic drug	Unremarkable	Withdraw, reduce or substitute if possible
Inherited syndrome	Morbid obesity, onset in childhood	Dysmorphic features	Genetic testing
	Hyperphagia	Other features of syndromes	Referral to specialist
	Developmental delay (often)		
	Other features of syndrome		
Hypothyroidism	Modest weight gain	Hypothyroid signs	TSH raised
	Hypothyroid symptoms	Growth arrest (children)	Free thyroxine low
			Autoantibody screen
Cushing syndrome	Facial changes	Cushingoid features	Urinary free cortisol raised
	Central obesity	Hypertension	Cortisol raised, not suppressed by dexamethasone
	Limb weakness	Proximal myopathy	Imaging of pituitary, adrenals

Table 15.9 Diagnostic features and further investigations for comorbidities of obesity.

Comorbidity	History	Examination	Further investigations
Type 2 diabetes	Diabetic symptoms	Acanthosis nigricans	Fasting glucose
	Diabetic complications	Diabetic complications	OGTT
			HOMA or QUICKI (measures of insulin resistance)
Cardiovascular disease	Angina	Arrhythmia	ECG
	Dyspnoea	Hypertension	Echocardiogram
	Palpitations	Heart failure	ETT
	Stroke	Peripheral pulses weak, bruits	24-h ambulatory blood pressure
	Claudication	Peripheral oedema	24-h Holter monitoring
	Ankle swelling		Coronary and peripheral angiography
Dyslipidaemia	Unremarkable	Unremarkable	Fasting lipids
Obesity-related liver disease	Unremarkable	Unremarkable	Liver function tests
			Liver imaging
			Liver biopsy
Obstructive sleep apnoea	Snoring, apnoea	Neck circumference >40 cm	Sleep studies and overnight pulse oximetry
	Daytime sleepiness (Epworth score)	Hypertension	Trial of CPAP
Gastro-oesophageal reflux	Heartburn	Unremarkable	Endoscopy
	Dyspepsia		
	Dysphagia (suspect carcinoma)		
Gallstones	Fatty food intolerance	Tender in right hypochondrium	Ultrasound or other imaging
	Dyspepsia		
PCOS	Irregular or absent periods	Hirsutism (not masculinization)	Ovarian ultrasound
	Infertility	Acanthosis nigricans	Hormonal profile (LH, FSH, progesterone, testosterone)
	Hirsutism		
Osteoarthritis	Pain	Osteoarthritic changes and deformities	X-ray
	Limitation of movement		Aspirate effusion (exclude gout)
Acanthosis nigricans	Asymptomatic	Typical lesions (indicate insulin resistance)	Fasting glucose and insulin
			OGTT
			HOMA or QUICKI

CPAP: continuous positive airway pressure; ETT: exercise tolerance test; HOMA: homeostatic model assessment; OGTT: oral glucose tolerance test; QUICKI: quantitative insulin sensitivity check index (see Chapter 3).

risk for cardiovascular disease and type 2 diabetes (Rosengren, Wedel and Wilhelmsen, 1999; Manson *et al.*, 1995; Colditz *et al.*, 1995; Schienkiewitz *et al.*, 2006).

Family history of obesity

This history may reveal a familial tendency to obesity, and occasionally a Mendelian pattern suggestive of an inherited cause. A positive family history of type 2 diabetes is an important predictor of this disease (see Chapter 9).

Lifestyle

Food and drink intake

Given the importance of overconsumption in causing obesity, and of energy restriction in managing the condition, the patient's dietary habits need to be carefully documented. Key information includes:

- the pattern of meals and snacks, including binges and nocturnal eating;
- timing, places and triggers of eating;
- types of food and the frequency of eating them;
- portion sizes;
- drinks, especially sweetened and alcoholic beverages.

This information is best obtained by a dietician, using techniques such as the 24-hour recall ('What did you eat in the last 24 hours?'), food-frequency questionnaires and 3- or 7-day food frequency diaries (Van Gaal, 1998; see Chapter 3). It must be remembered that obese people tend to underestimate their energy intake; helping them to appreciate this can be important in the successful management of obesity. The consumption of sweetened carbonated drinks and alcohol, both of which can substantially increase total energy intake, should be specifically detailed.

The patient's level of understanding of nutrition and healthy eating will determine whether basic or more advanced nutritional education should be provided (Kushner and Roth, 2003). It is also useful to determine who in the family buys and prepares food, and whether the patient enjoys cooking.

Physical activity

Physical activity is the most variable determinant of total energy expenditure and thus of overall energy balance; conversely, inactivity is an important contributor to lifestyle-related obesity. Physical inactivity is also an independent predictor of cardiovascular disease (Li *et al.*, 2006) and premature death (Hu *et al.*, 2004; Stevens *et al.*, 2002; Van Gaal, Mertens and De Block, 2006). The level of physical activity can modify the risks of obesity; in most studies, being active attenuated (but did not abolish) the adverse impact of obesity on coronary-heart disease, whereas being lean did not diminish the increased risk of being inactive (Li *et al.*, 2006).

The patient's current and previous level of physical activity should be determined, together with time spent on sedentary activities such as watching television or playing computer games. Transport to and from work or school, and practical barriers to active transport (walking or cycling), daily exercise and sport should also be explored. This information will point to the importance of inactivity in the subject's obesity and will also guide individualized recommendation for exercise.

Smoking

Smoking is relevant to the management of obesity for several reasons. It enhances the risks of cardiovascular disease and also of various malignancies, including some to which obesity also predisposes (e.g. colorectal carcinoma). The health risks of smoking and obesity appear to be at least additive, and smoking may exacerbate various obesity-related abnormalities such as insulin resistance, low HDL cholesterol and pro-inflammatory cytokine release (Van Gaal, Mertens and De Block, 2006). Ultimately, the combination of smoking and obesity further shortens life expectancy: on average, obese smokers die between 5 and 13 years before their non-smoking counterparts (Peeters *et al.*, 2003; Stevens *et al.*, 2002).

Smoking is associated with a lower fat mass and body weight, due partly to increased energy expenditure and decreased food intake through indirect and direct actions of nicotine (see Chapter 21). On average, middle-aged and older smokers have been shown to weigh 3–4 kg less than matched non-smokers, although weight differences are small (or non-existent) among adolescents and young adults (Bray, 2004). The lower BMI and higher mortality among smokers are partly responsible for the low extreme of the U-shaped relationship between BMI and risk of death (Chapter 9).

Conversely, smoking cessation often leads to weight gain. Several large prospective studies have shown that those who stop smoking gain on average 4–5 kg. Weight increase is more pronounced in women, younger subjects, Black people, heavy smokers and those whose initial weight is relatively low; overall, some 20% of those who stop smoking gain 10 kg or more (Bray, 2004). This is due to increased energy intake (especially of sweet and fat-rich foods), together with loss of the catabolic actions of nicotine. Smokers commonly view weight gain as a serious consequence of stopping smoking, and it is probably a major disincentive for many; some young people, especially women, may use smoking as a means to limit weight gain.

The benefits of stopping smoking undoubtedly outweigh any detrimental effects of post-cessation weight gain, and on balance, smoking cessation should take priority.

Medication

Current and previous medications, and their temporal relationship with obesity, should be documented. The main obesogenic drugs are shown in Table 15.2. If possible, obesogenic drugs should be withdrawn or their dosage reduced, or replaced by alternatives that do not cause weight gain (see Table 17.6).

Patients taking atypical (second-generation) antipsychotic drugs deserve particular attention. Those with schizophrenia, the most common indication for these agents, have an increased risk of developing both diabetes and cardiovascular disease (Lean and Pajonk, 2003), and commonly have an unhealthy lifestyle (smoking, poor diet, inactivity and alcohol excess). Weight can increase rapidly with atypical antipsychotic drugs and may not reach a plateau for a year or more (American Diabetes Association, 2004). Patients therefore need to be counselled and monitored before and during treatment and, if possible, drugs that are less likely to cause weight gain and glucose intolerance should be

prescribed (American Diabetes Association, 2004; Van Gaal, 2006).

Psychological status

The impact of obesity on an individual's psychological state is highly variable (see Chapter 14). Psychiatric disorders may occur, with depression being commonest in women, subjects with extreme obesity, those who actively seek treatment, and patients with binge-eating disorder (Fabricatore and Wadden, 2004). All obese people should therefore be screened for depression and anxiety, and specifically for eating disorders (Chapter 20), because all these conditions can impair the patient's quality of life and can also interfere with successful management. Many studies have attempted to identify psychological factors that predict success or failure of obesity management programmes, but no consistently useful guidelines have yet emerged (Teixeira et al., 2005).

Assessment of motivation

The patient's motivation and readiness for change are crucial determinants of the outcome of obesity management, and should be evaluated before starting treatment. This can be done using the American National Heart, Lung and Blood Institute (NHLBI) clinical guidelines (Hill and Wyatt, 2002; National Institutes of Health, 2000) (see Table 15.10).

The 'Transtheoretical' or 'Stages of Change' model proposes that, at any time, the patient is in one of six discrete phases of change: precontemplation, contemplation, preparation, action, maintenance and relapse (Prochaska, DiClemente and Norcross, 1992). Determining the patient's current stage of change using the features shown in Table 15.10 is helpful in tailoring the nature and intensity of the advice and the level of intervention.

There is often a marked mismatch between the patient's expectations – for example to lose most of the excess weight within a few weeks or months – and the reality of available weight-loss treatments, especially those based on lifestyle and pharmacotherapy (Foster et al., 1997). Unrealistic expectations will result in disappointment and frustration, even if clinically useful amounts of weight are lost (Kushner and Roth, 2003).

Table 15.10 Patient readiness checklist formulated by the American National Heart, Lung and Blood Institute (NHBLI) to assess an obese subject's motivation and readiness for lifestyle change.

Motivation and support

- How important is it for you to lose weight now?
- Have you tried to lose weight before? Which factors led to success? What made weight loss difficult? (e.g. *cost, peer pressure, no family support*)
- Is your decision to lose weight your own, or for someone else?
- Is your family supportive?
- Who, if anyone, supports your decision to lose weight?
- What do you consider the benefits of weight loss?
- What would you have to sacrifice? What are the disadvantages?

Stressful life events

- Are there events in your life now that might make losing weight especially difficult? (e.g. *work responsibilities, family commitments*)
- If now is not a convenient time, what would it take for you to be ready to lose weight? When do you think you might be ready to begin losing weight?

Psychiatric issues

- What is your mood like most of the time? Do you feel you have enough energy to lose weight? (*May need to assess for depression*)
- Do you feel that you eat what most people would consider a large amount of food in a short period of time? Do you feel out of control during this time? (*May need to assess for binge eating disorders*)
- Do you ever make yourself vomit, use laxatives, or take excessive physical activity to control your weight? (*May need to assess for bulimia nervosa*)

Time availability and constraints

- How much time can you devote to physical activity per week?
- Do you believe that you can make time to record how much you eat?
- Can you take time out to relax and engage in personal activities?

Weight-loss goals and expectations

- How much weight do you expect to lose?
- How fast do you expect to lose weight?
- What other benefits do you expect from losing weight?

'Stages of change' model to assess readiness

Stage	Characteristic
Precontemplation	Unaware of problem, no interest in change
Contemplation	Aware of problem, beginning to think of changing
Preparation	Realizes benefits of making changes and thinking about how to change
Action	Actively taking steps toward change
Maintenance	Initial treatment goals reached

Review of systems

This review should cover the main comorbidities of obesity, described above.

- *Type 2 diabetes.* Classical diabetic symptoms (polyuria, nocturia, thirst, blurred vision) may be present, although many patients are asymptomatic. Symptoms of diabetic complications may occasionally be present in undiagnosed cases.
- *Cardiovascular disease.* Symptoms of angina, heart failure, stroke and peripheral vascular disease should be sought. Their absence does not exclude increased or even high cardiovascular risk.
- *Obstructive sleep apnoea.* Patients often complain of daytime sleepiness (quantified using the Epworth Sleepiness Scale: Table 13.3 on page 328) and poor concentration; their partners may report the suggestive features of loud snoring with frequent episodes of apnoea (lasting 10 seconds or more) and awakening.
- *Gastrointestinal tract.* Heartburn and acid reflux suggest gastroesophageal reflux; dysphagia, with pain or difficulty on swallowing, requires the active exclusion of oesophageal carcinoma. Indigestion with fatty foods may be due to gallstones. Altered bowel habit or rectal bleeding may suggest colorectal carcinoma.
- *Reproductive system.* Menstrual irregularity (or anovulation), with or without infertility, may be due to PCOS.
- *Musculoskeletal system.* Pain and limitation of movement in the knees and hips suggests osteoarthritis, which may also involve the hands. Gout may also present with a painful swollen knee joint, or as the classical podagra affecting the first metatarsophalangeal joint.

Clinical examination

A thorough clinical examination is required to evaluate adiposity and its impact – which can potentially involve all the systems of the body.

General features

The examination may reveal clinical signs suggesting endocrine or genetic causes of obesity, features such as acanthosis nigricans (Figure 13.7 on page 331), or evidence of obesity-associated complications including malignancy.

Quantifying obesity

Ideally, the assessment of obesity should include a reliable measurement of the amount and distribution of body fat. The available methods are described in Chapter 3. In routine clinical practice, simple anthropometric measurements are adequate in most cases for stratifying risk and determining management. More sophisticated methods are available for specific indications; some are expensive, time-consuming and largely restricted to research applications.

Body Mass Index (BMI)

BMI has been used in international guidelines to define overweight and obesity and is widely used for diagnostic and management purposes, as well as to identify priorities for intervention (World Health Organization, 1997) (Table 15.11). It is calculated by dividing the weight (in kg) by the square of the height (in metres). Clinical protocols should therefore record weight, height and the resulting BMI.

BMI is generally regarded as a surrogate measure of body fat, but it does not provide precise information about body composition or the regional distribution of body fat (Prentice and Jebb, 2001). BMI overestimates body fat in muscular people, while it can underestimate fat content in older people who have lost muscle mass. Also, BMI does not take into account variations in body fat due to gender, age or ethnic origin (Gallagher *et al.*, 1996; Fernandez *et al.*, 2003; Bedogni *et al.*, 2001). The conventional BMI thresholds underestimate cardiovascular and metabolic risk in Asian populations, probably because they have a relatively higher body fat content at a given BMI, compared with the Caucasian reference population (Deurenberg-Yap and Deurenberg, 2003). Accordingly, modified BMI cut-off values have been proposed for Asian populations, with obesity defined as a BMI $>25 \, kg/m^2$ (Kanazawa *et al.*, 2002; see Chapter 9).

Waist circumference and WHR

The distribution of body fat, as well as its total amount, is important in determining the health

Table 15.11 Classification of overweight and obesity by BMI and waist circumference, and the associated level of health risk.

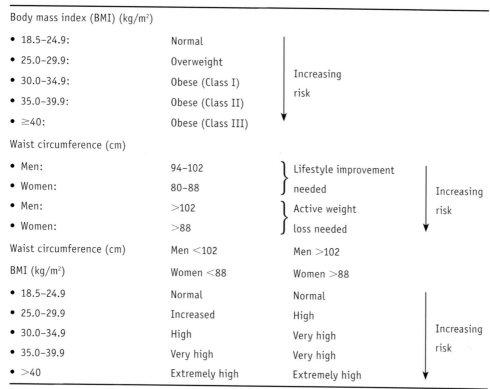

Body mass index (BMI) (kg/m²)

• 18.5–24.9:	Normal	
• 25.0–29.9:	Overweight	
• 30.0–34.9:	Obese (Class I)	Increasing risk
• 35.0–39.9:	Obese (Class II)	
• ≥40:	Obese (Class III)	

Waist circumference (cm)

• Men:	94–102	Lifestyle improvement needed	
• Women:	80–88		Increasing risk
• Men:	>102	Active weight loss needed	
• Women:	>88		

Waist circumference (cm)	Men <102	Men >102	
BMI (kg/m²)	Women <88	Women >88	
• 18.5–24.9	Normal	Normal	
• 25.0–29.9	Increased	High	
• 30.0–34.9	High	Very high	Increasing risk
• 35.0–39.9	Very high	Very high	
• >40	Extremely high	Extremely high	

The level of risk conferred by the combination of high BMI and increased waist circumference is shown below. From NIH/NHLBI Practical Guide (2000), adapted from World Health Organization (1997).

risks associated with obesity. There is abundant evidence that central or truncal obesity (and especially fat accumulating in and around the abdominal cavity) carries greater cardiovascular and metabolic risk than does 'lower-body' adiposity in the gluteo-femoral distribution (Vague, 1947; Kissebah et al., 1982; Larsson et al., 1984; Lapidus et al., 1984; Van Gaal and Mertens, 1998). Indeed, measures of central obesity such as the waist:hip ratio (WHR) and waist circumference are more powerful predictors than BMI of the risks of developing type 2 diabetes, dyslipidaemia, hypertension and atherosclerosis, and ultimately of premature death (Wang et al., 2005; Han et al., 1995; Janssen, Katzmarzyk and Ross, 2002; Shen et al., 2006). It has been shown that the amount of visceral fat is associated with the greatest health risk (Van Gaal, Mertens and De Block, 2006; Després and Lemieux, 2006). Waist circumference is highly correlated with total body fat (Lean, Han and Deurenberg, 1996) and BMI (Lean, Han and

Morrison, 1995) and may reflect visceral fat mass more closely than WHR (Pouliot et al., 1994), but neither measure distinguishes between accumulations of deep visceral or subcutaneous abdominal fat; this requires the imaging techniques described below.

Waist circumference and/or WHR should therefore be recorded routinely in obese patients. The waist circumference is generally measured using a horizontal tape at the midpoint between the iliac crest and the lower rib margin at the end of gentle expiration (Figure 15.3), and the hip circumference at the level of the greater trochanters (Klein et al., 2007). Training and attention to detail are important to ensure consistent readings.

Waist circumference or WHR can be used to stratify risk and guide management (see Table 15.11), and both are adequate in routine clinical practice. Waist circumference is useful in patients with a BMI of up to 35 kg/m², but seems to add little to the risk prediction

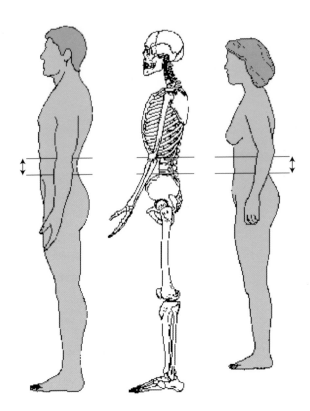

Figure 15.3 Anatomical landmarks for measuring waist circumference: the mid-point between the iliac crest and the lower rib margin. From National Institutes of Health (2000).

value of BMI for subjects whose BMI exceeds this limit (National Institute of Health, 2000; Chan *et al.*, 1994). The most widely-used cut-off thresholds for waist circumference are those derived from European populations by Han *et al.* (1995) (Table 15.11). Above values of 88 cm in women and 102 cm in men, cardiovascular risk increases rapidly, and active weight reduction is indicated. Below values of 80 cm (women) or 94 cm (men), risk is low and weight loss is not generally required. Monitoring and lifestyle improvement are recommended at intermediate levels. As discussed in Chapter 9, ethnic variations in body fat content mean that the risk thresholds for waist circumference are lower in Asian populations, and work is in progress to define other population-specific cut-off values for waist circumference (Alberts *et al.*, 2006; Albu *et al.*, 1997; Hayashi *et al.*, 2007; Kadowaki *et al.*, 2006).

Interestingly, an increased hip circumference has been suggested to protect against cardiovascular risk, perhaps especially in women (Seidell *et al.*, 2001; Lissner *et al.*, 2001; Snijder *et al.*,

2003a,b). Both fat and muscle mass in the upper leg may contribute to this effect, and regional differences in fat metabolism have been implicated (Snijder *et al.*, 2004; Lemieux, 2004). In theory, this could distort the relationship between health risk and WHR, although the INTERHEART study has identified WHR as the best adiposity marker for the risk of acute myocardial infarction (Yusuf *et al.*, 2005).

Body composition and fat mass

Body fat mass, fat-free mass (FFM; lean mass) and water content can be measured in various ways including underwater weighing (Siri, 1961), isotope dilution (Jebb and Elia, 1993; Vansant and Muls, 2002), air displacement plethysmography (e.g. using the BodPod apparatus) and bioelectrical impedance (bioimpedance). Serial scans of the whole body using dual-energy X-ray absorptiometry (DEXA) (Pietrobelli *et al.*, 2005), CT or MR imaging can also be used to reconstruct fat and lean tissue masses (see Chapter 3).

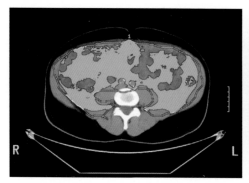 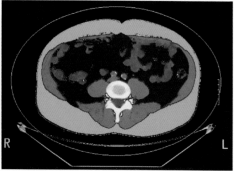

Figure 15.4 Transverse section of the abdomen at the level of L4/L5, imaged by CT scanning. Left: the cross-sectional area of visceral adipose tissue (VAT), highlighted in yellow, is measured to the inner boundary of the abdominal muscle layer. Right: the subcutaneous fat layer is highlighted.

Of these techniques, bioimpedance is widely available, relatively inexpensive and easy to use in routine clinical practice. Overall, bioimpedance-based estimates of fat mass, FFM and body water content correlate reasonably well with 'gold standard' methods such as underwater weighing. However, the predictive equations used to convert differences in whole-body electrical resistance into body composition may significantly underestimate body fat content, especially in subjects with morbid obesity (Kyle *et al.*, 2004).

In general, these techniques are not needed for routine assessment or follow up of obese patients, but may be useful in those with unusual body build or muscularity.

Measurements of visceral adipose tissue

The amount of visceral adipose tissue (VAT) is a strong predictor of cardiovascular and overall health risk (Van Gaal, Mertens and De Block, 2006; Després and Lemieux, 2006), and can be measured using sophisticated imaging techniques based on reconstructing multiple slices imaged by CT or MR (van der Kooy and Seidell, 1993; Lebovitz and Banerji, 2005). To limit cost and radiation exposure, the cross-sectional area of intra-abdominal fat on a single transverse CT slice at a standardized level (L4/L5) has been used as a surrogate for total visceral fat mass (Kvist *et al.*, 1988; Shen *et al.*, 2003) (Figure 15.4). Various cut-off values for VAT cross-sectional area (at L4/L5) have been proposed, according to their relationships with different health risks (Wajchenberg, 2000). These are summarized in Table 15.12. In general, cardiovascular risk appears to increase for both men and women if VAT area exceeds $110 \, cm^2$, with increases in metabolic risk and premature mortality at values of over $130 \, cm^2$.

Recent studies suggest that the correlation with total visceral fat volume is stronger if visceral fat area is measured at 10 cm above L4/L5 in men and 5 cm above L4/L5 in women (Shen *et al.*, 2004). Kuk *et al.* (2006a, 2006b) have shown that visceral fat area remains significantly associated with features of the metabolic syndrome, regardless of the exact level of measurement.

Table 15.12 Proposed cut-off values for visceral adipose tissue (VAT) cross-sectional area, measured at L4/L5, and the associated health risks.

Population	VAT area (cm²)	Risk	Reference
Women (pre- and post-menopause)	>110	CHD	Williams *et al.* (1996)
Men	>131	CHD	
Men and women	>100	CHD	Després and Lamarche (1993)
Men and women	>130	Metabolic syndrome	Wajchenberg (2000)
Men (middle-aged to old)	>130	Premature death	Kuk *et al.* (2006a, 2006b)

Cardiovascular system

Examination should include pulse, blood pressure (measured with an appropriately large cuff), palpation and auscultation of the heart for left ventricular hypertrophy and signs of heart failure, and checking the carotid and peripheral arteries for bruits or decreased pulses. Significant abnormalities (e.g. impaired left ventricular function) may not be detectable in clinical examination.

Other systems

The following systems should also be checked:

- *Respiratory system*. A neck circumference exceeding 40 cm indicates increased risk of OSA. Examination of the lungs is generally unremarkable.
- *Gastrointestinal system*. Gallstones and obesity-related liver disease are usually undetectable clinically but the abdomen and associated lymph nodes should be examined for signs of cirrhosis or intra-abdominal malignancy.
- *Reproductive system*. Hirsutism and acanthosis nigricans are both consistent with PCOS, but severe masculinization (male-pattern baldness, deep voice, clitoromegaly) suggests an alternative cause of androgen excess, such as an ovarian or adrenal tumour. The breasts should be examined, although small tumours are easily missed in large breasts.
- *Musculoskeletal system*. Typical osteoarthritic features may be present in the hands, with pain and limitation of movement in the knees and hips.

Screening investigations

The following investigations should ideally be performed in all obese subjects:

- *Fasting plasma glucose* (see Table 15.4).
- *Fasting plasma lipids*, with LDL, HDL and total cholesterol and triglycerides. The typical dyslipidaemia of obesity is a moderately raised LDL and a low HDL cholesterol (often with a normal total cholesterol) and moderately raised triglycerides (Chapter 10). Presence of these abnormalities increases the level of cardiovascular risk in an obese subject;

indeed, Lemieux *et al.* (2000) have suggested that high cardiovascular risk can be identified simply by a waist circumference that exceeds 90 cm in men (or 85 cm in women) and triglyceride concentration of >2.0 mmol/l. Plasma lipid screening may also reveal other relevant abnormalities, such as familial hyperlipidaemia or dyslipidaemia due to alcohol excess or hypothyroidism.

- *Liver function tests*, especially transaminase levels. The most common cause of moderately elevated transaminase levels in obese subjects is hepatic steatosis, but it must be remembered that these may be normal, even in some cases with advanced inflammation and fibrosis.
- *TSH and free thyroxine levels*. These should be measured if hypothyroidism is suspected, with a lower threshold of suspicion in middle-aged and older women.
- *ECG*. This may show signs of ischaemia or previous myocardial infarction, but is relatively insensitive for the latter. In obese subjects, the ECG may be falsely suggestive of inferior myocardial ischaemia or even ischaemia (see Chapter 12).

Further investigations

These are indicated to diagnose or evaluate specific comorbidities of obesity.

- *OGTT*. This is needed to identify IGT, and some cases of diabetes, and should be undertaken in subjects with normal fasting plasma glucose concentrations who are felt to be at increased risk of glucose intolerance. Criteria are suggested in Table 15.13.

Table 15.13   Criteria for performing an oral glucose tolerance test (OGTT) in obese subjects.

BMI >35 kg/m^2
Waist circumference >102 cm (men) or >88 cm (women)
Hypertension
Dyslipidaemia
Acanthosis nigricans
Family history of type 2 diabetes
History of gestational diabetes, or delivery of a baby weighing >4.5 kg

- *Liver imaging* (ultrasound, CT or MRI), if liver function tests are deranged or gallstones are suspected. This will show steatosis and comorbidities such as cirrhosis and hepatocellular carcinoma, but there are no consistent diagnostic features of hepatic inflammation and fibrosis. Liver biopsy may be required to stage obesity-related liver disease (Targher, 2007); indications for this are described in Chapter 11. Patients with cirrhosis should be monitored regularly for oesophageal varices (endoscopy) and hepatocellular carcinoma (CEA).
- *Sleep studies (polysomnography)*, including overnight pulse oximetry, are needed to diagnose OSA and should be followed by a trial of continuous positive airways pressure ventilation (CPAP), (see Chapter 13).
- *Cardiological investigations* include, as appropriate, echocardiography to investigate possible heart failure (this may reveal various subclinical abnormalities of systolic and diastolic function); exercise tolerance testing; coronary and peripheral angiography; 24-hour ambulatory blood pressure monitoring (in patients with variable or borderline hypertension, especially those at risk of cardiovascular disease); Doppler imaging of carotid and peripheral arteries. Measuring of the media-intima thickness of the carotid arteries has been proposed as a predictor of coronary heart disease but largely remains a research procedure (Kotsis *et al.*, 2006).
- *Gastrointestinal investigations* include gallbladder imaging for gallstones; upper gut endoscopy, in subjects with symptoms of reflux and especially dysphagia; bowel endoscopy for possible colorectal carcinoma.
- *Mammographic screening* should be considered for post-menopausal women and perhaps those over the age of 40 years.

Assessment of the overweight patient

Assessment of the overweight is an essential part of the 'secondary' prevention of obesity, that is, preventing overweight individuals from becoming obese (see Chapter 22). As discussed above, many of the health risks of obesity – including type 2 diabetes, cardiovascular disease and various malignancies – begin to appear at overweight levels of BMI. Moreover, weight gain in early adult life, even if within the normal body weight range, increases the risk of developing type 2 diabetes and cardiovascular disease (Willett *et al.*, 1995).

It follows that, where resources allow, overweight people should be evaluated, and offered appropriate lifestyle advice to prevent them from progressing to obesity and ideally to return them to normal weights. The protocol suggested above can also be applied in these cases.

References

Alberti, K.G., Zimmet, P. and Shaw, J. (2006) Metabolic syndrome-a new world-wide definition. A Consensus Statement from the International Diabetes Federation. *Diabetic Medicine: A Journal of the British Diabetic Association*, **23** (5), 469–80.

Albu, J.B., Murphy, L., Frager, D.H. *et al.* (1997) Visceral fat and race-dependent health risks in obese nondiabetic premenopausal women. *Diabetes*, **46** (3), 456–62.

American Diabetes Association, American Psychiatric Association, American Association of Clinical Endocrinologists, North American Association for the Study of Obesity 2004 'Consensus development conference on antipsychotic drugs and obesity and diabetes' *Diabetes Care*, 27 (2), 596–601.

American Diabetes Association (2007) Diagnosis and classification of diabetes mellitus. *Diabetes Care*, **30** (Suppl 1), S42–7.

Assmann, G., Cullen, P. and Schulte, H. (2002) Simple scoring scheme for calculating risk of acute coronary events based on the 10-y follow up of the prospective cardiovascular Münster (PROCAM) study. *Circulation*, **105** (3), 310–5.

Balkau, B. and Charles, M.A. (1999) Comment on the provisional report from the WHO consultation. European Group for the Study of Insulin Resistance (EGIR). *Diabetic Medicine: A Journal of the British Diabetic Association*, **16** (5), 442–3.

Barnard, R.J., Aronson, W.J., Tymchuk, C.N. and Ngo, T.H. (2002) Prostate cancer: another aspect of the insulin-resistance syndrome? *Obesity Reviews*, **3** (4), 303–8.

Bedogni, G., Pietrobelli, A., Heymsfield, S.B. *et al.* (2001) Is body mass index a measure of adiposity in elderly women? *Obesity Research*, **9** (1), 17–20.

Bliddal, H. and Christensen, R. (2006) The management of osteoarthritis in the obese patient: practical considerations and guidelines for therapy. *Obesity Reviews*, **7** (4), 323–31.

Boyko, E.J., Fujimoto, W.Y., Leonetti, D.L. and Newell-Morris, L. (2000) Visceral adiposity and risk of type 2 diabetes: a prospective study among Japanese Americans. *Diabetes Care*, **23** (4), 465–71.

Bray, G.A. (2002) The underlying basis for obesity: relationship to cancer. *The Journal of Nutrition*, **132** (11 suppl), 3451S–5S.

Bray, G.A. (2004) Classification and evaluation of the overweight patient, in *Handbook of Obesity. Clinical Applications*, 2nd edn (eds G.A. Bray and C. Bouchard), Marcel Dekker, Inc., New York, pp. 1–33.

Chan, J.M., Rimm, E.B., Colditz, G.A. *et al.* (1994) Obesity, fat distribution, and weight gain as risk factors for clinical diabetes in men. *Diabetes Care*, **17** (9), 961–9.

Chung, W.K. and Leibel, R.L. (2005) Molecular physiology of syndromic obesities in humans. *Trends in Endocrinology and Metabolism*, **16** (6), 267–72.

Coggon, D., Reading, I., Croft, P. *et al.* (2001) Knee osteoarthritis and obesity. *International Journal of Obesity*, **25** (5), 622–7.

Colditz, G.A., Willett, W.C., Rotnitzky, A. and Manson, J.E. (1995) Weight gain as a risk factor for clinical diabetes mellitus in women. *Annals of Internal Medicine*, **122** (7), 481–6.

Després, J.P. and Lamarche, B. (1993) Effects of diet and physical activity on adiposity and body fat distribution: implications for the prevention of cardiovascular disease. *Nutrition Research Reviews*, **6**, 137–59.

Després, J.P. and Lemieux, I. (2006) Abdominal obesity and metabolic syndrome. *Nature*, **444** (7121), 881–7.

Deurenberg-Yap, M. and Deurenberg, P. (2003) Is a re-evaluation of WHO body mass index cut-off values needed? The case of Asians in Singapore. *Nutrition Reviews*, **61** (5), S80–7.

Einhorn, D., Reaven, G.M., Cobin, R.H. *et al.* (2003) American College of Endocrinology position statement on the insulin resistance syndrome. *Endocrine Practice*, **9** (3), 237–52.

Erlinger, S. (2000) Gallstones in obesity and weight loss. *European Journal of Gastroenterology and Hepatology*, **12** (12), 1347–52.

Fabricatore, A.N. and Wadden, T.A. (2004) Psychological aspects of obesity. *Clinics in Dermatology*, **22** (4), 332–7.

Farooqi, I.S. (2005) Genetic and hereditary aspects of childhood obesity. *Best Practice and Research Clinical Endocrinology, and Metabolism* **19** (3), 359–74.

Farooqi, S. and O'Rahilly, S. (2006) Genetics of obesity in humans. *Endocrine Reviews*, **27** (7), 710–8.

Fernandez, J.R., Heo, M., Heymsfield, S.B. *et al.* (2003) Is percentage body fat differentially related to body mass index in Hispanic Americans, African Americans, and European Americans? *The American Journal of Clinical Nutrition*, **77** (1), 71–5.

Ford, E.S. (2005) Risks for all-cause mortality cardiovascular disease, and diabetes associated with the metabolic syndrome: a summary of the evidence. *Diabetes Care*, **28** (7), 1769–78.

Foster, G.D., Wadden, T.A., Vogt, R.A. and Brewer, G. (1997) What is a reasonable weight loss? Patients' expectations and evaluations of obesity treatment outcomes. *Journal of Consulting and Clinical Psychology*, **65** (1), 79–85.

Frayn, K.N., Arner, P. and Yki-Jarvinen, H. (2006) Fatty acid metabolism in adipose tissue, muscle and liver in health and disease. *Essays in Biochemistry*, **42**, 89–103.

Friedenreich, C. and Orenstein, M. (2002) Physical activity and cancer prevention: ethiological evidence and biological mechanisms. *The Journal of Nutrition*, **132** (11 suppl), 3456S–64S.

Gallagher, D., Visser, M., Sepulveda, D. *et al.* (1996) How useful is body mass index for comparison of body fatness across age, sex, and ethnic groups? *American Journal of Epidemiology*, **143** (3), 228–39.

Gambineri, A., Pelusi, C., Vicennati, V. *et al.* (2002) Obesity and the polycystic ovary syndrome. *International Journal of Obesity and Related Metabolic Disorders*, **26** (7), 883–96.

Gami, A.S., Caples, S.M. and Somers, V.K. (2003) Obesity and obstructive sleep apnea. *Endocrinology and Metabolism Clinics of North America*, **32** (4), 869–94.

Garcia Hidalgo, L. (2002) Dermatological complications of obesity. *American Journal of Clinical Dermatology*, **3** (7), 497–506.

Gelber, A.C., Hochberg, M.C., Mead, L.A. *et al.* (1999) Body mass index in young men and the risk of subsequent knee and hip osteoarthritis. *The American Journal of Medicine*, **107** (6), 542–8.

Grant, L.M. and Lisker-Melman, M. (2004) Nonalcoholic fatty liver disease. *Annals of Hepatology*, **3** (3), 93–9.

Grundy, S.M. (2006) Does a diagnosis of the metabolic syndrome have value in clinical practice? *The American Journal of Clinical Nutrition*, **83** (6), 1248–51.

Grundy, S.M., Cleeman, J.I., Daniels, S.R. *et al.*, American Heart Association and National Heart, Lung, and Blood Institute (2005) Diagnosis and management of the metabolic syndrome: an American Heart Association/National Heart, Lung, and Blood Institute (2005) Scientific Statement. *Circulation*, **112** (17), 2735–52.

Haffner, S.M., Lehto, S., Ronnemaa, T. *et al.* (1998) Mortality from coronary heart disease in subjects with type 2 diabetes and in nondiabetic subjects with and without prior myocardial infarction. *The New England Journal of Medicine*, **339** (4), 229–34.

Han, T.S., van Leer, E.M., Seidell, J.C. and Lean, M.E. (1995) Waist circumference action levels in the identification of cardiovascular risk factors:

prevalence study in a random sample. *British Medical Journal (Clinical Research Edition)*, **311** (7017), 1401–5.

Hayashi, T., Boyko, E.J., McNeely, M.J. *et al.* (2007) Minimum waist and visceral fat values for identifying Japanese Americans at risk for the metabolic syndrome. *Diabetes Care*, **30** (1), 120–7.

Hill, J.O. and Wyatt, H. (2002) Outpatient management of obesity: a primary care perspective. *Obesity Research*, **10** (suppl 2), 124S–30S.

Hu, F.B., Willett, W.C., Li, T. *et al.* (2004) Adiposity as compared with physical activity in predicting mortality among women. *The New England Journal of Medicine*, **351** (26), 2694–703.

IARC (2002) *IARC Handbooks of Cancer Prevention, Vol 6. Weight Control and Physical Activity*, IARC Press, Lyon.

Janssen, I., Katzmarzyk, P.T. and Ross, R. (2002) Body mass index, waist circumference, and health risk: evidence in support of current NIH guidelines. *Archives of Internal Medicine*, **162** (18), 2074–9.

Jebb, S.A. and Elia, M. (1993) Techniques for the measurement of body composition: a practical guide. *International Journal of Obesity and Related Metabolic Disorders*, **17** (11), 611–21.

Jinks, C., Jordan, K. and Croft, P. (2006) Disabling knee pain – another consequence of obesity: results from a prospective cohort study. *BMC Public Health*, **6**, 258–65.

Kadowaki, T., Sekikawa, A., Murata, K. *et al.* (2006) Japanese men have larger areas of visceral adipose tissue than Caucasian men in the same levels of waist circumference in a population-based study. *International Journal of Obesity*, **30** (7), 1163–5.

Kahn, R., Buse, J., Ferrannini, E. and Stern, M. (2005) The metabolic syndrome: time for a critical appraisal. Joint statement from the American Diabetes Association and the European Association for the Study of Diabetes. *Diabetes Care*, **28** (9), 2289–304.

Kanazawa, M., Yoshiike, N., Osaka, T. *et al.* (2002) Criteria and classification of obesity in Japan and Asia-Oceania. *Asia Pacific Journal of Clinical Nutrition*, **11** (suppl 8), S732–7.

Kissebah, A.H., Vydelingum, N., Murray, R. *et al.* (1982) Relation of body fat distribution to metabolic complications of obesity. *The Journal of Clinical Endocrinology and Metabolism*, **54** (2), 254–60.

Klein, S., Allison, D.B., Heymsfield, S.B. *et al.* (2007) Waist circumference and cardiometabolic risk: a consensus statement from Shaping America's Health: Association for Weight Management and Obesity Prevention; NAASO, the obesity society; the American Society for Nutrition and the American Diabetes Association. *Obesity*, **15** (5), 1061–7.

Knudsen, N., Laurberg, P., Rasmussen, L.B. *et al.* (2005) Small differences in thyroid function may be important for body mass index and the occurrence of obesity in the population. *The Journal of Clinical Endocrinology and Metabolism*, **90** (7), 4019–24.

Kotsis, V.T., Stabouli, S.V., Papamichael, C.M. and Zakopoulos, N.A. (2006) Impact of obesity in intima media thickness of carotid arteries. *Obesity*, **14** (10), 1708–15.

Kuk, J.L., Church, T.S., Blair, S.N. and Ross, R. (2006) Does measurement site for visceral and abdominal subcutaneous adipose tissue alter associations with the metabolic syndrome? *Diabetes Care*, **29** (3), 679–84.

Kuk, J.L., Katzmarzyk, P.T., Nichaman, M.Z. *et al.* (2006) Visceral fat is an independent predictor of all-cause mortality in men. *Obesity*, **14** (2), 336–41.

Kushner, R.F. and Roth, J.L. (2003) Assessment of the obese patient. *Endocrinology and Metabolism Clinics of North America*, **32** (4), 915–33.

Kvist, H., Chowdhury, B., Grangård, U. *et al.* (1988) Total and visceral adipose-tissue volumes derived from measurements with computed tomography in adult men and women: predictive equations. *The American Journal of Clinical Nutrition*, **48** (6), 351–61.

Kyle, U.G., Bosaeus, I., De Lorenzo, A.D. *et al.* and ESPEN (2004) Bioelectrical impedance analysis-part II: utilization in clinical practice. *Clinical Nutrition*, **23** (6), 1430–53.

Lapidus, L., Bengtsson, C., Larsson, B. *et al.* (1984) Distribution of adipose tissue and risk of cardiovascular disease and death: a 12 year follow up of participants in the population study of women in Gothenburg, Sweden. *British Medical Journal*, **289** (6454), 1257–61.

Larsson, B., Svärdsudd, K., Welin, L. *et al.* (1984) Abdominal adipose tissue distribution, obesity, and risk of cardiovascular disease and death: 13 year follow up of participants in the study of men born in 1913. *British Medical Journal*, **288** (6428), 1401–4.

Lean, M.E., Han, T.S. and Deurenberg, P. (1996) Predicting body composition by densitometry from simple anthropometric measurements. *The American Journal of Clinical Nutrition*, **63** (1), 4–14.

Lean, M.E., Han, T.S. and Morrison, C.E. (1995) Waist circumference as a measure for indicating need for weight management. *British Medical Journal (Clinical Research Edition)*, **311** (6998), 158–61.

Lean, M.E.J. and Pajonk, F.G. (2003) Patients on atypical antipsychotic drugs. Another high-risk group for type 2 diabetes. *Diabetes Care*, **26** (5), 1597–605.

Lebovitz, H.E. and Banerji, M.A. (2005) Point: visceral adiposity is causally related to insulin resistance. *Diabetes Care*, **28** (9), 2322–5.

Lemieux, I. (2004) Energy partitioning in gluteal-femoral fat: does the metabolic fate of triglycerides affect coronary heart disease risk? *Arteriosclerosis, Thrombosis, and Vascular Biology*, **24** (5), 795–7.

Lemieux, I., Pascot, A., Couillard, C. *et al.* (2000) Hypertriglyceridemic waist: A marker of the athero-genic metabolic triad (hyperinsulinemia; hyperapo-lipoprotein B; small, dense LDL) in men? *Circulation*, **102** (2), 179–84.

Li, T.Y., Rana, J.S., Manson, J.E. *et al.* (2006) Obesity as compared with physical activity in predicting risk of coronary heart disease in women. *Circulation*, **113** (4), 499–506.

Lissner, L., Bjorkelund, C., Heitmann, B.L. *et al.* (2001) Larger hip circumference independently predicts health and longevity in a Swedish female cohort. *Obesity Research*, **9** (10), 644–6.

Manson, J.E., Willett, W.C., Stampfer, M.J. *et al.* (1995) Body weight and mortality among women. *The New England Journal of Medicine*, **333** (11), 677–85.

McMillan, D.C., Sattar, N. and McArdle, C.S. (2006) ABC of obesity. Obesity and cancer. *British Medical Journal (Clinical Research Edition)*, **333** (7578), 1109–11.

McNeill, A.M., Rosamond, W.D., Girman, C.J. *et al.* (2005) The metabolic syndrome and 11-year risk of incident cardiovascular disease in the Atherosclerosis Risk in Communities study. *Diabetes Care*, **28** (2), 385–90.

McTiernan, A. (2000) Associations between energy balance and body mass index and risk of breast carcinoma in women from diverse racial and ethnic backgrounds in the U.S. *Cancer*, **88** (5 Suppl), 1248–55.

Murphy, K., Calle, E.E., Rodriguez, C. *et al.* (2000) Body mass index and colon cancer mortality in a large prospective study. *American Journal of Epidemiology*, **152** (9), 847–54.

Mutch, D.M. and Clément, K. (2006) Genetics of human obesity. *Best Practice and Research. Clinical Endocrinology and Metabolism*, **20** (4), 647–64.

Nathan, D.M., Buse, J.B., Davidson, M.B. *et al.* (2006) Management of hyperglycemia in type 2 diabetes: A consensus algorithm for the initiation and adjustment of therapy: a consensus statement from the American Diabetes Association and the European Association for the Study of Diabetes. *Diabetes Care*, **29** (8), 1963–72.

National Cholesterol Education Program (NCEP) Expert Panel on Detection, Evaluation, and Treatment of High Blood Cholesterol in Adults (Adult Treatment Panel III) 2002 'Third Report of the National Cholesterol Education Program (NCEP) Expert Panel on Detection, Evaluation, and Treatment of High Blood Cholesterol in Adults (Adult Treatment Panel III)(NCEP-ATPIII) Final report.' *Circulation*, 106 (25), 3143–421.

National Institutes of Health (2000) *The practical guide: identification, evaluation, and treatment of overweight and obesity in adults.* Washington NIH publ no 00-4084, pp. 1–258.

Peeters, A., Barendregt, J.J., Willekens, F. *et al.* and NEDCOM, the Netherlands Epidemiology and Demography Compression of Morbidity Research Group (2003) Obesity in adulthood and its consequences for life expectancy: a life-table analysis. *Annals of Internal Medicine*, **138** (1), 24–32.

Pietrobelli, A., Boner, A.L. and Tatò, L. (2005) Adipose tissue and metabolic effects: new insight into measurements. *International Journal of Obesity*, **29** (suppl 1), S97–100.

Pouliot, M.C., Després, J.P., Lemieux, S. *et al.* (1994) Waist circumference and abdominal sagittal diameter: best simple anthropometric indexes of abdominal visceral adipose tissue accumulation and related cardiovascular risk in men and women. *The American Journal of Cardiology*, **73** (1), 460–8.

Prentice, A.M. and Jebb, S.A. (2001) Beyond body mass index. *Obesity Reviews*, **2** (3), 141–7.

Prochaska, J.O., DiClemente, C.C. and Norcross, J. (1992) In search of how people change. *American Psychologist*, **47**, 1102–14.

Reaven, G.M. (1988) Banting lecture 1988. Role of insulin resistance in human disease. *Diabetes*, **37** (12), 1595–607.

Rose, P.G. (1996) Endometrial carcinoma. *The New England Journal of Medicine*, **335** (9), 640–9.

Rosengren, A., Wedel, H. and Wilhelmsen, L. (1999) Body weight and weight gain during adult life in men in relation to coronary heart disease and mortality. A prospective population study. *European Heart Journal*, **20** (4), 269–77.

Rotterdam ESHRE/ASRM-Sponsored PCOS Consensus Workshop Group (2004) Revised 2003 consensus on diagnostic criteria and long-term health risks related to polycystic ovary syndrome. *Fertility and Sterility*, **81** (1), 19–25.

Scheinfeld, N.S. (2004) Obesity and dermatology. *Clinics in Dermatology*, **22** (4), 303–9.

Schienkiewitz, A., Schulze, M.B., Hoffmann, K. *et al.* (2006) Body mass index history and risk of type 2 diabetes: results from the European Prospective Investigation into Cancer and Nutrition (EPIC)-Potsdam Study. *The American Journal of Clinical Nutrition*, **84** (2), 427–33.

Seidell, J.C., Perusse, L., Després, J.P. and Bouchard, C. (2001) Waist and hip circumferences have independent and opposite effects on cardiovascular disease risk factors: the Quebec Family Study. *The American Journal of Clinical Nutrition*, **74** (3), 315–21.

Shamsuzzaman, A.S., Gersh, B.J. and Somers, V.K. (2003) Obstructive sleep apnea: implications for cardiac and vascular disease. *The Journal of the American Medical Association*, **290** (14), 1906–14.

Shen, W., Punyanitya, M., Chen, J. *et al.* (2006) Waist circumference correlates with metabolic syndrome indicators better than percentage fat. *Obesity*, **14** (4), 727–36.

Shen, W., Punyanitya, M., Wang, Z. *et al.* (2004) Visceral adipose tissue: relations between single-slice areas and total volume. *The American Journal of Clinical Nutrition*, **80** (2), 271–8.

Shen, W., Wang, Z., Punyanita, M. *et al.* (2003) Adipose tissue quantification by imaging methods: a proposed classification. *Obesity Research*, **11** (1), 5–16.

Siri, W.E. (1961) Body composition from fluid spaces and density: analysis of methods, in *Techniques for Measuring Body Composition* (eds J. Brozek and A. Henschel), National Academy of Sciences NRC, Washington DC, pp. 223–44.

Snijder, M.B., Dekker, J.M., Visser, M. *et al.* (2003a) Associations of hip and thigh circumferences independent of waist circumference with the incidence of type 2 diabetes: the Hoorn Study. *The American Journal of Clinical Nutrition*, **77** (5), 1192–7.

Snijder, M.B., Dekker, J.M., Visser, M. *et al.* (2003b) Larger thigh and hip circumferences are associated with better glucose tolerance: the Hoorn study. *Obesity Research*, **11** (1), 104–11.

Snijder, M.B., Dekker, J.M., Visser, M. *et al.* (2004) Trunk fat and leg fat have independent and opposite associations with fasting and postload glucose levels: the Hoorn Study. *Diabetes Care*, **27** (2), 372–7.

Stern, M.P., Williams, K., Gonzalez-Villalpando, C. *et al.* (2004) Does the metabolic syndrome improve identification of individuals at risk of type 2 diabetes and/or cardiovascular disease? *Diabetes Care*, **27** (11), 2676–881.

Stevens, J., Cai, J., Evenson, K.R. and Thomas, R. (2002) Fitness and fatness as predictors of mortality from all causes and from cardiovascular disease in men and women in the lipid research clinics study. *American Journal of Epidemiology*, **156** (9), 832–41.

Targher, G. (2007) Non-alcoholic fatty liver disease, the metabolic syndrome and the risk of cardiovascular disease: the plot thickens. *Diabetic Medicine: A Journal of the British Diabetic Association*, **24** (1), 1–6.

Teixeira, P.J., Going, S.B., Sardinha, L.B. and Lohman, T.G. (2005) A review of psychosocial pre-treatment predictors of weight control. *Obesity Reviews*, **6** (1), 43–65.

Tominaga, M., Eguchi, H., Manaka, H. *et al.* (1999) Impaired glucose tolerance is a risk factor for cardiovascular disease, but not impaired fasting glucose. The Funagata Diabetes Study. *Diabetes Care*, **22** (6), 920–4.

Unwin, N., Shaw, J., Zimmet, P. and Alberti, K.G. (2002) Impaired glucose tolerance and impaired fasting glycaemia: the current status on definition and intervention. *Diabetic Medicine: A Journal of the British Diabetic Association*, **19** (9), 708–23.

Vague, J. (1947) Sexual differentiation. A factor affecting the forms of obesity. *Presse Medicale (Paris, France: 1983)*, **30**, 339–40.

van der Kooy, K. and Seidell, J.C. (1993) Techniques for the measurement of visceral fat: a practical guide. *International Journal of Obesity and Related Metabolic Disorders*, **17** (4), 187–96.

Van Gaal, L.F. (1998) Dietary treatment of obesity, in *Handbook of Obesity* (eds G.A. Bray, C. Bouchard and W.P.T. James), Marcel Dekker, New York, pp. 875–90.

Van Gaal, L.F. (2006) Long-term health considerations in schizophrenia: metabolic effects and the role of abdominal adiposity. *European Neuropharmacology*, **16** (Suppl 3), S142–8.

Van Gaal, L.F. and Mertens, I. (1998) Effects of obesity on cardiovascular system and blood pressure control, digestive disease and cancer, in *Clinical Obesity* (eds P. Kopelman and M. Stock), Blackwell Science, Oxford, pp. 205–25.

Van Gaal, L.F., Mertens, I.L. and De Block, C.E. (2006) Mechanisms linking obesity with cardiovascular disease. *Nature*, **444** (7121), 875–80.

Vansant, G. and Muls, E. (2002) Assessment of the obese patient, in *Managing Obesity and Cardiovascular Disease* (ed. J. Shepherd), Science Press.

Verrijken, A., Demunck, S., Mertens, I. and Van Gaal, L. (2006) Overgewicht, obesitas en kanker. *Tijdschr voor Geneeskunde*, **62** (18), 1304–11.

Wajchenberg, B.L. (2000) Subcutaneous and visceral adipose tissue: their relation to the metabolic syndrome. *Endocrine Reviews*, **21** (6), 697–738.

Wang, Y., Rimm, E.B., Stampfer, M.J. *et al.* (2005) Comparison of abdominal adiposity and overall obesity in predicting risk of type 2 diabetes among men. *The American Journal of Clinical Nutrition*, **81** (3), 555–63.

Wearing, S.C., Hennig, E.M., Byrne, N.M. *et al.* (2006) Musculoskeletal disorders associated with obesity: a biomechanical perspective. *Obesity Reviews*, **7** (3), 239–50.

Willett, W.C., Manson, J.E., Stampfer, M.J. *et al.* (1995) Weight, weight change, and coronary heart disease in women. Risk within the 'normal' weight range. *The Journal of the American Medical Association*, **273** (6), 461–5.

Williams, M.J., Hunter, G.R., Kekes-Szabo, T. *et al.* (1996) Intra-abdominal adipose tissue cut-points related to elevated cardiovascular risk in women. *International Journal of Obesity*, **20** (7), 613–7.

Wilson, P.W., D'Agostino, R.B., Levy, D. *et al.* (1998) Prediction of coronary heart disease using risk factor categories. *Circulation*, **97** (18), 1837–47.

World Health Organization (1997) *Obesity, Preventing and Managing the Global Epidemic: Report of a WHO Consultation on Obesity*, World Health Organization, Geneva, Switzerland.

World Health Organization (1999) *Definition, Diagnosis and Classification of Diabetes Mellitus and its Complications: Report of a WHO Consultation*, WHO: WHO/NCD/NCS 99.2, Geneva, Switzerland.

Yusuf, S., Hawken, S., Ounpuu, S. *et al.* and INTER-HEART Study Investigators (2005) Obesity and the risk of myocardial infarction in 27,000 participants from 52 countries: a case-control study. *Lancet*, **366** (9497), 1640–9.

Managing Obesity: General Approach and Lifestyle Intervention

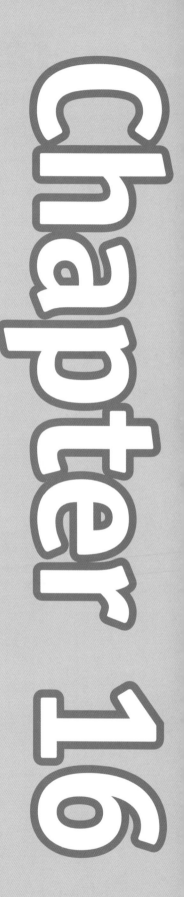

Key points

- Obesity management aims to reduce morbidity and mortality, while improving psychosocial well-being. Interventions are costly and time-consuming and should be targeted at individuals most likely to benefit.

- Obesity should be treated actively in subjects with BMI $\geq$30 kg/m^2 (or BMI $\geq$27 kg/m^2 with diabetes or other serious comorbidities of obesity) and/or a waist circumference better $\geq$102 cm (men) or 88 cm (women). The initial aim is to reduce weight by 5–10%.

- Weight loss of 10% or more can bring consistent improvements in blood pressure, blood lipids and glycaemic control in diabetic subjects (with fasting glucose falling by 2–3 mmol/l and HbA$_{1c}$ by 1% or more). Modest weight loss also decreases global cardiovascular risk by 40–50% and the risk of progressing from impaired glucose tolerance (IGT) to type 2 diabetes by up to 60%. The risk of premature death decreases by 20–33%.

- Substantial weight loss (30% or more), achieved by bariatric surgery, can reverse established type 2 diabetes in up to 80% of cases, correct sleep apnoea and, at least initially, restore normal blood pressure in 60–70% of subjects with hypertension.

- Adherence to weight-management programmes is generally poor but may be improved by involving the patient's family, tailoring advice to the individual, and using small-group education and social cognitive approaches. Internet-based counselling may also help.

- Lifestyle improvement, with healthy eating and increased physical activity, forms the basis of all weight-management programmes. The aim is to lose 0.5–1 kg/week initially, mobilizing adipose tissue preferentially.

- Total energy intake should be reduced by 500–1000 kcal/day. Fat intake should be limited to provide <30% of total energy, and saturated fats replaced by unsaturated. Carbohydrate (at least 55% of total energy intake) should comprise mainly starches and fibre, while avoiding simple sugars and sweetened drinks. Alcohol consumption should be restricted to healthy drinking limits or lower, and salt intake to <6 g/day.

- Very low calorie diets (VLCD), providing <800 kcal/day, can achieve rapid weight loss (averaging 20 kg over 12 weeks), but weight is often regained thereafter. Lifestyle support and behavioural therapy can improve the outcome. VLCD are indicated when rapid weight loss is needed on medical grounds but should only be used for 12–16 weeks; side effects include protein catabolism and gallstone formation.

- Numerous fad diets have been marketed, often with little or no scientific basis. Success is determined by the extent and duration of energy intake restriction, rather than any specific features of the diets. Some are nutritionally unbalanced and potentially dangerous.

- Increasing physical exercise is an important aspect of obesity management and helps to maintain energy expenditure and prevent weight regain after weight loss. This also reduces cardiovascular risk and that of premature death. Obese subjects should aim for at least 30 min every day of brisk walking or other moderate exercise.

Chapter 16   **Managing Obesity: General Approach and Lifestyle Intervention**

Susanne Wiesner and Jens Jordan

The ultimate goal of obesity treatment is to reduce morbidity and mortality while improving psychological well-being and social function. As well as reducing adiposity, risk reduction may also require other interventions such as lipid-lowering and antihypertensive therapy. At present, it is unclear to what extent some of the available weight-loss interventions can achieve all these goals in a satisfactory proportion of patients, because there is a lack of long-term outcome data from large, controlled clinical trials. Thus, much current clinical practice derives from pathophysiological considerations, epidemiological observations and data from trials that have assessed surrogate end-points.

This chapter describes the rationale and indications for obesity treatment, the selection of patients and treatment targets. The focus is on lifestyle interventions, which are the mainstay of all obesity treatment programmes, notably dietary modification and ways to increase physical exercise. Most obese people find it difficult to adopt and maintain these changes in the long term, and therefore require additional measures. Anti-obesity drugs and bariatric surgery are covered specifically in Chapters 17 and 18.

Selection of patients for obesity management

Obesity interventions are time-consuming and costly, and should therefore be offered to selected patients who will benefit from them, so that healthcare resources are used effectively and responsibly. In general, treatment is targeted at populations and individuals who are at increased risk of morbidity and mortality associated with their obesity. The greater the

risk, the greater should be the absolute benefit from an intervention. It follows that the treatment of obesity should be tailored to the individual's risk profile. The health hazards of obesity are described in detail in Chapters 9–14. The current rationale for treatment targets is mostly based on reducing the risk for type 2 diabetes and the cardiovascular abnormalities that are commonly associated with obesity in the so-called 'metabolic syndrome'.

Various measures can be used for risk stratification. Those applicable to clinical practice need to be easy to perform and inexpensive, and clinical decisions about selecting patients for obesity treatment have generally been based mainly on simple anthropometric measures. Detailed analyses of morbidity and mortality by many groups during the 1980s confirmed that a high body mass index (BMI) was an important risk factor (Chapter 9). This led the World Health Organization (WHO) in the early 1990s to define overweight as a BMI $\geq25\,\text{kg/m}^2$ and obesity as a BMI $\geq30\,\text{kg/m}^2$ (Hubert et al., 1983; Manson et al., 1995). These thresholds relate to increased levels of health risk, and indeed of premature death: life expectancy is reduced by 7.1 years for females and 5.9 years for males in obese non-smokers, as compared with subjects with a normal BMI (Peeters et al., 2003). These cut-off values have been used extensively to guide therapy.

However, BMI alone may not be sufficient to predict risk accurately in an individual patient. Waist circumference measurements can provide additional information, because there is a correlation between waist circumference and visceral fat mass that is an important determinant of cardiovascular and metabolic risk (see Chapters 9 and 10). It has been shown that risk (especially

Obesity: Science to Practice   Edited by Gareth Williams and Gema Frühbeck
© 2009 John Wiley & Sons, Ltd

Table 16.1 Indications for active management of obesity.

Waist circumference	Body mass index	Comorbidities
≥102 cm (men)	—	—
≥88 cm (women)	—	—
	≥30 kg/m²	—
	27–30 kg/m²	Diabetes
		Hypertension

cardiovascular) is significantly increased when waist circumference exceeds 102 cm in men and 88 cm in women (Lean, Han and Morrison, 1995; Formiguera and Canton, 2004).

Current guidelines suggest that obesity should be treated actively in patients with a BMI >30 kg/m² and/or waist circumference >102 cm in men or >88 cm in women. Individuals with a BMI >25 kg/m² and/or a waist circumference >94 cm in men and >80 cm in women may be considered for less intensive intervention and lifestyle advice (Manson *et al.*, 2004). Patients with established cardiovascular or metabolic comorbidities such as type 2 diabetes mellitus, dyslipidaemia or hypertension require a more

aggressive approach and are generally selected for active treatment if their BMI exceeds 27 kg/m². These indications are summarized in Table 16.1. Given the rapid increase in obesity prevalence, more refined methodologies are needed to select obese patients for treatment, and to identify those who will derive the most benefit.

An algorithm for the general evaluation and management of the obese patient is suggested in Figure 16.1.

Treatment targets

Intentional weight loss has been shown to improve many medical complications associated with obesity (Table 16.2). These improvements are broadly related to the magnitude of weight loss and are most convincing with the large reductions of excess weight that can be achieved with bariatric surgery (see Chapter 18). Nonetheless, even modest weight loss achieved by lifestyle improvement with or without pharmacotherapy may produce substantial benefits on cardiovascular and metabolic risk, as shown in the following section. Accordingly, a 5% or 10% reduction from the initial body weight is usually

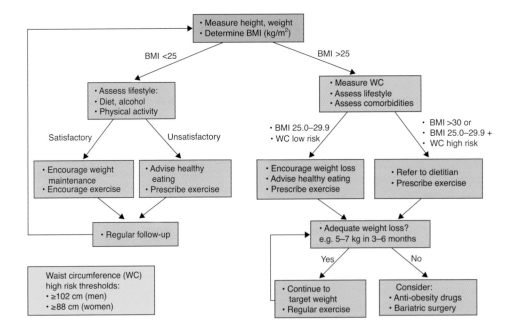

Figure 16.1 Algorithm for the basic evaluation and management of the overweight and obese patient.

Table 16.2 Benefits of weight loss.

Moderate weight loss: 5–10%

Achievable by lifestyle changes with or without pharmacotherapy

- Improved insulin sensitivity
- Reduce risk of IGT progressing to type 2 diabetes
- Lower plasma glucose and HbA_{1c} levels in diabetes
- Significant reduction in triglycerides (with >5% weight loss)
- Significant reduction in LDL cholesterol (with >10% weight loss)
- Improved liver function tests in non-alcoholic fatty liver disease
- Lower diastolic and systolic blood pressure
- Decreased total cardiovascular risk
- Reduction in all-cause mortality

Substantial weight loss: >30%

Achievable by bariatric surgery

- Improvement or reversal of established type 2 diabetes
- Improvement or normalization of hypertension
- Improvement or cure of sleep apnoea
- Reduction in premature mortality

regarded as a successful outcome in an individual patient (Klein and Canton, 2001).

Success can also be defined for a treatment programme rather than individual patient. It has been suggested that a successful treatment programme should retain at least 80% of the enrolled patients after one year, and that of those, 75% should have lost at least 5% of their initial body weight and 50% over 10%.

Effects of weight loss on comorbidities and mortality

Numerous studies have shown promising improvements with weight loss in surrogate end-points such as hyperglycaemia, blood lipid levels and blood pressure.

Weight loss of 10% or more improves insulin sensitivity and, in subjects with established type 2 diabetes, may reduce fasting blood glucose by 2–3 mmol/l and HbA_{1c} by 1% or more – effects that are comparable with those of oral hypoglycaemic agents. The glucose-lowering effect is less consistent with weight loss of 5–10%. Minor weight loss can be beneficial in preventing type 2 diabetes from developing in obese subjects. For example, data from the Framingham study suggest that the risk of diabetes decreased by half in subjects losing >6.8 kg of body weight (Moore *et al.*, 2000). Lifestyle changes resulting in relatively modest weight loss (~5%) have also been shown to decrease by up to 60% the risk of subjects with impaired glucose tolerance (IGT) progressing to type 2 diabetes (see Chapter 22).

Major weight loss is particularly effective in improving glucose metabolism. Over 80% of obese patients with type 2 diabetes who lost 30% of initial body weight after gastric bypass surgery achieved normal fasting blood glucose, insulin and glycated haemoglobin concentrations (Pories *et al.*, 1995; see Chapter 18).

Dyslipidaemia and associated cardiovascular risk also improve with modest weight loss. For example, the Framingham Offspring Study showed that approximately 2.3 kg of weight loss over 16 years was associated with a 40–50% reduction in total cardiometabolic risk conferred by systolic blood pressure, serum triglyceride levels, raised total cholesterol and reduced HDL cholesterol, and fasting blood glucose, in both women and men (Wilson *et al.*, 1999). The largest reductions in serum triglycerides, total cholesterol and LDL cholesterol occurred in the first 4–8 weeks of weight loss (Rössner *et al.*, 2000). Patients may have to maintain a 5% weight loss to experience a sustained reduction in triglyceride levels, and a 10% weight loss for a sustained fall in LDL cholesterol improvement (Rössner *et al.*, 2000; Rössner and Bjorvell, 1987; Ryttig, Flaten and Rössner, 1997). Serum HDL cholesterol concentrations decrease initially during active weight loss, but increase thereafter when subjects are at a stabilized reduced weight; this is probably related to the increased activity of lipoprotein lipase (an insulin-sensitive enzyme), leading to enhanced hydrolysis of VLDL cholesterol and transfer of lipids to HDL cholesterol (Dattilo and Kris-Etherton, 1992).

Evidence suggests that weight loss also lowers blood pressure, at least initially, but that this improvement may not be maintained. The Trials of Hypertension Prevention Phase II study showed a dose-response relationship between weight loss and blood pressure after 36 months of treatment (Stevens *et al.*, 2001), with an average weight loss of 8.8 kg being associated with a 7/5 (systolic/diastolic) mm Hg reduction in blood pressure. Major weight loss induced by bariatric surgery has been shown to improve or completely resolve hypertension in approximately two-thirds of patients (Foley *et al.*, 1992; Carson *et al.*, 1994), but this depressor response may not be sustained: eight years after surgery, 35% of the patients who had lost substantial amounts of weight were again hypertensive (Sjöström *et al.*, 2000). A large weight reduction during the first year tended to be accompanied by lower systolic and diastolic pressures, whereas weight increases during the last seven years were significantly related to higher blood pressure at eight years (Sjöström *et al.*, 2000). Thus, blood pressure may return to baseline values when weight loss reaches a plateau or weight begins to increase again.

Other complications of obesity benefit from various degrees of weight loss. A reduction of 34% in weight improves sleep apnoea in patients with BMI >40 kg/m^2 (Sugerman *et al.*, 1992; Barvaux, Aubert and Rodenstein, 2000; Charuzi *et al.*, 1985; Schwartz *et al.*, 1991; Sugerman *et al.*, 1988). Loss of 10% or more in body weight often normalizes liver function tests in subjects with non-alcoholic fatty liver disease (Chapter 11), while decreasing liver fat content and improving histological features of steatohepatitis (Palmer and Schaffner, 1990; Eriksson, Eriksson and Bondesson, 1986; Ranlov and Hardt, 1990).

The ultimate impact of weight loss on the excess mortality associated with obesity remains uncertain. For example, in epidemiological studies, intentional weight loss of any amount was associated with a 20% reduction in all-cause mortality (Williamson *et al.*, 1995), while intentional weight loss of 9–13 kg was associated with an approximately 33% reduction in premature mortality in overweight individuals with diabetes (Williamson *et al.*, 2000).

Whether or not survival is improved by weight loss achieved through lifestyle or pharmacological interventions has not yet been proven in randomized controlled trials. This is an important gap in knowledge, because presumed benefits in terms of morbidity and mortality for therapeutic interventions cannot be extrapolated from epidemiological observations or from studies that assess only surrogate end-points. To date, anti-obesity drug trials have been limited by their high attrition rates and lack of long-term morbidity and

mortality data (Padwal and Majumdar, 2007). Ongoing studies are aiming to test whether anti-obesity drugs (rimonabant and sibutramine) improve both morbidity and mortality in obese patients with high cardiovascular risk (Coutinho and Majumdar, 2007; Aylwin and Al-Zaman, 2008). Recently, major weight loss induced by bariatric surgery has been shown to decrease long-term mortality (particularly deaths from diabetes, heart disease, and cancer) in severely obese patients (Peeters *et al.*, 2007; Adams *et al.*, 2007).

Practical obesity management

Recognising that obesity is an important risk factor that requires treatment is an essential first step for both healthcare practitioners and the general population. The American National Heart Lung and Blood Institute (NHLBI) of the National Institute of Health (NIH) offers useful advice on identifying and treating overweight and obese patients (NHLBI, 2000). Relatively simple measures may help to persuade patients to become interested in adopting lifestyle changes that will improve or prevent obesity. Only 3–4 minutes of advice about physical activity, integrated into a routine consultation, can encourage sedentary patients to become more active (Albright *et al.*, 2000). The National Centre for Chronic Disease Prevention and Health Promotion (NCCDP) has developed material to help clinicians to counsel their patients about fitting more physical activity into their lives (Table 16.3) This is freely available at: www.cdc.gov/nccdphp/dnpa/physical/recommendations/index.htm. Once patients are involved, they may become more motivated to undertake more intensive weight-loss interventions.

Commercial slimming clubs, such as Weight Watchers, are established in many countries. It has not been demonstrated whether or not these organizations are more or less successful in achieving long-term weight loss than programmes devised by multidisciplinary clinical teams.

Adherence to weight-reduction programmes

To achieve lasting weight control, patients have to adhere to intensive weight-loss programmes in the long term, indeed for life. Unfortunately,

Table 16.3 Summary of NCCDP advice for encouraging physical exercise (available at www.cdc.gov/nccdphp/dnpa/physical/recommendations/index.htm).

It is never too late to start an active lifestyle.

Physical activity does not need to be hard to produce benefits.

Daily, moderate exercise can bring health benefits and improve quality of life.

This applies irrespective of age, or how unfit the subject feels, or for how long they have been inactive.

Adults should try to engage in moderate physical activities for at least 30 minutes on 5 or more days of the week, or in vigorous physical activity for 20 minutes or more on at least 3 days per week.

People participating regularly in physical activities should be encouraged and supported in their efforts to continue.

People should set realistic personal goals, including a variety of activities.

Practical recommendations on how to increase physical activity, based on current activity level:

If you...	Then...
Do not currently engage in regular physical activity	Begin with a few minutes of physical activity each day, gradually building up to 30 minutes or more of moderate activities.
Are active, but below the recommended levels	Try to adopt more consistent activity such as moderate physical activity for 30 minutes or more on 5 or more days of the week, or vigorous physical activity for 20 minutes or more on 3 or more days of the week.
Already do moderate activities for at least 30 minutes on 5 or more days of the week	You may achieve even greater health benefits by increasing the duration or intensity of those activities.
Already regularly engage in vigorous activities for 20 minutes or more on 3 or more days of the week	Continue to do so.

adherence is relatively low, even in a research setting. Drop-out rates during clinical trials are typically 30–40%. Some patients may be unable to afford the high costs of weight-loss programmes that require medication or high-quality food – a particular problem in low-income families who are at increased risk of obesity. Occasional patients may default because they do not understand the rationale of the programme (Teixeira et al., 2005). Interventions have been developed for a general practice setting that are less demanding for patients and healthcare providers; these can improve the practitioners' knowledge of the principles of obesity management, yet may not achieve adequate or lasting weight loss (Adamson and Mathers, 2004). Thus, adherence to relatively intensive weight-loss programmes needs to be improved, rather than decreasing the intensity of the intervention.

Adherence may be improved when weight-loss programmes involve the family, are conducted in small groups of patients, are sensitive to cultural considerations, and tailor advice appropriately to the target group. Social cognitive therapies may also be helpful in improving adherence (Levy et al., 2007). Indeed, patients may require assistance in developing their own behavioural change strategies and goal-setting. Recent investigations have shown that such measures can be distributed through the Internet. In one study, weight loss improved when e-mail counselling was added to a simple, Internet-based weight-loss programme (Tate, Jackvony and Wing, 2003) (Figure 16.2). Such a combination of virtual counsellors, backed up by tailored advice through intermittent contact with human counsellors, may be able to deliver social cognitive interventions to larger numbers of patients while containing costs.

Finally, adherence to weight-loss interventions may be improved when patients who are not responding sufficiently to life-style interventions are entered into pharmacotherapy or bariatric surgery programmes, according to current guidelines (Rössner et al., 2000; Wadden et al., 2005; Fried et al., 2007).

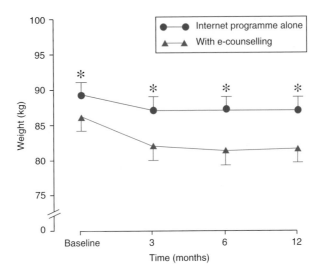

Figure 16.2 Behavioural counselling delivered by e-mail achieved significantly greater weight loss than an Internet-based education programme alone. *: $p < 0.05$ for the difference between the two interventions. From Tate, Jackvony and Wing (2003), with permission of the editor of *JAMA*.

Lifestyle modification

This comprises both a reduction in energy intake and increased physical activity, with the aim of inducing a consistent energy deficit that will cause the preferential mobilization of triglyceride in adipose tissue rather than the catabolism of other tissues. The relative proportions of decreased food intake and increased physical activity should be carefully tailored to the individual patient's needs.

Energy intake

The initial aim is generally to reduce total energy intake by 600–1000 kcal/day. Targets for individual patients may differ according to their specific needs. Practical dietary guidelines are summarized in Table 16.4 and Figure 16.3.

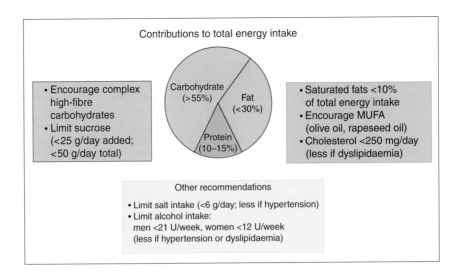

Figure 16.3 Current dietary guidelines for managing obesity. MUFA: monounsaturated fatty acids.

Table 16.4 Current dietary guidelines for obese subjects.

Nutrient	Recommended intake
Total energy	500–1000 kcal/day reduction from usual intake
	• The impact of alcohol calories on the total caloric intake needs to be assessed and appropriately controlled
Total fat	≤30% of total calories
	• Fat-modified foods may provide a helpful strategy for lowering total fat intake but will only be effective if they are also low in calories and there is no compensation of calories from other foods
Saturated fatty acids	8–10% of total calories • Reduce to <7% of total calories in patients with hypercholesterolaemia
Monounsaturated fatty acids	Up to 15% of total calories
Polyunsaturated fatty acids	Up to 10% of total calories
Cholesterol	<300 mg/day
	• Reduce to <200 mg/day in patients with hypercholesterolaemia
Protein	Approximately 15% of total calories
	• Proteins should be derived mainly from lean animal sources or plants.
Carbohydrates	≥55% of total calories
	• Mostly derived from complex carbohydrates
	• Limit intake of simple sugars (sugary drinks, sweets and foods sweetened with sucrose or fructose-rich corn syrup)
Fibre	>15 g per 1000 kcal of energy intake
	• Present in vegetables, whole grains, legumes and fruits
	• A diet high in fibre promotes satiety at higher levels of calorie and fat intake and helps to reduce blood cholesterol
Sodium chloride	<100 mmol/day (equivalent to 6 g of sodium chloride)
	• Decrease added salt when cooking
	• Watch food labelling for salt content
Calcium	1000–1500 mg/day
	• During weight loss, adequate calcium intake should be maintained, especially in women at risk of osteoporosis

Dietary fat: quantity and quality

Ingestion of a high-fat diet is an independent risk factor for overweight and obesity (Astrup, 2001). Fat is the most energy-dense macronutrient (containing 9 kcal/g) and has relatively low satiating capacity (see Chapter 8). The widespread availability of fat-rich, energy-dense foods is undoubtedly an important factor in the overall spread of obesity, although its role in an individual's weight gain will vary according to the person's environment and genetic background (see Chapter 8).

In addition, some subjects prone to obesity show a reduced ability to oxidize dietary and endogenous fat and thus lay down excess triglyceride in adipose tissue (Giacco et al., 2004). Similarly, obese subjects who have a relatively low lipid oxidation rate during a weight-reduction programme are more likely to regain weight in the future (Valtuena, Salas-Salvado and Lorda, 1997). By contrast, fat oxidation is relatively increased in obese individuals whose weight is stable, and this mechanism may help to limit further weight gain (Raben *et al.*, 1994; Schutz, 1995; Golay *et al.*, 1997; Ravussin and Smith, 2002).

Current guidelines are to limit the energy intake from fats to less than 30% of total energy intake (NHLBI, 2000) (see Table 16.4).

Ingestion of dietary fats may also affect cardiovascular and metabolic risk factors, in part independently of body weight. Importantly, the fatty-acid composition of the diet may markedly influence insulin sensitivity and blood lipid levels. In healthy subjects, ingesting variable amounts of fat (between 20 and 40% of total energy intake) does not significantly affect insulin sensitivity (Swinburn *et al.*, 1991; Borkman *et al.*, 1991; Bisschop *et al.*, 2001; Garg, Grundy and Unger, 1992; Hughes *et al.*, 1995; Sarkkinen *et al.*, 1996), whereas a selective increase in saturated fat intake may impair insulin action (Maron, Fair and Haskell, 1991; Parker *et al.*, 1993; Mayer *et al.*, 1993; Feskens, Loeber and Kromhout, 1994; Marshall, Bessesen and Hamman, 1997; Mooy *et al.*, 1998; Mayer-Davis *et al.*, 1997). Numerous studies have shown positive correlations between saturated fat intake and circulating insulin levels (an index of insulin resistance), independently of body fat mass (Maron, Fair and Haskell, 1991; Parker *et al.*, 1993; Mayer *et al.*, 1993; Feskens, Loeber and Kromhout, 1994; Marshall, Bessesen and Hamman, 1997; Mooy *et al.*, 1998; Mayer-Davis *et al.*, 1997). Moreover, increasing unsaturated fat intake is associated with improved insulin sensitivity (Pelikanova *et al.*, 1989; Borkman *et al.*, 1993; Vessby, Tengblad and Lithell, 1994; Pan *et al.*, 1995), particularly when total fat intake is relatively low (Vessby *et al.*, 2001). The mechanisms linking dietary fat composition to insulin sensitivity are under active investigation and may involve changes in the fatty-acid composition of cell membranes, which is known to influence insulin signalling (Inokuchi, 2006). In diabetic patients, diets rich in omega-6-polyunsaturated fatty acids improve insulin sensitivity (Summers *et al.*, 2002), whereas foods rich in omega-3-fatty acids diets do not (Borkman *et al.*, 1991). These findings have also been confirmed in healthy, non-diabetic subjects (Borkman *et al.*, 1991; Vessby *et al.*, 2001; Rivellese *et al.*, 1996).

Fatty acid composition also has powerful effects on lipoprotein metabolism. In the presence of insulin resistance, replacing saturated fats with unsaturated leads to lower LDL and VLDL lipoprotein concentrations (Swinburn *et al.*, 1991). Increasing the intake of long-chain omega-3-fatty acids effectively lowers triglyceride levels, even though insulin sensitivity does not change (Harris, 1997); however, this may also increase LDL cholesterol in hyperlipidaemic and in normolipaemic subjects (Rivellese *et al.*, 2003). Finally, increasing the intake of monounsaturated fatty acids may lower blood pressure (Stamler, Caggiula and Grandits, 1997; Trevisan *et al.*, 1990).

Together, these observations suggest that fatty-acid composition may be as important as reducing the total fat content of the diet in reducing cardiovascular and metabolic risk in the treatment of obesity. Ultimately, it may become feasible to tailor the unsaturated fatty acid composition of the diet to the individual patient's risk profile.

Dietary carbohydrate

Excessive carbohydrate ingestion can promote weight gain, and overconsumption of sugar-rich, energy-dense foods and soft drinks is an important contributor to obesity in children and adolescents (Ludwig, Peterson and Gortmaker, 2001).

Current guidelines aim to limit the amount of simple sugars in the diet (including sugary drinks, and sweets and foods sweetened with sucrose or fructose-rich corn syrup), while encouraging the intake of complex starches and fibre. Total carbohydrate intake must be considered within the reduction in overall energy intake and should account for at least 55% of the total (Table 16.4).

As with fats, the carbohydrate composition of the diet may also be important. One factor that has attracted interest is the variable speed of intestinal absorption of different carbohydrates. Simple sugars are more rapidly absorbed than complex carbohydrates, so that foods containing equal amounts of total carbohydrate may vary considerably in the blood glucose responses that they elicit after a meal (Jenkins *et al.*, 1983; Jenkins *et al.*, 1987). This has led to the concept of the glycaemic index or glycaemic load that is the ratio between the blood glucose curve area of the test substance, as compared with that after ingesting 50 g of glucose (Foster-Powell, Holt and Brand-Miller, 2002). Meals with a low glycaemic index, mainly containing slowly absorbed carbohydrates, produce more prolonged postprandial satiety (Leathwood and Pollet, 1988; Holt *et al.*, 1992) and may also have different effects on insulin and incretin hormones. The effect was postulated to be beneficial in the prevention of obesity, but this has not been proven in long-term studies (Astrup *et al.*, 2000). The Carbohydrate Ratio Management in European National (CARMEN) diets study tested the impact of complex versus simple carbohydrates in a fat-reduced diet (comprising 25–28% of total energy intake) with a control group (35% of total energy intake). After six months, a significant reduction in body weight and fat mass was observed in both high carbohydrate diets as compared with the control diet, whereas no marked effect of the type of carbohydrate on loss of body weight or fat was observed (Saris *et al.*, 2000). The glycaemic index has other limitations – for example, it can be altered by preparation and cooking methods and by mixing with other foods – and should only be applied to comparisons of foods within the same food group, that is fruits and vegetables, breads and cereals (Jarvi *et al.*, 1999).

Acute postprandial increases in glucose levels have been suggested to contribute to cardiovascular complications (Leiter *et al.*, 2005); whether or not this effect could be exploited by selecting foods with a low glycaemic index deserves further study.

A recent study observed a positive association between carbohydrate consumption and plasma leptin concentrations during energy restriction (Jenkins *et al.*, 1997). The macronutrient content of the diet may therefore modulate the activity of the leptinergic pathway, although the relevance of this to the regulation of energy balance in common human obesity is not clear (Chapter 6).

Protein intake

Current guidelines for protein intake are shown in Table 16.4. These are somewhat empirical. Protein malnutrition ensues when protein intake is reduced below an individual's threshold, which varies considerably. It has been suggested that a moderately increased protein intake may be harmful in otherwise healthy subjects. Even though this suggestion remains controversial, several current guidelines suggest an upper limit

of daily protein intake that is well below actual protein ingestion levels for many people.

Some studies suggest that replacing some dietary carbohydrate with protein might improve body composition changes during energy restriction (with better preservation of lean tissue), as compared with fat-restricted, high-carbohydrate diets (Layman *et al.*, 2003). A small study in hyperinsulinaemic obese men found that an energy-reduced diet with a relatively high protein content was more effective in reducing body weight than a carbohydrate-rich diet (Baba *et al.*, 1999).

A high-protein diet may also help to maintain the resting metabolic rate, which falls during energy restriction in proportion to the inevitable loss of lean tissue (Torbay, Baba and Sawaya, 2002; see Chapter 7). This phenomenon may be explained in part by the energy costs of nutrient absorption, processing and storage, which differ markedly between macronutrients (de Jonge and Bray, 1997). This energy requirement is highest for protein, comprising 25–30% of the ingested energy, followed by carbohydrates (6–8%) and finally fat (only 2–3%) (Nair, Halliday and Garrow, 1983; Jéquier and Bray, 2002). Protein intake sufficient to prevent negative nitrogen balance may be important to lessen the declines in both muscle mass (Demling and DeSanti, 2000) and energy expenditure that occur in conditions of overall energy deficit, including therapeutic weight-loss programmes (Whitehead, McNeill and Smith, 1996).

Several studies suggest that protein promotes satiety and reduces appetite as compared with fat or carbohydrates (Layman *et al.*, 2003; Westerterp-Plantenga *et al.*, 1999; Westerterp-Plantenga *et al.*, 2004; Poppitt, McCormack and Buffenstein, 1998; Latner and Schwartz, 1999; Stubbs *et al.*, 1996), although these findings have been contested (Raben *et al.*, 2003; Vozzo *et al.*, 2003). A diet rich in protein appears superior to conventional diets in improving insulin sensitivity (Layman *et al.*, 2003; Baba *et al.*, 1999; Foster *et al.*, 2003; Samaha *et al.*, 2003), with apparently no deleterious, short-term effects being reported on blood pressure (Foster *et al.*, 2003), total cholesterol and triglycerides (Layman *et al.*, 2003; Baba *et al.*, 1999; Foster *et al.*, 2003; Samaha *et al.*, 2003) or bone turnover (Farnsworth *et al.*, 2003; Skov *et al.*, 1999). However, it should be noted that many high-protein diets also have a very low carbohydrate content, a combination that leads in the first few days to rapid mobilization of hepatic glycogen and its associated water. The resulting diuresis can be misinterpreted as successful early weight loss, even though this is due mostly to loss of water and not fat (Coulston and Rock, 1994). These diets can lead to physiological ketosis when daily carbohydrate intake is less than 100 g.

Larger studies are warranted to evaluate the long-term effects of protein content on body composition and cardiometabolic risk during weight-loss programmes.

Other dietary components

Alcohol consumption should be limited to the current healthy drinking guidelines (21 units per week for men, 14 for women) or below, and salt intake to <6 g/day.

Specific diets

A sensible dietary programme, with the potential for success and minimal risk, includes some essential components. It should be well-balanced, moderately energy-restricted and nutritionally adequate to satisfy all macro- and micronutrient needs. It must be individualized, taking into consideration the patient's medical, social and cultural background. Wherever possible, food choices should try to meet the individual's tastes and preferences, with practical plans based on readily obtainable and socially acceptable foods. Finally, the programme must promote long-lasting changes in eating patterns that are conducive to improvement in overall health, and emphasize the need for permanent behavioural change.

Conventional low-calorie diets

These diets provide all essential micro- and macronutrients, and can therefore be applied in most patients with routine monitoring. The guidelines devised by Departments of Health in several Western countries (Table 16.4) define a conventional low-calorie diet as containing not more than 30% of total energy intake in the form of fat; it should be rich in complex carbohydrate and fibre, through increased intake of whole-grain cereals, vegetables and fruits (Shah et al., 1994). Typically, these diets have an energy content of 1200–1800 kcal/day

(4.8–7.2 MJ/day). Because energy requirements vary widely between subjects, it is best to estimate an individual's total energy requirements and then to subtract a chosen amount of energy – usually around 600 kcal/day (2.4 MJ/day). This energy deficit mobilizes triglyceride preferentially and mostly spares lean tissue and body protein. Weight loss is generally 0.5 kg per week initially.

Traditionally, the calorie deficit has been achieved mainly through reducing the dietary fat content. A comprehensive meta-analysis of 28 trials found that a 10% reduction in fat intake alone resulted in an average weight loss of 2.9 kg over six months (Bray and Popkin, 1998). Another meta-analysis pooled data from 16 studies comparing free consumption of low-fat diets with controls who followed their habitual diet or a free medium-fat diet; this found that reducing dietary fat without restricting total energy intake prevented weight gain in subjects of normal weight and produced weight loss in overweight subjects (Astrup et al., 2000). This conclusion is obviously relevant for public health campaigns to prevent overweight and obesity (Chapter 22).

Very low-calorie diets (VLCD)

These are diets defined as containing less than 800 kcal/day (3.4 kJ/day). They were devised in the 1920s to achieve larger and more rapid short-term weight loss than standard energy-restricted diets, while aiming to avoid the dangers and adverse effects of total fasting (National Task Force on the Prevention and Treatment of Obesity, 1993). VLCD can produce rapid weight losses. With good compliance, women lose on average 1.5–2 kg/week and men 2–2.5 kg/week, with an average weight loss of 20 kg over 12 weeks – as compared with an average weight loss of 8.5 kg over 20–24 weeks on a conventional low-calorie diet (Wadden, 1993). A weight loss of 1–2 kg/week is recommended during a VLCD, because faster loss suggests excessive breakdown of lean tissue, which could result in depletion of visceral tissue proteins, particularly detrimental in the case of the heart (Kanders and Blackburn, 1994). The standard duration of treatment with a VLCD is 12–16 weeks.

Although VLCD can produce greater initial weight loss than conventional low-calorie diets, this is not maintained over the long-term

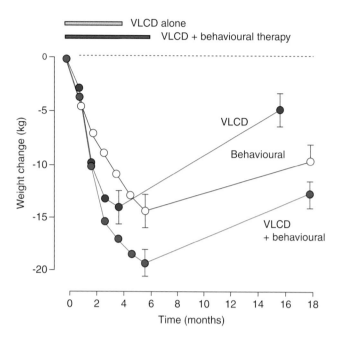

Figure 16.4 Weight loss achieved by a VLCD alone, behavioural therapy alone, and the two combined. Note the rapid weight regain after the end of the VLCD, and the enhanced weight loss and delayed regain when VLCD was supported by behavioural therapy. From Kanders and Blackburn (1994), in G.L. Blackburn and B.S. Kanders (eds). *Obesity: Pathophysiology, Psychology and Treatment*. Chapman & Hall, New York, USA, with permission of the editors.

(>1 year) because subjects tend to regain more weight after the VLCD ends (Metges and Barth, 2000) (Figure 16.4). VLCD alone are of comparable efficacy to behavioural therapy, but using the two together achieves significantly greater weight loss and delays weight regain (Figure 16.4). This emphasizes the importance of reinforcing lifestyle modification in VLCD programmes to promote long-term weight control (Kanders and Blackburn, 1994).

Current indications and contraindications for the use of VLCD are shown in Table 16.5. VLCD may be suitable for some patients with a BMI >30 kg/m² (or a BMI >27 kg/m² with significant comorbidities), who require rapid weight loss for medical reasons such as elective surgery or respiratory problems (National Task Force on the Prevention and Treatment of Obesity, 1993). At least in the short term, VLCD improve arterial hypertension (Eliahou *et al.*, 1992), lipoprotein profiles (Parenti *et al.*, 1992; Bryson *et al.*, 1996) and insulin sensitivity (Eliahou *et al.*, 1992). However, VLCD are not without risk. These diets may not contain all the essential nutrients in sufficient quantities, and rapid weight loss is potentially harmful because of enhanced

protein catabolism and electrolytic imbalance. Moreover, gallstone formation may be precipitated because the bile becomes supersaturated with cholesterol (Kanders and Blackburn, 1994). VLCD are therefore contraindicated in patients with significant heart disease (Fisler, 1992), cholelithiasis or cholecystitis (Anonymous, 2000), or renal failure (Pi-Sunyer, 1993). Relative contraindications include reduced bone density (Langlois *et al.*, 1996) and hyperuricaemia and clinical gout (Wadden, 1993). VLCD are also inappropriate for infants and children, elderly patients, and for pregnant or lactating women (Kanders and Blackburn, 1994). Common complaints include fatigue, dizziness, weakness, cold intolerance, muscle cramping, headaches, constipation, gastrointestinal distress, hair loss and dry skin.

Given the narrow margin for adequacy of nutrient and energy intake and the potential for serious side effects, VLCD should only be used when the patient can be carefully screened and monitored by an experienced physician (National Task Force on the Prevention and Treatment of Obesity, 1993; Wadden, 1993). Close medical supervision should include regular questioning

Table 16.5   Indications and contraindications for very low calorie diets (VLCD).

Indications

- BMI >30 kg/m^2 (or BMI >27 kg/m^2 with significant comorbidities), requiring rapid weight loss for medical reasons (e.g. elective surgery)
- Prior attempt with conventional low-calorie diet programme
- Commitment to close medical monitoring
- Start of simultaneous education on need for major lifestyle changes

Contraindications

- Pregnancy or lactation
- ≥65 or ≤12 years of age
- History of diabetic ketoacidosis
- Recent myocardial infarction (within previous 6 months)
- Active cardiac disease: arrhythmia, unstable angina, congestive heart failure
- Cerebrovascular disease
- Significantly impaired liver or renal function
- Malignancy
- Protein-wasting diseases (e.g. Cushing's disease, lupus erythematosus)
- Drug therapy causing protein wasting (e.g. steroids)
- History of eating and/or addictive disorders (e.g. bulimia, binge eating, alcoholism, drug abuse)
- Severe psychiatric disease
- Porphyria
- Cholelithiasis or cholecystitis
- Active or previous gout
- Electrolyte imbalances

about side effects, checking of body weight (and ideally body composition: see Chapter 3), blood pressure, heart rate, ECG and blood electrolytes. Patients taking medication for hypertension or diabetes should be carefully monitored because their regimen will probably need to be adjusted.

Other diets

Many diets, some obscure and imaginative, have been introduced over the years. These unconventional diets include the cabbage diet (also known as the Weight Watchers drop diet (Kron, 1996)), the Zone diet (Sears, 2000), the Sugar-Busters diet (Steward *et al.*, 1998), and the Atkins diet (Atkins, 1998). The key principles, claims and features of some popular diets are summarized in Table 16.6.

Many fad diets are aggressively marketed, with impressive but unsubstantiated claims that they produce prompt and substantial weight reduction and/or selectively remove fat from specific anatomical sites. Most have never been adequately evaluated for safety and efficacy in well-designed clinical studies. Weight can be lost if most of these diets are followed, simply because total energy intake is reduced below habitual intake. Several are very low in fat content, with <20% of energy intake from fat (e.g. the Ornish, Pritikin, Scarsdale, F-Plan, Rice and cabbage diets) and these drastically reduce total energy intake. Some have monotonous diet plans which, if followed, would be expected to lead to reduced energy intake because of the lack of dietary variety (see Chapter 8); examples are the cabbage and grapefruit diets. Others promote unusual food combinations or eating patterns (e.g. to avoid mixing proteins and carbohydrates), which are unfounded on any scientific evidence (e.g. the Zone and the

Table 16.6 Some popular diets and their key principles and features.

Diet	Principles and 'claims'	Key features
Ornish	Very low fat (<20%)	Omit oils, fats, nuts, refined CHO
		Avoid meat, poultry, fish
		Allow fat-free dairy products, egg whites
		Free fruit, vegetables, grain
Pritikin	Reduces whole-meal energy content	Avoid 'forbidden' fat
	Very low fat (<20%)	Allow pasta, potatoes, rice, fruit, poultry
Hip and Thigh	Very low fat (15–20%)	Omit oils, fats, nuts, seeds
	Varied meal plans	Allow fat-free dairy products, lean meat, starches
	Provides 1200 kcal/d	Free vegetables
	'Specific decrease in gluteofemoral fat'	
Scarsdale	Specific macronutrient proportions	High protein (43%); lean meat, fish
	Low fat (23%)	Moderate CHO (35%)
	Provides 1000 kcal/d	
F-Plan	High fibre (>35 g/d)	Free whole grains, baked potatoes, fruit, vegetables
	Provides 1250 kcal/d	
Rice	Rice and lacto-vegetarian	Rice, with other food items
	Very low fat (<5 g/d)	Low protein intake
		Limit salt intake
Weight Watchers	Calorie counting to limit total energy intake	Wholesome foods, including branded products
		Online calorie counting system
		Peer and mentor support, weekly meetings
Atkins	High fat	Free fat-rich foods
	Ketogenic	Limit CHO: <20 g/d initially, increasing to <100 g/d for maintenance
	Low CHO	
South Beach	'Healthy version of Atkins'	Similar to Atkins
	High fat; ketogenic	Allows more 'good' (low GI) CHO
	Low CHO	Eat until satisfied
Cabbage	7-day plan 'for rapid weight loss'	Cabbage and vegetable soup
	Very low fat	Limit meat, fish, fruit, brown rice
	High CHO, low protein	Omit alcohol, fizzy drinks
		High salt
Grapefruit	12-day plan 'for rapid weight loss'	Free grapefruit, with red onions, peppers, cabbage, carrots
	Very high CHO	Avoid white onions, potatoes, celery, meat, dairy products
	Low fat, low protein	

(continued)

Table 16.6   (*Continued*)

Diet	Principles and 'claims'	Key features
3-hour	Eating 3-hourly gives 'consistent blood sugar and heightened metabolism'	
	Decreases portion size, not calorie counting	Eat meals 3-hourly
		Always combine different food groups
		Allow junk foods
		Drink 8 glasses of water per day
Sugar Busters	'Cut toxic sugar to trim fat'	Allow stone-ground grains, high-fibre vegetables, some fruits
	Very high fat	Omit all refined sugars, flour, white rice, potatoes, corn
	Provides 1200 kcal/d	
Zone	High protein (40%)	All meals follow 40:30:30 proportions
	Fixed proportions of CHO (30%) and fat (30%)	Branded products (40:30:30) available
Rosedale	High fat	Allow fibrous green vegetables
	Very low CHO	Omit starches (for 3 weeks), bananas, oranges, grapes, potatoes
	Low protein	
	'Controls leptin'	
Hollywood	'Miracle juice to detoxify the body'	Juice containing fruits, antioxidants, vitamins, minerals
Beverly Hills	'Special foods contain enzymes that stop foods turning into fat'	
	Very low calorie	Fruit-only and vegetable-only days
	Provides 800 kcal/d	'Conscious combining' of different food types
	Low protein	

Notes: CHO: carbohydrate. Macronutrient contents are expressed as % of total daily energy intake.

3-hour diets). Several will inevitably lead to nutritional deficiencies (e.g. the Hollywood and Beverly Hills diets), while those that exclude basic food groups or induce ketogenesis may involve significant long-term health risks. Those that cannot currently be recommended because of potential health hazards include the Scarsdale, Pritikin, Atkins and Beverly Hills diets).

The Atkins diet can be appealing to obese patients, because there is rapid weight loss without hunger sensation during the first and most restrictive phase of the programme. This is probably because the ketones generated by the high-fat, low-carbohydrate diet tend to suppress appetite; the satiating effect of the high protein intake and/or limited food choices may also decrease energy intake. Also, as with VLCD, some of the initial weight loss is probably related to severe carbohydrate restriction, which depletes glycogen stores leading to excretion of glycogen-associated water.

The Atkins diet is not nutritionally balanced and is associated with ketosis, constipation, headaches and general fatigue. Other side effects include halitosis, muscle cramps and rashes (Metges and Barth, 2000; Steffen and Nettleton, 2006). Furthermore, this diet increases the protein load on the kidneys and induces mild acidosis, which can result in loss of bone mineral (Metges and Barth, 2000; Steffen and Nettleton, 2006). A systematic review of low-carbohydrate diets found that the weight loss achieved by the Atkins diet is related to the duration of the diet and the overall restriction

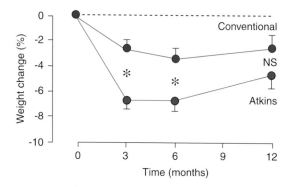

Figure 16.5 Weight loss during the Atkins diet (high fat, low carbohydrate) compared with a conventional weight management diet (low fat). Differences between the two interventions: * − $p < 0.05$; NS – not significant. From Foster *et al.* (2003), with permission of the editor of the *New England Journal of Medicine*.

of energy intake, but not to the restriction of carbohydrates (Astrup, Meinert Larsen and Harper, 2004). Two groups have reported longer-term randomized studies that compared instruction in the low-carbohydrate diet with a low-fat calorie-reduced diet in obese patients (Foster *et al.*, 2003; Stern *et al.*, 2004). Both trials showed better weight loss on the low-carbohydrate diet after 6 months, but no difference after 12 months (Figure 16.5).

Comparison of the Atkins, Ornish, Weight Watchers and Zone diets has shown that the amount of weight loss at one year for each diet was related to self-reported dietary adherence level but not to the type of diet (Dansinger *et al.*, 2005). All four diets significantly reduced the LDL/HDL cholesterol ratio by approximately 10%, with no significant effects on blood pressure or glucose, further suggesting that these effects are not related to decreased energy intake and not specifically to carbohydrate restriction. Longitudinal epidemiological studies have shown significantly lower risk of cardiovascular disease, stroke, cancer and other conditions associated with consumption of fruits, vegetables and whole-grains, which are noticeably reduced in low-carbohydrate diets (Steffen and Nettleton, 2006). Recent studies report that low-fat diets may confer greater cardiovascular protection than low-carbohydrate diets, with more favourable effects on endothelial function and metabolic risk markers (Phillips *et al.*, 2008; Tay *et al.*, 2008).

Long-term studies are needed to measure changes in nutritional status, body composition, kidney enzymes and markers of bone metabolism during the low-carbohydrate diets, as well as to assess fasting and postprandial cardiovascular risk factors and adverse effects. With the currently available information, low-carbohydrate diets should not be recommended.

Physical activity

Physical exercise is an important component of daily energy expenditure and the one that can be easily manipulated (see Chapters 3 and 7). Accordingly, exercise interventions are a crucial component of many weight-loss programmes. The goals are to improve overall health (especially metabolic and cardiovascular risk), encourage adherence to the weight-loss programme and help stabilize weight loss.

Physical exercise is a complex intervention. Therapeutic benefit may depend on the duration of exercise as well as its intensity; furthermore, different forms of exercise, such as strength training, endurance training or a combination of both, may elicit different responses. At present, most weight-loss programmes lack clarity in prescribing exercise to an individual obese patient – an issue that needs to be addressed.

Health benefits of physical exercise

Physical inactivity, which is particularly common among overweight and obese subjects, contributes to cardiovascular and metabolic risk as well as to obesity itself. For example, in the North American Nurses Health Study, the relative risk for developing type 2 diabetes among women in the highest quartile of physical activity was

26% lower than in those in the lowest activity quartile, after adjusting for age, BMI and other risk factors (Hu *et al.*, 1999).

Physical inactivity is also very costly for the healthcare system; physically inactive adults have significantly higher annual direct medical costs than those who are active (NHLBIEP, 1998; Colditz and Nettleton, 1999). Based on these observations, the direct costs of lack of physical activity, defined conservatively as absence of leisure-time physical activity, were approximately $24 billion or 2.4% of the US healthcare expenditure. Direct costs for obesity totalled $70 billion with costs attributable to inactivity and obesity accounting for 9.4% of the US healthcare expenditures.

Exercise interventions have been shown to improve cardiovascular and metabolic risk factors. A meta-analysis of 29 randomized controlled trials (involving 1533 hypertensive and normotensive participants) showed an average reduction in blood pressure of 5/3 mm Hg (systolic/diastolic) in subjects who enrolled in an aerobic exercise programme, as compared with inactive controls (Halbert *et al.*, 1997). Physical exercise has also been shown to increase insulin sensitivity (Rice *et al.*, 1999; De Feo *et al.*, 2003; Reynolds *et al.*,

2002; Goodpaster, Katsiaras and Kelley, 2003), cardiovascular fitness (Kraemer *et al.*, 1997) and fat oxidation (Van Aggel-Leijssen *et al.*, 2001; Schrauwen *et al.*, 1998; Binzen, Swan and Manore, 2001), independently of changes in body weight. In addition, visceral fat – the depot that is most strongly associated with cardiometabolic risk (Chapter 4) – can be specifically mobilized through regular physical training, independently of a change in body weight or overall body composition (Mayo, Grantham and Balasekaran, 2003; Irwin *et al.*, 2003) (Figure 16.6). Exercise is also associated with improvements in mood (Geliebter *et al.*, 1997), which may be particularly beneficial in obese patients given their increased risk of depressive disorders (Chapter 14).

As little as 30 minutes of moderate activity on most, if not all, days of the week (representing a total expenditure of 1000 kcal/week) has been shown to reduce all-cause mortality by 20–30% (Rockhill *et al.*, 2001). Further reductions in risk have been observed when exercise is increased to 1–2 hours per week.

Particular attention is now being devoted to the relative importance and independence of both 'fitness' and 'fatness' as risk factors for mortality (Stevens *et al.*, 2002; Stevens *et al.*,

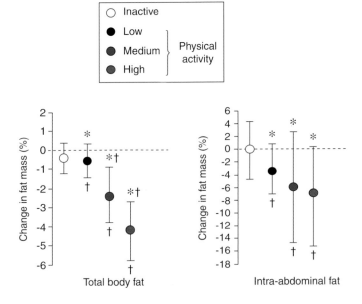

Figure 16.6 The effects of physical activity on total body and visceral fat mass. Both are mobilised in proportion to the average duration of physical activity per week during the weight-loss programme. Low, intermediate and high levels were <135 min/week, 136–195 min/week and >196 min/week, respectively, of moderate-intensity sport. Differences from baseline: * − $p < 0.05$; differences from inactive group: † − $p < 0.05$. From Irwin *et al.* (2003), with permission of the editor of *JAMA*.

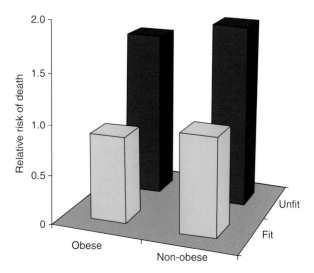

Figure 16.7 The interactions between 'fatness' and fitness in relation to all-cause mortality. Obesity was defined as a BMI >30 kg/m² and fitness as exceeding 9 minutes on a graded treadmill exercise test. From Pedersen (2007), with permission of the editor of the *Scandinavian Journal of Medicine and Science in Sports*.

2004; Pedersen, 2007; Sui *et al.*, 2007). Both fatness and poor fitness are predictors of premature mortality from all causes and from cardiovascular disease in men and women (Stevens *et al.*, 2002). Increasing levels of physical activity (whether self-reported or measured objectively) are associated with decreases in all-causes mortality, independently of body mass index (Stevens *et al.*, 2004; Pedersen, 2007). Being fit reduces, but does not completely reverse, the increased risk associated with excess adiposity (Figure 16.7). In older adults, poor fitness has been also shown to be a significant mortality predictor, independent of overall or abdominal adiposity (Sui *et al.*, 2007).

Figure 16.8 illustrates the 'physical activity pyramid' representing current recommendations for decreasing sedentarism and increasing both everyday energy expenditure and recreational physical activities. Practical exercise guidelines

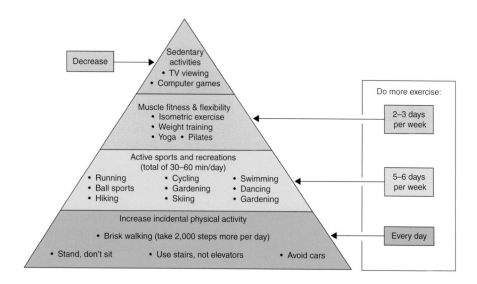

Figure 16.8 The 'pyramid' of physical activity recommendations for a healthy lifestyle.

Table 16.7 Summary of the current recommendations for increased physical exercise according to therapeutic goal.

For general health benefits:

- 30 minutes of moderate-intensity physical activity on most days of the week

- spread physical activity over at least 3 days per week, with no more than 2 consecutive days without exercise

- at least 150 minutes of moderate aerobic activity (or at least 90 minutes of vigorous activity) per week are needed to improve cardiorespiratory fitness, weight control and glycaemic control in diabetic subjects

To prevent weight gain and obesity:

- 60 minutes of moderate to vigorous activity on most days of the week

- activity can be spread through the day in bouts of 5–15 minutes

For maintaining weight loss:

- 60–90 minutes of moderate to vigorous activity each day

- more exercise may be needed to maintain substantial weight loss

for different indications – general health benefits, prevention of obesity and maintenance of weigh loss – are shown in Table 16.7.

Physical exercise in obesity management

The effect of exercise on body weight regulation is not solely explained by the increase in energy expenditure during exercise itself. Increases in energy expenditure also occur during the post-exercise recovery period (measured as excess post-exercise oxygen consumption) and may induce a short-term rise in basal metabolic rate for over 24 hours (Maehlum *et al.*, 1986; Borsheim and Bahr, 2003). Even though metabolic rate returns to baseline levels more rapidly in trained individuals (Frey, Byrnes and Mazzeo, 1993; Short and Sedlock, 1997), regular exercise bouts may produce small elevations in resting metabolic rate (Sjodin *et al.*, 1996; Melby *et al.*, 1993). By contrast, others have observed a decrease in resting metabolic rate with exercise training (Horton *et al.*, 1945; Westerterp *et al.*, 1994). Speakman and Selman (2003) have suggested

that down-regulation of uncoupling-protein 3 in muscle – perhaps to enhance mechanical efficiency during physical activity – is a possible reason for the apparent decline in resting metabolic rate. In addition, exercise training promotes skeletal muscle growth (Ryan, 2000), with strength training being particularly effective.

Many weight-loss programmes recommend that obese patients should train at a relatively low intensity in order to lose fat preferentially (so-called 'fat burner' regimens). This recommendation is based on the observation that fat oxidation declines progressively in favour of carbohydrate oxidation with increasing exercise intensity (Venables, Achten and Jeukendrup, 2005; see Chapter 3). However, despite the relative fall in fat oxidation at higher exercise intensities, the absolute quantity of fat oxidized may increase with the amount of work done. Thus, contrary to current assumptions, higher-intensity exercise might be more effective in obese patients, providing that exercise intensity is not limited by orthopaedic, cardiopulmonary or other health considerations. Furthermore, medium- to high-intensity exercise may be more effective in maintaining the increase in energy expenditure after the exercise ends (see above).

Prevention of overweight and obesity may require less exercise than its treatment (see Chapter 22). Recent research indicates that the energy expenditure equivalent to walking 6–7 miles/week (~30 min/day) appears to be a threshold level that prevents weight gain (Slentz *et al.*, 2004), although others have suggested that greater physical activity may be required (Sternfeld *et al.*, 2004). More physical activity (perhaps 60–90 min/day) than the current recommendation of 30 min/day may be necessary to maintain weight loss in people with a history of overweight and obesity (Erlichman, Kerbey and James, 2002; Fogelholm and Kukkonen-Harjula, 2000; Jeffery *et al.*, 2003; Jakicic *et al.*, 2003; Saris *et al.*, 2003).

Unfortunately, there is large discrepancy between these recommendations and real life. An American cross-sectional survey in 1996 showed that 25% of men and 43% of women reported trying to lose weight in the previous year, but that only 20% of these had followed the recommended nutritional and exercise strategies (Serdula *et al.*, 1999).

Physical exercise enhances weight loss when combined with dietary interventions. A meta-analysis of the effect of exercise, with or without dieting, on the body composition of overweight subjects found that men lost a further 3 kg over a 30-week period and women an additional 1.4 kg over 12 weeks (Garrow and Summerbell, 1995). Regular physical exercise may also help to maintain weight loss after dietary and other interventions. One potential mechanism is by offsetting the usual decline in resting metabolic rate following the inevitable reduction in fat-free mass that occurs in parallel with a fall in fat mass (Menozzi *et al.*, 2000). The reduction in fat-free mass varies between different dietary interventions, depending on macronutrient composition and energy content (Layman *et al.*, 2003; Farnsworth *et al.*, 2003), and cannot fully explain the reduction in resting metabolic rate (Torbay, Baba and Sawaya, 2002; Van Aggel-Leijssen *et al.*, 2002). Concomitant neuroendocrine disturbances may also be involved, such as falls in leptin levels (Doucet *et al.*, 2000; Harper *et al.*, 2002), thyroid status (Pelletier *et al.*, 2002) and sympathetic nervous system activity (Rosenbaum *et al.*, 2000). It is still unclear whether physical exercise can completely prevent the reduction in resting metabolic rate with weight loss. One study reported an increase in resting metabolic rate following strength training (Byrne and Wilmore, 2001), whereas another showed no change (Wilmore *et al.*, 1999), and two others found a decline (Van Aggel-Leijssen *et al.*, 2002; Byrne and Wilmore, 2001).

Exercise training without changes in energy intake produces rather small changes in body weight, although it can modify body composition. A substantial amount of exercise would be required if this were the sole strategy to decrease body fat. However, loss of weight and specifically of fat, can be promoted by the combination of aerobic exercise with a reduced-energy diet, and the beneficial effects of exercise may be explained in part by better maintenance of fat-free mass.

References

Adams, T.D., Gress, R.E., Smith, S.C. *et al.* (2007) Long-term mortality after gastric bypass surgery. *The New England Journal of Medicine*, **357**, 753–61.

Adamson, A.J. and Mathers, J.C. (2004) Effecting dietary change. *Proceedings of the Nutrition Society*, **63**, 537–47.

Albright, C.L., Cohen, S., Gibbons, L. *et al.* (2000) Incorporating physical activity advice into primary care: physician-delivered advice within the activity counseling trial. *American Journal of Preventive Medicine*, **18**, 225–34.

Andersen, T., Gluud, C., Franzmann, M.B. and Christoffersen, P. (1991) Hepatic effects of dietary weight loss in morbidly obese subjects. *Journal of Hepatology*, **12**, 224–9.

Anonymous (2000) Obesity: preventing and managing the global epidemic. Report of a WHO consultation. *World Health Organization: Technical Report Series*, **894**, i-253.

Astrup, A. (2001) Healthy lifestyles in Europe: prevention of obesity and type II diabetes by diet and physical activity. *Public Health Nutrition*, **4**, 499–515.

Astrup, A., Meinert Larsen, T. and Harper, A. (2004) Atkins and other low-carbohydrate diets: hoax or an effective tool for weight loss? *Lancet*, **364**, 897–9.

Astrup, A., Ryan, L., Grunwald, G.K. *et al.* (2000) The role of dietary fat in body fatness: evidence from a preliminary meta-analysis of ad libitum low-fat dietary intervention studies. *The British Journal of Nutrition*, **83** (Suppl 1), S25–32.

Aylwin, S. and Al-Zaman, Y. (2008) Emerging concepts in the medical and surgical treatment of obesity. *Frontiers of Hormone Research*, **36**, 229–59.

Baba, N.H., Sawaya, S., Torbay, N. *et al.* (1999) High protein vs high carbohydrate hypoenergetic diet for the treatment of obese hyperinsulinemic subjects. *International Journal of Obesity and Related Metabolic Disorders*, **23**, 1202–6.

Barvaux, V.A., Aubert, G. and Rodenstein, D.O. (2000) Weight loss as a treatment for obstructive sleep apnoea. *Sleep Medicine Reviews*, **4**, 435–52.

Binzen, C.A., Swan, P.D. and Manore, M.M. (2001) Postexercise oxygen consumption and substrate use after resistance exercise in women. *Medicine and Science in Sports and Exercise*, **33**, 932–8.

Bisschop, P.H., de, M.J., Ackermans, M.T. *et al.* (2001) Dietary fat content alters insulin-mediated glucose metabolism in healthy men. *The American Journal of Clinical Nutrition*, **73**, 554–9.

Borkman, M., Campbell, L.V., Chisholm, D.J. and Storlien, L.H. (1991) Comparison of the effects on insulin sensitivity of high carbohydrate and high fat diets in normal subjects. *The Journal of Clinical Endocrinology and, Metabolism*, **72**, 432–7.

Borkman, M., Storlien, L.H., Pan, D.A. *et al.* (1993) The relation between insulin sensitivity and the fatty-acid composition of skeletal-muscle phospholipids. *The New England Journal of Medicine*, **328**, 238–44.

Borsheim, E. and Bahr, R. (2003) Effect of exercise intensity, duration and mode on post-exercise oxygen consumption. *Sports Medicine*, **33**, 1037–60.

Bray, G.A. and Popkin, B.M. (1998) Dietary fat intake does affect obesity. *The American Journal of Clinical Nutrition*, **68**, 1157–73.

Bryson, J.M., King, S.E., Burns, C.M. et al. (1996) Changes in glucose and lipid metabolism following weight loss produced by a very low calorie diet in obese subjects. *International Journal of Obesity and Related Metabolic Disorders*, **20**, 338–45.

Byrne, H.K. and Wilmore, J.H. (2001) The effects of a 20-week exercise training program on resting metabolic rate in previously sedentary, moderately obese women. *International Journal of Sport Nutrition and Exercise Metabolism*, **11**, 15–31.

Capron, J.P., Delamarre, J., Dupas, J.L. et al. (1982) Fasting in obesity: another cause of liver injury with alcoholic hyaline? *Digestive Diseases and Sciences*, **27**, 265–8.

Carson, J.L., Ruddy, M.E., Duff, A.E. et al. (1994) The effect of gastric bypass surgery on hypertension in morbidly obese patients. *Archives of Internal Medicine*, **154**, 193–200.

Charuzi, I., Ovnat, A., Peiser, J. et al. (1985) The effect of surgical weight reduction on sleep quality in obesity-related sleep apnea syndrome. *Surgery*, **97**, 535–8.

Colditz, G.A. (1999) Economic costs of obesity and inactivity. *Medicine and Science in Sports and Exercise*, **11** (31 Suppl), S663–7.

Coulston, A.M. and Rock, C.L. (1994) Popular diets and use of moderate caloric restriction for the treatment of obesity, in *Obesity: Pathophysiology, Psychology, and Treatment* (eds G.L. Blackburn and B.S. Kanders), Chapman & Hall, New York, USA, pp. 185–95.

Coutinho, W.F. (2007) The obese older female patient: CV risk and the SCOUT study. *International Journal of Obesity (London)*, **2** (31 Suppl), S26–30.

Dansinger, M.L., Gleason, J.A., Griffith, J.L. et al. (2005) Comparison of the Atkins, Ornish, Weight Watchers, and Zone diets for weight loss and heart disease risk reduction: a randomized trial. *The Journal of the American Medical Association*, **293**, 43–53.

Dattilo, A.M. and Kris-Etherton, P.M. (1992) Effects of weight reduction on blood lipids and lipoproteins: a meta-analysis. *The American Journal of Clinical Nutrition*, **56**, 320–8.

de Jonge, L. and Bray, G.A. (1997) The thermic effect of food and obesity: a critical review. *Obesity Research*, **5**, 622–31.

De Feo, P., Di Loreto, C., Lucidi, P. et al. (2003) Metabolic response to exercise. *Journal of Endocrinological Investigation*, **26**, 851–4.

Demling, R.H. and DeSanti, L. (2000) Effect of a hypocaloric diet, increased protein intake and resistance training on lean mass gains and fat mass loss in overweight police officers. *Annals of Nutrition and Metabolism*, **44**, 21–9.

Doucet, E., St Pierre, S., Almeras, N. et al. (2000) Changes in energy expenditure and substrate oxidation resulting from weight loss in obese men and women: is there an important contribution of leptin? *The Journal of Clinical Endocrinology and Metabolism*, **85**, 1550–6.

Eliahou, H.E., Laufer, J., Blau, A. and Shulman, L. (1992) Effect of low-calorie diets on the sympathetic nervous system, body weight, and plasma insulin in overweight hypertension. *The American Journal of Clinical Nutrition*, **56**, 175S–8S.

Eriksson, S., Eriksson, K.F. and Bondesson, L. (1986) Nonalcoholic steatohepatitis in obesity: a reversible condition. *Acta Medica Scandinavica*, **220**, 83–8.

Erlichman, J., Kerbey, A.L. and James, W.P. (2002) Physical activity and its impact on health outcomes. Paper 2: Prevention of unhealthy weight gain and obesity by physical activity: an analysis of the evidence. *Obesity Reviews*, **3**, 273–87.

Farnsworth, E., Luscombe, N.D., Noakes, M. et al. (2003) Effect of a high-protein, energy-restricted diet on body composition, glycemic control, and lipid concentrations in overweight and obese hyperinsulinemic men and women. *The American Journal of Clinical Nutrition*, **78**, 31–9.

Feskens, E.J., Loeber, J.G. and Kromhout, D. (1994) Diet and physical activity as determinants of hyperinsulinemia: the Zutphen Elderly Study. *American Journal of Epidemiology*, **140**, 350–60.

Fisler, J.S. (1992) Cardiac effects of starvation and semistarvation diets: safety and mechanisms of action. *The American Journal of Clinical Nutrition*, **56**, 230S–4S.

Fogelholm, M. and Kukkonen-Harjula, K. (2000) Does physical activity prevent weight gain – a systematic review. *Obesity Reviews*, **1**, 95–111.

Foley, E.F., Benotti, P.N., Borlase, B.C. et al. (1992) Impact of gastric restrictive surgery on hypertension in the morbidly obese. *American Journal of Surgery*, **163**, 294–7.

Formiguera, X. and Canton, A. (2004) Obesity: epidemiology and clinical aspects. *Best Practice and Research Clinical Gastroenterology*, **18**, 1125–46.

Foster, G.D., Wyatt, H.R., Hill, J.O. et al. (2003) A randomized trial of a low-carbohydrate diet for obesity. *The New England Journal of Medicine*, **348**, 2082–90.

Foster-Powell, K., Holt, S.H. and Brand-Miller, J.C. (2002) International table of glycemic index and glycemic load values: 2002. *The American Journal of Clinical Nutrition*, **76**, 5–56.

Frey, G.C., Byrnes, W.C. and Mazzeo, R.S. (1993) Factors influencing excess postexercise oxygen consumption in trained and untrained women. *Metabolism: Clinical and Experimental*, **42**, 822–8.

Fried, M., Hainer, V., Basdevant, A. et al. (2007) Interdisciplinary European guidelines on surgery of severe obesity. *International Journal of Obesity (London)*, **31**, 569–77.

Garett, N.A., Brasure, M., Schmitz, K.H. et al. (2004) Physical inactivity: direct cost to a health plan. *American Journal of Preventive Medicine*, **27**, 304–9.

Garg, A., Grundy, S.M. and Unger, R.H. (1992) Comparison of effects of high and low carbohydrate diets on plasma lipoproteins and insulin sensitivity in patients with mild NIDDM. *Diabetes*, **41**, 1278–85.

Garrow, J.S. and Summerbell, C.D. (1995) Meta-analysis: effect of exercise, with or without dieting, on the body composition of overweight subjects. *European Journal of Clinical Nutrition*, **49**, 1–10.

Geliebter, A., Maher, M.M., Gerace, L. *et al.* (1997) Effects of strength or aerobic training on body composition, resting metabolic rate, and peak oxygen consumption in obese dieting subjects. *The American Journal of Clinical Nutrition*, **66**, 557–63.

Giacco, R., Clemente, G., Busiello, L. *et al.* (2004) Insulin sensitivity is increased and fat oxidation after a high-fat meal is reduced in normal-weight healthy men with strong familial predisposition to overweight. *International Journal of Obesity and Related Metabolic Disorders*, **28**, 342–8.

Golay, A. and Bobbioni, E. (1997) The role of dietary fat in obesity. *International Journal of Obesity and Related Metabolic Disorders*, **21** (Suppl 3), S2–11.

Goodpaster, B.H., Katsiaras, A. and Kelley, D.E. (2003) Enhanced fat oxidation through physical activity is associated with improvements in insulin sensitivity in obesity. *Diabetes*, **52**, 2191–7.

Halbert, J.A., Silagy, C.A., Finucane, P. *et al.* (1997) The effectiveness of exercise training in lowering blood pressure: a meta-analysis of randomised controlled trials of 4 weeks or longer. *Journal of Human Hypertension*, **11**, 641–9.

Harper, M.E., Dent, R., Monemdjou, S. *et al.* (2002) Decreased mitochondrial proton leak and reduced expression of uncoupling protein 3 in skeletal muscle of obese diet-resistant women. *Diabetes*, **51**, 2459–66.

Harris, W.S. (1997) n-3 fatty acids and serum lipoproteins: animal studies. *The American Journal of Clinical Nutrition*, **65**, 1611S–6S.

Holt, S., Brand, J., Soveny, C. and Hansky, J. (1992) Relationship of satiety to postprandial glycaemic, insulin and cholecystokinin responses. *Appetite*, **18**, 129–41.

Horton, T.J., Drougas, H.J., Sharp, T.A. *et al.* (1945) Energy balance in endurance-trained female cyclists and untrained controls. *Journal of Applied Physiology (Bethesda, MD, 1985)*, **76**, 1936–40.

Hu, F.B., Sigal, R.J., Rich-Edwards, J.W. *et al.* (1999) Walking compared with vigorous physical activity and risk of type 2 diabetes in women: a prospective study. *The Journal of the American Medical Association*, **282**, 1433–9.

Hubert, H.B., Feinleib, M., McNamara, P.M. and Castelli, W.P. (1983) Obesity as an independent risk factor for cardiovascular disease: a 26-year follow-up of participants in the Framingham Heart Study. *Circulation*, **67**, 968–77.

Hughes, V.A., Fiatarone, M.A., Fielding, R.A. *et al.* (1995) Long-term effects of a high-carbohydrate diet and exercise on insulin action in older subjects with impaired glucose tolerance. *The American Journal of Clinical Nutrition*, **62**, 426–33.

Inokuchi, J. (2006) Insulin resistance as a membrane microdomain disorder. *Biological and Pharmaceutical Bulletin*, **29**, 1532–7.

Irwin, M.L., Yasui, Y., Ulrich, C.M. *et al.* (2003) Effect of exercise on total and intra-abdominal body fat in postmenopausal women. A. randomized controlled trial. *The Journal of the American Medical Association*, **289**, 323–30.

Jakicic, J.M., Marcus, B.H., Gallagher, K.I. *et al.* (2003) Effect of exercise duration and intensity on weight loss in overweight, sedentary women: a randomized trial. *The Journal of the American Medical Association*, **290**, 1323–30.

Jarvi, A.E., Karlstrom, B.E., Granfeldt, Y.E. *et al.* (1999) Improved glycemic control and lipid profile and normalized fibrinolytic activity on a low-glycemic index diet in type 2 diabetic patients. *Diabetes Care*, **22**, 10–8.

Jeffery, R.W., Wing, R.R., Sherwood, N.E. and Tate, D.F. (2003) Physical activity and weight loss: does prescribing higher physical activity goals improve outcome? *The American Journal of Clinical Nutrition*, **78**, 684–9.

Jenkins, A.B., Markovic, T.P., Fleury, A. and Campbell, L.V. (1997) Carbohydrate intake and short-term regulation of leptin in humans. *Diabetologia*, **40**, 348–51.

Jenkins, D.J., Wolever, T.M., Jenkins, A.L. *et al.* (1983) The glycaemic index of foods tested in diabetic patients: a new basis for carbohydrate exchange favouring the use of legumes. *Diabetologia*, **24**, 257–64.

Jenkins, D.J., Wolever, T.M., Kalmusky, J. *et al.* (1987) Low-glycemic index diet in hyperlipidemia: use of traditional starchy foods. *The American Journal of Clinical Nutrition*, **46**, 66–71.

Jéquier, E. (2002) Pathways to obesity. *International Journal of Obesity and Related Metabolic Disorders*, **26** (Suppl 2), S12–7.

Kanders, B.S. and Blackburn, G.L. (1994) Very-low-calorie diets for the treatment of obesity, in *Obesity: Pathophysiology, Psychology, and Treatment* (eds G.L. Blackburn and B.S. Kanders), Chapman & Hall, New York, USA, pp. 197–216.

Klein, S. (2001) Outcome success in obesity. *Obesity Research*, **9** (Suppl 4), 354S–8S.

Kraemer, W.J., Volek, J.S., Clark, K.L. *et al.* (1997) Physiological adaptations to a weight-loss dietary regimen and exercise programs in women. *Journal of Applied Physiology (Bethesda, MD, 1985)*, **83**, 270–9.

Langlois, J.A., Harris, T., Looker, A.C. and Madans, J. (1996) Weight change between age 50 years and old age is associated with risk of hip fracture in white women aged 67 years and older. *Archives of Internal Medicine*, **156**, 989–94.

Latner, J.D. and Schwartz, M. (1999) The effects of a high-carbohydrate, high-protein or balanced lunch upon later food intake and hunger ratings. *Appetite*, **33**, 119–28.

Layman, D.K., Boileau, R.A., Erickson, D.J. *et al.* (2003) A reduced ratio of dietary carbohydrate to protein improves body composition and blood lipid profiles during weight loss in adult women. *The Journal of Nutrition*, **133**, 411–7.

Lean, M.E., Han, T.S. and Morrison, C.E. (1995) Waist circumference as a measure for indicating need for weight management. *British Medical Journal (Clinical Research Edition)*, **311**, 158–61.

Leathwood, P. and Pollet, P. (1988) Effects of slow release carbohydrates in the form of bean flakes on the evolution of hunger and satiety in man. *Appetite*, **10**, 1–11.

Leiter, L.A., Ceriello, A., Davidson, J.A. *et al.* and International Prandial Glucose Regulation Study Group (2005) Postprandial glucose regulation: new data and new implications. *Clinical Therapeutics*, **27** (Suppl B), S42–56.

Levy, R.L., Finch, E.A., Crowell, M.D. *et al.* (2007) Behavioral intervention for the treatment of obesity: strategies and effectiveness data. *The American Journal of Gastroenterology*, **102**, 2314–21.

Ludwig, D.S., Peterson, K.E. and Gortmaker, S.L. (2001) Relation between consumption of sugar-sweetened drinks and childhood obesity: a prospective, observational analysis. *Lancet*, **357**, 505–8.

Luyckx, F.H., Desaive, C., Thiry, A. *et al.* (1998) Liver abnormalities in severely obese subjects: effect of drastic weight loss after gastroplasty. *International Journal of Obesity and Related Metabolic Disorders*, **22**, 222–6.

Maehlum, S., Grandmontagne, M., Newsholme, E.A. and Sejersted, O.M. (1986) Magnitude and duration of excess postexercise oxygen consumption in healthy young subjects. *Metabolism: Clinical and Experimental*, **35**, 425–9.

Manson, J.E., Skerrett, P.J., Greenland, P. and VanItallie, T.B. (2004) The escalating pandemics of obesity and sedentary lifestyle. A call to action for clinicians. *Archives of Internal Medicine*, **164**, 249–58.

Manson, J.E., Willett, W.C., Stampfer, M.J. *et al.* (1995) Body weight and mortality among women. *The New England Journal of Medicine*, **333**, 677–85.

Maron, D.J., Fair, J.M. and Haskell, W.L. (1991) Saturated fat intake and insulin resistance in men with coronary artery disease. The Stanford Coronary Risk Intervention Project Investigators and Staff. *Circulation*, **84**, 2020–7.

Marshall, J.A., Bessesen, D.H. and Hamman, R.F. (1997) High saturated fat and low starch and fibre are associated with hyperinsulinaemia in a non-diabetic population: the San Luis Valley Diabetes Study. *Diabetologia*, **40**, 430–8.

Mayer, E.J., Newman, B., Quesenberry, C.P., Jr and Selby, J.V. (1993) Usual dietary fat intake and insulin concentrations in healthy women twins. *Diabetes Care*, **16**, 1459–69.

Mayer-Davis, E.J., Monaco, J.H., Hoen, H.M. *et al.* (1997) Dietary fat and insulin sensitivity in a tri-ethnic population: the role of obesity. The Insulin Resistance Atherosclerosis Study (IRAS). *The American Journal of Clinical Nutrition*, **65**, 79–87.

Mayo, M.J., Grantham, J.R. and Balasekaran, G. (2003) Exercise-induced weight loss preferentially reduces abdominal fat. *Medicine and Science in Sports and Exercise*, **35**, 207–13.

Melby, C., Scholl, C., Edwards, G. and Bullough, R. (1993) Effect of acute resistance exercise on postexercise energy expenditure and resting metabolic rate. *Journal of Applied Physiology (Bethesda, MD, 1985)*, **75**, 1847–53.

Menozzi, R., Bondi, M., Baldini, A. *et al.* (2000) Resting metabolic rate, fat-free mass and catecholamine excretion during weight loss in female obese patients. *The British Journal of Nutrition*, **84**, 515–20.

Metges, C.C. and Barth, C.A. (2000) Metabolic consequences of a high dietary-protein intake in adulthood: assessment of the available evidence. *The Journal of Nutrition*, **130**, 886–9.

Moore, L.L., Visioni, A.J., Wilson, P.W. *et al.* (2000) Can sustained weight loss in overweight individuals reduce the risk of diabetes mellitus? *Epidemiology*, **11**, 269–73.

Mooy, J.M., Grootenhuis, P.A., de Vries H. *et al.* (1998) Determinants of specific serum insulin concentrations in a general Caucasian population aged 50 to 74 years (the Hoorn Study). *Diabetic Medicine: A Journal of the British Diabetic Association*, **15**, 45–52.

Morris, K.L. and Zemel, M.B. (1999) Glycemic index, cardiovascular disease, and obesity. *Nutrition Reviews*, **57**, 273–76.

Nair, K.S., Halliday, D. and Garrow, J.S. (1983) Thermic response to isoenergetic protein, carbohydrate or fat meals in lean and obese subjects. *Clinical Science (London, England: 1979)*, **65**, 307–12.

National Heart Lung and Blood Institute (NHLBI). The Practical Guide Identification, Evaluation, and Treatment of Overweight and Obesity in Adults. NIH Publication Number 00-4084 October 2000. Available at http://www.nhlbi.nih.gov/guidelines/obesity/prctgd_c.pdf (last accessed 14 July 2008).

NHLBIEB (National Heart, Lung, and Blood Institutes Expert Panel) (1998) Clinical Guidelines on the Identification, Evaluation, and Treatment of Overweight and Obesity in Adults – The Evidence Report. *Obesity Research*, **6** (Suppl 2), 51S–209S.

National Task Force on the Prevention and Treatment of Obesity, National Institutes of Health (1993) Very low-calorie diets. *The Journal of the American Medical Association*, **270**, 967–74.

Padwal, R.S. and Majumdar, S.R. (2007) Drug treatments for obesity: orlistat, sibutramine, and rimonabant. *Lancet*, **369**, 71–7.

Palmer, M. and Schaffner, F. (1990) Effect of weight reduction on hepatic abnormalities in overweight patients. *Gastroenterology*, **99**, 1408–13.

Pan, D.A., Lillioja, S., Milner, M.R. *et al.* (1995) Skeletal muscle membrane lipid composition is related to adiposity and insulin action. *The Journal of Clinical Investigation*, **96**, 2802–8.

Parenti, M., Babini, A.C., Cecchetto, M.E. *et al.* (1992) Lipid, lipoprotein, and apolipoprotein assessment during an 8-wk very-low-calorie diet. *The American Journal of Clinical Nutrition*, **56**, 268S–70S.

Parker, D.R., Weiss, S.T., Troisi, R. *et al.* (1993) Relationship of dietary saturated fatty acids and body habitus to serum insulin concentrations: the Normative Aging Study. *The American Journal of Clinical Nutrition*, **58**, 129–36.

Pedersen, B.K. (2007) Body mass index-independent effect of fitness and physical activity for all-cause mortality. *Scandinavian Journal of Medicine and Science in Sports*, **17**, 196–204.

Peeters, A., Barendregt, J.J., Willekens, F. *et al.* (2003) Obesity in adulthood and its consequences for life expectancy: a life-table analysis. *Annals of Internal Medicine*, **138**, 24–32.

Peeters, A., O'Brien, P.E., Laurie, C. *et al.* (2007) Substantial intentional weight loss and mortality in the severely obese. *Annals of Surgery*, **246**, 1028–33.

Pelikanova, T., Kohout, M., Valek, J. *et al.* (1989) Insulin secretion and insulin action related to the serum phospholipid fatty acid pattern in healthy men. *Metabolism: Clinical and Experimental*, **38**, 188–92.

Pelletier, C., Doucet, E., Imbeault, P. and Tremblay, A. (2002) Associations between weight loss-induced changes in plasma organochlorine concentrations, serum T(3) concentration, and resting metabolic rate. *Toxicological Sciences*, **67**, 46–51.

Phillips, S.A., Jurva, J.W., Syed, A.Q. *et al.* (2008) Benefit of low-fat over low-carbohydrate diet on endothelial health in obesity. *Hypertension*, **51**, 376–82.

Pi-Sunyer, F.X. (1993) Medical hazards of obesity. *Annals of Internal Medicine*, **119**, 655–60.

Poppitt, S.D., McCormack, D. and Buffenstein, R. (1998) Short-term effects of macronutrient preloads on appetite and energy intake in lean women. *Physiology and Behavior*, **64**, 279–85.

Pories, W.J., Swanson, M.S., MacDonald, K.G. *et al.* (1995) Who would have thought it? An operation proves to be the most effective therapy for adult-onset diabetes mellitus. *Annals of Surgery*, **222**, 339–50.

Raben, A., Andersen, H.B., Christensen, N.J. *et al.* (1994) Evidence for an abnormal postprandial response to a high-fat meal in women predisposed to obesity. *The American Journal of Physiology*, **267**, E549–59.

Raben, A., Gerholm-Larsen, L., Flint, A. *et al.* (2003) Meals with similar energy densities but rich in protein, fat, carbohydrate, or alcohol have different effects on energy expenditure and substrate metabolism but not on appetite and energy intake. *The American Journal of Clinical Nutrition*, **77**, 91–100.

Ranlov, I. and Hardt, F. (1990) Regression of liver steatosis following gastroplasty or gastric bypass for morbid obesity. *Digestion*, **47**, 208–14.

Ravussin, E. and Smith, S.R. (2002) Increased fat intake, impaired fat oxidation, and failure of fat cell proliferation result in ectopic fat storage, insulin resistance, and type 2 diabetes mellitus. *Annals of the New York Academy of Sciences*, **967**, 363–78.

Reynolds, T.H., Brown, M.D., Supiano, M.A. and Dengel, D.R. (2002) Aerobic exercise training improves insulin sensitivity independent of plasma tumor necrosis factor-alpha levels in older female hypertensives. *Metabolism: Clinical and Experimental*, **51**, 1402–6.

Rice, B., Janssen, I., Hudson, R. and Ross, R. (1999) Effects of aerobic or resistance exercise and/or diet on glucose tolerance and plasma insulin levels in obese men. *Diabetes Care*, **22**, 684–91.

Rivellese, A.A., Maffettone, A., Iovine, C. *et al.* (1996) Long-term effects of fish oil on insulin resistance and plasma lipoproteins in NIDDM patients with hypertriglyceridemia. *Diabetes Care*, **19**, 1207–13.

Rivellese, A.A., Maffettone, A., Vessby, B. *et al.* (2003) Effects of dietary saturated, monounsaturated and n-3 fatty acids on fasting lipoproteins, LDL size and post-prandial lipid metabolism in healthy subjects. *Atherosclerosis*, **167**, 149–58.

Rockhill, B., Willett, W.C., Manson, J.E. *et al.* (2001) Physical activity and mortality: a prospective study among women. *American Journal of Public Health*, **91**, 578–83.

Rosenbaum, M., Hirsch, J., Murphy, E. and Leibel, R.L. (2000) Effects of changes in body weight on carbohydrate metabolism, catecholamine excretion, and thyroid function. *The American Journal of Clinical Nutrition*, **71**, 1421–32.

Rössner, S. and Bjorvell, H. (1987) Early and late effects of weight loss on lipoprotein metabolism in severe obesity. *Atherosclerosis*, **64**, 125–30.

Rössner, S., Sjöström, L., Noack, R. *et al.* (2000) Weight loss, weight maintenance, and improved cardiovascular risk factors after 2 years treatment with orlistat for obesity. European Orlistat Obesity Study Group. *Obesity Research*, **8**, 49–61.

Ryan, A.S. (2000) Insulin resistance with aging: effects of diet and exercise. *Sports Medicine*, **30**, 327–46.

Ryttig, K.R., Flaten, H. and Rössner, S. (1997) Long-term effects of a very low calorie diet (Nutrilett) in obesity treatment. A prospective, randomized, comparison between VLCD and a hypocaloric diet + behavior modification and their combination. *International Journal of Obesity and Related Metabolic Disorders*, **21**, 574–9.

Samaha, F.F., Iqbal, N., Seshadri, P. *et al.* (2003) A low-carbohydrate as compared with a low-fat diet in severe obesity. *The New England Journal of Medicine*, **348**, 2074–81.

Saris, W.H., Astrup, A., Prentice, A.M. *et al.* (2000) Randomized controlled trial of changes in dietary carbohydrate/fat ratio and simple vs complex carbohydrates on body weight and blood lipids: the CARMEN study. The Carbohydrate Ratio Management in European National diets. *International Journal of Obesity and Related Metabolic Disorders*, **24**, 1310–8.

Saris, W.H., Blair, S.N., Van Baak, M.A. *et al.* (2003) How much physical activity is enough to prevent unhealthy weight gain? Outcome of the IASO 1st Stock Conference and consensus statement. *Obesity Reviews*, **4**, 101–14.

Sarkkinen, E., Schwab, U., Niskanen, L. *et al.* (1996) The effects of monounsaturated-fat enriched diet and polyunsaturated-fat enriched diet on lipid and glucose metabolism in subjects with impaired glucose tolerance. *European Journal of Clinical Nutrition*, **50**, 592–8.

Schrauwen, P., Lichtenbelt, W.D., Saris, W.H. and Westerterp, K.R. (1998) Fat balance in obese subjects: role of glycogen stores. *The American Journal of Physiology*, **274**, E1027–33.

Schutz, Y. (1995) Macronutrients and energy balance in obesity. *Metabolism: Clinical and Experimental*, **44**, 7–11.

Schwartz, A.R., Gold, A.R., Schubert, N. *et al.* (1991) Effect of weight loss on upper airway collapsibility in obstructive sleep apnea. *The American Review of Respiratory Disease*, **144**, 494–8.

Serdula, M.K., Mokdad, A.H., Williamson, D.F. *et al.* (1999) Prevalence of attempting weight loss and strategies for controlling weight. *The Journal of the American Medical Association*, **282**, 1353–8.

Shah, M., McGovern, P., French, S. and Baxter, J. (1994) Comparison of a low-fat, ad libitum complex-carbohydrate diet with a low-energy diet in moderately obese women. *The American Journal of Clinical Nutrition*, **59**, 980–4.

Short, K.R. and Sedlock, D.A. (1997) Excess postexercise oxygen consumption and recovery rate in trained and untrained subjects. *Journal of Applied Physiology (Bethesda, MD, 1985)*, **83**, 153–9.

Sjodin, A.M., Forslund, A.H., Westerterp, K.R. *et al.* (1996) The influence of physical activity on BMR. *Medicine and Science in Sports and Exercise*, **28**, 85–91.

Sjöström, C.D., Peltonen, M., Wedel, H. and Sjöström, L. (2000) Differentiated long-term effects of intentional weight loss on diabetes and hypertension. *Hypertension*, **36**, 20–5.

Skov, A.R., Toubro, S., Ronn, B. *et al.* (1999) Randomized trial on protein vs carbohydrate in ad libitum fat reduced diet for the treatment of obesity. *International Journal of Obesity and Related Metabolic Disorders*, **23**, 528–36.

Slentz, C.A., Duscha, B.D., Johnson, J.L. *et al.* (2004) Effects of the amount of exercise on body weight, body composition, and measures of central obesity: STRRIDE – a randomized controlled study. *Archives of Internal Medicine*, **164**, 31–9.

Speakman, J.R. and Selman, C. (2003) Physical activity and resting metabolic rate. *Proceedings of the Nutrition Society*, **62**, 621–34.

Stamler, J., Caggiula, A.W. and Grandits, G.A. (1997) Relation of body mass and alcohol, nutrient, fiber, and caffeine intakes to blood pressure in the special intervention and usual care groups in the Multiple Risk Factor Intervention Trial. *The American Journal of Clinical Nutrition*, **65**, 338S–65S.

Steffen, L.M. and Nettleton, J.A. (2006) Carbohydrates: how low can you go? *Lancet*, **367**, 880–1.

Stern, L., Iqbal, N., Seshadri, P. *et al.* (2004) The effects of low-carbohydrate versus conventional weight loss diets in severely obese adults: one-year follow-up of a randomized trial. *Annals of Internal Medicine*, **140**, 778–85.

Sternfeld, B., Wang, H., Quesenberry, C.P., Jr *et al.* (2004) Physical activity and changes in weight and waist circumference in midlife women: findings from the Study of Women's Health Across the Nation. *American Journal of Epidemiology*, **160**, 912–22.

Stevens, J., Cai, J., Evenson, K.R. and Thomas, R. (2002) Fitness and fatness as predictors of mortality from all causes and from cardiovascular disease in men and women in the lipid research clinics study. *American Journal of Epidemiology*, **156**, 832–41.

Stevens, J., Evenson, K.R., Thomas, O. *et al.* (2004) Associations of fitness and fatness with mortality in Russian and American men in the lipids research clinics study. *International Journal of Obesity and Related Metabolic Disorders*, **28**, 1463–70.

Stevens, V.J., Obarzanek, E., Cook, N.R. *et al.* (2001) Long-term weight loss and changes in blood pressure: results of the Trials of Hypertension Prevention, phase II. *Annals of Internal Medicine*, **134**, 1–11.

Stubbs, R.J., van Wyk, M.C., Johnstone, A.M. and Harbron, C.G. (1996) Breakfasts high in protein, fat or carbohydrate: effect on within-day appetite and energy balance. *European Journal of Clinical Nutrition*, **50**, 409–17.

Sugerman, H.J., Baron, P.L., Fairman, R.P. *et al.* (1988) Hemodynamic dysfunction in obesity hypoventilation syndrome and the effects of treatment with surgically induced weight loss. *Annals of Surgery*, **207**, 604–13.

Sugerman, H.J., Fairman, R.P., Sood, R.K. *et al.* (1992) Long-term effects of gastric surgery for treating respiratory insufficiency of obesity. *The American Journal of Clinical Nutrition*, **55**, 597S–601S.

Sui, X., LaMonte, M.J., Laditka, J.N. et al. (2007) Cardiorespiratory fitness and adiposity as mortality predictors in older adults. *The Journal of the American Medical Association*, **298**, 2507–16.

Summers, L.K., Fielding, B.A., Bradshaw, H.A. et al. (2002) Substituting dietary saturated fat with polyunsaturated fat changes abdominal fat distribution and improves insulin sensitivity. *Diabetologia*, **45**, 369–77.

Swinburn, B.A., Boyce, V.L., Bergman, R.N. et al. (1991) Deterioration in carbohydrate metabolism and lipoprotein changes induced by modern, high fat diet in Pima Indians and Caucasians. *The Journal of Clinical Endocrinology and, Metabolism*, **73**, 156–65.

Tate, D.F., Jackvony, E.H. and Wing, R.R. (2003) Effects of Internet behavioral counseling on weight loss in adults at risk for type 2 diabetes: a randomized trial. *The Journal of the American Medical Association*, **289**, 1833–6.

Tay, J., Brinkworth, G.D., Noakes, M. et al. (2008) Metabolic effects of weight loss on a very-low-carbohydrate diet compared with an isocaloric high-carbohydrate diet in abdominally obese subjects. *Journal of the American College of Cardiology*, **51**, 59–67.

Teixeira, P.J., Going, S.B., Sardinha, L.B. and Lohman, T.G. (2005) A. review of psychosocial pre-treatment predictors of weight control. *Obesity Reviews*, **6**, 43–65.

Torbay, N., Baba, N.H. and Sawaya, S. (2002) High protein vs high carbohydrate hypoenergetic diet in treatment of obese normoinsulinemic and hyperinsulinemic subjects. *Nutrition Research*, **22**, 587–98.

Trevisan, M., Krogh, V., Freudenheim, J. et al. (1990) Consumption of olive oil, butter, and vegetable oils and coronary heart disease risk factors. The Research Group ATS-RF2 of the Italian National Research Council. *The Journal of the American Medical Association*, **263**, 688–92.

Valtuena, S., Salas-Salvado, J. and Lorda, P.G. (1997) The respiratory quotient as a prognostic factor in weight-loss rebound. *International Journal of Obesity and Related Metabolic Disorders*, **21**, 811–17.

Van Aggel-Leijssen, D.P., Saris, W.H., Hul, G.B. and Van Baak, M.A. (2001) Short-term effects of weight loss with or without low-intensity exercise training on fat metabolism in obese men. *The American Journal of Clinical Nutrition*, **73**, 523–31.

Van Aggel-Leijssen, D.P., Saris, W.H., Hul, G.B. and Van Baak, M.A. (2002) Long-term effects of low-intensity exercise training on fat metabolism in weight-reduced obese men. *Metabolism: Clinical and Experimental*, **51**, 1003–10.

Venables, M.C., Achten, J. and Jeukendrup, A.E. (2005) Determinants of fat oxidation during exercise in healthy men and women: a cross-sectional study. *Journal of Applied Physiology (Bethesda, MD, 1985)*, **98**, 160–7.

Vessby, B., Tengblad, S. and Lithell, H. (1994) Insulin sensitivity is related to the fatty acid composition of serum lipids and skeletal muscle phospholipids in 70-year-old men. *Diabetologia*, **37**, 1044–50.

Vessby, B., Unsitupa, M., Hermansen, K. et al. (2001) Substituting dietary saturated for monounsaturated fat impairs insulin sensitivity in healthy men and women: The KANWU Study. *Diabetologia*, **44**, 312–19.

Vozzo, R., Wittert, G., Cocchiaro, C. et al. (2003) Similar effects of foods high in protein, carbohydrate and fat on subsequent spontaneous food intake in healthy individuals. *Appetite*, **40**, 101–7.

Wadden, T.A. (1993) Treatment of obesity by moderate and severe caloric restriction. Results of clinical research trials. *Annals of Internal Medicine*, **119**, 688–93.

Wadden, T.A., Van Itallie, T.B. and Blackburn, G.L. (1990) Responsible and irresponsible use of very-low-calorie diets in the treatment of obesity. *The Journal of the American Medical Association*, **263**, 83–5.

Wadden, T.A., Berkowitz, R.I., Womble, L.G. et al. (2005) Randomized trial of lifestyle modification and pharmacotherapy for obesity. *The New England Journal of Medicine*, **353**, 2111–20.

Westerterp, K.R., Meijer, G.A., Schoffelen, P. and Janssen, E.M. (1994) Body mass, body composition and sleeping metabolic rate before, during and after endurance training. *European Journal of Applied Physiology and Occupational Physiology*, **69**, 203–8.

Westerterp-Plantenga, M.S., Lejeune, M.P., Nijs, I. et al. (2004) High protein intake sustains weight maintenance after body weight loss in humans. *International Journal of Obesity and Related Metabolic Disorders*, **28**, 57–64.

Westerterp-Plantenga, M.S., Rolland, V., Wilson, S.A. and Westerterp, K.R. (1999) Satiety related to 24 h diet-induced thermogenesis during high protein/carbohydrate vs high fat diets measured in a respiration chamber. *European Journal of Clinical Nutrition*, **53**, 495–502.

Whitehead, J.M., McNeill, G. and Smith, J.S. (1996) The effect of protein intake on 24-h energy expenditure during energy restriction. *International Journal of Obesity and Related Metabolic Disorders*, **20**, 727–32.

Williamson, D.F., Pamuk, E., Thun, M. et al. (1995) Prospective study of intentional weight loss and mortality in never-smoking overweight US white women aged 40–64 years. *American Journal of Epidemiology*, **141**, 1128–41.

Williamson, D.F., Thompson, T.J., Thun, M. et al. (2000) Intentional weight loss and mortality among overweight individuals with diabetes. *Diabetes Care*, **23**, 1499–504.

Wilmore, J.H., Despres, J.P., Stanforth, P.R. et al. (1999) Alterations in body weight and composition consequent to 20 wk of endurance training: the HERITAGE Family Study. *The American Journal of Clinical Nutrition*, **70**, 346–52.

Wilson, P.W., Kannel, W.B., Silbershatz, H. and D'Agostino, R.B. (1999) Clustering of metabolic factors and coronary heart disease. *Archives of Internal Medicine*, **159**, 1104–9.

Chapter 17

Pharmacological Approaches for Treating Obesity

Key points

- Anti-obesity drugs can cause weight loss by decreasing hunger and food intake, stimulating energy expenditure, or by inhibiting the intestinal absorption of dietary fats. Some centrally-acting appetite-suppressants also increase energy expenditure.

- Many anti-obesity drugs have been withdrawn or clinical development halted because of poor efficacy and/or severe side effects, including amphetamines (high risk of dependence), fenfluramine (risk of pulmonary hypertension and valvular heart disease) and β_3 adrenergic agonists (poor efficacy and sympathetic side effects). Thyroxine should not be used to treat obesity in euthyroid subjects because of adverse effects including cardiac arrhythmias.

- Novel approaches under active investigation include inhibitors of the neuropeptide Y (NPY) Y5 receptor, which mediates NPYs powerful hyperphagic action; agonists at the melanocortin MC4 receptor, which decreases feeding; and receptor antagonists of ghrelin, an appetite-stimulating gut peptide. As yet, these have not yielded effective and safe drugs suitable for use in humans.

- Anti-obesity drugs are not a cure, but aim to supplement lifestyle education and change. Weight loss of <5% of the pre-treatment level is unlikely to bring clinical benefits, whereas loss of ≥10% can decrease the risk of obesity-related comorbidities, notably type 2 diabetes and cardiovascular disease.

- Treatment with an anti-obesity drug can be considered in patients with BMI ≥30 kg/m², or BMI ≥27 kg/m² together with one or more obesity-related comorbidities (e.g. type 2 diabetes, hypertension, dyslipidaemia or coronary-heart disease). Lifestyle modification (energy intake restriction and increased physical activity) should have been tried for three months and shown to achieve inadequate weight loss. Compliance with drug therapy and continuing lifestyle modification are essential.

- Orlistat is a semi-synthetic inhibitor of gut lipases, which decreases the absorption of dietary fat by up to 30%. Dosage is 120 mg thrice daily. Side effects are the consequences of fat malabsorption, notably steatorrhoea and (potentially) deficiencies of fat-soluble vitamins.

- Sibutramine acts centrally to inhibit the reuptake of both serotonin and noradrenaline, thus enhancing the action of both these appetite-suppressing monoamines. Dosage is 10 or 15 mg once daily. Problems include sympathomimetic effects such as tachycardia and dry mouth and occasionally hypertension.

- Rimonabant is a centrally-acting antagonist at the cannabinoid CB1 receptor, which mediates the appetite-stimulating action of endocannabinoids released in the brain. Dosage is 20 mg once daily. Side effects include severe psychiatric problems (depression and anxiety), nausea and dizziness. Licensing approval for rimonabant was withdrawn in Europe in late 2008.

- The three drugs in current use – orlistat, sibutramine and rimonabant – all achieve ≥10% weight loss after one year's treatment in up to one-third of cases. Weight tends to be regained during prolonged treatment, and generally returns to baseline values if the drug is withdrawn. Reductions in waist circumference, indicating a decrease in visceral fat mass, are generally seen. Modest improvements in obesity-related metabolic and cardiovascular risk factors – hyperglycaemia, dyslipidaemia and hypertension – often occur.

- Many drugs cause weight gain, notably corticosteroids, progesterone contraceptives, certain anti-convulsant and anti-psychotic agents, β-blockers, and sulphonylureas and insulin. These should be prescribed with particular care, or alternatives used, in obese subjects.

Chapter 17 Pharmacological Approaches for Treating Obesity

John Wilding

Effective management of obesity requires individuals to make changes to their dietary intake, physical activity and lifestyle that must be sustained over a long period. These changes must overcome powerful biological signals that have evolved to counteract the threat of negative energy balance, and a social context that discourages healthy eating and physical activity. Accordingly, it is perhaps unsurprising that most weight-loss programmes – apart from specialist centres treating carefully selected patients – achieve disappointing results, with an average weight loss of only 4 kg after a year or more (Diabetes Prevention Program Research Group, 2002; Tuomilheto et al., 2001; Avenell et al., 2004; The Treatment of Mild Hypertension Research Group, 1991; Curioni and Lourenco, 2005).

The need for effective management of obesity is of ever increasing importance because of the global spread of obesity and its sequelae, notably type 2 diabetes and cardiovascular complications – which threaten to reverse the recent trend to decreasing incidence of coronary-heart disease in many Western nations (Olshansky et al., 2005). Many of the comorbidities of obesity have been shown by epidemiological research and short-term studies to be improved by weight loss (Goldstein, 1992), while the favourable outcomes of bariatric surgery for morbid obesity point to long-term benefits of sustained weight loss (Sjöström et al., 2004). It is therefore reasonable to consider whether anti-obesity drugs may be used to supplement lifestyle modification to achieve and maintain long-term weight loss.

This chapter describes the historical, pharmacological and clinical aspects of drugs used to treat obesity, focusing on agents in current use, but also looking to potential therapeutic approaches in the future.

Historical context

The history of drugs to treat obesity is long and littered with agents that have failed to live up to expectation, or have been withdrawn or had their use severely restricted because of adverse side effects. Structures and basic pharmacological actions of some compounds in previous or current use are shown in Figure 17.1.

The earliest drugs were approved as 'adjuncts to the management of obesity', acknowledging that medication was intended to supplement rather than replace lifestyle changes. These included amphetamine and desoxyephedrine (approved in the United States in 1947), and 'amphetamine congeners' such as phentermine, diethylpropion, phenmetrazine, benzphetamine and phendimetrazine, which were claimed to have less potential for dependence and were approved during the 1950s (Colman, 2005). At that time, there were no randomized controlled trials, and documentation of adverse effects was woefully inadequate by modern standards; these drugs were widely advertised and prescribed (Figure 17.2).

During the 1960s, a second wave of anti-obesity drugs entered clinical practice, including mazindol (an inhibitor of noradrenaline reuptake) and fenfluramine, a serotonin-releasing agent. Amendments to the FDA registration process in 1962 required evidence of efficacy from well-controlled investigations, although the data supporting the use of these drugs were largely derived from short-term studies of 12 weeks' duration or less. In 1970, all anti-obesity drugs were required to show statistical superiority over placebo in formal clinical trials. The use of these agents declined steadily during the 1970s and 1980s, because of concerns over the potential for dependence (amphetamines

Obesity: Science to Practice   Edited by Gareth Williams and Gema Frühbeck
© 2009 John Wiley & Sons, Ltd

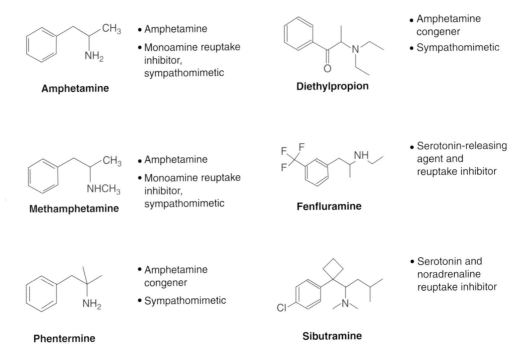

Figure 17.1 Structures and pharmacological actions of some commonly used anti-obesity drugs from the past and present.

were increasingly used as recreational drugs of abuse) and the emerging recognition that certain appetite-suppressing drugs could cause the rare complication of primary pulmonary hypertension (Abenhaim *et al.*, 1996).

In the early 1990s, a combination of phentermine and fenfluramine experienced an extensive but brief revival in the USA, with much media interest. 'Phen/fen' was shown to produce weight loss of up to 5kg over four years, in a single study of 121 patients, of whom only 43% completed the trial (Weintraub *et al.*, 1992a,b,c,d,e). Dexfenfluramine, the dextro-isomer of fenfluramine, was licensed in Europe in 1995 and in the USA in 1996, largely on the basis of a large 12-month randomized controlled trial that demonstrated both superiority over placebo and also that most of patients achieved the all-important 5% weight loss that had become an FDA approval criterion in 1995 (Guy-Grand *et al.*, 1989). Dexfenfluramine was also the first agent shown to confer some benefits on other risk factors such as hypertension, dyslipidaemia and hyperglycaemia (Willey, Molyneaux and Yue, 1994); nevertheless, continuing concerns over

pulmonary hypertension restricted treatment to only three months. The use of these agents came to an abrupt halt in 1997 when carcinoid-like cardiac valve disease was demonstrated in patients exposed to fenfluramine and dexfenfluramine, particularly when taken in combination with phentermine (Connolly *et al.*, 1997). This adverse reaction remains unexplained, but may relate to the drugs' ability to release serotonin from other tissues, including endothelial cells and platelets. Although subsequent reports have suggested that the risk is lower than originally reported, fenfluramine and dexfenfluramine were withdrawn by the manufacturers, and are unlikely to return to clinical use (Sachdev *et al.*, 2002).

Phentermine and diethylpropion remain available in Europe (largely due to a legal loophole, and without enthusiasm from the regulatory authorities) and in the USA. Restrictions on their prescription remain in place, and continuing concerns over potential dependence, lack of long-term efficacy data and the risk of primary pulmonary hypertension have substantially reduced their use.

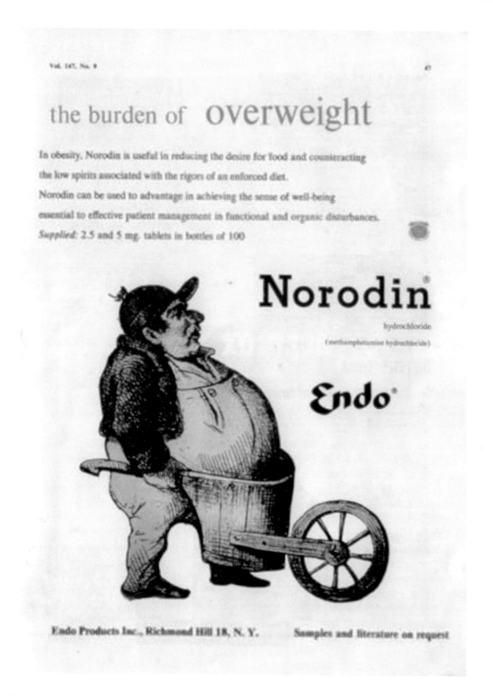

Figure 17.2 Advertisement, from medical journals in 1958, for metamphetamine.

Other agents that have been used for the treatment of obesity – but without a specific licence in most countries – include phenylpropanolamine (a sympathomimetic amine previously found in common cold remedies) (Caffry, Kissileff and Thornton, 1987), a combination of ephedrine and caffeine (Astrup *et al.*, 1992), and thyroxine. All induce a degree of weight loss by enhancing sympathetic activity and thus energy expenditure, but all are non-selective and suffer from sympathomimetic side effects. Phenylpropanolamine was withdrawn because of an increased risk of stroke in young women, and ephedrine/caffeine because of unresolved concerns about safety and lack of efficacy. The medical establishment abandoned thyroxine as a treatment for obesity in euthyroid subjects in the 1920s, but it has still been used for this purpose; iatrogenic hyperthyroidism can cause life-threatening (and medicolegally indefensible) arrhythmias.

This historical background highlights the great challenges faced by researchers and the pharmaceutical industry when attempting to develop safe and effective anti-obesity drugs. It has also shaped the context in which new drugs are evaluated and regulatory decisions made. Key considerations include the drug's efficacy in reducing weight and whether this is clinically significant, its ability to maintain weight loss, its impact on the comorbidities of obesity, and the balance between its benefits and any adverse effects.

Defining the efficacy of anti-obesity drugs

Many epidemiological studies and clinical trials indicate that weight loss improves the health of obese people, but the debate continues as to how much weight must be lost to achieve significant clinical benefits. There is no simple answer to this question: an individual's weight-loss goal may depend on factors such as the starting weight and the nature of comorbidities, while the patient's expectations may differ markedly from those of health professionals. The tissue composition of weight loss is also important, because anti-obesity drugs should selectively reduce adipose rather than lean tissue, and ideally target visceral fat. Many drugs also have clinical benefits or adverse effects that may modify the effect of weight loss on co-morbidities, notably diabetes and vascular disease. These issues, together with continuing ambiguities around some of the evidence for the benefits of weight loss, complicate the evaluation of a drug's efficacy and benefit/risk profile.

Overall, epidemiological studies that examined intentional and non-intentional weight loss, together with intervention trials, suggest that weight loss of at least 5–10% of the initial level is needed to provide consistent and clinically relevant improvements in obesity-related risk factors and comorbidities, notably type 2 diabetes and cardiovascular disease (Diabetes Prevention Program Research Group, 2002; Williamson et al., 1995; Williamson et al., 2000). For patients with established type 2 diabetes, at least 10% weight loss is generally required to achieve meaningful improvements in glycaemic control, such as a significant reduction in HbA_{1c} levels of the magnitude seen with oral hypoglycaemic drugs (Wing, 1989). Effects are less impressive in patients with longer-duration diabetes and those requiring insulin. Long-term maintenance of greater degrees of weight loss (15–25%) can dramatically improve type 2 diabetes – indeed, bariatric surgery can induce remission in 80–90% of cases (Kushner and Noble, 2006) – but this is beyond the scope of current anti-obesity drugs.

Significant reductions in cardiovascular morbidity and mortality were also seen with long-term weight loss of ≥5%, in the North American Nurses and Physicians Health Studies (Williamson et al., 1995). Further analysis suggests that this also applies to diabetic subjects (Williamson et al., 2000). Epidemiological evidence also suggests that overall cancer risk is reduced by between 11 and 25% in subjects who are able to achieve and maintain a weight loss of 10% (Williamson et al., 1995; Parker and Folsom, 2003).

Lesser degrees of weight loss may produce tangible clinical benefits in certain settings, such as impaired glucose tolerance (IGT), hypertension and dyslipidaemia. Four major studies have examined the impact of lifestyle intervention (mild dietary restriction, increased physical activity) on the progression of IGT. The studies, carried out in Finland, USA, China and India, all found that ~4% weight loss achieved by lifestyle modification and sustained for 4–6 years was associated with a 50–60% reduction in the risk of developing type 2 diabetes during this period (Diabetes Prevention Program Research Group, 2002; Tuomilheto et al., 2001). Dyslipidaemia and hypertension also improved. The Treatment of Hypertension Study (Stevens et al., 2001) also demonstrated significant reductions in blood pressure (averaging 5 and 7 mm Hg in systolic and diastolic values, respectively) in the subset of hypertensive subjects who maintained weight loss of ~5% for three years.

Regulatory criteria

The regulatory authorities in both the USA (the FDA) and Europe have set conservative criteria for the degree of weight loss required for an anti-obesity drug to be considered clinically effective, and both also require a demonstrable reduction in comorbid risk factors. European and American regulatory criteria differ in some respects and both are under review. The current European criteria require weight loss of at least 10% from baseline after 12 months treatment, which has to be statistically greater than placebo. The FDA demands 5% greater weight loss than placebo after 12 months' duration. American (but not European) guidelines require weight loss during the trial's run-in period to be excluded from the total weight loss achieved, which is obviously relevant to the overall 10% weight-loss target. For both, long-term efficacy must be demonstrated, with maintenance of weight loss for two years or more. There must also be improvements that are both statistically significant and clinically relevant in secondary endpoints such as cardiovascular risk factors, and specific studies must be conducted in subgroups of patients at particular risk, such as those with diabetes, hypertension and hyperlipidaemia.

Ultimately, only long-term outcome studies can determine whether a pharmacological treatment produces worthwhile clinical benefits, especially decreased mortality and morbidity. Such studies pose huge logistical problems because of the large numbers of patients required and the difficulty of retaining them in the trial, the need for complete follow up on relevant outcomes in all patients, and the necessarily long duration (perhaps ten years or more). The vast costs involved are challenging for research funders, especially the pharmaceutical industry, because the outcomes may be uncertain. Few such studies have been undertaken.

Potential targets for intervention

Recent years have seen rapid growth in the scientific understanding of energy balance regulation (Chapter 6), and this has helped identify many new potential targets for anti-obesity drugs. In theory, a drug treatment for obesity may reduce energy intake (decreasing appetite and/or enhancing satiety), reduce nutrient absorption, or increase energy expenditure or substrate utilization; in practice, some agents have effects on more than one aspect of energy balance regulation (Figure 17.3).

The central nervous system (CNS)

The CNS plays a key role in appetite regulation. It integrates peripheral information about body

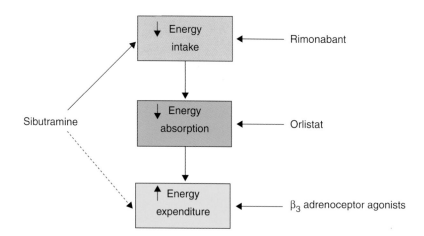

Figure 17.3 Principal targets for anti-obesity drugs, with examples of agents that exploit these mechanisms.

fat stores, together with satiety signals from the gastrointestinal tract and taste/hedonic signals, to determine how much and what type of food is eaten (Chapter 6). The CNS also contributes to the regulation of nutrient absorption, metabolism and overall energy expenditure. At a higher level, the brain controls food-seeking behaviour and prioritizes this among the animal's other activities. These high-order coordinating roles are reflected in the complexity of the systems that have evolved to regulate energy balance in higher mammals, including humans (see Figure 17.4).

Many brain areas are involved but the main integrating centre is the hypothalamus, at the base of the brain. Hypothalamic neurones contain over 50 neurotransmitters that can modulate energy balance, and so are a rich source of potential drug targets. However, there are two

important notes of caution. First, consistent with the crucial importance of energy balance to the survival of any organism, there is considerable 'redundancy' (i.e. functional overlap) among these systems; thus, interfering with a single neurotransmitter is unlikely to produce profound effects on energy balance because of compensatory changes that will be triggered in one or more other pathways in response to weight loss. Second, particular neurotransmitters and the neural systems that express them also influence many other vital functions; for example, some of the major appetite-regulating pathways also affect reproductive function, perhaps to ensure that an individual can reproduce only when energy reserves are sufficient to support the demands of a growing fetus and to feed the young. There are also important

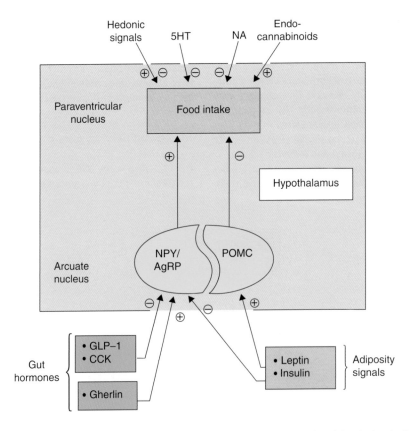

Figure 17.4 Overview of appetite control mechanisms, showing the interplay of peripheral signals (including gut hormones and the adiposity signals, leptin and insulin) and other central influences and neurotransmitters within the arcuate-paraventricular pathway in the hypothalamus. 5HT: serotonin; AgRP: agouti gene-related peptide; CCK: cholecystokinin; GLP-1: glucagon-like peptide-1; NA: noradrenaline; NPY: neuropeptide Y; POMC: proopiomelanocortin.

interactions with other physiological functions such as control of blood pressure, fluid balance and temperature regulation. These problems create considerable challenges for drug hunters trying to find a 'magic bullet' that selectively targets body weight. Some of the most promising CNS neurotransmitters and systems are shown in Table 17.1.

Monoamines

The early anorectic agents, notably the amphetamines and amphetamine congeners, act predominantly in the CNS. These drugs are sympathomimetic amines, and simulate the effect of noradrenaline released in the hypothalamus and elsewhere (see Figure 17.10 on page 437). This causes fat mobilization and weight loss by inducing an overall energy deficit; appetite is suppressed while energy expenditure increases, in keeping with the concept that most endogenous neurotransmitters that decrease appetite also enhance the energy deficit by stimulating energy expenditure, and vice versa (Bray, 1991).

The recognition that serotonin is important in inhibiting food intake and restraining body weight came with the development of fenfluramine, a non-selective serotonin-releasing agent. Subsequent research, using a combination of pharmacological tools and genetic manipulation of the various serotonin receptor subtypes, has identified the $5HT_{2c}$ and $5HT_{1b}$ receptors as likely mediators of serotonin's hypophagic action (Vickers et al., 2003; Halford et al., 2005) (see Figure 17.10 on page 437). Many monoamine reuptake inhibitors have been tested for efficacy as weight-reducing drugs; these appear to act independently of the $5HT_{2c}$ and $5HT_{1b}$ receptors to inhibit reuptake, thus increasing the availability of serotonin to act at these receptors. The antidepressant drugs, sertraline and fluoxetine, have been shown in randomized clinical trials to produce some weight loss (Goldstein et al., 1994), although tolerance develops to this effect and weight loss is not sustained. By contrast, sibutramine, originally developed as an antidepressant (King and Devaney, 1988), is largely devoid of antidepressant properties, but was subsequently shown to cause weight loss in obesity (Bray et al., 1996); it is currently the only licensed agent in this class.

Dopamine D2 receptors may also contribute to the regulation of food intake (Hawkins, Barkemeyer and Tulley, 1986), with the D2 receptor subtype specifically implicated in 'reward' and hedonic eating behaviour. As yet, however, no agent in this class has emerged as a likely drug candidate. The widespread distribution of dopamine throughout the CNS, and the observation that dopamine agonism may contribute to the dependency and abuse potential of amphetamines, make this an unattractive target.

Orexigenic peptide neurotransmitters

Much recent interest has focused on 'orexigenic' peptide neurotransmitters that stimulate appetite (Wilding, 2002). Many of these are involved in now well-characterized circuits that mediate the effects of leptin on energy balance (see Chapter 6). These include neuropeptide Y (NPY), galanin and melanin concentrating hormone (MCH).

Of these, the NPY Y5 receptor has been considered the most promising target. NPY is one of the most powerful appetite-stimulating substances known and seems to mediate hunger and hyperphagia in various animal models, including certain genetically-obese syndromes; moreover, the Y5 receptor appears specific for NPYs orexigenic action (Hwa et al., 1999; Marsh et al., 1998). However, genetic knockout of either NPY or the Y5 receptor does not create a lean phenotype, and the validity of this target has been further questioned by variable results of Y5 blockade in both animal models and early human studies (Marsh et al., 1998). For example, the selective Y5 antagonist (MIK-0557) failed to achieve significant weight loss in early clinical trials.

The other orexigenic peptides remain potential but speculative targets, with no drugs yet reaching clinical development. Orexin A (also termed hypocretin 1) was originally named for its appetite-stimulating action (Sakurai et al., 1998), but this property is relatively weak and it is now thought to have a more important role in regulating the sleep-wake cycle – which also makes this system unattractive for anti-obesity drug development (Brisbare-Roch et al., 2007). Opioid peptides, particularly those acting on μ and κ opioid receptor subtypes, also stimulate food intake. Antagonists at these receptors are therefore potential anti-obesity agents, but the ubiquitous nature of opioid peptide systems and their involvement in nociceptive and other functions may limit their clinical utility (Koch et al., 1995).

Table 17.1 CNS neurotransmitters as potential anti-obesity drug targets.

Neurotransmitter	Sites of:			Effects on:			Compounds and actions
	Production	Action	Receptor	Food intake	Energy expenditure		
Serotonin (5HT)	Midbrain (raphe nuclei)	Hypothalamus (PVN)	$5HT_{1b}$ $5HT_{1c}$	↓↓	↑		• 5HT release (fenfluramine) • 5HT reuptake inhibitor (sibutramine)
Noradrenaline (NA)	Medulla (CA1-5 nuclei)	Hypothalamus (PVN)	α_2	↓↓	↑		• Mimic NA (amphetamines) • NA reuptake inhibitor (sibutramine)
α-MSH, β-MSH	Hypothalamus (ARC)	Hypothalamus (PVN)	MC4-R	↓↓	↑		• *MC4-R agonists*
Neuropeptide Y (NPY)	Hypothalamus (ARC)	Hypothalamus (PVN)	Y5	↑↑↑	↓		• *Y5 antagonist*
Orexin A	Hypothalamus (LHA)	Hypothalamus (PVN, etc.)	ORX-1	↑	—		• *ORX-1 antagonist*
Endocannabinoids	Widespread	Hypothalamus (other regions)	CB1	↑↑	—		• CB1 antagonist (rimonabant)

Notes: Target compounds that have not yet yielded effective drugs are shown in italics.

Abbreviations: ARC: arcuate nucleus (in rat; human equivalent is the tubero-infundibular nucleus); LHA: lateral hypothalamic area; NA: noradrenaline PVN: paraventricular nucleus.

The endocannabinoid system

The endocannabinoid system, although discovered only relatively recently, has already produced one drug that has reached clinical practice, with several others in development. The appetite-stimulating properties of cannabis have been recognized for many years but were unexplained until the cloning of the CB1 and CB2 cannabinoid receptors that recognize tetrahydrocannabinol, the active ingredient. Further work led to the discovery of the endocannabinoids, endogenous lipid neurotransmitters that are also agonists at cannabinoid receptors; they stimulate feeding via the CB1 receptor, and are now known to be involved in the physiological regulation of energy balance (Gerard et al., 1991; Shire et al., 1996).

Endocannabinoids are synthesized on demand within neurones from arachidonic acid, and include anandamide and 2-arachidonoglycerol (2-AG) (Kirkham, 2005). The endocannabinoid–CB1 system has been implicated in mediating the effects of leptin on food intake, and also in the hedonic aspects of eating (Higgs, Williams and Kirkham, 2003; Di Marzo et al., 2001). Animals with genetic and dietary obesity show increased endocannabinoid activity (as evidenced by increased release of 2-AG within the brain), while mice with genetic knockout of the CB1 receptor are lean and resistant to dietary obesity (Di Marzo et al., 2001; Trillou et al., 2004; Trillou et al., 2003). CB1 receptors are widespread throughout the body, and have also been implicated in regulating nutrient absorption in the gut as well as lipid and glucose metabolism – observations that further increase the system's appeal as a therapeutic target in obesity (Spoto et al., 2006; Bluher et al., 2006; Engeli et al., 2005) (Figure 17.5). CB1 receptors are also involved in a number of other processes, and are now thought important in regulating mood, which probably explains some of the serious adverse psychiatric effects (depression and anxiety) of CB1 blockade. CB2 receptors (Shire et al., 1996) are less well characterized, but appear to have a role in immune function and peripheral pain sensation.

Anorexigenic peptide neurotransmitters

Many peptides synthesized in the CNS have been shown to reduce food intake and/or increase energy expenditure in various animal models (see Figure 17.4). These include the proopiomelanocortin (POMC) products, α-melanocyte

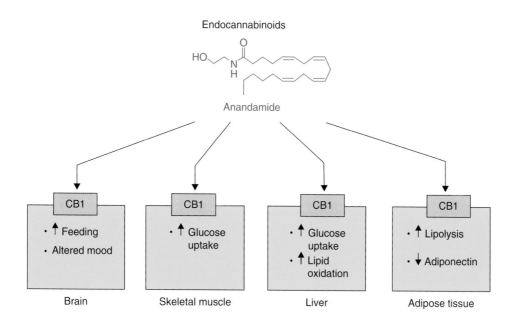

Endocannabinoids

Anandamide

CB1	CB1	CB1	CB1
• ↑ Feeding • Altered mood	• ↑ Glucose uptake	• ↑ Glucose uptake • ↑ Lipid oxidation	• ↑ Lipolysis • ↓ Adiponectin
Brain	Skeletal muscle	Liver	Adipose tissue

Figure 17.5 Central and peripheral actions of endocannabinoids, showing the receptors that mediate these effects. The structure of one of the major endocannabinoids, anandamide, is shown.

stimulating hormone (α-MSH) and β-MSH, and also neurotensin, all of which are involved in the leptin signalling pathway (Sahu, 1998). The POMC products (melanocortins), and the melanocortin receptors (especially MC4-R) through which they reduce feeding, are potentially promising targets, because this pathway is now known to be important in humans: mutations in POMC and MC4-R constitute one of the most common defined genetic causes of obesity (Krude and Gruters, 2000). However, pharmacological development of small peptide agonists that can gain access to relevant sites within the CNS is likely to prove challenging, and melanocortins also influence reproductive and other functions. No compound manipulating this pathway has yet reached clinical development.

Many gut-derived peptides, such as cholecystokinin, glucagon-like-peptide 1 and ghrelin, are also found in the CNS; these are discussed below.

Peripheral signals from the gut

The short-term regulation of energy intake is dominated by signals from the gut that help both to initiate and terminate meals. Most work has focused on satiety. Cholecystokinin (CCK) was the first recognized satiety signal, and research has confirmed that physiological blood concentrations of CCK (reached after eating) decrease hunger in humans (Ballinger et al., 1994; Dourish, Rycroft and Iversen, 1989). However development of a CCK-1 receptor antagonist was recently stopped after showing disappointing efficacy in phase 2 trials.

Several other gut hormones have also been found to be important in mediating post-prandial satiety. These include a cleavage fragment of peptide YY (PYY$_{3-36}$), pancreatic polypeptide, glucagon-like peptide-1 (GLP-1), and the proglucagon product, oxyntomodulin (Batterham et al., 2002; Cohen et al., 2003; Nakajima et al., 1994). GLP-1 and its synthetic analogues have been shown to reduce food intake in humans; the effect is modest, although the resultant weight loss may augment the insulin-releasing (incretin) effect of GLP-1 to improve glycaemic control in type 2 diabetic subjects (Edwards et al., 2001; Nauck et al., 2007). It is not yet known whether inhibitors of dipeptidyl peptidase IV (DPP-IV), the enzyme that degrades GLP-1 in

the circulation, may also enhance satiety and decrease food intake, but unlike many other treatments for type 2 diabetes, these drugs do not cause weight gain in clinical trials (Bonora, 2007). Small-molecule agonists are difficult to develop, but other gut-derived satiety peptides may become targets for new therapeutic agents. It remains to be seen whether a single drug would produce enough weight loss to obtain registration as a treatment for obesity.

The gut also produces an orexigenic peptide, namely the growth hormone-releasing peptide, ghrelin, which acts via the growth hormone secretagogue (GHS) receptor (Kamegai et al., 2000). The finding that ghrelin is predominantly expressed in the stomach soon led to the discovery that it was a potent stimulus to food intake; circulating ghrelin levels are high before meals and fall subsequently, suggesting a physiological role in meal initiation (Shintani et al., 2001). Circulating concentrations of ghrelin are low in obesity (English et al., 2002); nonetheless, ghrelin antagonists may be worth exploring, because the relevant receptors are mostly situated peripherally (the effects of ghrelin are abolished by vagotomy), and the drug would not necessarily need to enter the CNS to reduce food intake. Another product of the ghrelin gene, obestatin, was initially reported to decrease food intake (Zhang et al., 2005), but this has not been substantiated.

Inhibiting nutrient absorption

Iatrogenic malabsorption of nutrients is part of the rationale for successful bariatric surgical operations, and sets the precedent for pharmacological intervention. Fat malabsorption is the most logical target because of the high energy density (9 kcal/g) of lipids. This has been achieved by blocking intestinal lipases and is the mode of action of orlistat (see Figure 17.6). Another strategy under investigation is to block the process of fat absorption in the enterocyte, by preventing the resynthesis of triglyceride and formation of chylomicrons; it remains to be seen whether this will be viable in practice. In general, problems with the steatorrhoea that results from inhibiting fat absorption have limited widespread acceptance of these drugs.

Carbohydrate malabsorption can also be induced pharmacologically, for example with the

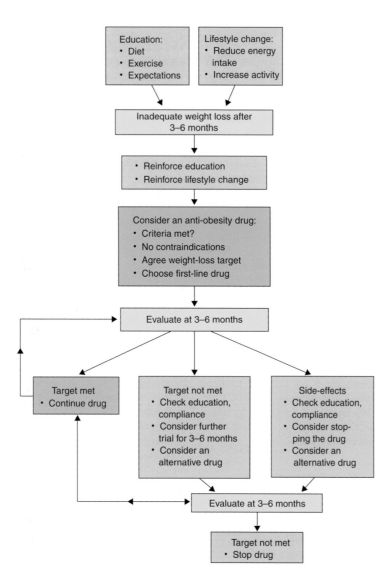

Figure 17.6 Flow-chart showing a suggested approach to the use of anti-obesity drugs in clinical practice.

α-glucosidase inhibitor, acarbose. However, this drug does not cause weight loss, although it can slightly improve blood glucose control in diabetes (Holman, Cull and Turner, 1999).

Energy expenditure and substrate utilization

Energy expenditure comprises three main components: basal energy expenditure, the thermic effect of food and voluntary activity (see Chapters 3 and 7). Basal energy expenditure comprises about two-thirds of total energy expenditure in most sedentary humans and is broadly proportional to lean body mass; however, it can be increased by as much as 30% by thyroid hormones or direct activation of the sympathetic nervous system, and is therefore a potential target for pharmacological intervention (Arch, 2002). As described above, thyroid hormones or pure sympathomimetic agents can be effective, but produce unacceptable and potentially dangerous adverse effects. More subtle approaches to enhance energy expenditure must therefore be considered. Energy is produced as ATP in the mitochondria; ultimately, any drug that increases energy expenditure must either reduce the efficiency with which ATP is produced (for example, by uncoupling oxidative phosphorylation), or increase ATP utilization (for example, through 'futile' metabolic cycles).

For many years, the 'magic bullet' of obesity management was thought to be drugs that could increase thermogenic activity by selective activation of the β_3 adrenoceptor that is closely linked to uncoupling of oxidative phosphorylation in the brown adipose tissue of rodents (Arch and Wilson, 1996) (see Chapters 4 and 5). Subsequent realization that this mechanism is less important in humans, and the failure in clinical trials of drugs that had been developed specifically to target the rodent β_3 receptor, have tempered enthusiasm for this approach.

Other proposed treatments that increase fat oxidation include a growth hormone fragment (AOD9604), but clinical results with this agent have so far been disappointing (Ng et al., 2000). Various knockout mice with targeted deletions involving specific biochemical pathways either have a lean phenotype or are resistant to diet-induced obesity, and several activators or inhibitors of key enzymes have been identified as potential anti-obesity agents; however, none has yet reached clinical development.

Targeting specific genetic defects

Modern pharmacology can allow the design of specific agents to treat obesity that has a known and specific cause, even if that approach may not be generally effective. The most dramatic example is leptin, which has little impact in most obese individuals, but is highly effective in the extremely rare cases with genetic leptin deficiency (Farooqi et al., 1999) (see Figure 21.1 on page 510). Specific treatments may ultimately be developed to treat other genetic defects once these are characterized, but the practical challenges may remain considerable.

Indications for pharmacotherapy in obesity

Not all obese patients want, or will benefit from, drug treatment; it is important to target those who are most likely to benefit, to recognize when

treatment is not working, and discontinue the drug if this is the case. Effective pharmacotherapy for obesity requires the individualized evaluation of comorbidities and assessment of specific contraindications. It is essential to balance the benefits of therapy against its potential risks, side effects and costs at the outset and throughout treatment.

Indications for pharmacotherapy in obesity are summarized in Table 17.2. At present, drug treatment can be considered in patients with BMI $\geq 30\,kg/m^2$ who are well motivated, but have failed to achieve a target weight loss of 10% despite supervised efforts to modify their lifestyle through diet, exercise and behavioural change over a period of 3–6 months. It is important to consider the presence of other medical conditions that might be related to obesity, or that might alter the risk-benefit ratio when considering the use of a particular drug. Under some circumstances, it may be appropriate to prescribe drugs to overweight patients with BMI $\geq 27\,kg/m^2$ who also have one or more comorbidities that are likely to improve with weight loss (e.g. diabetes, hypertension, dyslipidaemia), but only if that is allowed within the product licence of the drug. Drug therapy should be avoided in patients who have evidence of an eating disorder such as bulimia.

Programmes of weight management must include clearly defined procedures for monitoring progress. It is recommended that patients

Table 17.2 Indications for pharmacotherapy in obesity.

Clinically significant obesity:

- BMI $\geq 30\,kg/m^2$, or
- BMI $\geq 25\,kg/m^2$ with ≥ 1 obesity-related comorbidity

Failure of adequate trial (3–6 months) of lifestyle and dietary modifications

- Weight loss $< 1\,kg/month$

Prepared to accept ongoing education, lifestyle and modification

Prepared to adhere to drug therapy

No specific contradictions:

- Sibutramine: refractory hypertension
- Rimonabant: depression, psychosis

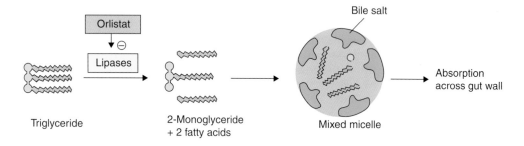

Figure 17.7 Mechanism of action of orlistat, an inhibitor of the pancreatic and intestinal lipases that hydrolyse dietary triglyceride into absorbable lipids.

prescribed anti-obesity drugs should be supervised at least monthly, with records of body weight, waist circumference, blood pressure and other relevant measures such as blood glucose and lipids. The initial target for patients treated with pharmacotherapy is 5% weight loss from the start of drug treatment over three months – which is implicit in the product licences for the currently licensed drugs.

Continuation of drug treatment should depend on the balance between the health benefits of maintained weight and the potential adverse effects of the drug. Treatment should be stopped if the patient has not lost weight during the first month or continues to gain weight despite drug treatment (Royal College of Physicians, 2003). Once a weight-loss target has been achieved, there should be an opportunity for re-negotiation of a new target, if indicated, and/or long-term monitoring with reinforcement. Drug treatment should not be considered ineffective because weight loss has stopped, providing that the lower weight is maintained.

After 3–6 months of pharmacotherapy, the effects on weight loss, body composition and cardiometabolic risk factor profile should be re-evaluated and the treatment aims redefined according to the therapeutic response and individual needs of the patient. Because of the paucity of robust data on long-term efficacy and safety, present guidelines are that drug treatment should not be continued for longer than two years; there is no evidence base to support subsequent courses of treatment.

As the currently approved drugs act through completely different mechanisms, combination therapy could in theory enhance weight loss. However, limited clinical trials with sibutramine and orlistat combined did not suggest a synergistic effect of the two drugs; indeed, a simple additive effect of the two drugs has not been clearly established (Wadden *et al.*, 2000; Kaya *et al.*, 2004). To date, no results on combinations with rimonabant are available.

The flow chart in Figure 17.7 summarizes the treatment protocol suggested above.

Currently available treatments

Orlistat

Pharmacology

Orlistat (tetrahydrolipstatin) is a semi-synthetic derivative of a naturally-occurring lipase inhibitor, lipstatin (Ransac *et al.*, 1991), originally isolated from the fungus *Streptomyces toxytricini*. Orlistat is a potent inhibitor of both pancreatic and intestinal lipases, blocking the hydrolysis of dietary triglyceride to glycerol and free fatty acids (FFA), the lipid products that can be absorbed from the gut lumen (see Figure 17.6). At therapeutic dosages, orlistat inhibits the absorption of about 30% of dietary triglyceride (Hussain *et al.*, 1994), which comprises >99% of dietary lipid. It is highly selective for lipases, having no appreciable activity against other digestive enzymes, and is not absorbed systemically. Most is excreted unchanged in the stools; trace amounts of its major metabolites (M1 and M3) can be detected in the circulation, but these have <0.1% of the potency of orlistat and no appreciable inhibition of systemic lipase activity has been detected (Zhi *et al.*, 1996). Its short half-life and mode of action mean that it needs to be taken thrice-daily, before meals.

Adverse effects

The main side effects of orlistat relate to the persistence of dietary triglyceride in the gut lumen, causing steatorrhoea, with loose oily motions, faecal urgency and sometimes incontinence (Drent *et al.*, 1995). These side effects are common early in treatment, but tend to resolve in patients who persevere with the drug, probably because of behavioural adaptation (avoiding fat-rich foods to escape the side effects), rather than any pharmacological tolerance (Sjöström *et al.*, 1998). The inhibition of fat absorption also impairs co-absorption of the fat-soluble vitamins A, E, D and K, resulting in a ~10% fall in their circulating levels during chronic treatment; in most patients, however, plasma vitamin concentrations remain within the reference ranges (Sjöström *et al.*, 1998; Melia, KossTwardy, Zhi, 1996). There is no evidence that parathyroid hormone levels or bone density are altered with orlistat treatment.

It is recommended that the INR is monitored carefully in patients taking warfarin, although there is no clear evidence that warfarin absorption or vitamin K-dependent clotting factors are specifically altered by orlistat (Ransac *et al.*, 1991). Orlistat does not have clinically significant interactions with other drugs, although potentiation of the action of pravastatin (but not other statins) has been noted.

Clinical efficacy in obesity

A number of clinical trials, ranging from a few months to two years in duration, have been conducted to establish the safety and efficacy of orlistat. Representative data are shown in Figures 17.8 and 17.9. Review of these trials shows that overall weight loss from the start of the treatment (at the standard dose of 120 mg thrice daily) averaged 8–10 kg during the first year, compared with approximately 4–6 kg weight loss with placebo. In the double-blind, randomized cross-over trial shown in Figure 17.8, some weight was regained during the second year in patients who continued orlistat, while weight returned to placebo levels in patients who switched from active treatment to placebo, confirming the role of the drug in maintaining weight loss (Davidson, 1997). The proportion of patients achieving 10% of body weight loss after the first year was 39%, compared with 18% of placebo-treated subjects (Sjöström *et al.*, 1998).

A recent meta-analysis, presented to the UKs National Institute for Health and Clinical Excellence (NICE), found that 54% of orlistat-treated patients lost ≥5% of weight after one year, compared with 39% of those taking placebo. Reductions in waist circumference of 2.6–6.4 cm over placebo, suggesting reductions in visceral fat, have also been shown in some of these

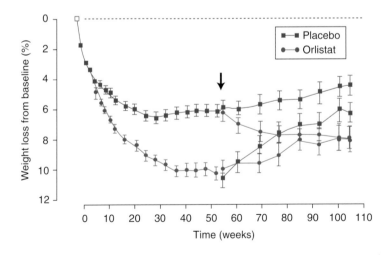

Figure 17.8 Effects of orlistat and placebo on body weight during a 2-year clinical trial. Patients were randomized after 1 year to continue with either orlistat or placebo. Note the fall in weight when orlistat was started, and the regain when it was withdrawn. Redrawn from Wadden *et al.*, 2000.

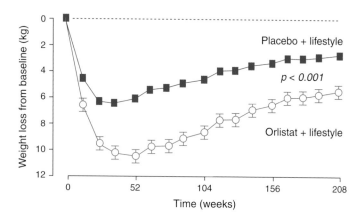

Figure 17.9 Effects of orlistat and placebo on body weight during the 4-year XENDOS study (Davidson, 1997).

studies (Davidson *et al.*, 1999; Torgerson *et al.*, 2004).

Clinical efficacy in special patient groups

Several clinical trials have examined the effects of orlistat in patients with diabetes and vascular risk factors (Hollander *et al.*, 1998; Miles *et al.*, 2001; Broom *et al.*, 2002). In general, weight loss with orlistat was consistent with that described above, although rather fewer patients achieved clinically significant weight loss. The analysis presented to NICE in the UK found that among subjects with comorbidities such as type 2 diabetes, 39% and 14% lost ≥5% and ≥10% of initial weight, compared to 15% and 4% if treated with placebo.

Orlistat treatment produces modest improvements in metabolic risk factors. Overall, total cholesterol fell by 0.21 mmol/l over 12 months, compared with an increase of 0.16 mmol/l for placebo, with similar changes seen in patients with diabetes and hypertension. Triglyceride levels were also reduced slightly (by 0.02 mmol/l, compared with a rise of 0.28 mmol/l for placebo). In type 2 diabetic patients taking various glucose-lowering treatments, HbA_{1c} fell on average by 0.62% with orlistat treatment, compared with a rise of 0.27% with placebo.

Blood pressure reductions were also seen, of approximately 3 mm Hg systolic and 2 mm Hg diastolic, compared with falls of 1 and 1 mm Hg with placebo (NICE, 2006). In hypertensive patients, blood pressure decreases were more impressive: systolic blood fell by 13 mm Hg for orlistat and 11 mm Hg for placebo, and diastolic by 11 mm Hg for orlistat and 9 mm Hg for placebo.

The only long-term outcome study to date (XENDOS) was conducted exclusively in Sweden and lasted four years (see Figure 17.9). Weight loss was consistent with that in other studies, and a statistically significant difference between active treatment and placebo was maintained throughout. Twenty percent of the patients had IGT, and among these, orlistat treatment reduced by 45% the risk of progressing to type 2 diabetes (Torgerson *et al.*, 2004) (Table 17.3).

The outcomes of the three currently available drugs in diabetic patients, drawn from individual trials and meta-analysis, are compared in Table 17.4.

In summary, orlistat appears to be an effective treatment for weight loss, achieving ≥10% weight loss in perhaps one-third of cases. It also confers relatively minor benefits on various vascular risk factors including hypertension, dyslipidaemia and diabetes, and may reduce progression to type 2 diabetes in patients with IGT over and above the effects of lifestyle intervention.

Interestingly, orlistat treatment barely achieves the 10% decrease in weight from baseline required by the European licensing authorities, while the meta-analysis estimate of mean weight loss falls short of the American requirement of 5% greater loss than with placebo; presumably the US licence was granted on the basis of data available at that time, perhaps mitigated by the drug's good safety profile and its overall benefits on vascular risk factors.

Recent cost-effectiveness analyses, carried out in the UK for the NICE submission, suggest

Table 17.3 Effects of orlistat on metabolic and cardiovascular risk factors in obesity subjects. Data from the Xendos study (Torgerson *et al.* 2004).

	Placebo	Orlistat	*p*-value
Systolic blood pressure (mm Hg)	−1.9	−2.6	<0.01
Diastolic blood pressure (mm Hg)	−3.4	−2.9	<0.01
Total cholesterol (% change)	−2.3	−7.9	<0.01
LDL-cholesterol (% change)	−5.1	−12.8	<0.01
HDL-cholesterol (% change)	+9.1	+6.5	<0.01
Triglycerides (% change)	+2.9	+2.4	<0.01
Glucose (mmol/l)	+0.2	+0.1	<0.01

Table 17.4 Effect of treatment with orlistat, sibutramine and rimonabant on weight and glycaemic control in obese patients with type 2 diabetes.

Drug	Placebo-subtracted weight loss	Placebo-subtracted effect on HbA$_{1c}$	Effect on HbA$_{1c}$ in subjects who lost ≥5% weight	Effect on HbA$_{1c}$ in subjects who lost ≥10% weight
Orlistat (3 studies)	2.7 kg	−0.4%	Not reported	Not reported
Sibutramine (8 studies)	4.5 kg	−0.3%	−0.7%	−1.1%
Rimonabant (1 study)	4.2 kg	−0.7%	Not reported[a]	Not reported[a]

[a]Regression analysis showed that reduction in HbA$_{1c}$ was proportional to weight loss.

that the cost per quality of life year gain QALY) is approximately £20 000, which would make orlistat a cost-effective treatment by accepted guidelines. It should be remembered, however, that costs increase with time, and modelling (based only on the XENDOS study and perhaps omitting some relevant outcomes) suggests that benefits were less clear for longer-term treatment.

Sibutramine

Pharmacology

Sibutramine inhibits the reuptake of both serotonin and noradrenaline into nerve terminals, thus enhancing the synaptic availability and action of both transmitters (Figure 17.10). Importantly, sibutramine differs pharmacologically from fenfluramine and dexafenfluramine, which are serotonin-releasing agents, and it does not bind significantly to dopamine receptors (Cheetham *et al.*, 1995). Sibutramine is rapidly metabolized to primary and secondary metabolites (M2 and M1, respectively), which are thought to be responsible for most of its pharmacological actions (Stock, 1997).

Originally tested as an anti-depressant, sibutramine was found to cause significant loss of body weight, but had no significant impact on mood (King and Devaney, 1988; Bray *et al.*, 1996). In animal models, sibutramine reduces both food intake and rate of weight gain, largely due to reductions in fat mass (Jackson *et al.*, 1997; Brown *et al.*, 2001). In humans, short-term clinical studies have shown that sibutramine decreases food intake and may also increase metabolic rate; overall, however, the contribution of any thermogenic effect to weight loss appears modest, and has not been apparent in all studies (Hansen *et al.*, 1999; Walsh, Leen and Lean, 1999; Seagle, Bessesen and Hill, 1998).

Clinical efficacy in obesity

Early studies demonstrated that sibutramine produced dose-dependent weight loss across the dosage range of 5–30 mg daily (Bray *et al.*, 1999). The clinically licensed doses of 10 or 15 mg once daily have been tested in several

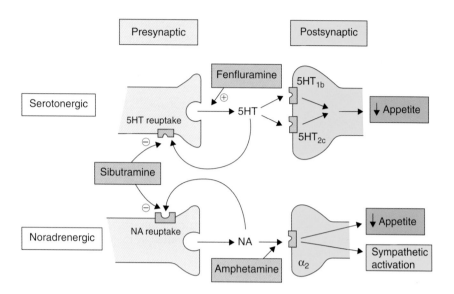

Figure 17.10 Different mechanisms of action of the centrally-acting appetite-suppressing drugs, sibutramine, fenfluramine and amphetamine. Those acting on the noradrenergic neurones to enhance or mimic the effect of noradrenaline (sibutramine, amphetamine) also cause sympathetic stimulation in addition to decreasing appetite.

clinical trials of up to two years' duration in patients with uncomplicated obesity. In the recent NICE systematic review and appraisal, the average absolute weight loss across studies after 12 months was 5.3 kg for sibutramine, compared with 0.5 kg for placebo. Weight is regained after stopping sibutramine treatment. One trial (STORM) suggested that sibutramine can maintain 5% weight loss in 69% of participants after 18 months; however, patients in this particular study who did not achieve 5% weight loss after six months on active treatment were excluded from the randomization and this may have overestimated the effects of

sibutramine (James *et al.*, 2000) (Figure 17.11). Changes in body fat have not been formally measured, but reductions of 7–9 cm in waist circumference point to decreases in visceral fat.

The main side effects associated with sibutramine are attributable to its central sympathomimetic actions, resulting from enhanced noradrenaline availability. These include increases in heart rate and blood pressure, constipation and dry mouth. Headaches also occur. In general, sibutramine could be considered well tolerated, and it does not appear to have any potential for abuse (Cole *et al.*, 1998).

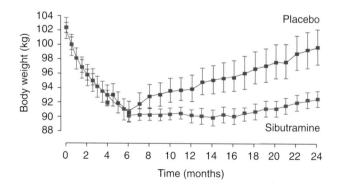

Figure 17.11 Effects of sibutramine and placebo on body weight during the 2-year STORM study (Bray *et al.*, 1996).

Clinical efficacy in special patient groups

Sibutramine has also been shown to be effective in patients with type 2 diabetes, whether treated with diet and physical activity alone, metformin or sulphonylureas (McNulty, Ur and Williams, 2003; Fujioka et al., 2000; Serrano-Rios, Meichionda and Moreno-Carretero, 2002). HbA_{1c} levels were reduced by 0.3%, and fasting glucose by approximately 0.4 mmol/l, as compared with placebo.

Modest improvements are seen in metabolic and vascular risk factors, typified by the outcomes of the 2-year STORM study (Bray et al., 1996) (Table 17.5). Total and LDL cholesterol were not significantly altered by sibutramine, but HDL cholesterol increased by approximately 0.12 mmol/l, compared with 0.03 mmol/l with placebo. Triglyceride levels were reduced by approximately 0.2 mmol/l compared to 0.01 mmol/l for placebo. The improved lipid profile is offset, however, by increases in both systolic and diastolic blood pressure that averaged ~2 mm Hg across studies; one trial in hypertensive patients found that systolic blood pressure was comparable with the placebo group, but that sibutramine increased diastolic pressure by ~3 mm Hg (Hazenberg, Wickens and Chong, 2001).

At present, there are no long-term data on the use of sibutramine but the ongoing Sibutramine Cardiovascular Outcome Trial (SCOUT) is testing whether sibutramine will reduce rates of vascular disease. This study has recruited over 9000 patients aged over 55 years, with significant risk factors for vascular disease including previous myocardial infarction, stroke, peripheral vascular disease and type 2 diabetes; it is expected to report in 2009.

The recent NICE reviews suggested that cost per QALY with sibutramine was approximately £16 000, and that it could therefore be regarded as cost-effective.

Rimonabant

Rimonabant is a highly selective antagonist at the cannabinoid 1 (CB1) receptor, and blocks the orexigenic effects of endocannabinoids (see Figure 17.5). It was previously licensed for use in Europe, but approval was withdrawn in late 2008 because of concern about its severe psychiatric side effects – which also prevented its consideration by the FDA (see below).

Pharmacology

Rimonabant has over 1000-fold selectivity at CB1 compared with CB2 receptors. It is rapidly absorbed after oral administration and it has a long half-life that is proportional to body weight; in obese patients, this is approximately 16 days. Rimonabant is largely metabolized in the liver by cytochrome CYP53A4 and inhibitors of this enzyme (e.g. ketoconazole) can double circulating rimonabant levels – an interaction that must be remembered in clinical practice.

Clinical efficacy in obesity

Rimonabant has been evaluated in the Rimonabant In Obesity (RIO) programme, which comprises four major trials involving over 6500 patients with simple or complicated obesity. All the studies tested doses of 5 mg and 20 mg

Table 17.5 Effects of sibutramine on metabolic and cardiovascular risk factors in obese subjects.

	Placebo	Sibutramine	p-value
Systolic blood pressure (mm Hg)	−2.4	+1.9	$p < 0.001$
Diastolic blood pressure (mm Hg)	−0.5	+3.4	$p < 0.001$
Total cholesterol (% change)	+3	+1	ns
LDL-cholesterol (% change)	+1	0	ns
HDL-cholesterol (% change)	+8	+16	$p < 0.001$
Triglycerides (% change)	−6	−25	$p < 0.001$
Fasting glucose (mmol/l)	+0.07	−0.06	ns

Data from the STORM study (Bray et al., 1996)
ns: not significant

daily; the 5-mg dose generally produced slightly greater weight loss than placebo, while consistent clinical effects were seen with 20 mg daily, which is the dose previously licensed in Europe. The results of the clinical trials (20 mg daily) were remarkably consistent, with a mean weight loss of almost 5 kg greater than with placebo in subjects with uncomplicated obesity, and almost 4 kg greater than placebo in those with type 2 diabetes. Overall, 27% of rimonabant-treated subjects lost ≥10% of body weight after one year (compared with 7% of those taking placebo), while 40–50% lost ≥5% (Bray *et al.*, 1999) (see Figure 17.12). As with other treatments, cessation of drug therapy results in weight regain over one year. Rimonabant treatment was also associated with 4–7 cm reductions in waist circumference.

There were also small but significant improvements in lipid profiles. After two years' treatment, HDL cholesterol increased by 7% compared with placebo, while triglycerides fell by 9%. Fasting plasma glucose fell by 0.8 mmol/l as compared with placebo (Pi-Sunyer *et al.*, 2006). Similar changes were seen in patients with pre-existing dyslipidaemia. Obese hypertensive patients showed a significant reduction in blood pressure, but comparable with that seen with placebo (Després, Golay and Sjöström, 2005). Interestingly, there were improvements in markers of systemic inflammation, with a fall of 0.6 mg in C-reactive protein and a 27% rise in adiponectin.

The RIO Diabetes Trial recruited patients with type 2 diabetes treated with either a sulphonylurea or metformin, most of whom were hypertensive. The mean fall in HbA$_{1c}$ was 0.6% with rimonabant compared with a 0.1% rise with placebo, and as with the other studies there was a significantly greater rise in HDL cholesterol and reduction in triglycerides, compared with placebo.

Adverse effects

The most common reported side effects during these placebo-controlled trials of rimonabant were nausea (13% of cases), dizziness (9% of cases) and diarrhoea (7%); the frequency of these complaints was generally 2–3 times that with placebo. However, the greatest concern is the potential for neuropsychiatric side effects, notably anxiety and depression. The CB1 receptor influences mood – albeit in a complex fashion, with effects on anxiety and depression reported with both agonists and antagonists – and so some impact on mental state was anticipated. Patients with depressive illness were largely excluded from studies of rimonabant, as with other obesity drug trials. A recent meta-analysis has shown that patients receiving rimonabant 20 mg daily were 2.5 times more likely to discontinue treatment because of depressive symptoms, and that anxiety scores (measured by the Hospital Anxiety and Depression Scale) were threefold higher, compared

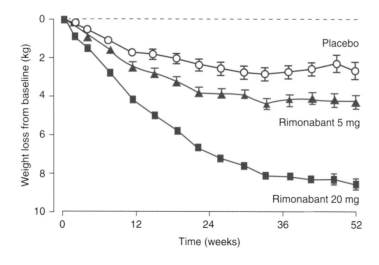

Figure 17.12 Effects of rimonabant and placebo on body weight during the 1-year RIO North America study (James *et al.*, 2000).

with placebo (Christensen *et al.*, 2007). The overall risk may be even higher in populations that did not exclude subjects with known psychiatric disease.

The manufacturer has withdrawn rimonabant from consideration by the FDA, because of concerns over depression and an apparent doubling in the risk of suicide attempts or suicidal ideation. For the same reason, European licensing approval for rimonabant was withdrawn in 2008.

Rimonabant shows some promise in limiting weight gain after stopping smoking. Long-term trials were until recently under way to test the impact of rimonabant on diabetes and cardiovascular disease. These, and all clinical trials of rimonabant, have now been discontinued.

Other treatments

Topiramate and zonisamide

Topiramate and zonisamide are both novel neurotherapeutic agents licensed as anticonvulsants;

Table 17.6   Drugs associated with weight gain: alternatives that do not cause weight gain are shown.

Class	Examples	Alternatives
Anticonvulsants	Sodium valproate	Topiramate
	Phenytoin	Zonisamide
	Gabapentin	
Antidepressants	Citalopram	Fluoxetine
	Mirtazepine	
Antipsychotics	Chlorpromazine	Quetiapine
	Clozapine	
	Haloperidol	
	Risperidone	
	Olanzepine	
	Sulpiride	
Beta-blockers	Atenolol	Depends on indication (consider alternative antihypertensives in obese subjects)
	Propranolol	
	Metoprolol	
Corticosteroids	Prednisolone	
	Dexamethasone	
Insulin	Most formulations	Insulin detemir
Sex steroids	Medroxyprogesterone acetate	Other contraceptive methods
Oral hypoglycaemic drugs	Glibenclamide	Metformin DPP-IV inhibitors (e.g. sitagliptin)
	Gliclazide	
	Pioglitazone	Injectable GLP-1 analogues (e.g. exenatide, liraglutide)
	Repaglinide	
	Rosiglitazone	
Protease inhibitors	Indinavir	
	Ritonavir	

See W.S. Leslie, C.R. Hankey and M.E.J. Lean (2007) 'Weight gain as an adverse effect of some commonly prescribed drugs: a systematic review'. *QJM*, 100, 395–404, with kind permission.

topiramate is also approved for treatment of refractory migraine. Following observations that their use resulted in weight loss in obese patients treated for epilepsy, both were tested as anti-obesity drugs, although neither is licensed for this indication.

Topiramate, a sulfamate-substituted poly-saccharide, has a wide range of effects reported in preclinical studies, including decreased food intake, enhanced energy expenditure and increased substrate utilization (Richard *et al.*, 2000). It was found to cause weight loss in a 6-month dose-ranging study and a subsequent 12-month trial, which also demonstrated beneficial effects on cardiovascular risk factors, including blood lipids and glucose and blood pressure (Bray *et al.*, 2003; Wilding *et al.*, 2004). Topiramate's development as an anti-obesity drug was halted because of unfavourable side effects, including paraesthesiae, mood changes (notably depressed mood and suicidal ideation) and cognitive dysfunction.

Zonisamide was tested in a single study, which showed 9.2 kg weight loss, compared with 1.2 kg with placebo over 32 weeks (Gadde *et al.*, 2003).

These agents should not be used specifically to treat obesity, but could be considered for obese patients with epilepsy or migraine – especially as alternative treatments (e.g. sodium valproate, see Table 17.6) can cause weight gain.

Use of anti-obesity drugs in children and adolescents

Increasing concerns over childhood obesity and the general effectiveness of non-pharmacological interventions in children have led to clinical trials of both orlistat and sibutramine in children and adolescents aged 12–18 years (Berkowitz *et al.*, 2006; Godoy-Matos *et al.*, 2005; Ozkan *et al.*, 2004; McDuffie *et al.*, 2002). The efficacy and adverse effect profiles appear similar to those in adult populations, and these drugs are beginning to be used in specialist centres as adjuncts to lifestyle and other strategies. As yet, there are no data concerning the use of rimonabant in people under the age of 18 years.

The long-term outcomes and risks of drug treatment begun during childhood and potentially continued into adult life are of obvious concern (see Chapter 21).

Drugs causing weight gain

It is important for clinicians to recognize that many commonly-used drugs may lead to weight gain (see Chapter 8). The possibility of iatrogenic obesity must always be considered when assessing an obese patient. Moreover, patients who need medication that can cause obesity must be informed of this risk and given appropriate support to help avoid weight gain; alternative agents may be available, or it may be possible to limit the dosage and/or duration of treatment.

The main classes of drugs associated with weight gain include corticosteroids, depot progesterone contraceptives, anticonvulsants and antipsychotic drugs, β-adrenoreceptor antagonists, several oral hypoglycaemic agents and insulin.

Details of these drugs are provided in Table 17.6, together with some suggested alternatives.

Future directions

Pharmacotherapy for obesity is a rapidly developing field, and the wide range of novel treatments under investigation include agents that influence nutrient absorption, gut hormones and analogues that promote satiety, centrally-acting drugs and others that alter substrate utilization. It is likely that some of these will eventually prove effective to a degree and safe enough to be offered to patients. The limited ability of each of the available drugs to achieve and maintain weight loss will make it important to test the potential of drug combinations to improve efficacy.

As better understanding is gained of the pathophysiology and genetic basics of obesity, it may eventually be possible to exploit clinical and/or genetic information to choose the most effective drug or drug combination for an individual patient For now, however, clinical judgment and careful evaluation of the outcomes will remain the best guide to determining which patients are likely to benefit from pharmacotherapy, and which agent to use.

References

Abenhaim, L., Moride, Y., Brenot, F. et al. (1996) Appetite-suppressant drugs and the risk of primary pulmonary hypertension. *New England Journal of Medicine*, **335** (9), 609–16.

Arch, J.R.S. (2002) beta(3)-adrenoceptor agonists: potential, pitfalls and progress. *European Journal of Pharmacology*, **440** (2–3), 99–107.

Arch, J.R.S. and Wilson, S. (1996) Prospects for beta(3)-adrenoceptor agonists in the treatment of obesity and diabetes. *International Journal of Obesity*, **20**, 191–9.

Astrup, A., Breum, L., Toubro, S. et al. (1992) The effect and safety of an ephedrine caffeine compound compared to ephedrine, caffeine and placebo in obese subjects on an energy restricted diet – a double-blind trial. *International Journal of Obesity*, **16** (4), 269–77.

Avenell, A., Broom, J., Brown, T.J. et al. (2004) Systematic review of the long-term effects and economic consequences of treatments for obesity and implications for health improvement. *Health Technology Assessment*, **8** (21), 1–182.

Ballinger, A.B., Mcloughlin, L., Medbak, S. and Clark, M.L. (1994) Cholecystokinin is a satiety hormone at physiological post prandial concentrations. *Gastroenterology*, **106**, 798.

Batterham, R.L., Cowley, M.A., Small, C.J. et al. (2002) Gut hormone PYY3-36 physiologically inhibits food intake. *Nature*, **418** (6898), 650–4.

Berkowitz, R.I., Fujioka, K., Daniels, S.R. et al. (2006) Effects of sibutramine treatment in obese adolescents – a randomized trial. *Annals of Internal Medicine*, **145** (2), 81–90.

Bluher, M., Engeli, S., Kloting, N. et al. (2006) Dysregulation of the peripheral and adipose tissue endocannabinoid system in human abdominal obesity. *Diabetes*, **55** (11), 3053–60.

Bonora, E. (2007) Antidiabetic medications in overweight/obese patients with type 2 diabetes: drawbacks of current drugs and potential advantages of incretin-based treatment on body weight. *International Journal of Clinical Practice*, **61**, 19–28.

Bray, G.A. (1991) Reciprocal relation between the sympathetic nervous system and food intake. *Brain Research Bulletin*, **27**, 517–20.

Bray, G.A., Blackburn, G.L., Ferguson, J.M. et al. (1999) Sibutramine produces dose-related weight loss. *Obesity Research*, **7**, 189–98.

Bray, G.A., Ryan, D.H., Gordon, D. et al. (1996) Double-blind randomized placebo-controlled trial of sibutramine. *Obesity Research*, **4**, 263–70.

Bray, G.A., Hollander, P., Klein, S. et al. (2003) A 6-month randomized, placebo-controlled, dose-ranging trial of topiramate for weight loss in obesity. *Obesity Research*, **11** (6), 722–33.

Brisbare-Roch, C., Dingemanse, J., Koberstein, R. et al. (2007) Promotion of sleep by targeting the orexin system in rats, dogs and humans. *Nature Medicine*, **13** (2), 150–5.

Broom, I., Wilding, J., Stott, P. and Myers, N. (2002) Randomised trial of the effect of orlistat on body weight and cardiovascular disease risk profile in obese patients: UK multimorbidity study. *International Journal of Clinical Practice*, **56** (7), 494–9.

Brown, M., Bing, C., King, P. et al. (2001) Sibutramine reduces feeding, body fat and improves insulin resistance in dietary-obese male Wister rats independently of hypothalamic neuropeptide Y. *British Journal of Pharmacology*, **132** (8), 1898–1900.

Caffry, E.W., Kissileff, H.R. and Thornton, J.C. (1987) Assessment of the effects of phenylpropanolamine on appetite and food intake. *Pharmacology, Biochemistry, and Behavior*, **26**, 321–5.

Cheetham, S.C., Kettle, C.J., Martin, K.F. and Heal, D.J. (1995) D-1 receptor-binding in rat striatum – modification by various d-1 and d-2 antagonists, but not by sibutramine hydrochloride, antidepressants or treatments which enhance central dopaminergic function. *Journal of Neural Transmission – General Section*, **102**, 35–46.

Christensen, R., Kristensen, P.K., Bartels, E.M. et al. (2007) Efficacy and safety of the weight-loss drug rimonabant: a meta-analysis of randomised trials. *Lancet*, **370**, 1706–13.

Cohen, M.A., Ellis, S.M., Le Roux, C.W. et al. (2003) Oxyntomodulin suppresses appetite and reduces food intake in humans. *Journal of Clinical Endocrinology and Metabolism*, **88** (10), 4696–701.

Cole, J.O., Levin, A., Beake, B. et al. (1998) Sibutramine: A new weight loss agent without evidence of the abuse potential associated with amphetamines. *Journal of Clinical Psychopharmacology*, **18**, 231–6.

Colman, E. (2005) Anorectics on trial: A half century of federal regulation of prescription appetite suppressants. *Annals of Internal Medicine*, **143** (5), 380–5.

Connolly, H.M., Crary, J.L., McGoon, M.D. et al. (1997) Valvular heart disease associated with fenfluramine-phentermine. *The New England Journal of Medicine*, **337** (9), 581–8.

Curioni, C.C. and Lourenco, P.M. (2005) Long-term weight loss after diet and exercise: a systematic review. *International Journal of Obesity and Related Metabolic Disorders*, **29**, 1168–71.

Davidson, M. (1997) A 2 year, US, randomized, controlled study of orlistat, a gastrointestinal lipase inhibitor, for obesity treatment. *Journal of The American Medical Association*, **96**, 4119.

Davidson, M.H., Hauptman, J., DiGirolamo, M. et al. (1999) Weight control and risk factor reduction in obese subjects treated for 2 years with orlistat – a randomized controlled trial. *Journal of The American Medical Association*, **281**, 235–42.

Despres, J.P., Golay, A. and Sjöström, L. (2005) Effects of rimonabant on metabolic risk factors in overweight patients with dyslipidemia. *New England Journal of Medicine*, **353** (20), 2121–34.

Di Marzo, V., Goparaju, S.K., Wang, L. *et al.* (2001) Leptin-regulated endocannabinoids are involved in maintaining food intake. *Nature*, **410** (6830), 822–5.

Diabetes Prevention Program Research Group (2002) Reduction in the incidence of type 2 diabetes with lifestyle intervention or metformin. *The New England Journal of Medicine*, **346**, 393–403.

Dourish, C.T., Rycroft, W. and Iversen, S.D. (1989) Postponement of satiety by blockade of cholecystokinin (CCK-B) receptors. *Science*, **245**, 1509–11.

Drent, M.L., Larsson, I., Williamolsson, T. *et al.* (1995) Orlistat (Ro-18-0647), a lipase inhibitor, in the treatment of human obesity – a multiple-dose study. *International Journal of Obesity*, **19**, 221–6.

Edwards, C.M.B., Stanley, S.A., Davis, R. *et al.* (2001) Exendin-4 reduces fasting and postprandial glucose and decreases energy intake in healthy volunteers. *American Journal of Physiology – Endocrinology and Metabolism*, **281** (1), E155–61.

Engeli, S., Bohnke, J., Feldpausch, M. *et al.* (2005) Activation of the peripheral endocannabinoid system in human obesity. *Diabetes*, **54** (10), 2838–43.

English, P.J., Ghatei, M.A., Malik, I.A. *et al.* (2002) Food fails to suppress ghrelin levels in obese humans. *Journal of Clinical Endocrinology and Metabolism*, **87** (6), 2984–7.

Farooqi, I.S., Jebb, S.A., Langmack, G. *et al.* (1999) Effects of recombinant leptin therapy in a child with congenital leptin deficiency. *New England Journal of Medicine*, **341** (12), 879–84.

Fujioka, K., Seaton, T.B., Rowe, E. *et al.* (2000) Weight loss with sibutramine improves glycaemic control and other metabolic parameters in obese patients with type 2 diabetes mellitus. *Diabetes Obesity & Metabolism*, **2** (3), 175–87.

Gadde, K.M., Franciscy, D.M., Wagner, H.R. and Krishnan, K.R.R. (2003) Zonisamide for weight loss in obese adults – a randomized controlled trial. *Journal of The American Medical Association*, **289** (14), 1820–5.

Gerard, C.M., Mollereau, C., Vassart, G. and Parmentier, M. (1991) Molecular-cloning of a human cannabinoid receptor which is also expressed in testis. *Biochemical Journal*, **279**, 129–34.

Godoy-Matos, A., Carraro, L., Vieira, A. *et al.* (2005) Treatment of obese adolescents with sibutramine: a randomized, double-blind, controlled study. *Journal of Clinical Endocrinology and Metabolism*, **90** (3), 1460–5.

Goldstein, D.J. (1992) Beneficial health-effects of modest weight-loss. *International Journal of Obesity*, **16**, 397–415.

Goldstein, D.J., Rampey, A.H., Enas, G.G. *et al.* (1994) Fluoxetine – a randomized clinical-trial in the treatment of obesity. *International Journal of Obesity*, **18**, 129–35.

Guy-Grand, B., Apfelbaum, M., Crepaldi, G. *et al.* (1989) International trial of long term dexfenfluramine in obesity. *Lancet*, **11** (2), 1142–5.

Halford, J.C.G., Harrold, J.A., Lawton, C.L. and Blundell, J.E. (2005) Serotonin (5-HT) drugs: Effects on appetite expression and use for the treatment of obesity. *Current Drug Targets*, **6** (2), 201–13.

Hansen, D.L., Toubro, S., Stock, M.J. *et al.* (1999) The effect of sibutramine on energy expenditure and appetite during chronic treatment without dietary restriction. *International Journal of Obesity*, **23**, 1016–24.

Hawkins, M.F., Barkemeyer, C.A. and Tulley, R.T. (1986) Synergistic effects of dopamine agonists and centrally administered neurotensin on feeding. *Pharmacology, Biochemistry, and Behavior*, **24**, 1195–201.

Hazenberg, B.P., Wickens, M. and Chong, E. (2001) Sibutramine vs placebo: Meta-analysis of mean changes in resting blood pressure in obese patients with hypertension. *Obesity Research*, **9**, 153S.

Higgs, S., Williams, C.M. and Kirkham, T.C. (2003) Cannabinoid influences on palatability: microstructural analysis of sucrose drinking after Delta(9)-tetrahydrocannabinol, anandamide, 2-arachidonoyl glycerol and SR141716. *Psychopharmacology*, **165** (4), 370–7.

Hollander, P.A., Elbein, S.C., Hirsch, I.B. *et al.* (1998) Role of orlistat in the treatment of obese patients with type 2 diabetes – a 1-year randomized double-blind study. *Diabetes Care*, **21**, 1288–94.

Holman, R.R., Cull, C.A. and Turner, R.C. (1999) A randomized double-blind trial of acarbose in type 2 diabetes shows improved glycemic control over 3 years (UK Prospective Diabetes Study 44). *Diabetes Care*, **22**, 960–4.

Hussain, Y., Guzelhan, C., Odink, J. *et al.* (1994) Comparison of the inhibition of dietary-fat absorption by full versus divided doses of orlistat. *Journal of Clinical Pharmacology*, **34**, 1121–5.

Hwa, J.J., Witten, M.B., Williams, P. *et al.* (1999) Activation of the NPYY5 receptor regulates both feeding and energy expenditure. *American Journal of Physiology – Regulatory, Integrative and Comparative Physiology*, **277** (5), R1428–34.

Jackson, H.C., Needham, A.M., Hutchins, L.J. *et al.* (1997) Comparison of the effects of sibutramine and other monoamine reuptake inhibitors on food intake in the rat. *British Journal of Pharmacology*, **121**, 1758–62.

James, W.P.T., Astrup, A., Finer, N. *et al.* (2000) Effect of sibutramine on weight maintenance after weight loss: a randomised trial. *Lancet*, **356** (9248), 2119–25.

Kamegai, J., Tamura, H., Shimizu, T. *et al.* (2000) Central effect of ghrelin, an endogenous growth hormone secretagogue, on hypothalamic peptide gene expression. *Endocrinology*, **141** (12), 4797–800.

Kaya, A., Aydin, N., Topsever, P. *et al.* (2004) Efficacy of sibutramine, orlistat and combination therapy on short-term weight management in obese patients. *Biomedicine & Pharmacotherapy*, **58** (10), 582–7.

King, D.J. and Devaney, N. (1988) Clinical pharmacology of sibutramine hydrochloride (BTS 54524), a new antidepressant, in healthy volunteers. *British Journal of Clinical Pharmacology*, **26** (5), 607–11.

Kirkham, T.C. (2005) Endocannabinoids in the regulation of appetite and body weight. *Behavioural Pharmacology*, **16** (5–6), 297–313.

Koch, J.E., Glass, M.J., Cooper, M.L. and Bodnar, R.J. (1995) Alterations in deprivation, glucoprivic and sucrose intake following general, mu and kappa opioid antagonists in the hypothalamic paraventricular nucleus of rats. *Neuroscience*, **66**, 951–7.

Krude, H. and Gruters, A. (2000) Implications of proopiomelanocortin (POMC) mutations in humans: the POMC deficiency syndrome. *Trends in Endocrinology and Metabolism*, **11** (1), 15–22.

Kushner, R.F. and Noble, C.A. (2006) Long-term outcome of bariatric surgery: an interim analysis. *Mayo Clinic Proceedings*, **81** (10), S46–51.

Leslie, W.S., Hankey, C.R. and Lean, M.E.J. (2007) Weight gain as an adverse effect of some commonly prescribed drugs: a systematic review. *QJM: An International Journal of Medicine*, **100**, 395–404.

Marsh, D.J., Hollopeter, G., Kafer, K.E. and Palmiter, R.D. (1998) Role of the Y5 neuropeptide Y receptor in feeding and obesity. *Nature Medicine*, **4** (6), 718–21.

McDuffie, J.R., Calis, K.A., Uwaifo, G.I. *et al.* (2002) Three-month tolerability of orlistat in adolescents with obesity-related comorbid conditions. *Obesity Research*, **10** (7), 642–50.

McNulty, S.J., Ur, E. and Williams, G. (2003) A randomized trial of sibutramine in the management of obese type 2 diabetic patients treated with metformin. *Diabetes Care*, **26** (1), 125–31.

Melia, A.T., KossTwardy, S.G. and Zhi, J.G. (1996) The effect of orlistat, an inhibitor of dietary fat absorption, on the absorption of vitamins A and E in healthy volunteers. *Journal of Clinical Pharmacology*, **36**, 647–53.

Miles, J.M., Aronne, L.J., Hollander, P. and Klein, S. (2001) Effect of orlistat in overweight and obese type 2 diabetes patients treated with metformin. *Diabetes*, **50**, A442–3.

Nakajima, M., Inui, A., Teranishi, A. *et al.* (1994) Effects of pancreatic polypeptide family peptides on feeding and learning behavior in mice. *Journal of Pharmacology and Experimental Therapeutics*, **268**, 1010–4.

Nauck, M.A., Duran, S., Kim, D. *et al.* (2007) A comparison of twice-daily exenatide and biphasic insulin aspart in patients with type 2 diabetes who were suboptimally controlled with sulfonylurea and metformin: a non-inferiority study. *Diabetologia*, **50** (2), 259–67.

Ng, F.M., Sun, J., Sharma, L. *et al.* (2000) Metabolic studies of a synthetic lipolytic domain (AOD9604) of human growth hormone. *Hormone Research*, **53** (6), 274–8.

NICE (2006) Obesity: the prevention, identification, assessment and management of overweight and obesity in adults and children. See http://www.nice.org.uk/CG043 (last accessed 16 July 2008).

Olshansky, S.J., Passaro, D.J., Hershow, R.C. *et al.* (2005) A potential decline in life expectancy in the United States in the 21st century. *New England Journal of Medicine*, **352** (11), 1138–45.

Ozkan, B., Bereket, A., Turan, S. and Keskin, S. (2004) Addition of orlistat to conventional treatment in adolescents with severe obesity. *European Journal of Pediatrics*, **163** (12), 738–41.

Parker, E.D. and Folsom, A.R. (2003) Intentional weight loss and incidence of obesity-related cancers: the Iowa Women's Health Study. *International Journal of Obesity*, **27** (12), 1447–52.

Pi-Sunyer, F., Aronne, L.J., Heshmati, H.M. *et al.* (2006) Effect of rimonabant, a cannabinoid-1 receptor blocker, on weight and cardiometabolic risk factors in overweight or obese patients – RIO-North America: a randomized controlled trial. *Journal of The American Medical Association*, **295** (7), 761–75.

Ransac, S., Gargouri, Y., Moreau, H. and Verger, R. (1991) Inactivation of pancreatic and gastric lipases by tetrahydrolipstatin and alkyl-dithio-5-(2-Nitrobenzoic acid) – a kinetic-study with 1,2- didecanoyl-sn-glycerol monolayers. *European Journal of Biochemistry*, **202**, 395–400.

Richard, D., Ferland, J., Lalonde, J. *et al.* (2000) Influence of topiramate in the regulation of energy balance. *Nutrition*, **16** (10), 961–6.

Royal College of Physicians (2003) Anti-obesity drugs: guidance on appropriate prescribing and management. Royal College of Physicians, London.

Sachdev, M., Miller, W.C., Ryan, T. and Jolis, J.G. (2002) Effect of fenfluramine-derivative diet pills on cardiac valves: a meta-analysis of observational studies. *American Heart Journal*, **144** (6), 1065–73.

Sahu, A. (1998) Evidence suggesting that galanin (GAL), melanin-concentrating hormone (MCH), neurotensin (NT), proopiomelanocortin (POMC) and neuropeptide Y (NPY) are targets of leptin signaling in the hypothalamus. *Endocrinology*, **139** (2), 795–8.

Sakurai, T., Arnemiya, T., Ihsii, M. *et al.* (1998) Orexins and orexin receptors: a family of hypothalamic neuropeptides and G protein coupled receptors that regulate feeding behaviour. *Cell*, **92**, 573–85.

Seagle, H.M., Bessesen, D.H. and Hill, J.O. (1998) Effects of sibutramine on resting metabolic rate and weight loss in overweight women. *Obesity Research*, **6**, 115–21.

Serrano-Rios, M., Meichionda, N. and Moreno-Carretero, E. (2002) Role of sibutramine in the treatment of obese type 2 diabetic patients receiving sulphonylurea therapy. *Diabetic Medicine*, **19** (2), 119–24.

Shintani, M., Ogawa, Y., Ebihara, K. *et al.* (2001) Ghrelin, an endogenous growth hormone secretagogue, is a novel orexigenic peptide that antagonizes leptin action through the activation of hypothalamic neuropeptide Y/Y1 receptor pathway. *Diabetes*, **50** (2), 227–32.

Shire, D., Calandra, B., RinaldiCarmona, M. *et al.* (1996) Molecular cloning, expression and function of the murine CB2 peripheral cannabinoid receptor. *Biochimica et Biophysica Acta – Gene Structure and Expression*, **1307** (2), 132–6.

Sjöström, L., Rissanen, A., Andersen, T. *et al.* (1998) Randomised placebo-controlled trial of orlistat for weight loss and prevention of weight regain in obese patients. *Lancet*, **352**, 167–72.

Sjöström, L., Lindroos, A.K., Peltonen, M. *et al.* (2004) Lifestyle, diabetes, and cardiovascular risk factors 10 years after bariatric surgery. *New England Journal of Medicine*, **351** (26), 2683–93.

Spoto, B., Fezza, F., Parlongo, G. *et al.* (2006) Human adipose tissue binds and metabolizes the endocannabinoids anandamide and 2-arachidonoylglycerol. *Biochimie*, **88** (12), 1889–97.

Stevens, V.J., Obarzanek, E., Cook, N.R. *et al.* (2001) Long-term weight loss and changes in blood pressure: results of the trials of hypertension prevention, phase II. *Annals of Internal Medicine*, **134** (1), 1–11.

Stock, M.J. (1997) Sibutramine: a review of the pharmacology of a novel anti-obesity agent. *International Journal of Obesity and Related Metabolic Disorders*, **21** (Suppl 1), S25–9.

The Treatment of Mild Hypertension Research Group (1991) The treatment of mild hypertension study. A randomized, placebo-controlled trial of a nutritional-hygienic regimen along with various drug monotherapies. *Archives of Internal Medicine*, **151** (7), 1413–23.

Torgerson, J.S., Hauptman, J., Boldrin, M.N. and Sjöström, L. (2004) XENical in the prevention of diabetes in obese subjects (XENDOS) study. *Diabetes Care*, **27** (1), 155–61.

Trillou, C.R., Arnone, M., Delgorge, C. *et al.* (2003) Anti-obesity effect of SR141716, a CB1 receptor antagonist, in diet-induced obese mice. *American Journal of Physiology –Regulatory, Integrative and Comparative Physiology*, **284** (2), R345–53.

Trillou, C.R., Delgorge, C., Menet, C. *et al.* (2004) CB1 cannabinoid receptor knockout in mice leads to leanness, resistance to diet-induced obesity and enhanced leptin sensitivity. *International Journal of Obesity*, **28** (4), 640–8.

Tuomilheto, J., Lindstrom, J., Erickson, J.G. *et al.* (2001) Prevention of type 2 diabetes mellitus by changes in lifestyle amongst subjects with impaired glucose tolerance. *The New England Journal of Medicine*, **344**, 1343–50.

Vickers, S.P., Easton, N., Webster, L.J. *et al.* (2003) Oral administration of the 5-HT2C receptor agonist, mCPP, reduces body weight gain in rats over 28 days as a result of maintained hypophagia. *Psychopharmacology*, **167** (3), 274–80.

Wadden, T.A., Berkowitz, R.I., Womble, L.G. *et al.* (2000) Effects of sibutramine plus orlistat in obese women following 1 year of treatment by sibutramine alone: a placebo-controlled trial. *Obesity Research*, **8** (6), 431–7.

Walsh, K.M., Leen, E. and Lean, M.E.J. (1999) The effect of sibutramine on resting energy expenditure and adrenaline-induced thermogenesis in obese females. *International Journal of Obesity*, **23**, 1009–15.

Weintraub, M., Sundaresan, P.R., Madan, M. *et al.* (1992a) Long-term weight control study. 1. (Weeks 0 to 34) – the enhancement of behavior-modification, caloric restriction, and exercise by fenfluramine plus phentermine versus placebo. *Clinical Pharmacology & Therapeutics*, **51** (5), 586–94.

Weintraub, M., Sundaresan, P.R., Schuster, B. *et al.* (1992b) Long-term weight control study. 2. (Weeks 34 to 104) – an open-label study of continuous fenfluramine plus phentermine versus targeted intermittent medication as adjuncts to behavior-modification, caloric eestriction, and exercise. *Clinical Pharmacology & Therapeutics*, **51** (5), 595–601.

Weintraub, M., Sundaresan, P.R., Schuster, B. *et al.* (1992c) Long-term weight control study. 3. (Weeks 104 to 156) – an open-label study of dose adjustment of fenfluramine and phentermine. *Clinical Pharmacology & Therapeutics*, **51** (5), 602–7.

Weintraub, M., Sundaresan, P.R., Schuster, B. *et al.* (1992d) Long-term weight control study. 4. (Weeks 156 to 190) – the 2nd double-blind phase. *Clinical Pharmacology & Therapeutics*, **51** (5), 608–14.

Weintraub, M., Sundaresan, P.R., Schuster, B. *et al.* (1992e) Long-term weight control study. 5. (Weeks 190 to 210) – follow-up of participants after cessation of medication. *Clinical Pharmacology & Therapeutics*, **51** (5), 615–8.

Wilding, J.P.H. (2002) Neuropeptides and appetite control. *Diabetic Medicine: a Journal of the British Diabetic, Association*, **19**, 619–27.

Wilding, J., Van Gaal, L., Rissanen, A. *et al.* (2004) A randomized double-blind placebo-controlled study of the long-term efficacy and safety of topiramate in the treatment of obese subjects. *International Journal of Obesity*, **28** (11), 1399–410.

Willey, K.A., Molyneaux, L.M. and Yue, D.K. (1994) Obese patients with type 2 diabetes poorly controlled by insulin and metformin: effects of adjunctive dexfenfluramine therapy on glycaemic control. *Diabetic*

Medicine: a Journal of the British Diabetic, Association **11**, 701–4.

Williamson, D.F., Pamuk, E., Thun, M. *et al.* (1995) Prospective study of intentional weight loss and mortality in never-smoking overweight US white women aged 40–64 years. *American Journal of Epidemiology*, **141**, 1128–41.

Williamson, D.F., Thompson, T.J., Thun, M. *et al.* (2000) Intentional weight loss and mortality among overweight individuals with diabetes. *Diabetes Care*, **23** (10), 1499–504.

Wing, R.R. (1989) Behavioral strategies for weight-reduction in obese type-ii diabetic-patients. *Diabetes Care*, **12**, 139–44.

Zhang, J.V., Ren, P.G., Avsian-Kretchmer, O., Luo *et al.* (2005) Obestatin, a peptide encoded by the ghrelin gene, opposes ghrelin's effects on food intake. *Science*, **310** (5750), 996–9.

Zhi, J.G., Melia, A.T., Funk, C. *et al.* (1996) Metabolic profiles of minimally absorbed orlistat in obese/overweight volunteers. *Journal of Clinical Pharmacology*, **36**, 1006–11.

Surgical Approaches to the Management of Obesity

Key points

- Modern bariatric surgical procedures are safe and effective and should be considered in selected patients with severe obesity who fail to lose sufficient weight through other means. Bariatric surgery is the only treatment for obesity that can reliably achieve major and lasting weight loss with sustained improvement of co-morbidities.

- 'Restrictive' procedures such as gastric banding create a small gastric pouch which fills rapidly and enhances satiety signals. 'Malabsorptive procedures' such as the jejunoileal bypass exclude ingested food from the absorptive surface of the jejunum and ileum. Gastric bypass and biliopancreatic diversion operations employ both strategies.

- Early operations were often effective but are now little used because of severe side-effects. A notable example was the jejunoileal bypass, which caused the 'blind loop' syndrome (abdominal bloating due to anaerobic bacterial overgrowth in the bypassed ileum), oxalate nephropathy and electrolyte and vitamin deficiencies.

- The Roux-en-Y gastric bypass (RYGBP) connects a small gastric pouch to the distal jejunum, with the proximal jejunum anastomosed to the lower ileum to bypass part of its absorptive area. The RYGBP is widely used and can be performed laparoscopically; it can achieve loss of 50–60% of excess weight for up to 5 years. Side-effects include deficiencies of iron, folate, calcium and vitamins (necessitating daily supplementation) and of protein; Wernicke's encephalopathy is a rare post-operative complication.

- Biliopancreatic diversion (BPD) avoids a static blind loop by anastomosing the proximal stomach to the ileum; the proximal small bowel, perfused by bile and pancreatic secretions, is connected to the distal ileum. With the BPD, 80% of excess weight can be lost initially. Deficiencies of fat-soluble vitamins, iron, calcium and protein may occur.

- Gastric banding uses bands to partition the upper stomach, creating a 15–25 ml pouch. Most operations are performed laparoscopically and employ inflatable bands connected to a subcutaneously-buried reservoir into which saline is injected to adjust the tension. Excess weight can be reduced by ~50%. Complications include slippage of the band (which can obstruct the stomach) and infection or leakage of the reservoir system.

- Most bariatric procedures are now performed laparoscopically, which considerably reduces surgical trauma, postoperative complications (especially thromboembolism), duration of hospitalisation, and perioperative mortality.

- Selection criteria for bariatric surgery are severe obesity (BMI $\geq$ 40 kg/m², or $\geq$ 35 kg/m² with serious comorbidity) that has resisted medical therapy; absence of treatable causes of obesity and of significant psychiatric disorder; acceptable operative risk; and the patient's acceptance of pre-operative education and life-long follow-up. An expert surgeon and a dedicated multi-disciplinary support team are essential.

- Successful bariatric surgery can markedly improve the comorbidities of obesity, with complete resolution of type 2 diabetes in up to 70% of cases, hypertension (over 40% of cases) and obstructive sleep apnoea (90% of cases). Quality of life often improves rapidly, and 10-year mortality is reduced by 30%. After several years, some patients regain weight, when comorbidities may recur.

Chapter 18 Surgical Approaches to the Management of Obesity

Mervyn Deitel

Severe obesity and its sequelae are serious, debilitating and progressive diseases that shorten life. In many cases, obesity is not amenable to lifestyle modification or pharmacotherapy (Bloomberg *et al.*, 2005; Stunkard and McLaren-Hume, 1959; Van Itallie, 1980; Wooley and Garner, 1991). Weight loss of 15 kg, which may be achieved by perhaps one-third of subjects treated with anti-obesity drugs, can bring significant clinical benefits to a patient weighing 95 kg, but may make little impact on someone weighing 190 kg. Moreover, most morbidly obese patients ultimately regain any weight that they lose through lifestyle or pharmacological management programmes. In such cases, weight-reducing or 'bariatric' surgery should be considered – indeed, it is the only therapy proven to achieve and maintain weight-loss and to improve the comorbidities of obesity in the long term (Buchwald and Williams, 2004; Deitel and Shahi, 1992).

This chapter describes the rationale, indications and outcomes of the various surgical procedures devised to induce weight loss. The main focus is on the operations most widely used today, notably gastric bypass and gastric banding. The historical background is also briefly reviewed, to show the dramatic evolution of this field and particularly the greatly improved efficacy and safety of modern techniques.

Rationale of bariatric surgical procedures

Bariatric operations cause weight loss through two broad mechanisms:

- Restrictive procedures reduce the effective volume of the stomach, thus enhancing normal satiety signals that terminate eating (see Chapter 6). The adult stomach has a resting volume of 300–500 ml and when fully distended can accommodate 1000 ml. Restrictive operations such as gastroplasty and gastric banding create a gastric pouch with a volume of only 25–50 ml. Other procedures that act by increasing satiety include the intragastric balloon.

- Malabsorptive procedures reduce the access of ingested food to the parts of the small bowel where absorption of nutrients takes place. The largest absorptive surface is in the jejunum and ileum, which are responsible for the uptake of dietary lipid products (triglycerides, glycerol), monosaccharides and aminoacids – and also of fluid, electrolytes and vitamins. The adult jejunum and ileum average 2.5 and 3.5 metres in length respectively; jejunoileal bypass (now largely abandoned) and duodenal switch operations reduce the effective absorptive surface of the small intestine by perhaps 90% and 85% respectively. Other procedures that induce a degree of malabsorption include the biliopancreatic diversion and gastric bypass operation; these and modern gastric bypass operations create a small gastric pouch and therefore also have a restrictive component. In the past five years, the first part of the duodenal switch (sleeve gastrectomy) has emerged as a first stage in high-risk patients and as a definitive procedure by some surgeons, and is essentially a restrictive operation.

Some bariatric procedures are effective through both these mechanisms (see Table 18.1).

History of bariatric surgery

The first operation performed specifically to induce weight loss in severely obese patients was extensive small bowel resection, carried out by

Obesity: Science to Practice Edited by Gareth Williams and Gema Frühbeck
© 2009 John Wiley & Sons, Ltd

Table 18.1 Bariatric procedures and their mechanisms of action.

	Malabsorptive	Restrictive
Abandoned procedures		
• Jejunoileal bypass	+++	−
Current procedures		
• Roux-en-Y gastric bypass		
– proximal anastomosis	++	++
– distal anastomosis	+++	++
• Biliopancreatic diversion	+++	+
• Duodenal switch	+++	+
• Gastroplasty (vertical banded)	−	+++
• Gastric banding	−	+++
• Sleeve gastrectomy	−	+++
Other bariatric procedures		
• Intragastric balloon		

Henrikson in five cases during the 1950s (Henrikson, 1952). This followed the clinical observation that small bowel resection, undertaken for other indications, caused severe malabsorption of fat and carbohydrate. Operative details and actual weight loss were not documented in this early series. The operation was soon abandoned: it was irreversible and caused intractable gastrointestinal losses of water, electrolytes, vitamins and protein.

Jejunocolic bypass was subsequently developed by Turnbull and by Payne (Deitel, 1989; Lewis, Turnbull and Page, 1966; Payne, DeWind and Commons, 1963). The proximal 37–35 cm of the jejunum was joined directly to the transverse colon, thereby excluding most of the small bowel. This procedure produced considerable weight loss, but also led to severe fluid and electrolyte losses and hepatic dysfunction (possibly due to choline deficiency). These side effects often necessitated reversal of the operation, when weight was regained.

Jejunoileal bypass

Jejunoileal bypass (JIB) was first described by Kremen in the 1950s (Kremen, Linner and Nelson,

1954) and subsequently modified, with numerous variations on the length of ileum bypassed and the configuration of the anastomosis (Buchwald, Schwartz and Varco, 1973; DeWind and Payne, 1976). It was abandoned, but was the precursor for the biliopancreatic diversion and the duodenal switch, which are in use. In Payne's procedure (Figure 18.1a), the proximal 35 cm of jejunum was anastomosed to the side (end-to-side) of the distal 10 cm of the ileum (Deitel *et al.*, 1993; Sylvan, Sjölund and Januger, 1995). In the Scott procedure (Salmon, 1971; Alden, 1977; Sylvan, Sjölund and Januger, 1995), the proximal 30 cm of jejunum was anastomosed end-to-end to the distal 25 cm of ileum. The bypassed jejunoileum was thus anastomosed end-to-side to the distal ileum, caecum or transverse or even sigmoid colon in these operations. All these operations created a 'blind loop' of bypassed jejunoileum, in which stasis favoured the overgrowth of predominantly anaerobic bacteria (Deitel, 1989). The 'blind loop syndrome' was responsible for many of the operation's adverse effects, described below.

Jejunoileal bypass could be effective, with up to 50% of excess weight being lost within 12 months (Deitel *et al.*, 1993; Sylvan, Sjölund and Januger, 1995). However, the operation required regular and expert follow up and was beset by frequent and potentially serious side effects. These included:

- Abdominal bloating due to gas production by anaerobes in the blind loop, especially with anastomosis of the bypassed bowel to the colon (Deitel *et al.*, 1993; Deitel, 1989; Scott *et al.*, 1977). Penicillins and other antibiotics that enhanced anaerobe overgrowth exacerbated these symptoms, which could be treated by broad-spectrum antibiotics (e.g. metronidazole and tetracyclines) that covered anaerobes.
- Oxalate stones and nephropathy (Clayman and Williams, 1971; Deitel *et al.*, 1993), due to excessive absorption of dietary oxalate. Oxalate is normally bound and rendered insoluble by ingested calcium; with the JIB, fat malabsorption raises intraluminal levels of free fatty acids that avidly bind calcium, thus leaving oxalate available for absorption in the ascending colon. Oxalate stone formation was discouraged by avoiding oxalate-rich foods (e.g. spinach, carrots and cocoa) and maintaining a high fluid intake, but still necessitated reversal of the operation in 6–12% of cases.

- Deficiencies of potassium, magnesium and zinc (all absorbed in the ileum), of fat-soluble vitamins (A, D, E and K that are co-absorbed with lipids), and of vitamin B12 (for operations that bypassed the terminal ileum).
- Liver dysfunction, apparently due to deficiency of choline, resulting from malabsorption of its precursor, methionine. This was an occasional problem but could largely be prevented by an adequate protein intake and/or methionine supplementation (including pre-digested collagen capsules); acute liver failure could be reversed by intravenous amino acid solutions (Heimberger *et al.*, 1975).
- Migratory arthritis and rarely dermatitis. This complication was due to a synovial hypersensitivity reaction to products of anaerobes absorbed from the blind loop (Wands *et al.*, 1976).

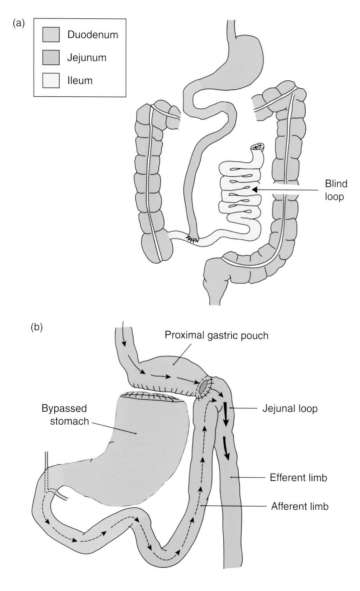

Figure 18.1 Bariatric surgical procedures now rarely performed. (a) Jejunoileal bypass. In the Payne version, the jejunum (35 cm) was anastomosed to the side of the last 10 cm of distal ileum, leaving a blind loop of bypassed ileum. (b) Gastric bypass. A proximal gastric pouch has been formed and anastomosed to a loop of jejunum; tension on the jejunal loop had the potential for the anastomosis to break down. (c) Horizontal gastroplasty. A proximal gastric pouch was created above horizontal lines of staples and the greater curvature outlet was formed by a suture around a bougie inserted during the operation.

(*continues*)

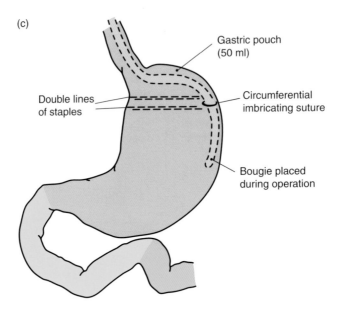

(c)

Gastric pouch
(50 ml)

Double lines
of staples

Circumferential
imbricating suture

Bougie placed
during operation

Figure 18.1 (*Continued*)

It responded to broad-spectrum antibiotics, whereas treatment with non-steroidal anti-inflammatory drugs or corticosteroids was ineffective.

The JIB has now been largely abandoned because of its side effects. Two modifications overcame the problems of bacterial overgrowth in the blind loop. In the JIB with ileogastrostomy, the distal end of the bypassed ileum was anastomosed to the side of the stomach, instead of being closed to create the blind loop; communication with the low pressure in the stomach helped to prevent stasis and therefore the growth of anaerobes (Cleator *et al.*, 2006; Rae and Cleator, 1993). An alternative is the biliointestinal bypass, in which the distal end of the bypassed ileum is anastomosed to the gall bladder, allowing biliary flow through the bypassed jejunoileum and preventing bacterial overgrowth (Eriksson, 1981). This operation is now rarely performed.

Gastric bypass

This procedure, first performed by Mason in the 1960s, developed from his observation that patients who had undergone subtotal gastrectomy (for peptic ulcer disease or cancer) lost weight post-operatively (Mason and Ito, 1967; Mason and Ito, 1978). This loop gastric bypass was the first 'restrictive' procedure and led ultimately to the Roux-en-Y gastric bypass, which remains the most widely used operation in the USA and parts of Europe (see below).

Mason's original operation involved creating a small (50 ml) horizontal gastric pouch at the fundus and anastomosing this to the jejunum, which was mobilized and brought up in a loop; the bypassed distal stomach was left *in situ* (Figure 18.1b). The restrictive gastric pouch permitted only small meals and induced premature satiety, while the unpleasant symptoms of the 'dumping syndrome' (caused by a high sugar load rapidly entering the jejunum) discouraged the ingestion of sugar-rich foods and drinks. This operation often achieved substantial weight loss, but suffered from two main side effects, namely gastritis due to bile refluxing into the gastric pouch from the jejunum, and the risk of the gastrojejunal anastomosis breaking down because the jejunal loop was under tension; the latter complication was potentially catastrophic because escape of the major digestive secretions caused peritonitis. These problems have been addressed in the modified operations in current use, described below.

Horizontal gastroplasty

During the mid-1970s, various gastric restrictive procedures were devised, in which the oesophagus

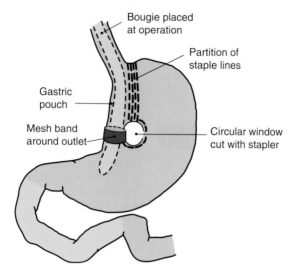

Bougie placed
at operation

Partition of
staple lines

Gastric
pouch

Mesh band
around outlet

Circular window
cut with stapler

Figure 18.2 Vertical banded gastroplasty. The vertical gastric pouch was created at the lesser curve, around a bougie inserted during the operation; the rest of the stomach was excluded by a line of staples, and the pouch outlet encircled by a mesh band. This procedure has now been frequently superseded by the adjustable gastric banding operation, performed laparoscopically.

led into a small upper gastric pouch that communicated with the body of the stomach through a narrow channel. The earliest operation, the horizontal gastroplasty, partitioned off most of the width of the proximal stomach with one or more lines of staples, producing a pouch of 50 ml capacity that communicated with the body of the stomach through an aperture with a diameter of 1 cm (Pace *et al.*, 1979). The aperture was reinforced by a circumferential imbricating (non-slipping) suture that was tightened around a bougie inserted into the stomach at operation. Several variations were developed, including that of Gomez (1980), shown in Figure 18.1c.

Horizontal gastroplasties initially achieved significant weight loss, but these procedures did not prevent the gastric pouch and its outlet from enlarging – when weight was soon regained and the benefits of the operation lost.

Vertical banded gastroplasty

In the early 1980s, Mason developed the vertical banded gastroplasty (VBG), in which the channel was constructed at the lesser curvature, where the muscle is thicker and more resistant to dilation (Mason, 1982). An antero-posterior window, enclosed by staples, was punched through the stomach using a circular stapler, and a vertical pouch was created with four parallel

rows of staples running from the window to the angle of His (Figure 18.2). The channel was made around a 1-cm diameter bougie, and the outlet reinforced by overlapping a strip of polypropylene mesh to produce a collar of 5 cm in circumference and 1.5 cm high (Deitel *et al.*, 1986; Mason, Doherty and Cullen, 1998).

The VBG permitted only small meals that had to be chewed well and eaten slowly, to prevent vomiting (Eckhout, Willbanks and Moore, 1981). Weight loss was initially satisfactory, averaging about 60% of excess weight after 12 months, but many patients tended to regain weight thereafter, and up to 25% had reached their preoperative weight within five years (Deitel and Shikora, 2002). Weight regain was due in some cases to maladaptive eating, for example consuming calorie-dense drinks that pass readily through the channel – which underlines the crucial importance of educating patients contemplating bariatric surgery to ensure their compliance. Patients with a gastroplasty require chewable or liquid vitamin supplements and sometimes liquid iron; red meat passes through the channel with difficulty and may be avoided by some patients. Non-steroidal anti-inflammatory drugs and irritating medications such as iron tablets should be avoided, because high concentrations of these agents in the narrow channel can cause local ulceration.

The VBG can be performed through a very short midline abdominal incision (Deitel *et al.*, 1986) and more recently laparoscopically (Näslund *et al.*, 1999), and is still in use. However, it has been largely superseded by the adjustable gastric banding operation.

Bariatric operations in current use

The operations described below account for the vast majority of new bariatric procedures. Despite considerable geographical variation, there is a general move towards the Roux-en-Y gastric bypass and adjustable gastric banding, performed laparoscopically.

Roux-en-Y gastric bypass (RYGBP)

This modification of the original loop gastric bypass (Figure 18.1b) was introduced by Griffen, Young and Stevenson (1977). The jejunum is divided and the distal end brought up as the 'Roux' or 'alimentary' limb to join the small

(25 ml) proximal gastric pouch. The proximal jejunum (the 'afferent' or 'biliopancreatic' limb) is anastomosed to the side of the jejunum distally; the small bowel distally is termed the 'common' limb (Figure 18.3). This Y-shaped configuration decreases the tension on the gastric anastomosis and therefore the risk of breakdown, while a long Roux loop of >40 cm also prevents bile reflux gastritis in the pouch. Longer Roux or biliopancreatic limbs (and therefore a shorter common limb) lead to greater malabsorption (Brolin *et al.*, 1992; Buchwald *et al.*, 2004; Fox, Fox and Oh, 1996; Miller and Goodman, 1989; Scrugs *et al.*, 1993). Symptoms of the dumping syndrome may occur, especially initially.

The Roux-en-Y gastric bypass (RYGBP) and its numerous variants remain the most common bariatric operations performed in the USA (Buchwald and Williams, 2004). Modifications aiming to prevent dilatation of the pouch and its outlet into the Roux loop include constructing the gastric pouch on the lesser curvature (taking advantage of the thicker muscle layer) and placing a polypropylene band around the pouch (Capella and Capella, 1999; Fobi *et al.*,

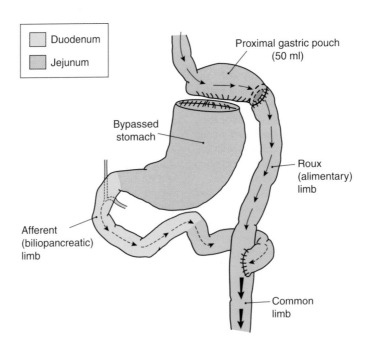

Figure 18.3 Roux-en-Y gastric bypass (RYGBP). The proximal gastric pouch is joined to an 'alimentary' limb of the distal end of the divided jejunum, through which food passes. The proximal cut end of jejunum (which, with the duodenum, forms the afferent limb that drains bile and pancreatic secretions) is then anastomosed to the side of the distal jejunum, creating a Y-shaped configuration that avoids tension on the gastrojejunal junction. Placing the end-to-side jejunoileal anastomosis more distally shortens the common limb and therefore further reduces the absorptive area accessible to ingested food.

2005; Torres, Oca and Garrison, 1983). The RYGBP is now usually performed laparoscopically (Higa, Boone and Ho, 2000; Rosenthal *et al.*, 2006; Wittgrove and Clark, 2000), but internal hernias (e.g. into the space behind the Roux loop) are a particular complication and may cause small bowel obstruction (Finnell *et al.*, 2006). The higher incidence of internal hernias with the laparoscopic RYGBP may occur because open surgery produces more adhesions that tend to prevent loops of bowel from lodging in these spaces.

Outcomes

After RYGBP, patients generally maintain a loss of 50–60% of excess weight in the long term, with a slight tendency to regain weight after five years, which is probably due to dilatation of the gastric pouch and its outflow (Deitel and Shikora, 2002; White *et al.*, 2005). As mentioned above, malabsorption and therefore weight loss are greater if the biliopancreatic limb is anastomosed more distally to create a shorter common limb. However, this 'far distal' Roux-en-Y configuration may

lead to aminoacid malabsorption and hypoalbuminaemia. All patients require long-term follow up with nutritional surveillance, and supplements of multivitamins (including B12 and folate), iron and calcium.

Biliopancreatic diversion

Biliopancreatic diversion (BPD) was a progression from the original jejunoileal bypass, by Scopinaro in the late 1970s, to avoid the blind loop and its complications (Scopinaro *et al.*, 1979). The bypassed small bowel, extending from the duodenum to the mid-ileum and termed the 'biliopancreatic limb', is anastomosed to the side of the lower ileum; the duodenal end is closed, but stasis is prevented by the flow of bile and pancreatic secretions. The 'alimentary limb' of ileum is connected to a 200–500 ml pouch of proximal stomach (Scopinaro *et al.*, 1998); the distal stomach has to be removed because of the high risk of marginal ulceration at the anastomosis (Figure 18.4). This procedure combines both restrictive and malabsorptive elements,

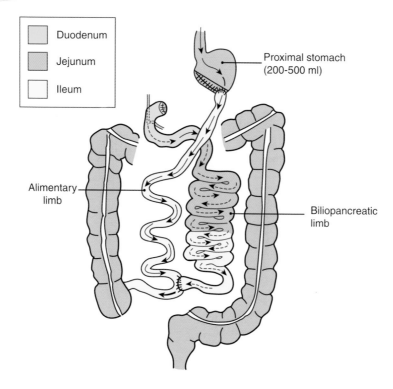

Figure 18.4 Biliopancreatic diversion (BPD). Distal gastrectomy creates a proximal gastric pouch that is joined to the distal 250 cm of ileum; 200 cm will form the alimentary limb. The biliopancreatic limb, carrying bile and pancreatic secretions, is anastomosed to the side of the distal 50 cm of ileum, creating the 50 cm common limb where nutrient absorption takes place.

with the gastric pouch (although this tends to dilate after several months) and absorption of fat and starches confined to the 50 cm of distal ileum ('common limb'). Cholecystectomy is required because the intestinal site of cholecystokinin (CCK) release is bypassed; reduced gall-bladder contractility leads to gallstone formation, which is also favoured by weight loss (Deitel and Petrov, 1987). The operation can be performed laparoscopically.

Outcome

BPD can achieve the greatest weight loss of any bariatric procedure, with up to 80% of excess weight lost initially. There is some tendency for weight to be regained subsequently, because the gastric pouch dilates with time (Scopinaro *et al.*, 1998). The operation does not suffer from problems of the blind loop syndrome. However, the procedure demands great surgical expertise and close long-term follow up is required because of the high risk of deficiencies

of vitamins (especially fat-soluble), iron and calcium; menstruating women are at particular risk of iron deficiency and occasionally require parenteral iron treatment (Bloomberg *et al.*, 2005; Deitel and Shikora, 2002). Protein intake should be high to prevent protein malnutrition and hypoalbuminaemia.

Duodenal switch

This further modification of the BPD is widely used (Baltasar *et al.*, 2001; Hess and Hess, 1998; Lagace *et al.*, 1995). Here, the greater curve of the stomach is resected, leaving the lesser curvature, pylorus and first part of duodenum in continuity as a tube for anastomosis to the alimentary limb of distal ileum. Thus, the proximal gastric pouch of the BPD is replaced by a lesser curvature gastric tube of 150–250 ml capacity that, at least initially, restricts food intake. The biliopancreatic limb is again joined to the distal ileum (Figure 18.5). By preserving the pylorus, the duodenal switch avoids both the dumping syndrome and marginal

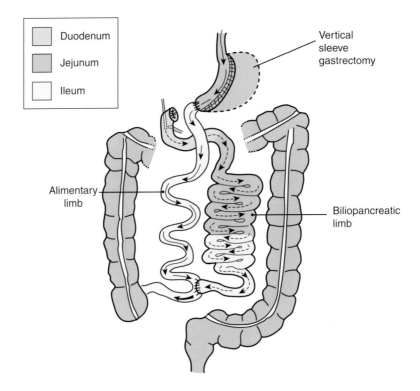

Figure 18.5 Duodenal switch. Removal of the greater curve portion of the stomach ('sleeve gastrectomy'), preserving the pylorus and first part of duodenum, creates a gastric pouch that is anastomosed end-to-end to the distal 200–250 cm of ileum, forming the alimentary limb. The biliopancreatic limb is then joined to the side of 75–100 cm of distal ileum, forming the common limb where nutrients are absorbed.

ulceration at the anastomosis of the first part of the duodenum to ileum. This operation can be carried out laparoscopically.

The outcome of duodenal switch is comparable to that of BPD, with about 75% of excess weight lost initially and maintained for up to five years; some regain tends to occur, but a 50% reduction of excess weight may still be seen after ten years (Buchwald *et al.*, 2004).

Sleeve gastrectomy

Vertical sleeve gastrectomy, the first step in the duodenal switch operation, is increasingly performed – usually laparoscopically – as a safer first-stage procedure in high-risk patients. The second stage (duodenal switch) can be performed later if weight loss is inadequate (Baltasar *et al.*, 2005). The operation has recently become popular as a definitive operation, creating a narrower lesser curvature channel. Although mainly restrictive, the sleeve gastrectomy may also speed transit through the gut (Melissas *et al.*, 2007).

Gastric banding

Gastric banding was developed during the 1970s so as to partition the stomach without stapling, creating a very small gastric pouch that restricted intake and induced satiety (Oria and Harboe, 2003). Early bands were simple mesh strips of polypropylene, Dacron, Teflon or silicone; bands impregnated with silicone caused little local tissue reaction and were easily removed, thus rendering the operation reversible (Kuzmak, 1991). The optimal circumference of these fixed bands was difficult to judge: those that were too tight caused intractable vomiting, whereas loose bands did not achieve adequate weight loss.

Inflatable, adjustable bands devised by Kuzmak in the USA (Kuzmak, 1992) and Forsell in Sweden (Forsell, Hallberg and Hellers, 1993) overcome this problem. The band is connected by tubing to a subcutaneous reservoir filled with sterile saline, implanted over the rectus abdominis muscle or lower sternum (Figures 18.6 and 18.7). Injection or withdrawal of saline in the reservoir (by medical staff) tightens or loosens the band (Belachew *et al.*, 1992; Belachew, Legrand and Vincent, 2001). Early bands were 9.5 cm in circumference and had to be placed using perigastric dissection, under the adipose tissue at the lesser curvature. Modern bands are larger (11 cm) and have a lower filling pressure. They can be inserted using the 'pars flaccida' approach, entering through

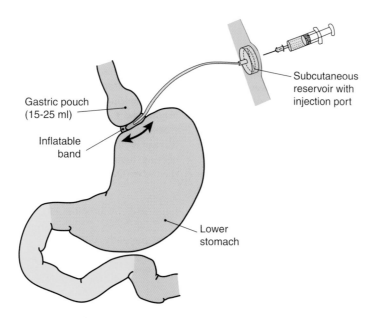

Figure 18.6 Adjustable gastric banding. An inflatable band, which can be tightened by injecting saline into a subcutaneously-implanted reservoir, is placed around the proximal stomach to create a tiny gastric pouch. The operation is usually performed laparoscopically (LAGB).

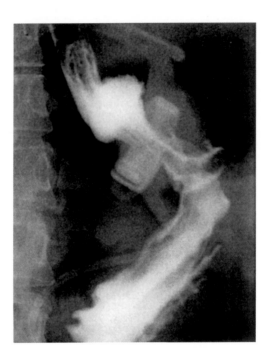

Figure 18.7 Laparoscopic adjustable gastric band (LAGB). This barium swallow shows a small (15 ml) pouch above the radio-opaque band, with contrast entering the distal stomach through a 12 mm diameter outlet.

the lesser omentum and dissecting along the crura of the diaphragm, outside the gastric fat (Forsell, 2000; Mittermair, Aigner and Nehoda, 2004; O'Brien *et al.*, 2005). The pars flaccida approach is technically simpler and carries a much lower risk of the band slipping.

Current operations place the band above the lesser sac, which also reduces the risk of slippage (O'Brien *et al.*, 2005); a 15–25 ml pouch is formed around a gastric balloon inflated via an orogastric tube, inserted at operation. The band is anchored anterior to the stomach with imbricating gastro-gastric sutures. The operation is readily performed laparoscopically (Figure 18.7), and its use has greatly increased since the 1990s; laparoscopic adjustable gastric banding (LAGB) is the most common bariatric procedure in Europe and Australia (Buchwald and Williams, 2004).

Outcomes

LAGB can be highly effective, reducing excess weight by an average of 45–50% at five years (see Figure 18.8). However, maladaptive eating (e.g. energy-dense milkshakes) can readily undermine its benefits and also lead to dilatation of the pouch. Some patients regain

weight after 24 months and a few progress to more invasive procedures such as the RYGBP (Mognol, Chosidow and Marmuse, 2004).

Early complications are less frequent with LAGB than with most other bariatric operations, but some specific complications can occur. The most common (up to 10% of cases) has been slippage of the band, especially downwards, when the distal stomach can herniate through the band; vomiting and obstruction of the stomach may follow. Rarely, the band can erode into the stomach. Other occasional complications include leakage or infection of the injection port or connecting tubing, and twisting and occlusion of the latter (Chevallier *et al.*, 2004).

Laparoscopic surgical techniques

Since the early 1990s, laparoscopic (minimally invasive) surgery has increasingly replaced open operations in many fields of surgery and, because of the higher operative risks in obese patients, is widely used for gastric banding and other bariatric procedures.

For laparoscopic surgery, a pneumoperitoneum is produced by insufflating the peritoneal cavity with CO_2, usually to a pressure of about 15 mm Hg.

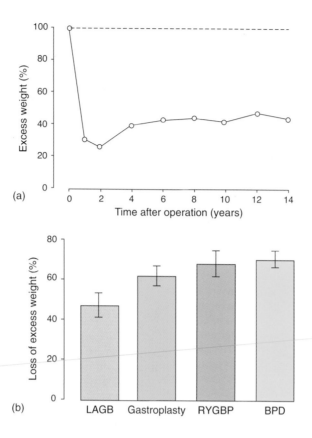

Figure 18.8 Weight loss achieved by bariatric procedures. (a) Average weight loss (expressed as percentage of initial excess weight) following gastric bypass surgery. Data from Pories *et al.* (1995). (b) Weight loss (expressed as percentage of initial excess) achieved by various bariatric operations. LAGB: laparoscopic adjustable gastric banding; RYGBP: Roux-en-Y gastric bypass; BPD: biliopancreatic diversion.

The operation is performed using highly special-ized instruments and visualized by a laparo-scopic camera connected to a video monitor; the camera and instruments are all inserted into the peritoneal cavity through trocar sites.

By avoiding the operative trauma and potential hernia complications of the traditional abdomi-nal incision and direct handling of the viscera, laparoscopic surgery causes much less morbidity and mortality than conventional open surgery; patients can be mobilized more rapidly after sur-gery, with earlier discharge from hospital, faster healing and an earlier return to work and normal activities.

Gastric banding and sleeve gastrectomy lend themselves particularly well to the laparoscopic approach, but every bariatric operation can be performed laparoscopically; however, these operations are technically demanding and require much training and experience. The benefits of laparoscopic surgery are very clear in this setting. As an example, open RYGBP generally requires a hospital stay of 5–6 days and car-ries an overall mortality rate of 1.5–2%; when performed laparoscopically, hospital stay is shortened to 2–3 days, and the mortality rate is <1% (Buchwald *et al.*, 2004).

Other bariatric approaches

Intragastric balloons

These were developed during the 1980s and were popular for about two years (Nieben and Harboe, 1982); because of poor long-term effi-cacy and complications, their use is now limited to particular short-term indications.

Early balloons were spherical or cylindrical, contained about 500 ml of air and floated on the gastric contents. Modern versions are spherical, made of silicone and filled with saline; they are placed under sedation, attached to an orogastric tube that is removed after filling the balloon.

By activating gastric stretch receptors (see Chapter 6), gastric balloons induce a sensation of satiety, but this is highly variable and generally short lived. Up to 10–15 kg can be lost within the first 3–6 months, but most patients regain weight thereafter; at 12 months, weight loss is comparable to that in sham-operated controls (McFarland, Grundy and Gazet, 1987).

The main complication is breakage, which occurred in about 7% of early balloons and led to their withdrawal. Breakage is potentially serious, because the deflated balloon can migrate into the small bowel and cause obstruction; methylene blue in saline is put into balloons, when green urine or blue stools would indicate rupture.

The newer, smooth, silicone spherical intragastric balloons have been used in recent years, mainly in Europe and Brazil (Sallet *et al.*, 2004; Totté *et al.*, 2001). The main indication is to achieve initial weight loss in extremely obese patients (BMI >50 kg/m²), in preparation for definitive bariatic surgery. This can greatly reduce the risks and technical difficulties of surgery, and also leads to rapid shrinkage of the characteristic fatty liver (see Chapter 11). The manufacturer recommends that use of the balloon is limited to six months.

Gastric pacing

The technology that underpins the compact electrical stimulators used for cardiac pacemakers and to treat conditions such as urinary incontinence and neuropathic pain has been exploited in the gastric electrical stimulator (GES). This subcutaneously-implanted unit (about $3 \times 2 \times 1$ cm) generates a train of electrical impulses that are delivered by two electrodes attached to the anterior surface of the stomach at the lesser curvature. Originally developed to treat diabetic gastroparesis, the GES has also been used for 'gastric pacing', superimposing artificial impulses on the normal autonomic signals that are generated by the gastric pacemaker in the proximal stomach, and which regulate contractility of the stomach. The resulting disordered motility induces a sensation of fullness (Cigaina *et al.*, 1996; Shikora, 2004). The electrical leads can be placed laparoscopically, but must be checked endoscopically during the procedure to ensure that the stomach has not been perforated. This procedure is currently experimental, and weight loss appears modest.

General aspects of bariatric surgery

Selection of patients

Table 18.2 shows selection criteria for bariatric surgery (Deitel and Shahi, 1992; Deitel and Shikora, 2002; NIHCDCDS, 1991). Crucially, all patients must be willing to comply with preoperative education, dietary advice and particularly life-long follow up. Patients with binge-eating disorder should be selected with care, because continuation of these behaviours (see Chapter 20) can undermine the efficacy and benefit of surgery. Those with significant psychiatric disease (especially psychosis) are generally avoided, although some have been successfully treated with the agreement and surveillance of their psychiatrist.

An experienced surgeon and anaesthetist should perform all these operations, supported by a dedicated multidisciplinary team skilled in preoperative education, postoperative care and long-term follow up.

Preoperative weight loss, perhaps including use of the intragastric balloon, has been shown to facilitate surgery by decreasing liver size and reducing operative risk (Fris, 2004). Smoking should stop at least one month before surgery, to decrease thrombosis risk and assist healing.

Review visits should be frequent (3- to 6-monthly) initially, becoming annual after a few

Table 18.2 Selection criteria for bariatric surgery.

- Severe obesity: BMI ≥ 40 kg/m², or BMI ≥ 35 kg/m² with serious comorbidity
- Failure of documented attempts of medical therapies over two years or more
- No endocrine or other potentially treatable cause of obesity (e.g. Cushing's syndrome)
- Acceptable operative risk
- Clearance by multidisciplinary team on medical, nutritional and psychological grounds
- Absence of significant psychiatric disorder
- Receptive to preoperative education
- Prepared to cooperate with life-long follow up

Guidelines modified from Deitel and Shahi (1992) and NIHCDCDS (1991).

years, but patients must agree to return if any potential problems arise (Deitel and Shahi, 1992). As well as the medical problems highlighted below, all patients should be monitored for social and psychological problems that may require support and intervention, although evidence suggests that some of these, such as depression, may improve substantially after successful bariatric surgery (see Chapter 14).

Plastic surgery may be considered to reduce the abdominal overhang (and frequently troublesome intertrigo) and redundant skin following marked weight loss; abdominal lipectomy, breast reduction or lift, and arm, thigh and buttock skin reductions may all be indicated (Fotopoulos, Kehagias and Kalfarentzos, 2000).

Efficacy and outcomes

Results of bariatric surgery vary widely between the various operations, individuals and centres. Typically, however, the most widely-used operations – Roux-en-Y gastric bypass (RYGBP) and laparoscopic adjustable gastric banding (LAGB) – can achieve a loss of 50–60% of excess weight, sustained in many cases for five years or longer, while BPD can be even more effective but requires greater surveillance (Figure 18.8). This degree of weight loss usually equates to absolute reductions of 30–60 kg. Weight is lost much more rapidly than with lifestyle modification and pharmacotherapy, which makes careful surveillance for nutritional problems all the more important.

Eventual regain of weight may be due to post-surgical changes (e.g. dilatation of the gastric pouch or channel in the RYGBP or LAGB), or to maladaptive eating. With LAGB, the band can be further tightened by injecting more saline into the subcutaneous reservoir, and this may improve weight loss.

Effects on diabetes and other comorbidities

As discussed in Chapter 17, sustained weight loss of 10% or more of initial weight can significantly alleviate some of the comorbidities of obesity (Busetto et al., 2000; Goldstein, 1991; Kuhlmann, Falcone and Wolf, 2000). The weight loss achieved by bariatric surgery often exceeds this threshold, and far outstrips the effects of pharmacotherapy, even in the 30% or so of patients taking anti-obesity drugs who will lose ≥10% of weight. Accordingly, there can be a marked improvement in several important comorbidities (Table 18.3), notably type 2 diabetes, coronary-heart disease, gastro-oesophageal reflux, infertility, joint pain and depression (Cowan and Buffington, 1998; Deitel et al., 1988; Dhabuwala, Cannan and Stubbs, 2000; Herrera and Deitel, 1991; Lankford,

Table 18.3 Impact of gastric bypass on comorbidities in severely obese patients.

		Post-operative (%)		
	Preoperative (n)	Resolved	Improved	Unchanged
Diabetes				
• Taking oral hypoglycaemics	12	92	8	—
• Taking insulin	6	17	—	—
• Diet-controlled	1	100	—	—
Lipid abnormalities				
• Hypercholesterolaemia	84	27	30	8
• Hypertriglyceridaema	61	49	7	8
• Abnormal cholesterol HDL ratio	94	45	15	2
Hypertension	42	43	31	24
Asthma	34	50	26	15
Obstructive sleep apnoea	12	92	8	—

Data from 157 subjects. Preoperative cholesterol levels, triglyceride levels and cholesterol/HDL ratios were available in 144, 141 and 139 patients respectively. Adapted from Dhabuwala, Cannan and Stubbs (2000).

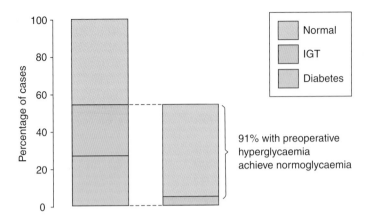

Figure 18.9 Resolution of diabetes (type 2) and impaired glucose tolerance (IGT) following gastric bypass surgery. In total, 55% of subjects were hyperglycaemic before surgery; one year after the procedure, only 4% remained hyperglycaemic. Data from Pories *et al.* (1995).

Proctor and Richard, 2005; McGoey *et al.*, 1990; Sjöström *et al.*, 1999; Van Itallie, 1980; White *et al.*, 2005). Few other interventions in medicine can claim to bring benefits to such a wide range of diseases.

The beneficial impact on type 2 diabetes and impaired glucose tolerance (IGT) is particularly noteworthy. Hyperglycaemia improves rapidly after gastric restrictive operations (e.g. LAGB) and especially malabsorptive procedures (e.g. RYGBP and biliopancreatic diversion) – indeed, faster than might be predicted from the rate of weight loss and reduction in fat mass (Cleator *et al.*, 2006; Deitel *et al.*, 1986). With restrictive operations, the marked decrease in energy intake after surgery (often to as low as 500–700 kcal/day initially, partly because of post-operative oedema in the gastric pouch) may contribute, as may rapid mobilization of triglyceride from the liver (decreasing hepatic insulin resistance). Following malabsorptive procedures, decreased absorption of carbohydrates may play a role; other potential factors include enhanced secretion of glucagon-like peptide-1 (GLP-1) by the L-cells of the distal ileum, due to increased stimulation by unabsorbed nutrients reaching this part of the bowel (Valverde *et al.*, 2005; Deitel, 2008). GLP-1 is an incretin hormone that directly stimulates the release of insulin from the pancreatic β cells; it also increases satiety through both central and peripheral mechanisms (see Chapter 6).

Overall, meta-analysis of various bariatric operations (notably RYGBP, LAGB and especially biliopancreatic diversion) shows that up to 85% of patients with established type 2 diabetes show an improvement, while 77% become normoglycaemic within one year (Buchwald *et al.*, 2004). Of those with IGT initially, almost all revert to normoglycaemia (see Figure 18.9). Resolution of diabetes is particularly striking with the biliopancreatic diversion, following which 97% of patients with established diabetes become normoglycaemic and no longer need anti-diabetic medication (Marinari *et al.*, 2000); the resolution rate is lower (48%) with LAGB (Buchwald *et al.*, 2004).

Meta-analysis suggests that, overall, hypertension resolves in over 60% of patients undergoing bariatric surgery, with over 80% following BPD; blood pressure often tends to rise again after five years (Buchwald *et al.*, 2004).

Quality of life often improves significantly, and within three months (see Chapter 14). The large Swedish Obese Subjects study, involving over 2000 patients treated with bariatric surgery and 2000 receiving conventional management, has recently reported that the risk of death was reduced by 30% over an average follow up period of ten years, in subjects treated surgically (Sjöström *et al.*, 2007) (Figure 18.10).

Complications of bariatric surgery

Obese patients undergoing surgery are at increased risk of thromboembolism (deep vein thrombosis, pulmonary embolism) (MacLean *et al.*, 1997; Sapala *et al.*, 1998). and wound and post-operative chest infections – further rationale for laparoscopic surgery, wherever possible.

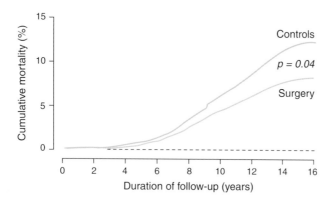

Figure 18.10 Bariatric surgery reduces the risk of death. These data, with a mean follow up of ten years, show that cumulative mortality was reduced by up to 30% after 16 years. From L. Sjöström *et al.* (2007) 'Effects of bariatric surgery on mortality in Swedish Obese Subjects'. *New England Journal of Medicine*, 357, 741–52, with kind permission.

Appropriate prophylaxis with heparin, advice to stop smoking and monitoring for infections are all therefore essential.

Specific complications of the various operations have been described above and, in some cases (notably the jejunoileal bypass), have led to the procedure being abandoned. General nutritional problems, resulting from the combination of greatly decreased fluid and food intake, altered diet and malabsorption, need to be anticipated and promptly treated (Bloomberg *et al.*, 2005; Deitel and Shikora, 2002; Rhode and MacLean, 2000).

Dehydration

Mild dehydration is common in the early postoperative phase after all bariatric operations and is due mainly to decreased fluid intake. After gastric restrictive procedures, patients have particular difficulty in drinking enough as they adapt to very small gastric capacities, while malabsorptive procedures cause frequent watery stools that cause significant fluid loss. Post-operative vomiting or diarrhoea may further exacerbate dehydration. Fluid status and plasma electrolytes must all be closely monitored after surgery. Patients can also be instructed to use thirst (and perhaps urine colour) to guide fluid intake.

All patients should follow a high-protein diet (60–80 grams daily); it may be difficult to maintain this intake, especially for patients who can no longer eat meat, and protein supplements may need to be prescribed. Protein malnutrition is an uncommon complication of gastric restrictive procedures, including the proximal RYGBP. For malabsorptive operations, such as the distal RYGBP and biliopancreatic diversion, protein may also be lost in the stool. Higher protein intake may be necessary and should be guided by serum albumin levels.

Vitamins and minerals

Purely restrictive operations do not alter nutrient movement through the upper gut, and vitamin and mineral deficiencies are therefore uncommon. However, they may develop because of changes in the quantity and composition of the diet. As mentioned above, patients who cannot eat red meat are at greater risk of iron deficiency.

Proximal RGYBP increases the risk of deficiencies of iron, folate, calcium, vitamin B12 and vitamin D. Dietary changes contribute, while bypassing most of the stomach, the duodenum and the proximal jejunum – crucial for absorption of iron, vitamin B12 and calcium. Most patients can be maintained with adequate diet and daily supplementation with iron gluconate (325 mg/day, more in menstruating women and patients who consume little meat), 500–600 µg of vitamin B12, 1 mg of folate and 500–1000 mg of calcium daily. Patients with significant vomiting, poor food intake or vomiting in child-bearing age may require additional vitamins and iron.

Serum levels of iron, calcium, folate and vitamin B12 should be monitored twice-yearly.

It is important to watch for patients with continued post-operative vomiting who may develop Wernicke's encephalopathy, with loss of balance, disturbed gait and nystagmus. This must be treated immediately by intravenous or intramuscular vitamin B1 (thiamine), followed by oral thiamine, to prevent permanent neurological damage. Folic acid must be administered to women who may become pregnant, to avoid neural tube defects in their children. After gastric restrictive procedures, pregnancy should be delayed until after the period of rapid weight loss, generally one year. After the malabsorptive procedures, pregnancy is best delayed, if possible, to 18 months, when weight loss has stabilized. Up to that point, a reliable means of birth control may be used. Oral contraceptives may be absorbed erratically and thus lose efficacy following malabsorptive operations. Other medications such as thyroid and warfarin also may be absorbed unpredictably after malabsorptive procedures.

Conclusions

Surgery is continually undergoing evolution, development and improvement, and bariatric surgery is no exception (Deitel, 1996). The procedures in use today are based on sound physiological rationale, are highly effective and carry low risks of morbidity and mortality – even in high-risk patients. This situation is very different from the early history of bariatric surgery, which has adversely coloured perceptions of its risks and benefits for patients, health professionals and the general public. A widespread lack of understanding and sympathy for the obese has also contributed (see Chapter 14).

Bariatric surgery has now come of age and should be considered, in selected cases, as part of the modern management of obesity.

References

Alden, J.F. (1977) Gastric and jejunoileal bypass: a comparison in the treatment of morbid obesity. *Archives of Surgery (Chicago, Ill: 1960)*, **112**, 799–806.

Baltasar, A., Bou, R., Bengochea, M. *et al.* (2001) Duodenal switch: an effective therapy for morbid obesity – intermediate results. *Obesity Surgery*, **11**, 54–8.

Baltasar, A., Serra, C., Perez, N. *et al.* (2005) Laparoscopic sleeve gastrectomy: a multi-purpose bariatric operation. *Obesity Surgery*, **15**, 1124–8.

Belachew, M., Legrand, M., Vincent, V. *et al.* (1992) Laparoscopic placement of adjustable silicone gastric band in the treatment of morbid obesity. *Obesity Surgery*, **5**, 66–9.

Belachew, M., Legrand, M.J. and Vincent, V. (2001) History of Lap-Band®: from dream to reality. *Obesity Surgery*, **11**, 297–302.

Bloomberg, R.D., Fleishman, A., Nalle, J.E. *et al.* (2005) Nutritional deficiencies following bariatric surgery: what have we learned? *Obesity Surgery*, **15**, 145–54.

Brolin, R.E., Kenler, H.A., Gorman, J.H. and Cody, R.P. (1992) Long-limb gastric bypass in the superobese. A prospective randomized study. *Annals of Surgery*, **215**, 387–395.

Buchwald, H., Avodor, Y., Braunwald, E. *et al.* (2004) Bariatric surgery. A systematic review and meta-analysis. *The Journal of the American Medical Association*, **292**, 1724–37.

Buchwald, H., Schwartz, M.Z. and Varco, R.L. (1973) Surgical treatment of obesity. *Advances in Surgery*, **7**, 235–55.

Buchwald, H. and Williams, S.E. (2004) Bariatric surgery worldwide 2003. *Obesity Surgery* **14**, 1157–64.

Busetto, L., Pisent, C., Rinaldi, D. *et al.* (2000) Variation in lipid levels in morbidly obese patients operated with the LAP-BAND® adjustable gastric banding system: effects of different levels of weight loss. *Obesity Surgery*, **10**, 569–77.

Capella, J.F. and Capella, R.F. (1999) Gastro-gastric fistulas and marginal ulcers in gastric bypass procedures for weight reduction. *Obesity Surgery*, **9**, 22–7.

Chevallier, J.-M., Zinzindohoue, F., Douard, R. *et al.* (2004) Complications after laparoscopic adjustable gastric banding for morbid obesity: experience with 1,000 patients over 7 years. *Obesity Surgery*, **14**, 407–14.

Cigaina, V., Pinato, G.P., Rigo, V. *et al.* (1996) Gastric peristalsis control by in situ electrical stimulation: preliminary study. *Obesity Surgery*, **6**, 247–9.

Clayman, R.V. and Williams, R.D. (1971) Oxalate urolithiasis following jejunoileal bypass. *Surgical Clinics of North America*, **59**, 1071–7.

Cleator, I.G.M., Birmingham, C.L., Kovacevic, S. *et al.* (2006) Long-term effect of ileogastrostomy surgery for morbid obesity on diabetes mellitus and sleep apnea. *Obesity Surgery*, **16**, 1337–41.

Cowan, G.S.M.J., Jr, and Buffington, C.K. (1998) Significant changes in blood pressure, glucose and lipids with gastric bypass surgery. *World Journal of Surgery*, **22**, 987–92.

DeWind, L.T. and Payne, J.H. (1976) Intestinal bypass surgery for morbid obesity: long-term results. *The Journal of the American Medical Association*, **236**, 2298–301.

Deitel, M. (1989) Jejunocolic and jejunoileal bypass: an historical perspective, in *Surgery for the Morbidly Obese Patient* (ed. M. Deitel), FD-Communications, Toronto, pp. 81–90. (ISBN 0-8121-1136-2)

Deitel, M. (1996) The development of general surgical operations, and weight-loss operations. *Obesity Surgery*, **6**, 206–12.

Deitel, M. (2008) Surgery for diabetes at lower BMI: some caution. *Obesity Surgery*, **18**, 1211–4.

Deitel, M., Jones, B.A., Petrov, I. *et al.* (1986) Vertical banded gastroplasty: results in 233 patients. *Canadian Journal of Surgery*, **29**, 322–4.

Deitel, M. and Petrov, I. (1987) Incidence of symptomatic gallstones after bariatric surgery. *Surgery Gynecology & Obstetrics*, **164**, 549–53.

Deitel, M. and Shahi, B. (1992) Morbid obesity: selection of patients for surgery. *Journal of the American College of Nutrition*, **11**, 457–66.

Deitel, M., Shahi, B., Anand, P.K. *et al.* (1993) Long-term outcome in a series of jejuno-ileal bypass patients. *Obesity Surgery*, **3**, 247–52.

Deitel, M. and Shikora, S.A. (2002) The development of the surgical treatment of morbid obesity. *Journal of the American College of Nutrition*, **5**, 365–71.

Deitel, M., Stone, E., Kassam, H.A. and Wilk, E. (1988) Gynecologic-obstetric changes after loss of massive excess weight following bariatric surgery. *Journal of the American College of Nutrition*, **7**, 147–53.

Dhabuwala, A., Cannan, R.J. and Stubbs, R.S. (2000) Improvement in co-morbidities following weight loss from gastric bypass surgery. *Obesity Surgery*, **10**, 428–35.

Eckhout, G.V., Willbanks, O.L. and Moore, J.T. (1981) Vertical ring gastroplasty for obesity: five year experience with 1463 patients. *American Journal of Surgery*, **141**, 343–9.

Eriksson, F. (1981) Bilio-intestinal bypass. *International Journal of Obesity*, **5**, 437–47.

Finnell, C.W., Madan, A.K., Tichansky, D.S. *et al.* (2006) Non-closure of defect during laparoscopic Roux-en-Y gastric bypass. *Obesity Surgery*, **16**, 145–8.

Fobi, M.A.L., Lee, H., Felahy, B. *et al.* (2005) Choosing an operation for weight control, and the transected banded gastric bypass. *Obesity Surgery*, **15**, 114–21.

Forsell, P. (2000) Experience with the Swedish adjustable gastric band in the treatment of morbid obesity, in *Update: Surgery for the Morbidly Obese Patient* (eds M. Deitel and G.S.M. Cowan Jr), FD-Communications, Toronto, pp. 359–78. (ISBN 0-9684426-1-7)

Forsell, P., Hallberg, D. and Hellers, G. (1993) A gastric band with adjustable inner diameter for obesity surgery. *Obesity Surgery*, **3**, 303–6.

Fotopoulos, L., Kehagias, I. and Kalfarentzos, F. (2000) Dermolipectomies following weight loss after surgery for morbid obesity. *Obesity Surgery*, **10**, 451–9.

Fox, S.R., Fox, K.M. and Oh, K.H. (1996) The gastric bypass for failed bariatric surgical procedures. *Obesity Surgery*, **6**, 145–50.

Fris, R. (2004) Preoperative low energy diet diminishes liver size. *Obesity Surgery*, **14**, 1165–70.

Goldstein, D.J. (1991) Beneficial health effects of modest weight loss. *International Journal of Obesity*, **16**, 397–415.

Gomez, C.A. (1980) Gastroplasty in the surgical treatment of morbid obesity. *The American Journal of Clinical Nutrition*, **33**, 406–15.

Griffen, W.O., Young, V.L. and Stevenson, C.C. (1977) A prospective comparison of gastric and jejunoileal bypass procedures for morbid obesity. *Annals of Surgery*, **186**, 500–9.

Heimberger, S.L., Steiger, E., Lo Gerfo, P. *et al.* (1975) Reversal of severe fatty hepatic infiltration after intestinal bypass for morbid obesity by calorie-free amino acid infusion. *American Journal of Surgery*, **129**, 229–35.

Henrikson, V. (1952) Kan tunnfarmsresektion forsvaras som terapi mot fettsot? *Nordisk Medicin*, **47**, 44–77.

Herrera, M.F. and Deitel, M. (1991) Cardiac function in massively obese patients and the effect of weight loss. *Canadian Journal of Surgery*, **34**, 431–4.

Hess, D.S. and Hess, D.W. (1998) Biliopancreatic diversion with a duodenal switch. *Obesity Surgery*, **8**, 267–82.

Higa, K.D., Boone, K.B. and Ho, T. (2000) Complications of the laparoscopic Roux-en-Y gastric bypass: 1,040 patients – What have we learned? *Obesity Surgery*, **10**, 509–13.

Kremen, A.J., Linner, J.H. and Nelson, C.H. (1954) An experimental evaluation of the nutritional importance of proximal and distal small intestine. *Annals of Surgery*, **140**, 439–44.

Kuhlmann, H.W., Falcone, R.A. and Wolf, A.M. (2000) Cost-effective bariatric surgery in Germany today. *Obesity Surgery*, **10**, 549–52.

Kuzmak, L.I. (1991) A review of seven years experience with silicone gastric banding. *Obesity Surgery*, **1**, 403–8.

Kuzmak, L.I. (1992) Stoma adjustable silicone gastric banding. *Problems in General Surgery*, **9**, 298–317.

Lagace, M., Marceau, P., Marceau, S. *et al.* (1995) Biliopancreatic diversion with a new type of gastrectomy: some previous conclusions revisited. *Obesity Surgery*, **5**, 411–8.

Lankford, D.A., Proctor, C.D. and Richard, R. (2005) Continuous positive airway pressure (CPAP) changes in bariatric patients undergoing rapid weight loss. *Obesity Surgery*, **15**, 336–41.

Lewis, L.A., Turnbull, R.B., Jr, and Page, H. (1966) Effects of jejunocolic shunt on obesity, serum lipoproteins, lipids and electrolytes. *Archives of Internal Medicine*, **117**, 4–16.

MacLean, L.D., Rhode, B.M., Nohr, C. *et al.* (1997) Stomal ulcer after gastric bypass. *Journal of the American College of Surgeons*, **185**, 1–7.

Marinari, G.M., Papadia, F.S., Briatore, L. *et al.* (2000) Type 2 diabetes and weight loss following biliopancreatic diversion for obesity. *Obesity Surgery*, **16**, 1440–4.

Mason, E.E. (1982) Vertical banded gastroplasty. *Archives of Surgery*, **117**, 701–6.

Mason, E.E., Doherty, C. and Cullen, J.J. (1998) Vertical gastroplasty: evaluation of vertical banded gastroplasty. *World Journal of Surgery*, **22**, 919–24.

Mason, E.E. and Ito, I. (1967) Gastric bypass in obesity. *Surgical Clinics of North America*, **47**, 1345–51.

Mason, E.E. and Ito, C. (1978) Graded gastric bypass. *World Journal of Surgery*, **2**, 341–7.

McFarland, R., Grundy, A. and Gazet, J.-C. (1987) The intragastric balloon: a novel idea proved ineffective. *The British Journal of Surgery*, **74**, 137–9.

McGoey, B.V., Deitel, M., Saplys, R.J. *et al.* (1990) Effects of weight loss on musculoskeletal pain in the morbidly obese. *The Journal of Bone and Joint Surgery*, **72-B**, 322–3.

Melissas, J., Koukouraki, S., Askoxylakis, J. *et al.* (2007) Sleeve gastrectomy – a restrictive procedure? *Obesity Surgery*, **17**, 57–62.

Miller, D.K. and Goodman, G.N. (1989) Gastric bypass procedures, in *Surgery for the Morbidly Obese Patient* (ed. M. Deitel), FD-Communications, Toronto, pp. 124–7. (ISBN 0-8121-1136-2)

Mittermair, R.P., Aigner, F. and Nehoda, H. (2004) Results and complications after laparoscopic adjustable gastric banding in super-obese patients, using the Swedish band. *Obesity Surgery*, **14**, 1327–30.

Mognol, P., Chosidow, D. and Marmuse, J.-P. (2004) Laparoscopic conversion of laparoscopic gastric banding to Roux-en-Y gastric bypass: a review of 70 patients. *Obesity Surgery*, **14**, 1349–53.

Näslund, E., Freedman, J., Lagergren, J. *et al.* (1999) Three-year results of laparoscopic vertical banded gastroplasty. *Obesity Surgery*, **9**, 369–73.

National Institutes of Health Consensus Development Conference Draft Statement (NIHCDCDS) (1991) Gastrointestinal surgery for severe obesity. *Obesity Surgery*, **1**, 257–65.

Nieben, O.G. and Harboe, H. (1982) Intragastric balloons as an artificial bezoar for treatment of obesity. *Lancet*, **1**, 198–9.

O'Brien, P.E., Dixon, J.B., Laurie, C. *et al.* (2005) A prospective randomized trial of placement of the laparoscopic adjustable band: comparison of the perigastric and pars flaccida pathways. *Obesity Surgery*, **15**, 820–6.

Oria, H.E. and Harboe, H. (2003) Marcel Molina: the loss of a pioneer. *Obesity Surgery*, **13**, 806–7.

Pace, W.G., Martin, E.W., Jr, Tetirick, T. *et al.* (1979) *Annals of Surgery*, **190**, 392–400.

Payne, J.H., DeWind, L.T. and Commons, R.R. (1963) Metabolic observations in patients with jejunocolic shunts. *American Journal of Surgery*, **106**, 273–89.

Pories, W.J., Swanson, M.S., MacDonald, K.G. *et al.* (1995) Who would have thought it: an operation proves to be the most effective therapy for adult-onset diabetes mellitus. *Annals of Surgery*, **222**, 339–520.

Rae, A.J. and Cleator, I.G.M. (1993) Quality of life assessment of ileogastrostomy. *Obesity Surgery*, **3**, 360–4.

Rhode, B.M. and MacLean, L.D. (2000) Vitamin and mineral supplementation after gastric bypass, in *Update: Surgery for the Morbidly Obese Patient* (eds M. Deitel and G.S.M. Cowan Jr), FD-Communications, Toronto, pp. 161–70. (ISBN 0-9684426-1-7)

Rosenthal, R.J., Szomstein, S., Kennedy, C.I. *et al.* (2006) Laparoscopic surgery for morbid obesity: 1,001 consecutive bariatric operations performed at the bariatric institute, Cleveland Clinic Florida. *Obesity Surgery*, **16**, 119–24.

Sallet, J.A., Marchesini, J.B., Paiva, D.S. *et al.* (2004) Brazilian multicenter study of the intragastric balloon. *Obesity Surgery*, **14**, 991–8.

Salmon, P.A. (1971) The results of small intestine bypass operations for the treatment of obesity. *Surgery Gynecology & Obstetrics*, **132**, 965–79.

Sapala, J.A., Wood, M.H., Sapala, M.A. and Flake, T.M., Jr, (1998) Marginal ulcer after gastric bypass: a prospective 3-year study of 173 patients. *Obesity Surgery*, **8**, 505–16.

Scopinaro, N., Adami, G.F., Marinari, G.M. *et al.* (1998) Biliopancreatic diversion. *World Journal of Surgery*, **22**, 936–46.

Scopinaro, N., Gianetta, E., Civalleri, D. *et al.* (1979) Biliopancreatic bypass for obesity: II Initial experience in man. *The British Journal of Surgery*, **66**, 618–20.

Scott, H.W., Jr, Dean, R.H., Shull, H.J. and Gluck, F. (1977) Results of jejunoileal bypass in 200 patients with morbid obesity. *Surgery Gynecology & Obstetrics*, **145**, 661–3.

Scrugs, D.M., Cowan, G.S.M., Jr, Klesges, L. *et al.* (1993) Weight loss and calorie intake after regular and extended gastric bypass. *Obesity Surgery*, **3**, 233–8.

Shikora, S.A. (2004) Implantable gastric stimulation for the treatment of severe obesity. *Obesity Surgery*, **14**, 545–8.

Sjöström, C.D., Lissner, L., Wedel, H. and Sjöström, L. (1999) Reduction in incidence of diabetes, hypertension and lipid disturbance after intentional weight loss induced by bariatric surgery: the SOS intervention study. *Obesity Research*, **7**, 477–84.

Sjöström, L., Nabro, K., Sjöström, C.D. *et al.* (2007) Effects of bariatric surgery on mortality in Swedish Obese Subjects. *New England Journal of Medicine*, **357**, 741–52.

Stunkard, A. and McLaren-Hume, M. (1959) The results of treatment for obesity. *Archives of Internal Medicine*, **103**, 79–85.

Sylvan, A., Sjölund, B. and Januger, K.G. (1995) Favorable long-term results with end-to-side jejunoileal bypass. *Obesity Surgery*, **5**, 357–63.

Torres, J.C., Oca, C.F. and Garrison, R.N. (1983) Gastric bypass Roux-en-Y gastrojejunostomy from the lesser curvature. *Southern Medical Journal*, **76**, 1217–21.

Totté, E., Hendrickx, L., Pauwels, R. and Van Hee, R. (2001) Weight reduction by means of intragastric device: Experience with the BioEnterics intragastric balloon. *Obesity Surgery*, **11**, 519–23.

Valverde, I., Puente, J., Martin-Duce, A. *et al.* (2005) Changes in glucagon-like peptide-1 (GLP-1) secretion after biliopancreatic diversion or vertical banded gastroplasty. *Obesity Surgery*, **15**, 387–97.

Van Itallie, T.B. (1980) Morbid obesity: a hazardous disorder that resists conservative treatment. *The American Journal of Clinical Nutrition*, **33**, 358–63.

Wands, J.R., LaMont, J.T., Mann, E. and Isselbacher, K.J. (1976) Arthritis associated with intestinal-bypass procedure for morbid obesity. *The New England Journal of Medicine*, **294**, 121–4.

White, S., Brooks, E., Jurikova, L. and Stubbs, R.S. (2005) Long-term outcomes after gastric bypass. *Obesity Surgery*, **15**, 155–63.

Wittgrove, A.C. and Clark, G.W. (2000) Laparoscopic gastric bypass, Roux-en-Y – 500 patients: technique and results, with 3–60 month follow-up. *Obesity Surgery*, **10**, 233–9.

Wooley, S.C. and Garner, D.M. (1991) Obesity treatment: the high cost of false hope. *Journal of the American Dietetic Association*, **91**, 1248–51.

Special Considerations in Managing Obesity

Key points

- Weight gain is a side effect of many drugs, notably glucocorticoids, insulin and oral hypoglycaemic agents (not metformin), antipsychotic and antiepileptic drugs. Low dosages or non-obesogenic alternatives should be used if possible, with lifestyle modification to encourage weight loss.

- Endocrine diseases causing obesity include Cushing syndrome and hypothalamic damage. Weight gain, usually milder, also occurs with hypothyroidism, hypopituitarism and hyperprolactinaemia. Weight generally falls with successful treatment of the underlying condition.

- Many subjects who stop smoking gain weight, with over 10% gaining 11 kg or more; both increased food intake and a fall in energy expenditure contribute. Weight gain can be limited by prior counselling and lifestyle measures; bupropion and rimonabant may help, although weight generally rebounds after withdrawal of nicotine replacement. Stopping smoking should have a higher priority than losing weight.

- Eating disorders may accompany obesity and can complicate its management. Binge-eating disorder, which affects up to 30% of obese subjects, may respond to psychotherapy, notably cognitive behavioural therapy; anti-obesity drugs or bariatric surgery may be indicated in some cases. Night-eating syndrome appears less amenable to treatment.

- Depression in obese subjects may improve with exercise and weight loss, especially with behavioural therapy. Some antidepressants cause weight gain, and rimonabant is contraindicated in depressed subjects because it increases the risk of severe episodes and of suicidal tendencies.

- Complications of pregnancy are more common in obese women and their children. Weight should be reduced before conception, perhaps with metformin or anti-obesity drugs; the latter should not be used during pregnancy. Screening for gestational diabetes and hypertension is crucial. Elective caesarean section may be needed for large babies, and antithrombotic measures are indicated after delivery. Breastfeeding is encouraged and reduces the child's later risk of obesity.

- Type 2 diabetes in obese patients should be treated to conventional targets for glycaemic control (HbA1c $<7\%$), blood pressure ($<130/80$ mm Hg) and blood lipids. Healthy eating and increased exercise that achieves 5–10% weight loss may lower HbA1c by 1% or more in established diabetic patients, and markedly decreases the risk of subjects with IGT becoming diabetic; blood pressure and lipids also improve.

- Energy intake should be restricted by 500–1000 kcal/day, and fat intake to $<30\%$ of total energy intake. Complex, fibre-rich carbohydrates are encouraged, while simple sugar, alcohol and salt intakes are reduced. Physical activity should be increased, ideally to 30–60 min of moderate exercise each day.

- Anti-obesity drugs can reduce weight by 10% or more in about one-third of obese type 2 diabetic patients, often with clinically useful improvements in HbA1c, blood pressure and lipids. Bariatric surgery can be considered for diabetic subjects with BMI ≥ 35 kg/m²; gastric bypass surgery can reverse established diabetes in up to 80% of cases.

- Insulin, sulphonylureas and thiazolidinediones cause increased adiposity through their anabolic and lipogenic actions. Metformin and GLP-1 analogues do not cause weight gain. Weight gain can be limited by combining insulin with metformin; the increase in fat mass appears to be less with insulin detemir.

- Dyslipidaemia in obesity typically comprises raised triglyceride levels and low HDL cholesterol. It should be actively treated to reduce cardiovascular risk. Dyslipidaemia may improve with lifestyle modification alone but statins and/or fibrates are often required.

- Obese subjects are increasingly trying complementary and alternative therapies, but few of these have been evaluated rigorously enough to demonstrate efficacy or safety. Regular long-term yoga can help to reduce weight and maintain weight loss.

Chapter 19

Special Considerations in Managing Obesity

Mimi Chen and Robert Andrews

This chapter deals with several special considerations in the practical management of obesity. These include the treatment of secondary obesity due to obesogenic drugs, genetic syndromes and endocrine diseases, and intercurrent conditions such as smoking, eating disorders and pregnancy in the obese subject. The co-morbidities of obesity, notably type 2 diabetes, cardiovascular disease and dyslipidaemia, are also covered. The chapter concludes with a section on the alternative and complementary therapies that many obese people try in an attempt to lose weight.

Managing causes of secondary obesity

Drug-induced obesity

Several drugs used to treat chronic diseases can induce obesity; indeed, it is reported that 9% of adults attribute weight gain to current or previous medication (Vossenaar et al., 2004). The major obesogenic drugs are listed in Table 19.1 and their mechanisms of action are discussed further in Chapter 8. Weight gain can be due to various mechanisms, notably increased appetite (e.g. corticosteroids) or reduced metabolic rate (β-adrenoceptor blockers). In some cases, weight loss may have occurred as a result of the underlying disease, and recovery with effective treatment will include weight regain. However, weight gain is mostly due to increased fat mass, rather than restoration of the lean tissue that is generally depleted by chronic illness, and can confer the adverse effects of obesity.

If these drugs are to be prescribed, the potential for weight gain should be discussed with the patients before starting therapy, and effective advice and support to avoid weight gain should be provided, together with access to a dietitian. This approach should help to minimize weight gain, as well as improve compliance with treatment. Additional measures may be needed to minimize or reverse weight gain.

Corticosteroids

Corticosteroids are widely prescribed, and chronic therapy (>3 weeks) with high dosages (>5 mg/day of prednisolone or equivalent) causes many adverse effects. These include suppression of the Hypothalamic-pituitary-adrenal (HPA) axis and Cushing's syndrome, with accumulation and redistribution of fat into abdominal depots, glucose intolerance, osteoporosis, hypertension and increased risk of cardiovascular disease, and changes in mental state. Weight gain is due to a combination of increased food intake as a result of increased appetite (perhaps from suppression of the anorexigenic hypothalamic peptide, CRF), and fluid retention induced by enhanced sodium reabsorption.

The risks and benefits of corticosteroids must always be carefully considered, and long-term therapy only used where there is convincing evidence of benefit. Specific treatment goals should be identified and objective criteria used to assess the response. Treatment should be stopped if the treatment goals are not met or if complications arise, and if possible when maximum benefit has been achieved.

As weight gain and other side effects are dependent on circulating glucocorticoid concentrations, non-systemic preparations should be used where possible to deliver therapeutic local concentrations while minimizing systemic exposure. Topical preparations containing urea, dimethyl sulphoxide or salicylic acid, or those applied to skin under occlusive dressings, enhance systemic absorption and should be avoided. When systemic corticosteroids are

Obesity: Science to Practice   Edited by Gareth Williams and Gema Frühbeck
© 2009 John Wiley & Sons, Ltd

Table 19.1   Drugs that induce obesity, and their mechanisms of action.

Class and drug	Increased appetite	Decreased energy expenditure	Other obesogenic effects
Glucocorticoids	++	+	• ↑ Adipocyte differentiation • ↑ Visceral fat depot • ↑ Glucose intolerance
Antidiabetic drugs			
• Insulin	−	−	• Anabolic effects
• Sulphonylureas	±	−	• Abolish glycosuria
• Thiazolidinediones	−	−	• ↑ Adipocyte differentiation
Antipsychotic drugs			
• 'Atypical', for example clozapine	++	+	−
• Classical, for example haloperidol	++	+	−
Antidepressants			
• Tricyclics	++	+	−
Antiepileptic drugs			
• Carbamazepine	++	−	−
• Gabapentin	++	−	−
β-blockers			
• Propranolol	−	++	−
Endocrine drugs			
• Progestagens	+	−	−
• Tamoxifen	−	−	• ↑ Total body fat • ↑ Hepatic triglyceride accumulation
Miscellaneous			
• Antihistamines	+	+	−
• Cyproheptadine	++	−	−
• Pizotifen	++	−	−

required, alternate-day treatment or pulsed intravenous therapy may aid in reducing weight gain (Mentink *et al.*, 2006). Giving once-daily doses of short-acting corticosteroids causes less HPA suppression and in theory should result in less weight gain. Where possible, medications that inhibit cytochrome p450 3A4 should not be co-prescribed, because these can impair the metabolism of corticosteroids and thus increase their serum levels.

In theory, sibutramine and metformin could help both to limit and treat corticosteroid-induced weight gain, but this possibility has not yet been tested in clinical trials (Alisky, 2007).

Antidiabetic drugs

Insulin treatment, especially if intensive, can cause weight gain in both type 1 and type 2 diabetic patients. This is due partly to the anabolic effects of insulin, and sometimes to hunger and hyperphagia induced by hypoglycaemia. Weight can increase by 4 kg or more.

Sulphonylureas and glitinides, which stimulate insulin secretion, have similar effects, and weight can rise by 4–5 kg. Thiazolidinediones increase fat mass (especially subcutaneous) by causing pre-adipocytes to differentiate into adipocytes, and also cause sodium and water retention; weight often increases by 2–3 kg.

Drugs such as exenatide that mimic or enhance the action of GLP-1 (which induces satiety as well as insulin release) are less prone to cause weight gain. Metformin does not increase weight and can be useful as monotherapy in treating diabetes in obese subjects; dosages of insulin and other drugs can often be reduced if metformin is added.

Antipsychotic drugs

Several of these drugs increase fat mass and weight through the combination of decreased physical activity (due to their sedative effects) and increased appetite due to their blockade of dopamine, serotonin and histamine receptors (Bernstein, 1987; Baptista, 1999; see Chapter 8). Weight tends to rise during the first two months of treatment, commonly reaching a plateau of 3 kg or more after several months.

Weight gain is greatest with atypical neuroleptics such as clozapine, olanzapine, sertindole and zotepine, followed by classical neuroleptics such as chlorpromazine, thioridazine and haloperidol. Ziprasidone and possibly aripiprazole appear to induce little or no weight gain and, if appropriate, should be tried as first-line therapy. The lowest effective doses of clozapine and olanzapine should be used, because weight gain with these agents seems to be dose related. If low doses are ineffective, changing to aripiprazole may help in limiting weight gain. Switching from an obesogenic drug to another that causes less weight gain may produce significant reductions in body weight.

Supervised exercise programmes, dietary restriction and cognitive programmes have all been shown to limit weight gain when patients begin antipsychotic therapy, and can also help to reduce weight in individuals already taking these drugs (Werneke, Taylor and Sanders, 2002). Pharmacotherapy appears less successful. Serotonin reuptake inhibitors (fluoxetine, sertraline and paroxetine) have not been found to limit weight gain (Bustillo et al., 2003); nizatidine (a histamine H-2 receptor antagonist) may do so initially but this effect dwindles after

16 weeks and patients then gain weight (Cavazzoni et al., 2003). Sibutramine and topiramate are effective in limiting weight gain and in helping patients already established on medication to lose weight, but are poorly tolerated (McElroy et al., 2007). Topiramate should only be used in patients who require treatment for epilepsy (see Chapter 17).

Other drugs

Antiepileptic drugs (carbamazepine and gabapentin) can cause significant weight gain that can reach several kilograms and often damages compliance; an alternative is topiramate, which causes weight loss but which, because of its side effects, should not be used to treat obesity in its own right.

β-adrenoceptor blockers often increase weight and insulin resistance, due to inhibition of sympathetically mediated thermogenesis and decreased physical movement. This side-effect can preclude their use in treating hypertension or coronary heart disease in obese patients.

Endocrine diseases

Hypothyroidism often presents with weight gain, although overt obesity does not usually develop. Weight is lost over weeks and months once thyroxine replacement is started.

Cushing's syndrome is characterized by marked central obesity, a round face and fat deposition over the lower cervical spine ('buffalo hump'). Hypertension, glucose intolerance and proximal myopathy are common (see Figure 19.1). With successful treatment of hypercortisolism, the excess adipose tissue is mobilized, with remodelling of the facies.

Hypothalamic and pituitary disorders

The hypothalamus is important in controlling appetite and body weight (Chapter 6). Damage to this area as a result of tumours, surgery or radiotherapy has long been recognized as a cause of hyperphagia and weight gain (hypothalamic obesity). There are very few published studies and no consensus regarding optimal weight management strategies for individuals with hypothalamic obesity. They are usually unresponsive to diet, physical activity and most pharmacologic interventions (Eyal et al., 2006).

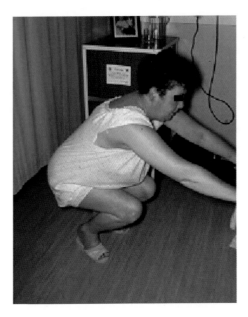

Figure 19.1 Cushing disease, presenting with weight gain and thigh weakness due to proximal myopathy (illustrated here by the patient's inability to rise from a squatting position). Weight loss followed successful removal of the ACTH-secreting pituitary adenoma. Image reproduced courtesy of Professor Gareth Williams, University of Bristol.

Octreotide, a somatostatin analogue that blocks the hypersecretion of insulin occurring in this condition, has been shown to produce a modest reduction in weight (Lustig *et al.*, 2003). In a few reported cases, bariatric surgery appears to be safe and effective (Inge *et al.*, 2007).

Various pituitary diseases can also lead to obesity, although this is not as severe as with hypothalamic damage. Hyperprolactinaemia, due to a prolactinoma or transection or compression of the pituitary stalk, is associated with modest weight gain, and treatments that lower prolactin levels result in weight loss (Greenman, Tordjman and Stern, 1998).

Hypopituitary patients continue to gain weight and up to one-half of them develop obesity, even with adequate hormonal replacement therapy including growth hormone replacement (Gotherstrom *et al.*, 2001). Long-term studies have revealed that adults with conventionally treated hypopituitarism also have increased cardiovascular mortality rates (Rosen and Bengtsson, 1990). The high prevalence of obesity and cardiovascular risk factors in hypopituitarism requires effective weight loss management in these patients. Unlike patients

with hypothalamic damage, these patients lose a similar amount of weight with diet, exercise, drug and surgical therapies as those with simple obesity (Mersebach *et al.*, 2004). They can therefore be managed in the conventional manner.

Syndromic obesity

The various genetic obesity syndromes, often presenting with morbid obesity in childhood, are described in Chapter 21. These may present considerable challenges in management.

The most common genetic cause of morbid obesity is the Prader-Willi syndrome (PWS), which is characterized by behavioural problems, food foraging and hyperphagia leading to early-onset childhood obesity; mental retardation and hypogonadism are also features. Limiting food intake through close supervision is the key strategy for controlling weight.

Anti-obesity drugs have so far had only limited success in PWS. Sibutramine or orlistat have not been systematically studied, but some data suggest that they can be helpful and are worth trying. Decreased appetite and reduced weight have also been observed with essentially anecdotal trials of topiramate and metformin (Butler, 2006). Bariatric surgery has been shown to be effective, but should only be considered in severe cases when serious obesity-related comorbidities are present and when rapid weight loss is needed (Stevenson *et al.*, 2007).

Management of intercurrent conditions in obesity

Smoking and smoking cessation

Cigarette smoking is the single most important preventable cause of death and illness in the developed world, while cessation is associated with substantial health benefits. However, only 40–70% of smokers ever attempt to stop, and fear of gaining weight is the most common explanation for not trying (Filozof, Fernández Pinilla and Fernández-Cruz, 2004). Weight gain is also cited as a major reason for relapsing after stopping smoking.

Most people who stop smoking will gain less than 4.5 kg but up to 13% of people may gain as much as 11 kg (Figure 19.2). Low socioeconomic class, higher BMI, age <55 years, African-American origin and heavy cigarette consumption

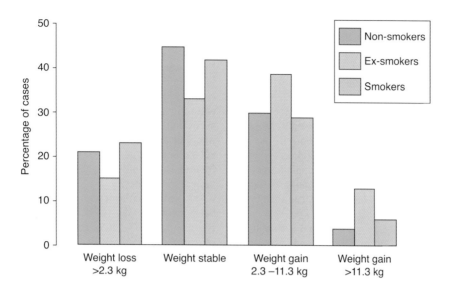

Figure 19.2 Weight gain following smoking cessation. In this study, 13% of ex-smokers gained 11 kg or more. From Swan and Carmelli (1995), with permission of the editor of the *American Journal of Pathology*.

(>25 per day) are all associated with greater weight gain (Filozof, Fernández Pinilla and Fernández-Cruz, 2004). Some studies (e.g. Swan and Carmelli, 1995), but not others (Dale *et al.*, 1998), have reported that women gain more weight than men. Twin studies suggest that genetic factors are important in determining the degree of weight gain (Swan and Carmelli, 1995).

Most weight gain occurs in the first two months after cessation, and is largely due to increased body fat. Causes include increased energy intake (especially of sweet, energy-dense foods), decreased energy expenditure (by about 9%), decreased physical activity and increased lipoprotein lipase activity. Nicotine reduces food intake, possibly by inhibiting hypothalamic NPY neurones, and smokers also have a raised resting metabolic rate; on average, they weight 3–4 kg less than matched non-smokers.

Measures to prevent weight gain after smoking cessation (e.g. by dieting simultaneously) were previously thought to undermine the attempt to stop smoking (Perkins, 1994; Hall *et al.*, 1992), but this concern appears unfounded. Many studies have reported similar (Norregaard *et al.*, 1996) or even higher (Danielsson, Rössner and Westin, 1999) success rates for smoking cessation when this is combined with strategies for weight loss. The benefits of stopping smoking generally outweigh the adverse effects of the resulting weight gain, and stopping smoking should be the priority.

Exercise can help to minimize cigarette craving and withdrawal symptoms, and roughly halves the weight gain. It also increases the chances of quitting and thus should be recommended to all patients who are trying to stop smoking (Ussher, 2005). Greater benefits are seen when exercise is combined with a cognitive-behavioural smoking cessation programme (Marcus *et al.*, 1999).

Bupropion, an atypical antidepressant that blocks nicotinic receptors, has been reported to reduce weight gain slightly after stopping smoking, with a suggestion that this effect is maintained after the drug is stopped (Hays *et al.*, 2001). However, more recent studies have yielded divergent effects; no significant increase in smoking cessation rates among subjects treated with bupropion (Simon *et al.*, 2006) as opposed to a significant effect of bupropion on smoking cessation but not on weight gain (Fossati *et al.*, 2007). In obese patients, bupropion might be considered to supplement lifestyle changes and counselling. The starting dosage is 150 mg once daily for 6 days, increasing to a maximum of 150 mg twice daily for 7–9 weeks.

Nicotine replacement therapy is commonly given in combination with counselling for smoking cessation. Nicotine is available as a skin patch, inhaler, gum and nasal spray, and limits weight gain after stopping smoking. Nicotine gum is the most effective, showing a dose-dependent relationship between gum use and weight loss. However, once nicotine replacement is stopped, the patient gains about the same amount of weight as if nicotine replacement had not been given (Gross et al., 1989). Fluoxetine has similar effects, reducing post-cessation weight gain in a dose-related manner, but dose-dependent weight rebound follows its discontinuation (Borrelli et al., 1999). These drugs can be useful by allowing patients to concentrate on stopping smoking rather than preventing weight gain; when the habit is successfully broken, they can then focus on limiting weight gain.

Rimonabant, a selective type 1 cannabinoid (CB1) receptor antagonist, is used as an anti-obesity drug (see Chapter 17). It may assist with smoking cessation, increasing the likelihood of stopping by approximately 50%. Post-cessation weight gain is also considerably less, but it is not known whether this effect is maintained when treatment is discontinued (Cahill and Ussher, 2007). Rimonabant is potentially a second-line agent, although concerns about its psychiatric side effects (notably depression and suicide risk) have prevented its approval for clinical use in the USA and now Europe.

To date, the possibility that sibutramine or orlistat might limit weight gain after smoking cessation has not been formally studied.

Eating disorders

Clinically significant eating disorders may accompany obesity and are frequently overlooked by families, carers and even healthcare workers. Importantly, their presence often reduces the effectiveness of long-term obesity management. Eating disorders should therefore be actively sought, and their treatment form part of the overall obesity management plan.

The two most common eating disorders are Binge Eating Disorder (BED) and Night-time Eating Syndrome (NES) (Stunkard, 2003). These are described in detail in Chapter 20. This section focuses on their management and outcomes.

Binge Eating Disorder (BED)

BED is characterized by recurrent binge eating, but without the inappropriate compensatory weight-control methods, such as self-induced vomiting, excessive exercise, that are found in bulimia nervosa (American Psychiatric Association, 1994). It affects about 5% of the general population, rising to 17% among the obese and to 30% in those participating in weight reduction programmes (Spitzer et al., 1993). Patients who manage to stop binge eating lose more weight or are at least able to maintain their weight loss for longer than those who fail to stop (Grilo, Masheb and Wilson, 2005a; Golay et al., 2005). Thus, BED should be treated as part of the management package for patients with obesity.

The main treatments for BED are cognitive behavioural therapy (CBT), interpersonal psychotherapy (IPT), drug therapy and various combinations of psychotherapy with drugs.

CBT is usually administered on an individual basis at regular intervals as part of a structured weight reduction programme. The aim is to improve and maintain motivation, self-monitoring and problem solving. Currently, CBT is regarded as the best established intervention for BED (National Institute for Clinical Excellence, 2004; Wilson and Fairburn, 2000), but there are no convincing data that it promotes weight loss on its own.

IPT is another type of psychotherapy, which focuses on problem resolution within four social domains: grief, interpersonal role disputes, role transitions, and interpersonal deficits. It can be as effective as CBT in stopping binges and thus helps to maintain weight loss, but again has not been shown to decrease weight in its own right (Wilfley et al., 2002).

A few small trials have evaluated antidepressants (both SSRIs and monomine oxidase inhibitors) or anti-obesity drugs (sibutramine and topiramate) in BED. All showed a significant fall in the frequency of binge episodes and weight loss of 2–7 kg, with sibutramine and topiramate being the most effective (Carter et al., 2003; Appolinario et al., 2003). However, all these studies were small and under six month's duration; use of these drugs in BED therefore remains limited to specialist clinics.

More recently, CBT has been used in combination with exercise or drugs (orlistat, sibutamine or imipramine). These approaches result in greater weight loss and more improvements in abnormal eating behaviour than these modalities on their own (Grilo, Masheb and Salant, 2005b; Golay et al., 2005; Devlin et al., 2005; Pendleton et al., 2002; Levin, Marcus and Mouton, 1996; Laederach-Hofmann et al., 1999).

There is no consensus as to whether bariatric surgery should be offered to these patients. It does not cure the underlying eating disorder and in some cases has been reported to worsen BED. Nevertheless, the average weight loss after surgery is broadly similar in patients with BED to that in unaffected obese subjects. An exception is patients with powerful cravings for sweet food, who lose little weight (Burgmer *et al.*, 2005); if surgery is offered to these patients, it should be combined with CBT and monitored closely to discourage abnormal behaviours such as overconsumption of sweetened, energy-dense drinks.

Night-time eating syndrome (NES)

NES is a distinct entity that consists of morning anorexia, evening hyperphagia and insomnia. Its prevalence in obese individuals is reported to be as high as 27%, compared with only 1.5% in non-obese individuals (Rand, Macgregor and Stunkard, 1997). Both CBT and IPT are commonly employed in the management of NES, but they appear to be less effective than in the treatment of BED.

Small trials have suggested that high-dose sertraline (50–200 mg) may be beneficial in treating NES, with a reduction in energy consumed in the evening and an average weight loss of 3 kg (O'Reardon, Stunkard and Allison, 2004; O'Reardon *et al.*, 2006). These findings need to be validated in a larger population before the routine use of this drug can be recommended.

Limited evidence suggests that the outcome of bariatric surgery is not adversely affected by the presence of NES, and that nocturnal eating may become less frequent post-operatively, possibly due to improvements in both sleep quality and symptoms of depression (Powers *et al.*, 1999).

Psychological and psychiatric disorders

Obesity can cause a negative emotional effect and is linked with disorders including low self-esteem, body image dissatisfaction, depression, anxiety disorders (Simon *et al.*, 2006), self-harm and borderline personality symptomatology (Sansone, Sansone and Fine, 1995; see Chapter 14). These disorders may lead to other physical and mental illnesses (Stewart-Brown, 1998). It is thus crucial that warning signs and symptoms of psychological and psychiatric disorders are recognized and treated without delay as part of the general management of obesity. In particular, patients taking rimonabant must be monitored carefully, because they have a nearly twofold higher risk of developing severe anxiety or depression (Christensen *et al.*, 2007; see Chapter 17).

Weight reduction itself, even moderate, can lead to improvements in depression (Dymek *et al.*, 2001; Gladis *et al.*, 1998) and in psychological well-being (Rippe *et al.*, 1998). Thus, treatments that tend to help to improve mood as well as decrease weight offer particular advantages; examples are exercise and behavioural therapy.

Regular exercise should be encouraged in such individuals, principally to generate a feeling of well-being rather than to improve fitness (Martinsen and Stephens, 1994). Exercise has been shown to be as effective as drugs at improving mood, as well as reducing the risk of depression associated with obesity (The Mental Health Foundation, 2005). It also helps to maintain weight loss, as compared with individuals who do not exercise regularly (Pendleton *et al.*, 2002).

Behavioural therapy (BT), which is based on the idea that behaviour is learned and reinforced by particular social circumstances, can also be used in this setting. BT helps to promote positive attitudes and encourages healthy eating patterns, but also appears ineffective at inducing weight loss on its own (University of York, 1997). CBT and IPT are as effective as antidepressants in the management of depression in obese individuals (Agosti and Ocepek-Welikson, 1997; Stunkard, 2003), but again there is no evidence that these reduce weight.

Antidepressants and anti-psychotics are frequently prescribed for more severe psychiatric problems resistant to other therapies. The tendency of some of these drugs (especially atypical antipsychotics) to cause weight gain has been mentioned above.

Rimonabant (not now licensed in either USA or Europe) is contraindicated in subjects with mental disorders. Furthermore, sibutramine should not be given to patients taking SSRIs, monoamine oxidase inhibitors or lithium. Bariatric surgery with gastric banding has been shown to be less effective in patients with significant psychiatric disease, presumably because of poor compliance (Kinzl *et al.*, 2006).

Pregnancy

As described in Chapter 13, pregnancy can be hazardous for obese mothers and their children. Obese women are more susceptible to complications during both pregnancy and labour, while children of obese mothers are more likely to suffer congenital abnormalities or die *in utero* or within the first year (Linne, 2004). For this reason, pre-conception assessment and counselling, followed by careful monitoring throughout pregnancy, are strongly advised for patients with a BMI >30 kg/m² (see Table 19.2).

Pre-conception management

Information should be provided about the possible complications of obesity, and the woman encouraged to undergo a weight reduction programme, including diet, exercise, behavioural treatment and perhaps pharmacological therapy, before attempting to become pregnant.

Orlistat can be used to reduce weight before conception. As well as being safe and effective, it can also help to normalize ovulation and menstruation, thus improving fertility, and perhaps lessen the risk of gestational diabetes. Metformin can improve insulin sensitivity and induce ovulation.

The number of women of child-bearing age undergoing bariatric surgery (Chapter 18) is increasing. Previous concerns that these operations might be associated with anaemia, intrauterine growth retardation or neural tube defects in pregnancy (Woodard, 2004) have not been confirmed by recent studies (Dao *et al.*, 2006). Women who have undergone a bariatric procedure should be advised to delay pregnancy for 12–18 months after surgery, to avoid becoming pregnant during the period of rapid weight loss.

Table 19.2 Hazards and management of pregnancy in obese women.

Stage	Hazards	Management
Pre-conception	Reduced fertility	Counselling and lifestyle advice
		Routine obesity management
		Metformin
Pregnancy (mother)	Gestational diabetes	Screen for hyperglycaemia
	Hypertension	Monitor blood pressure
	Pre-eclampsia	Monitor urinary albumin
	Maternal death	Treat cardiovascular risk factors
		Limit weight gain (without using anti-obesity drugs)
		Promote exercise and healthy diet
Pregnancy (fetus)	Congenital defects	Ultrasound scanning
	Macrosomia	Monitor fetal growth
	Birth injury	Monitor fetal heart rate and movements
	Intrauterine death	
Labour	Prolonged labour	Consider elective caesarean section
	Birth injury	Fetal monitoring
Postnatal	Venous thrombosis	Early mobilization
	Continuing obesity	Anti-thrombotic measures
		Review by obesity specialist
		Promote breastfeeding
Follow-up	Maternal obesity	Review by obesity specialist
	Child's obesity	Promote breastfeeding

Antenatal management

Weight and BMI must be carefully measured at the first antenatal visit. Women with a BMI >40 kg/m^2 are at the highest risk and require specialist referral. Ultrasound scans should be carried out early for accurate dating of pregnancy, because these patients are likely to have had irregular menses and it may be difficult to determine the fundal height. Screening for glucose intolerance should be carried out at presentation or in the first trimester and repeated later in pregnancy if the initial screening test is positive, especially in women at increased risk of gestational diabetes (Table 19.3). According to the WHO criteria, gestational diabetes is diagnosed if fasting plasma glucose exceeds 7.0 mmol/l, or if the value 2 hours after an oral challenge of 75 g glucose is over 7.8 mmol/l (WHO, 1999). Blood pressure should be monitored closely throughout, using an appropriately sized cuff, because obese women are at increased risk of pre-eclampsia (Cedergren, 2004; see Chapter 12).

Patients should be referred for dietary assessment and advice. The aim is to limit weight gain to 7–11 kg for overweight women and to 7 kg for obese women (Institute of Medicine, 1990). Weight loss is not advocated; for this reason, anti-obesity drugs have not been used, and they should be discontinued if an obese woman becomes pregnant. Energy restricted diets can be used, but low protein diets should not because these may be harmful to the developing fetus (Kramer and Kakuma, 2003). Exercise should be encouraged, because this can help to limit weight gain as well as improve cardiovascular fitness.

Table 19.3 Clinical risk factors for gestational diabetes.

Obesity

Family history of diabetes

Previous diabetes (associated with oral contraceptive usage or pregnancy)

Previous macrosomic infant, unexplained stillbirth or neonatal death during previous pregnancy

Glycosuria on two or more occasions during current pregnancy

High-risk ethnic group (Asian, Afro-Caribbean)

Women with a gastric band should be monitored throughout pregnancy by their surgeon, because band adjustment may be required. Finally, nutritional and vitamin supplements may be necessary, because deficiencies of iron, vitamin B12, folate and calcium can occur after bariatric surgery (Poitou Bernert et al., 2007).

Management of labour

An elective caesarean section should be considered if the estimated fetal weight at term is over 5 kg in women without diabetes (Spellacy et al., 1985), or over 4.5 kg in women with diabetes (Lipscomb, Gregory and Shaw, 1995). During labour, if not contraindicated, elective placement of an epidural catheter should be considered in women with a BMI >35 kg/m^2, with the aim of decreasing anaesthetic and perinatal complications associated with any emergency regional or general anaesthesia that may be needed. If a caesarean section is required, an experienced senior obstetrician and anaesthetist should carry this out; a neonatologist should also be present. Prophylactic antibiotics should be given.

Obese patients are at increased risk of thromboembolic disease (Cedergren, 2004). After normal vaginal delivery, early mobilization, hydration and anti-thrombotic stockings should be promoted. If labour is prolonged or a caesarean section has been performed, then thomboprophylaxis with subcutaneous heparin should be considered.

Nutrition and exercise counselling should be continued after the pregnancy and breastfeeding should be encouraged, because this has been shown to reduce the risk of obesity during infancy and childhood (see Chapter 21). Consultation with an obesity specialist should be encouraged before attempting another pregnancy.

Managing type 2 diabetes in obese patients

The increasingly common combination of obesity with type 2 diabetes can be difficult to manage effectively. In theory, treating obesity should also increase insulin sensitivity and lower glycaemia, while also improving obesity related co-morbidities such as dyslipidaemia and hypertension. Indeed, modest weight loss of 5–10%

of initial weight can lower blood glucose by 2–3 mmol/l and glycated haemoglobin (HbA1c) by 1% or more, effects that are comparable to those achieved by oral hypoglycaemic agents. Unfortunately, this degree of weight loss is rarely achieved through lifestyle modification alone, and the individual glycaemic response to weight loss is highly variable.

Obese patients with type 2 diabetes must be fully evaluated for cardiovascular and other risks when first seen, and regularly reviewed thereafter. Screening and further investigations are described in Chapter 15.

Management of obese type 2 diabetic patients begins with lifestyle modification, and proceeds in the majority of cases who do not achieve satisfactory glycaemic control to treatment with glucose lowering and perhaps anti-obesity drugs. Some patients will meet the criteria for

bariatric surgery, and this can lead to substantial weight loss and marked falls in blood glucose or even complete resolution of established type 2 diabetes.

Algorithms for treating overweight and hyperglycaemia in obese type 2 diabetic patients are suggested in Figures 19.3 and 19.4. General treatment targets are the same as for all patients with type 2 diabetes (Table 19.4).

Lifestyle modification

This combines an energy restricted diet with increased physical exercise, and has long been the starting point for managing both obesity and type 2 diabetes, even though success is likely to be limited in a routine clinical setting.

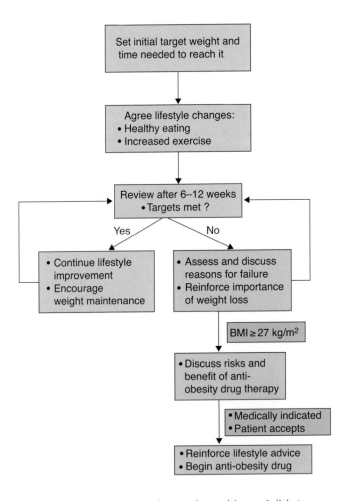

Figure 19.3 Algorithm for treating overweight in obese patients with type 2 diabetes.

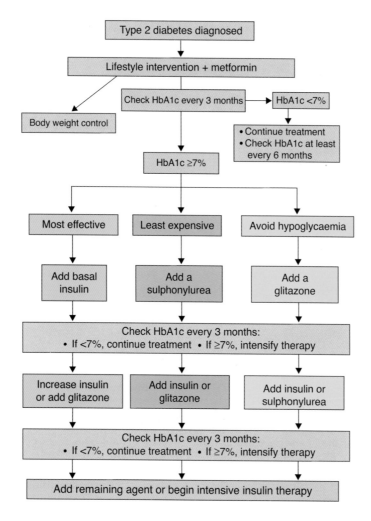

Figure 19.4 Algorithm for treating hyperglycaemia in obese patients with type 2 diabetes. Modified from consensus statements by the American Diabetes Association and the European Association for the Study of Diabetes. See Nathan *et al.* (2008) *Diabetes Care* 31: 173–95.

Diet

Standard dietetic guidelines (Figure 19.5 and Table 19.5) should be followed. Total energy intake should be reduced by 500 kcal/day (or up to 1000 kcal/day), with the emphasis on reducing dietary fat and substituting complex carbohydrate and fibre. The traditional 'low sugar' diabetic diet, originally based on oversimplistic assumptions about the impact of ingested sugar on blood glucose, is obsolete and, by favouring a higher fat intake, may have worsened obesity, insulin resistance and cardiovascular risk.

Energy restriction (rather than manipulating macronutrient composition) is the key determinant of fat loss and of improvements in insulin sensitivity and blood glucose. Reducing energy intake by 500–1000 kcal/day will initially induce weight loss of 0.5–1 kg per week. This mostly represents mobilization of fat; faster weight loss may involve catabolism of protein and muscle, and the rate should not exceed 2 kg per week. Weight loss will stabilize, generally after 3–6 months, in patients who remain compliant, and some will lose 5–10%, levels at which consistent improvements in blood glucose, lipids and blood pressure are often seen.

Total fat intake should be reduced to provide 25–30% of total energy intake and should comprise mainly monounsaturated or polyunsaturated

Table 19.4   Treatment targets for type 2 diabetes, as proposed by the American Diabetes Association and endorsed by other national diabetes organizations.

Glycaemic control	Normal	Goal	Additional action needed
HbA1c (%)	<6.0	<7.0	>8.0
Venous plasma glucose			
• Fasting (mmol/l)	≤6.2	5.2–7.3	<5.0 or >8.8
Self-monitored blood glucose			
• Average preprandial (mmol/l)	≤5.6	4.4–6.7	<4.5 or >7.8
• Average bedtime (mmol/l)	<6.2	5.6–7.8	<6.2 or >8.9
Body mass index (kg/m²)			
• Men	<25		
• Women	<25		
Blood lipids (mmol/l)	Low risk	Borderline	High risk
• LDL-cholesterol	<2.60	2.60–3.35	>3.35
• HDL-cholesterol[a]	>1.15	0.90–1.15	<0.90
• Triglycerides	<2.30	2.30–4.50	>4.50
Blood pressure (mm Hg)	<130 and 80		

HDL: high-density lipoprotein; LDL: low-density lipoprotein.
HbA_{1c} concentrations should be measured using a Diabetes Control and Complications Trial (DCCT)-aligned assay.
[a]For women, the HDL-cholesterol values should be increased by 0.26 mmol/l.

fat; saturated fat should provide <10% of total energy intake. For patients with raised LDL cholesterol, saturated fat intake should be further reduced to <7% of energy intake, and dietary cholesterol to <200 mg/day.

Carbohydrate should provide the bulk of energy intake (50–55%), particularly fruit, vegetables and starchy foods rich in complex carbohydrates and fibre (the intake of which should exceed 14 g/1000 kcal consumed).

Contributions to total energy intake

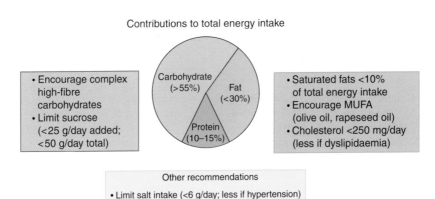

Figure 19.5 General dietary recommendations for obese patients with type 2 diabetes, as endorsed by the American Diabetes Association and other national diabetes organizations.

Table 19.5   Practical advice for healthy eating.

Quench thirst with water or other sugar-free drinks

Eat regular meals, avoiding fried and very sugary foods

Eat plenty of vegetables

Have high fibre and low glycaemic index foods (e.g. whole grains, legumes or brown rice) as the main part of each meal

Eat plenty of whole fruit

Limit consumption of animal products rich in saturated fat (e.g. red meat, eggs, liver and high fat dairy products).

Choose lean meat, fish, poultry (without skin) and low fat dairy products

For snacks between meals, avoid biscuits, cake or confectionery and use nuts and fruits instead

Use natural liquid vegetable oils for cooking, baking and frying

Choose small portions, especially when eating in a restaurant. Do not overeat

Limit alcohol to 1 unit per day for women and 1–2 units per day for men

Avoid adding salt to food or in cooking

Alcohol (which contains 7 kcal/g) should be restricted to healthy drinking limits (21 units/week for men, 14 units/week in women) or lower. As well as providing excess energy, alcohol can be hazardous in patients taking insulin or sulphonylureas, because it blocks the acute increase in hepatic glucose production that enables recovery from hypoglycaemia.

'Diabetic' sweets and foods containing sorbitol (a cause of diarrhoea) or artificial sweeteners are expensive and best avoided.

Exercise

Physical activity should be increased, ideally to 30–60 minutes of moderate exercise (brisk walking or equivalent) on most or all days of the week.

Exercise should be tailored to the individual's daily routine and capability, with due attention to co-morbidities such as osteoarthritis or cardiovascular disease. Those with angina, hypertension or cardiovascular risk factors should be screened with an ECG, and an exercise tolerance test if appropriate.

Outcomes of lifestyle modification

Lifestyle modification has a poor record of success in obese diabetic patients. Few manage to lose 10% of weight, and only a small percentage will achieve lasting glycaemic control with these measures alone. This is probably due to the effects of continuing weight gain superimposed on the progressive decline in β-cell function in type 2 diabetes that has been clearly demonstrated by the UK Prospective Diabetes Study (UKPDS) and other longitudinal studies (see Chapter 10). The outcomes are better for patients who have longer and more frequent contact with dietitians.

All patients should persevere with lifestyle improvement, even if progressing to treatment with anti-obesity or glucose-lowering drugs. A checklist for reviewing progress at each encounter with the patient is shown in Figure 19.6.

Anti-obesity drugs

The three anti-obesity drugs in current use – orlistat, sibutramine and rimonabant (not now licensed in USA or Europe) – have all been evaluated in obese type 2 diabetic subjects. The outcomes are summarized in Table 19.6.

Each drug can achieve weight loss of 10% or more in about one-third of cases, with concomitant improvements in HbA1c (by up to 1%) and in fasting blood glucose (2–3 mmol/l). These effects are apparently related to the degree of weight loss, although there is some evidence that rimonabant may have an additional, independent insulin-sensitizing action (see Chapter 17).

Pharmacotherapy with any of these drugs can be considered in type 2 diabetic patients whose BMI exceeds 27 kg/m^2, following the guidelines outlined in Chapter 17. Contraindications for the individual drugs must be observed: depression and psychiatric illness for rimonabant, and uncontrolled hypertension for sibutramine. Long-term efficacy and safety data are lacking but treatment is often continued beyond two years if there is still evidence of benefit; stopping the drug is usually followed by weight gain. General guidance is given in Figure 19.7.

Each of these drugs can be combined with oral hypoglycaemic agents or insulin, and can lead to variable improvements in blood glucose, HbA1c,

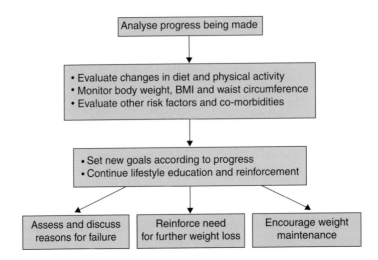

Figure 19.6 Checklist for reviewing progress at each encounter with an obese patient with type 2 diabetes.

blood lipids and blood pressure in patients who lose >5% of weight.

Glucose lowering drugs

Lifestyle changes, with or without anti-obesity drugs, are often insufficient to achieve and maintain adequate glycaemic control (Table 19.4). Some subjects may be eligible for bariatric surgery (see below), but most will require glucose lowering drugs. The main agents used are shown in Table 19.7.

Using these drugs in obese patients often poses a therapeutic dilemma, because insulin and most other glucose lowering drugs will increase fat mass, sometimes markedly, and can potentially worsen other obesity related co-morbidities. However, an important priority is to meet glycaemic control criteria (Table 19.4) as far as possible, so as to reduce the risk of diabetic microvascular complications such as retinopathy

and nephropathy. This is particularly important for obese children with type 2 diabetes, who appear to be at high risk of microvascular disease, and for Asian subjects who are especially susceptible to nephropathy (see Chapters 9 and 21). Weight gain can be minimized by using metformin and specific insulin regimens, and by reinforcing lifestyle advice about healthy eating and exercise.

Metformin

Metformin, a biguanide, lowers blood glucose primarily by inhibiting hepatic gluconeogenesis, the main source of the liver's glucose production that underpins basal hyperglycaemia in type 2 diabetes. It does not increase insulin levels and therefore does not induce hypoglycaemia. Importantly, it does not cause weight gain; the UK Prospective Diabetes Study (UKPDS, 1998) found that obese type 2 diabetic

Table 19.6 Effects of anti-obesity drugs on weight and glycaemic control in type 2 diabetes. See Chapter 17 for details of the studies.

Drug	Placebo-subtracted weight loss	Placebo-subtracted effect on HbA1c	Effect on HbA1c in 5% weight loss responders	Effect on HbA1c in 10% weight loss responders
Orlistat (3 studies)	2.7 kg	−0.4%	Not reported	Not reported
Sibutramine (8 studies)	4.5 kg	−0.3%	−0.7%	−1.1%
Rimonabant (1 study)	4.2 kg	−0.7%	Not reported[a]	Not reported[a]

[a]Regression analysis showed that reduction in HbA1c was proportional to weight loss.

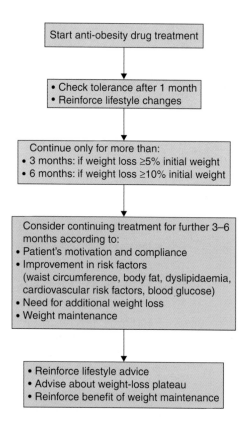

Start anti-obesity drug treatment

↓

• Check tolerance after 1 month
• Reinforce lifestyle changes

↓

Continue only for more than:
• 3 months: if weight loss ≥5% initial weight
• 6 months: if weight loss ≥10% initial weight

↓

Consider continuing treatment for further 3–6 months according to:
• Patient's motivation and compliance
• Improvement in risk factors
  (waist circumference, body fat, dyslipidaemia, cardiovascular risk factors, blood glucose)
• Need for additional weight loss
• Weight maintenance

↓

• Reinforce lifestyle advice
• Advise about weight-loss plateau
• Reinforce benefit of weight maintenance

Figure 19.7 General guidance for using anti-obesity drugs in patients with type 2 diabetes.

patients taking metformin lost 1–2 kg over six years, compared with weight gain of 4–5 kg with sulphonylureas and 10 kg with insulin. Furthermore, subjects taking metformin showed reductions in diabetes-related deaths, notably from cardiovascular disease, compared with the other treatments.

For these reasons, metformin is first-line glucose lowering therapy for obese type 2 diabetic patients. It can be effectively combined with insulin, often reducing the insulin dosage and therefore the risk of hypoglycaemia and weight gain. Metformin (850 mg) is usually taken twice daily with the morning and evening meals, and is generally well tolerated, apart from mostly mild gastrointestinal side effects, including nausea, abdominal discomfort and diarrhoea. The risk of lactic acidosis, although very low (incidence, 0.03 episodes per 1000 patient-years), contraindicates its use in patients with significant renal, cardiac, liver or respiratory failure.

Sulphonylureas and meglitinide analogues

Sulphonylureas (e.g. gliclazide, glibenclamide and glimepiride) stimulate insulin secretion. They bind to a specific sulphonylurea receptor (SUR-1) associated with the ATP-sensitive K⁺ channel in the β-cell membrane, closing the channel; this raises the intracellular K^+ concentration, depolarising the β-cell membrane and triggering the exocytosis of insulin. Sulphonylureas typically lower blood glucose by 2–3 mmol/l and HbA1c by 1% or more.

Because they induce hyperinsulinaemia, sulphonylureas cause hypoglycaemia. Glibenclamide has a prolonged action profile and is particularly hazardous, especially in the elderly and those with renal impairment (which, if significant, is a contraindication for these drugs). Sulphonylureas also cause significant weight gain, due to the anabolic effects of hyperinsulinaemia and the reduction of energy losses through glycosuria. In the UKPDS, weight gain averaged 4–5 kg over six years (UKPDS, 1998). Accordingly, they are second-line oral therapy for obese type 2 diabetic subjects, and often used together with metformin.

Meglitinide and its analogues (repaglinide and nateglinide) also bind to the SUR-1 receptor and stimulate insulin secretion. Their capacity to lower glucose and cause hypoglycaemia and weight gain are comparable to those of the sulphonylureas (Purnell and Weyer, 2003); they are used similarly, but are more expensive.

Thiazolidinediones (TZDs)

These drugs (e.g. rosiglitazone and pioglitazone) activate the PPAR-γ receptor that regulates numerous genes involved in lipid metabolism. The net effect is to lower circulating free fatty acid (FFA) levels which are related to insulin resistance (see Chapter 10). This improves insulin sensitivity and glucose utilization; hepatic glucose production and blood glucose levels fall (Yki-Järvinen, 2004). TZDs may also improve β-cell function and survival by clearing intracellular lipid deposits (Chapter 10). They generally lower blood glucose levels by 2–3 mmol/l and HbA1c by about 1%.

TZDs stimulate preadipocyte differentiation and lipogenesis, especially in subcutaneous depots; this is the main cause of weight gain (typically 2–3 kg) during treatment. Visceral fat mass does not increase, and overall insulin

Table 19.7 Main features of glucose-lowering drugs and their effects on weight.

Drug	Effect on weight	Advantages	Disadvantages
Metformin	Neutral	Cheap	• Gastrointestinal side-effects
		Decreased cardiac risk	• Lactic acidosis (rare)
Sulphonylureas	Increase	Cheap	• Hypoglycaemia
Thiazolidinediones	Increase	Improved lipids (pioglitazone)	• Fluid retention
		Potential decreased myocardial infarction risk (pioglitazone)	• Increased risk of congestive heart failure (rosiglitazone and pioglitazone)
			• Increased risk of myocardial infarction (rosiglitazone)
			• Increased risk of bone fractures
			• Expensive
Acarbose	Neutral		• Gastrointestinal side-effects
			• Modest glucose lowering action
			• Expensive
Meglitinide analogues	Increase	Short duration	• Hypoglycaemia
			• Expensive
Pramlintide	Loss		• Given by injection
			• Gastrointestinal side-effects
			• Expensive
Exenatide, liraglutide	Loss		• Given by injection
			• Gastrointestinal side-effects
			• Expensive
Insulin	Increase (less with detemir)	Cheap	• Hypoglycaemia
		Powerful glucose-lowering action	• Given by injection

sensitivity improves. TZDs also cause sodium and water retention, and rosiglitazone and pioglitazone are associated with an increased risk of cardiac failure. Recent data also indicate a 30–40% excess risk of myocardial infarction with rosiglitazone; accordingly, it should be avoided in patients with active coronary-heart disease or high cardiovascular risk in reducing weight gain (Nissen and Walski, 2007).

Other drugs

Below is a list of some other glucose lowering drugs:

• *Acarbose.* This inhibits the α-glucosidase in the intestinal mucosa that hydrolyses polysaccharides to yield absorbable monosaccharides. It has a modest glucose lowering effect, and prominent gastrointestinal side effects due to persistence of undigested sugars in the bowel.

• *GLP-1 mimics and enhancers.* Glucagon-like peptide-1 (GLP-1) is an incretin hormone (i.e. it stimulates insulin secretion in response to food ingestion) that is released from the small intestine after eating. It also enhances satiety both through central actions on the hypothalamus and by delaying gastric emptying, thus enhancing the activity of gastric stretch receptors (see Chapter 6). These potentially beneficial actions can be exploited either by GLP-1 analogues, or by prolonging the survival of endogenous

GLP-1 in the circulation. *Exenatide*, a GLP-1 analogue and mimetic, can lower HbA1c by up to 1% and body weight by 4–5 kg after 18 months of treatment (Barnett, 2007). It is expensive and has to be injected subcutaneously. Inhibitors of dipeptidyl peptidase IV (DPP-IV), which degrades circulating GLP-1, enhance the hormone's normal actions. *Sitagliptin* and *vildagliptin* reduce HbA1c by up to 1% and do not alter weight (Elrishi *et al.*, 2007). All these compounds can cause nausea and vomiting, presumably related to gastric stasis.

- *Pramlintide*. This is a synthetic analogue of the β-cell peptide amylin, which is normally co-secreted with insulin. Its actions include mild satiety (like GLP-1, through central effects and delayed gastric emptying) and inhibition of excessive glucagon secretion after meals. It produces modest falls in HbA1c (<1%) and body weight (2–3 kg). It is expensive and is injected subcutaneously; side effects include mild nausea and vomiting, but it does not induce hypoglycaemia. It may be used to reduce insulin dosages (Edelman, Darsow and Frias, 2006).

Insulin

Insulin is the last therapeutic resort for type 2 diabetic patients who fail to respond to lifestyle improvement and oral agents. It can always lower blood glucose if enough is given; very large dosages (>150 units per day) may be required in morbidly obese and very insulin-resistant patients, and many obese subjects need dosages exceeding 1 U/kg/day to achieve acceptable glycaemic control.

Hypoglycaemia and increased adiposity are the main problems in using insulin to treat obese type 2 diabetic patients. Hypoglycaemia is particularly troublesome with intensive regimens (especially multiple daily injections), with high dosages, and when insulin is combined with sulphonylureas. Weight gain is typically 4–5 kg. This is attributed mainly to the anabolic and lipogenic effects of insulin (see Chapter 4), and initially to decreasing losses of glucose in the urine, which can amount to several hundred kcal per day in poorly controlled subjects. Hypoglycaemia also induces intense hunger, and food intake can increase significantly in patients with frequent episodes.

Numerous insulin regimes have been proposed to treat type 2 diabetes, either alone or in combination with one or more oral hypoglycaemic agents. Metformin synergises effectively with insulin, often allowing a reduction in insulin dosage and therefore in the potential for both hypoglycaemia and weight gain. The combination of insulin with sulphonylureas is obesogenic, and co-administration of insulin and TZDs is not advised because the risk of cardiac failure related to TZDs appears to be increased.

Insulin regimens that are reported to control glycaemia effectively and with limited weight gain include:

- Once daily long acting insulin, especially contained with mealtime dosages of metformin (Yki-Järvinen, 2001). The long-acting analogue detemir is particularly associated with little or no weight gain; the reason is unknown but may relate to enhancement of insulin's central anorexigenic action (see Chapter 6).
- Rapid-acting insulin analogues injected at mealtimes, together with metformin (Poulsen *et al.*, 2003).

Bariatric surgery

The operations and their outcomes are described in Chapter 18. Various procedures can achieve substantial weight loss (up to 80% of excess weight), notably the biliopancreatic diversion (BPD), Roux-en-Y gastric bypass (RYGBP) and gastric banding. Blood glucose levels fall dramatically, and normoglycaemia can be restored in up to 80% of cases with IGT or even established type 2 diabetes treated with BPD or RYGBP (Buchwald *et al.*, 2004) (Figure 19.8). Patients with long-standing diabetes and those taking high insulin dosages are less likely to respond. Some patients eventually regain some weight after the post-operative fall (see Chapter 18), and glucose intolerance and ultimately overt diabetes may return. Successful bariatric surgery also improves hypertension, dyslipidaemia and sleep apnoea (Maggard *et al.*, 2005) (Figure 19.8).

General indications for bariatric surgery are discussed in Chapter 18. Obese subjects with type 2 diabetes could be considered if their BMI exceeds 35 kg/m²; if their obesity is likely to be the main impediment to achieving good glycaemic control and has resisted other measures; or if other serious obesity related co-morbidities are present.

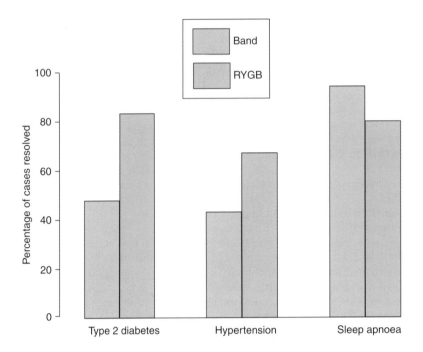

Figure 19.8 Outcomes of bariatric surgery. Clinical resolution rates are shown for type 2 diabetes, hypertension, dyslipidaemia and sleep apnoea, achieved by gastric banding and Roux-en-Y gastric bypass (RYGBP). From H. Buchwald *et al.* (2004) 'Bariatric surgery: a systematic review and meta-analysis'. *Journal of the American Medical Association*, **292** (14), 1724–37, with kind permission.

Follow up and monitoring

Obese type 2 diabetic patients are at increased risk of cardiovascular disease and also the microvascular complications of diabetes. They therefore need regular follow up and surveillance as described in Chapter 15, together with regular checks for diabetic retinopathy and nephropathy, neuropathy and diabetic foot disease. Hypertension and dyslipidaemia are frequently associated, and must be sought and actively treated (see below).

Management of IFG and IGT

Impaired fasting glucose (IFG) and impaired glucose tolerance (IGT) are diagnosed as described in Chapter 3. Diagnostic criteria from fasting plasma glucose and the oral glucose tolerance test (OGTT) are shown in Table 19.8. These states are commonly associated with obesity. They represent glucose intolerance that falls short of diabetes, and they do not carry the risk of microvascular complications. However, they are clinically important because each

can progress to diabetes (about 3–6% of cases per year), and each confers an increased risk of cardiovascular disease.

Obese subjects found to have IFG or IGT should be counselled that they may become diabetic, and that lifestyle modification resulting in relatively modest weight loss (5–10%) can greatly decrease this risk. Reasonable recommendations, based on the Finnish Diabetes Prevention Study (Tuomilehto *et al.*, 2001) and others, include:

- Taking 150 minutes of moderate exercise (e.g. brisk walking) per week.
- Increasing the intake of dietary fibre (to over 14 g per 1000 kcal of total energy intake).
- Decreasing dietary fat intake, and especially saturated fat (to <10% of energy intake).

Similar measures have been shown to reduce the risk of subjects with IGT progressing to overt diabetes by 60% or more (Figure 19.9; see Chapter 23).

If these measures fail to reduce weight or normalize blood glucose, drug treatment could be considered with metformin (Knowler *et al.*, 2002),

Table 19.8 States of glucose tolerance defined by criteria set by the American Diabetes Association (1997) and World Health Organization (1999).

		2-h plasma glucose, mmol/l (mg/dl)		
		< 7.8 (140)	7.8–11.0 (140–199)	≥ 11.1 (200)
Fasting plasma glucose, mmol/l (mg/dl)	< 6.1 (110)	Normal	IGT	Diabetes on an isolated 2-h hyperglycaemia IPH (isolated postchallenge hyperglycaemia)
	6.1–6.9 (110–125)	IFG	IFG and IGT	
	≥ 7.0 (126)	Diabetes on an isolated fasting hyperglycaemia		Diabetes on both fasting and 2-h hyperglycaemia

IFG, impaired fasting glucose; IGT, impaired glucose tolerance; IPH, isolated postchallenge hyperglycaemia.

orlistat or acarbose (Chiasson *et al.*, 2002; Berne, 2005); all these drugs have been shown to decrease the progression from IGT to diabetes.

Patients with IFG or IGT should be screened for other cardiovascular risk factors and treated accordingly. Glycaemic status should be rechecked every 1–2 years.

Management of dyslipidaemia

As described in Chapter 10, obese subjects and especially those with type 2 diabetes often have the dyslipidaemia, moderately raised triglycerides and low HDL cholesterol, characteristic of

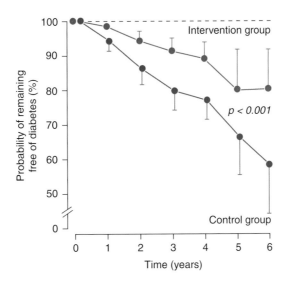

Figure 19.9 Lifestyle modification decreases the risk of subjects with IGT progressing to type 2 diabetes. In the Finnish Diabetes Prevention Study, risk at six years fell from 42% in controls to 20% with lifestyle intervention, a relative risk reduction of 60%. From J. Tuomilehto *et al.* (2001) 'Prevention of type 2 diabetes mellitus by changes in lifestyle among subjects with impaired glucose tolerance'. *The New England Journal of Medicine*, **344** (18), 1343–50, with permission of the editor.

the metabolic syndrome. Although apparently modest, this profile conceals a markedly pro-atherogenic series of lipid abnormalities that confers high cardiovascular risk and must therefore be treated actively.

Cardiovascular risk can be evaluated in various ways, including the Framingham risk calculators (Table 19.9). The presence of diabetes, smoking, hypertension (blood pressure ≥140/90 mm Hg, or use of antihypertensive medication), low HDL cholesterol (<1.1 mmol/l, or <40 mg/dl), or a positive family history of ischaemic heart disease (in a male first-degree relative ≤55 years of age, or in a female first-degree relative ≤65 years of age), all constitute major risk factors.

Patients found to have dyslipidaemia should begin with lifestyle modification if this is not already in place to manage their obesity. As described above, this focuses on the reduction of saturated fat and cholesterol intakes and increases in dietary fibre, together with increased physical activity. These measures should be tried alone for not more than three months, and if the targets below are not met, drug therapy should be started.

In individuals with diabetes over 40 years of age, who are without overt cardiovascular disease but have one or more major risk factors, the primary goal is to lower the LDL-cholesterol (LDL-C) level to <2.6 mmol/l (<100 mg/dl). If LDL-lowering drugs such as statins are used, a reduction of at least 30–40% in LDL-C levels should be obtained. If baseline LDL-C is <100 mg/dL, statin therapy should be started based on risk factor assessment and clinical judgment. A fibrate should be added if fasting triglyceride levels remain above 1.7 mmol/l (<150 mg/dl).

Complementary therapies and obesity

A substantial and growing number of people are turning to complementary and alternative medicine (CAM) to treat numerous conditions, including obesity (Kemper et al., 2007). These therapies are commonly viewed as natural and time-honoured treatments that can supplement or replace orthodox medicine. However, many CAM therapies are poorly standardized and heavily operator dependent, and very few have

Table 19.9 Framingham risk score (Grundy et al., 2006). This estimates the risk of 'hard' CHD end-points including myocardial infarction and death. Note that the Framingham score does not include LDL cholesterol; nonetheless, LDL cholesterol remains a primary therapeutic target. The table below shows the calculator (www.nhlbihin.net/atpiii/calculator) and the fields that are filled in with the subject's data.

Risk Assessment Tool for Estimating 10-year Risk of Developing Hard CHD (Myocardial Infarction and Coronary Death)

The *risk assessment tool* below uses recent data from the Framingham Heart Study to estimate 10-year risk for 'hard' coronary heart disease outcomes (myocardial infarction and coronary death). This tool is designed to estimate risk in adults aged 20 and older who do not have heart disease or diabetes.

Age: ☐ years

Gender: Female/Male

Total cholesterol: ☐ mg/dL

HDL cholesterol: ☐ mg/dL

Smoker: No/Yes

Systolic blood pressure: ☐ mm/Hg

Currently on medication for high blood pressure? No/Yes

Calculate 10-Year Risk

- *Total and HDL cholesterol*: values should be the average of at least two measurements.

- *Smoker*: The designation 'smoker' means any cigarette smoking in the past month.

- *Systolic blood pressure*: The value obtained at the time of assessment, regardless of whether the person is taking antihypertensive therapy (treated hypertension carries residual risk).

been tested rigorously enough to demonstrate efficacy and safety.

A recent survey in the USA reported that 36% of respondents had tried CAM in the previous 12 months, with 3% using therapies for weight loss. The most common were non-prescription supplements, including Ayurvedic herbal preparations, Chitosan (chitin from crustaceans), *Ephedra sinica* (a shrub that yields the sympathomimetic agent, ephedrine) and chromium picolinate. Other measures included yoga, meditation, massage, acupuncture, Eastern martial arts (*Tai chi* and *Qi gong*), hypnotherapy and homeopathy (Sharpe *et al.*, 2007).

Few good quality trials have attempted to evaluate whether CAM therapies genuinely induce weight loss and are safe, and the nature of some of these interventions makes conventional study design (e.g. placebo-control and double-blinding) difficult to apply (Pittler and Ernst, 2004). As some of the literature is not in English, it is possible that some evidence may have eluded reviews or meta-analyses (Pham *et al.*, 2005).

A few limited studies of non-prescription supplements have reported statistically significant weight loss compared with placebo, but the effects appear very modest (<0.2 kg) and require confirmation (Pittler and Ernst, 2004).

Prolonged administration or high doses of some preparations can lead to adverse effects, including psychiatric and gastrointestinal symptoms and palpitations with ephedrine containing products.

Hypnotherapy has been reported to cause additional weight reduction of 5–6 kg when used as an adjunct to dietary advice (Stradling *et al.*, 1998) or in combination with CBT (Allison and Faith, 1996).

Acupuncture is demonstrably effective in alleviating postoperative pain, nausea and vomiting, and in chemotherapy related nausea and vomiting (Birch *et al.*, 2004). It is believed to alter central nervous system neurotransmitter levels, inducing the release of endorphins and monoamines involved in reward pathways (Lacey, Tershakovec and Foster, 2003). Acupuncture has been tried for weight reduction (Vickers, Wilson and Kleijnen, 2002), often in combination with conventional medicines. In particular, auricular acupuncture, in which beads or needles are applied to specific points on the ears, is supposed to induce satiety. Rigorous evaluation is awaited.

Regular, long-term yoga exercises have been shown to produce moderate weight loss and improve weight maintenance (Yang, 2007; Kristal *et al.*, 2005) (Figure 19.10). *Qi gong* improves

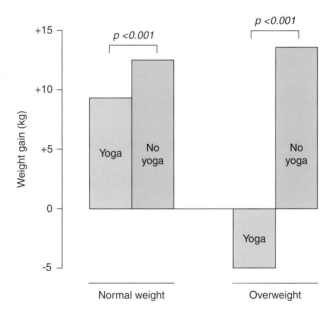

Figure 19.10 Yoga, practised regularly for at least four years, can enhance and maintain weight loss. Subjects were recruited from the Vitamin and Lifestyle (VITAL) study of over 15 500 adults. From A.R. Kristal *et al.* (2005) 'Yoga practice is associated with attenuated weight gain in healthy, middle-aged men and women'. *Alternative Therapies in Health and Medicine*, **11** (4), 28–33, with permission of the editor.

well being but has no effect on weight (Xin, 2007; Elder *et al.*, 2007). Meditation based treatments are currently being studied for weight control in obese individuals (Ospina *et al.*, 2007). There is no robust evidence that homoeopathic treatments induce significantly greater weight loss than placebo.

References

Agosti, V. and Ocepek-Welikson, K. (1997) The efficacy of imipramine and psychotherapy in early-onset chronic depression: a reanalysis of the National Institute of Mental Health Treatment of Depression Collaborative Research Program. *Journal of Affective Disorders*, **43**, 181–6.

Alisky, J.M. (2007) Phentermine, sibutramine and metformin could be used for the prevention and treatment of steroid-induced weight gain. *Medical Hypotheses*, **68** (2), 460–1.

Allison, D.B. and Faith, M.S. (1996) Hypnosis as an adjunct to cognitive behavioural psychotherapy for obesity: a meta-analytical reappraisal. *Journal of Consulting and Clinical Psychology*, **64**, 513–6.

American Diabetes Association (1997) Expert Committee on the Diagnosis and Classification of Diabetes Mellitus: Report of the Expert Committee on the Diagnosis and Classification of Diabetes. *Diabetes Care* **30**, 1183–119.

American Psychiatric Association (1994) Diagnostic and Statistical Manual of Mental Disorders. Fourth Edition. Published by American Psychiatric Association.

Appolinario, J.C., Bacaltchuk, J., Sichieri, R. *et al.* (2003) A randomized, double-blind, placebo-controlled study of sibutramine in the treatment of binge-eating disorder. *Archives of General Psychiatry*, **60** (11), 1109–16.

Baptista, T. (1999) Body weight gain induced by antipsychotic drugs. *Acta Psychiatrica Scandinavica*, **100**, 3–16.

Barnett, A. (2007) Exenatide. *Expert Opinion on Pharmacotherapy*, **8** (15), 2593–608.

Berne, C., the Orlistat Swedish Type 2 diabetes Study Group (2005) A randomized study of orlistat in combination with a weight management programme in obese patients with type 2 diabetes treated with metformin. *Diabetic Medicine: A Journal of the British Diabetic Association*, **22** (5), 612–8.

Bernstein, J.G. (1987) Induction of obesity by psychotropic drugs. *Annals of the New York Academy of Sciences*, **499**, 203–15.

Birch, S., Hesselink, J.K., Jonkman, F.A.M. *et al.* (2004) Clinical research on acupuncture: part 1. What have reviews of the efficacy and safety of acupuncture told us so far? *Journal of Alternative and Complementary Medicine*, **10** (3), 468–80.

Borrelli, B., Spring, B., Niaura, R. *et al.* (1999) Weight suppression and weight rebound in ex-smokers treated with fluoxetine. *Journal of Consulting and Clinical Psychology*, **76**, 124–31.

Buchwald, H., Avidor, Y., Braunwald, E. *et al.* (2004) Bariatric surgery: a systematic review and meta-analysis. *Journal of the American Medical Association*, **292** (14), 1724–37.

Burgmer, R., Grigutsch, K., Zipfel, S. *et al.* (2005) The influence of eating behavior and eating pathology on weight loss after gastric restriction operations. *Obesity Surgery*, **15** (5), 684–91.

Bustillo, J.R., Lauriello, J., Parker, K. *et al.* (2003) Treatment of weight gain with fluoxetine in olanzapine-treated schizophrenic outpatients. *Neuropsychopharmacology*, **28** (3), 527–9.

Butler, M.G. (2006) Management of obesity in Prader-Willi syndrome. *Nature Clinical Practice Endocrinology and Metabolism*, **2** (11), 592–3.

Cahill, K. and Ussher, M. (2007) Cannabinoid type 1 receptor antagonists (rimonabant) for smoking cessation. *Cochrane Database of Systematic Reviews*, (4), CD00535.

Carter, W.P., Hudson, J.I., Lalonde, J.K. *et al.* (2003) Pharmacologic treatment of binge eating disorder. *International Journal of Eating Disorders*, **34** (suppl), S74–88.

Cavazzoni, P., Tanaka, Y., Roychowdhury, S.M. *et al.* (2003) Nizatidine for prevention of weight gain with olanzapine: a double-blind placebo-controlled trial. *European Neuropsychopharmacology: The Journal of the European, College of Neuropsychopharmacology*, **13** (2), 81–5.

Cedergren, M.I. (2004) Maternal morbid obesity and the risk of adverse pregnancy outcome. *Obstetrics and Gynecology*, **103** (2), 219–24.

Chiasson, J.L., Josse, R.G., Gomis, R. *et al.*, STOP-NIDDM Trail Research Group (2002) Acarbose for prevention of type 2 diabetes mellitus: the STOP-NIDDM randomised trial. *Lancet*, **359** (9323), 2072–7.

Christensen, R., Kristensen, P.K., Bartels, E.M. *et al.* (2007) Efficacy and safety of the weight-loss drug rimonabant: a meta-analysis of randomised trials. *The Lancet*, **370** (9600), 1706–13.

Dale, L.C., Schroeder, D.R., Wolter, T.D. Croghan, I.T., Hurt, R.D. and Offord, K.P. (1998) Weight change after smoking cessation using variable doses of transdermal nicotine replacement. *Journal of General Internal Medicine*, **13**, 9–15.

Danielsson, T., Rössner, S. and Westin, A. (1999) Open randomised trial of very low energy diet together with nicotine gum for stopping smoking in women who gained weight in previous attempts to quit. *British Medical Journal (Clinical Research Edition)*, **319**, 490–4.

Dao, T., Kuhn, J., Ehmer, D. *et al.* (2006) Pregnancy outcomes after gastric-bypass surgery. *American Journal of Surgery*, **192** (6), 762–6.

Devlin, M.J., Goldfein, J.A., Petkova, E. *et al.* (2005) Cognitive behavioral therapy and fluoxetine as adjuncts to group behavioral therapy for binge eating disorder. *Obesity Research*, **13**, 1077–88.

Dymek, M.P., le Grange, D., Neven, K. and Alverday, J. (2001) Quality of life and psychosocial adjustment in patients after Roux-en-Y gastric bypass: a brief report. *Obesity Surgery*, **11**, 32–9.

Edelman, S.V., Darsow, T. and Frias, J.P. (2006) Pramlintide in the treatment of diabetes. *International Journal of Clinical Practice*, **60** (12), 1647–53.

Elder, C., Ritenbaugh, C., Mist, S. *et al.* (2007) Randomized trial of two mind-body interventions for weight-loss maintenance. *Journal of Alternative and Complementary Medicine*, **13**, 67–78.

Elrishi, M.A., Khunti, K., Jarvis, J. and Davies, M.J. (2007) The dipeptidyl-peptidase-4 (DPP4) inhibitors: a new class of oral therapy for patients with type 2 diabetes. *Practical Diabetes*, **24** (9), 474–82.

Eyal, O. *et al.* (2006) Obesity in patients with craniopharyngioma. *Endocrinologist*, **16**, 286–93.

Filozof, C., Fernández Pinilla, M.C. and Fernández-Cruz, A. (2004) Smoking cessation and weight gain. *Obesity Reviews*, **5** (2), 95–103.

Fossati, R., Apolone, G., Negri, E., Compagnoni, A., La Vecchia, C., Mangano, S., Clivio, L. and Garattini, S. (2007) for the General Practice Tobacco Cessation Investigators Group. A double-blind, placebo-controlled, randomized trial of bupropion for smoking cessation in primary care. *Arch Intern Med.* **167** (16), 1791–7.

Gladis, M.M., Wadden, T.A., Vogt, R. *et al.* (1998) Behavioral treatment of obese binge eaters: Do they need different care? *Journal of Psychosomatic Research*, **44**, 375–84.

Golay, A., Laurent-Jaccard, A., Habicht, F. *et al.* (2005) Effect of orlistat in obese patients with binge eating disorder. *Obesity Research*, **13**, 1701–8.

Gotherstrom, G., Svensson, J., Koranyi, J. *et al.* (2001) A prospective study of 5 years of GH replacement therapy in GH-deficient adults: sustained effects on body composition, bone mass, and metabolic indices. *The Journal of Clinical Endocrinology and Metabolism*, **86**, 4657–65.

Greenman, Y., Tordjman, K. and Stern, N. (1998) Increased body weight associated with prolactin secreting pituitary adenomas: weight loss with normalization of prolactin levels. *Clinical Endocrinology*, **48** (5), 547–53.

Grilo, C.M., Masheb, R.M. and Wilson, G.T. (2005a) Efficacy of cognitive behavioral therapy and fluoxetine for the treatment of binge eating disorder: a randomized double-blind placebo-controlled comparison. *Biological Psychiatry*, **57**, 301–9.

Grilo, C.M., Masheb, R.M. and Salant, S.L. (2005b) Cognitive behavioral therapy guided self-help and orlistat for the treatment of binge eating disorder: a randomized, double-blind, placebo-controlled trial. *Biological Psychiatry*, **57**, 1193–201.

Gross, J., Stitzer, M.L. and Maldonado, J. (1989) Nicotine replacement effects on postcessation weight gain. *Journal of Consulting and Clinical Psychology*, **57**, 87–92.

Hall, S.M., Tunstall, C.D., Vila, K.L. and Duffy, J. (1992) Weight gain prevention and smoking cessation: cautionary findings. *American Journal of Public Health*, **82**, 799–803.

Hays, J.T., Hurt, R.D., Rigotti, N.A. *et al.* (2001) Sustained-release bupropion for pharmacological relapse prevention after smoking cessation: a randomised controlled trial. *Annals of Internal Medicine*, **135**, 423–33.

Inge, T.H., Pfluger, P., Zeller, M. *et al.* (2007) Gastric bypass surgery for treatment of hypothalamic obesity after craniopharyngioma therapy. *Nature Clinical Practice Endocrinology and Metabolism*, **3** (8), 606–9.

Institute of Medicine (US) (1990) Nutritional status and weight gain, in *Nutrition During Pregnancy*, National Academy Press, Washington, DC, pp. 27–233.

Kemper, K.J., Dirkse, D., Eadie, D. and Pennington, M. (2007) What do clinicians want? Interest in integrative health services at a North Carolina academic medical centre. *BMC Complementary and Alternative Medicine*, **7**, 5.

Kinzl, J.F., Schrattenecker, M., Traweger, C. *et al.* (2006) Psychosocial predictors of weight loss after bariatric surgery. *Obesity Surgery*, **16** (12), 1609–14.

Knowler, W.C., Barrett-Connor, E., Fowler, S.E. *et al.*, Diabetes Prevention Program Research Group (2002) Reduction in the incidence of type 2 diabetes with lifestyle intervention or metformin. *The New England Journal of Medicine*, **346** (6), 393–403.

Kramer, M.S. and Kakuma, R. (2003) Energy and protein intake in pregnancy. *Cochrane Database of Systematic Reviews* (4), CD000032.

Kristal, A.R., Littman, A.J., Benitez, D. and White, E. (2005) Yoga practice is associated with attenuated weight gain in healthy, middle-aged men and women. *Alternative Therapies in Health and Medicine*, **11** (4), 28–33.

Lacey, J.M., Tershakovec, A.M. and Foster, G.D. (2003) Acupuncture for the treatment of obesity: a review of the evidence. *International Journal of Obesity*, **27**, 419–27.

Laederach-Hofmann, K., Graf, C., Horber, F. *et al.* (1999) Imipramine and diet counselling with psychological support in the treatment of obese binge eaters: a randomized, placebo-controlled double-blind study. *International Journal of Eating Disorders*, **26**, 231–44.

Levin, M.D., Marcus, M. and Mouton, P. (1996) Exercise in the treatment of binge eating disorder. *International Journal of Eating Disorders*, **19**, 171–7.

Linne, Y. (2004) Effects of obesity on women's reproduction and complications during pregnancy. *Obesity Reviews*, **5** (3), 137–43.

Lipscomb, K.R., Gregory, K. and Shaw, K. (1995) The outcome of macrosomic infants weighing at least 4500 grams: Los Angeles County + University of Southern California experience. *Obstetrics and Gynecology*, **85** (4), 558–64.

Lustig, R.H. *et al.* (2003) Octreotide therapy of pediatric hypothalamic obesity: a double-blind, placebo-controlled trial. *The Journal of Clinical Endocrinology and Metabolism*, **88**, 2586–92.

Maggard, M.A., Shugarman, L.R., Suttorp, M. *et al.* (2005) Meta-analysis: surgical treatment of obesity. *Annals of Internal Medicine*, **142** (7), 547–59.

Marcus, B.H., Albrecht, A.E., King, T.K. *et al.* (1999) The efficacy of exercise as an aid for smoking-cessation interventions in women: a randomised controlled trial. *Archives of Internal Medicine*, **159**, 1229–34.

Martinsen, E.W. and Stephens, T., (1994) Exercise and mental health in clinical and free-living populations, in *Advances in Exercise Adherence* (ed. R.K. Dishman), Human Kinetics, Champaign, IL, pp. 55–72.

McElroy, S.L., Frye, M.A., Altshuler, L.L. *et al.* (2007) A 24-week, randomized, controlled trial of adjunctive sibutramine versus topiramate in the treatment of weight gain in overweight or obese patients with bipolar disorders. *Bipolar Disorders*, **9** (4), 426–34.

Mentink, L.F., Mackenzie, M.W., Tóth, G.G. *et al.* (2006) Randomized controlled trial of adjuvant oral dexamethasone pulse therapy in pemphigus vulgaris: PEMPULS trial. *Archives of Dermatology*, **142** (5), 570–6.

Mersebach, H., Klose, M., Svendsen, O.L. *et al.* (2004) Combined dietary and pharmacological weight management in obese hypopituitary patients. *Obesity Research*, **12** (11), 1835–44.

Nathan, D.M., Buse, J.B., Davidson, M.B., Ferrannini, E., Holman, R.R., Sherwin, R. and Zinman, B. (2008) Management of hyperglycaemia in type 2 diabetes mellitus: a consensus algorithm for the initiation and adjustment of therapy: update regarding the thiazolidinediones. *Diabetologia* **51** (1), 8–11.

National Institute for Clinical Excellence (2004) CG9 Eating disorders: NICE guideline Published Jan 2004 by National Institute for Clinical Excellence. http://www.nice.org.uk/CG009NICEguideline.

Nissen, S.E. and Wolski, K. (2007) Effect of rosiglitazone on the risk of myocardial infarction and death from cardiovascular causes. *The New England Journal of Medicine*, **356** (24), 2457–71.

Norregaard, J., Jorgensen, S., Mikkelsen, K.L. *et al.* (1996) The effect of ephedrine plus caffeine on smoking cessation and postcessation weight gain. *Clinical Pharmacology and Therapeutics*, **60**, 679–86.

O'Reardon, J.P., Allison, K.C., Martino, N.S. *et al.* (2006) A randomized, placebo-controlled trial of sertraline in the treatment of night eating syndrome. *The American Journal of Psychiatry*, **163** (5), 893–8.

O'Reardon, J.P., Stunkard, A.J. and Allison, K.C. (2004) Clinical trial of sertraline in the treatment of night eating syndrome. *International Journal of Eating Disorders*, **35**, 16–26.

Ospina, M.B., Bond, T.K., Karkhaneh, M. *et al.* (2007) Meditation Practices for Health: State of the Research. Evidence Report/Technology Assessment No. 155. (Prepared by the University of Alberta), Agency for Healthcare Research and Quality. June.

Pendleton, V.R., Goodrick, G.K., Carlos Poston, W.S. *et al.* (2002) Exercise augments the effects of cognitive-behavioral therapy in the treatment of binge eating. *International Journal of Eating Disorders*, **31**, 172–84.

Perkins, K.E. (1994) Issues in the prevention of weight gain after smoking cessation. *Annals of Behavioral Medicine*, **16**, 46–52.

Pham, B., Klassen, T.P., Lawson, M.L. and Moher, D. (2005) Language of publication restrictions in systematic reviews gave different results depending on whether the intervention was conventional or complementary. *Journal of Clinical Epidemiology*, **58** (8), 769–76.

Pittler, M.H. and Ernst, E. (2004) Dietary supplements for body-weight reduction: a systematic review. *The American Journal of Clinical Nutrition*, **79**, 529–626.

Poitou Bernert, C., Ciangura, C., Coupaye, M. *et al.* (2007) Nutritional deficiency after gastric bypass: diagnosis, prevention and treatment. *Diabetes and Metabolism*, **33** (1), 13–24.

Poulsen, M.K., Henriksen, J.E., Hother-Nielsen, O. and Beck-Nielsen, H. (2003) The combined effect of triple therapy with rosiglitazone, metformin, and insulin aspart in type 2 diabetic patients. *Diabetes Care*, **26** (12), 3273–9.

Powers, P.S., Perez, A., Boyd, F. and Rosemurgy, A. (1999) Eating pathology before and after bariatric surgery: a prospective study. *International Journal of Eating Disorders*, **25**, 293–300.

Primary prevention of coronary heart disease: guidance from Framingham: a statement for healthcare professionals from the AHA Task Force on Risk Reduction. American Heart Association. Grundy, S.M., Balady, G.J., Criqui, M.H., Fletcher, G., Greenland, P., Hiratzka, L.F., Houston-Miller, N., Kris-Etherton, P., Krumholz, H.M., LaRosa, J., Ockene, I.S., Pearson, T.A., Reed, J., Washington, R., Smith, S.C. Jr. *Circulation*. 1998 May 12;97(18), 1876–87.

Purnell, J.Q. and Weyer, C. (2003) Weight effect of current and experimental drugs for diabetes mellitus: from promotion to alleviation of obesity. *Treatments in Endocrinology*, **2** (1), 33–47.

Rand, C.S., Macgregor, A.M.C. and Stunkard, A.J. (1997) The night eating syndrome in the general population and among postoperative obesity surgery patients. *International Journal of Eating Disorders*, **22** (1), 65–9.

Rippe, J.M., Price, J.M., Hess, S.A. *et al.* (1998) Improved psychological well-being, quality of life, and health practices in moderately overweight women participating in a 12-week structured weight loss program. *Obesity Research*, **6**, 208–18.

Rosen, T. and Bengtsson, B.A. (1990) Premature mortality due to cardiovascular disease in hypopituitarism. *Lancet*, **336**, 285–8.

Sansone, R.A., Sansone, L.A. and Fine, M.A. (1995) The relationship of obesity to borderline personality symptomatology, self-harm behaviours, and sexual abuse in female subjects in a primary care setting. *Journal of Personality Disorders*, **9**, 254–65.

Sharpe, P.A., Blanck, H.M., Williams, J.E. *et al.* (2007) Use of complementary and alternative medicine for weight control in the United States. *Journal of Alternative and Complementary Medicine*, **13** (2), 217–22.

Simon, G.E., Von Korff, M., Saunders, K. Miglioretti, D., Crane, P.K. van Belle, G. and Kessler R.C. (2006) Association between obesity and psychiatric disorders in the US adult population. *Archives of General Psychiatry*, **63**, 824–30.

Spellacy, W.N., Miller, S., Winegar, A. and Peterson, P.Q. (1985) Macrosomia – maternal characteristics and infant complications. *Obstetrics and Gynecology*, **66** (2), 158–61.

Spitzer, R.L., Yanovski, S., Wadden, B.T. *et al.* (1993) Binge eating disorder: its further validation in a multisite study. *International Journal of Eating Disorders*, **13**, 137–53.

Stevenson, D.A., Heinemann, J., Angulo, M. *et al.* (2007) Gastric rupture and necrosis in Prader-Willi syndrome. *Journal of Pediatric Gastroenterology and Nutrition*, **45** (2), 272–4.

Stewart-Brown, S. (1998) Emotional well-being and its relation to health: physical disease may well result from emotional distress. *British Medical Journal (Clinical Research Edition)*, **317**, 1608–9, (editorial).

Stradling, J., Roberts, D., Wilson, A. and Lovelock, F. (1998) Controlled trial of hypnotherapy for weight loss in patients with obstructive sleep apnoea. *International Journal of Obesity and Related Metabolic Disorders*, **22** (3), 278–81.

Stunkard, A.J. and Allison, K.C. (2003) Two forms of disordered eating in obesity: binge eating and night eating (review). *International Journal of Obesity*, **27**, 1–12.

Stunkard, A.J., Faith, M.S. and Allison, K.C. (2003) Depression and obesity. *Biological Psychiatry*, **54**, 330–7.

Swan, G. and Carmelli, D. (1995) Characteristics associated with excessive weight gain after smoking cessation in men. *American Journal of Public Health*, **85**, 73–7.

The Mental Health Foundation (2005) Up and running? Exercise therapy and the treatment of mild or moderate depression in primary care. March. (http://www.mentalhealth.org.uk/campaigns/exercise-and-depression/information-for-gps/ (last accessed 14 July 2008).

Tuomilehto, J., Lindström, J., Eriksson, J.G. *et al.*, Finnish Diabetes Prevention Study Group (2001) Prevention of type 2 diabetes mellitus by changes in lifestyle among subjects with impaired glucose tolerance. *The New England Journal of Medicine*, **344** (18), 1343–50.

UKPDS Study Group (1998) Effect of intensive blood-glucose control with metformin on complications in overweight patients with type 2 diabetes (UKPDS 34). UK Prospective Diabetes Study (UKPDS) Group. *Lancet*, **352** (9131), 854–65.

University of York (1997) Effective Health Care, the prevention and treatment of obesity. NHS Centre for Reviews and Disseminations. Bulletin on the effectiveness of health service interventions for decision makers. Vol 3, No 2.

Ussher, M. (2005) Exercise interventions for smoking cessation. *Cochrane Database of Systematic Reviews* (1), CD002295.

Vickers, A., Wilson, P. and Kleijnen, J. (2002) Acupuncture. Effectiveness bulletin. *Quality and Safety in Health Care*, **11**, 92–7.

Vossenaar, M., Anderson, A., Lean, M. and Ocke, M. (2004) Perceived reasons for weight gain in adulthood. *International Journal of Obesity*, **28** (S1), S67.

Werneke, U., Taylor, D. and Sanders, T.A. (2002) Options for pharmacological management of obesity in patients treated with atypical antipsychotics. *International Clinical Psychopharmacology*, **17** (4), 145–60.

Wilfley, D.E., Welch, R.R., Stein, R.I. *et al.* (2002) A randomized comparison of group cognitive-behavioral therapy and group interpersonal psychotherapy for the treatment of overweight individuals with binge-eating disorder. *Archives of General Psychiatry*, **59**, 713–21.

Wilson, G.T. and Fairburn, C.G. (2000) The treatment of binge eating disorder. *European Eating Disorders Review*, **8**, 351–4.

Woodard, C.B. (2004) Pregnancy following bariatric surgery. *Journal of Perinatal and Neonatal Nursing*, **18** (4), 329–40.

World Health Organization (1999) World Health Organization: Defination, diagnosis and classification of diabetes mellitus and its complications: Report of a WHO Consultation, Part 1. Diagnosis and classification of diabetes mellitus. Geneva, World Health Organization.

Xin, L., Miller, Y.D. and Brown, W.J. (2007) A qualitative review of the role of qigong in the management of diabetes. *The Journal of Alternative and Complementary Medicine*, **13** (4), 427–34.

Yang, K. (2007) A review of yoga programs for four leading risk factors of chronic diseases. *eCAM*, **4**(4), 487–91.

Yki-Järvinen, H. (2001) Combination therapies with insulin in type 2 diabetes. *Diabetes Care*, **24** (4), 758–67.

Yki-Järvinen, H. (2004) Thiazolidinediones. *The New England Journal of Medicine*, **351** (11), 1106–18.

Eating Disorders in Obesity

Key points

- Eating behaviour is often disturbed in obese subjects, and clinically diagnosable eating disorders are relatively common. Eating disorders can worsen obesity and complicate its management, and should therefore be actively sought, but the diagnoses are often missed.

- Binge eating disorder (BED), the commonest eating disorder in obesity, is defined by frequent episodes (at least two per week) of excessive eating, accompanied by feelings of loss of control, persisting for at least six months. There are no compensatory weight-reducing behaviours such as self-induced vomiting, abuse of laxatives or diuretics, or excessive exercise. BED may affect 9–19% of unselected obese subjects, but perhaps 30–50% of those who seek obesity treatment, including bariatric surgery. Males and middle-aged subjects are often affected.

- The cause of BED is unknown, but two different theories have been advanced. Restraint theory suggests that these are individuals who set themselves inflexible rules when trying to lose weight, and then react with an 'all-or-none' response of overeating when they break their own rules. Affect regulation theory postulates that binge eating is used to control negative mood states such as anger, anxiety and loneliness.

- During a single binge in BED, several hundred or several thousand kcal may be consumed, but BED may not be clinically apparent. Warning signs include an earlier onset and/or more rapid development of obesity, frequent weight fluctuations, distress when discussing weight, shape or eating, and admissions of loss of control or disgust after eating.

- Compared with obese subjects without BED, those who have BED have lower self-esteem, greater social and work dysfunction, and higher prevalences of major depression, anxiety and personality disorders.

- Binge eating in obese subjects may respond to cognitive behavioural therapy (CBT), but this may not achieve adequate weight loss. Anti-obesity drugs (e.g. sibutramine) appear less effective than CBT in treating binges, but obese subjects with BED show weight loss comparable to that in subjects without BED. A conventional behavioural weight-loss programme should also be employed in obese people with BED. Bariatric surgery can be considered but has yielded variable results.

- Night eating syndrome (NES) is defined by evening hyperphagia (consuming >25% of total daily energy intke after the evening meal) and/or eating for half or more of the time spent awake at night. Associated but non-diagnostic features include morning anorexia and delayed eating of the first daily meal. NES may affect 1.5% of unselected individuals of all weights, but 9–15% of obese subjects seeking active obesity treatment and 8–42% of those considering bariatric surgery. The onset of NES may be associated with depression, and poor self-esteem and depression are commoner than in unaffected obese subjects. Selective serotonin reuptake inhibitors (SSRIs) may be helpful.

- 'Body dissatisfaction' encompasses a spectrum of negative thoughts and feelings about body shape and weight. It is commoner among obese people, especially those who became obese (and were teased) during childhood, although the degree of dissatisfaction is not significantly correlated with BMI.

- Ideally, a structured psychological evaluation, using an investigator-based interview, should be performed at the start of treatment for all obese subjects. The Eating Disorder Examination (EDE), or a self-administered questionnaire version (EDE-Q), can be used to identify potential eating disorders and subjects who need referral to a clinical psychologist.

Chapter 20 Eating Disorders in Obesity

Susan M. Byrne and Emma R. Dove

Obese people often describe atypical behaviours and attitudes related to eating and weight, such as binge eating, body image disturbance and a pre-occupation with weight, shape and eating. These problems may contribute to the development and/or maintenance of obesity, and in some cases, symptoms are so significant that an eating disorder is clinically diagnosable. The most common eating disorders observed in obese individuals are Binge Eating Disorder (BED) and Night Eating Syndrome (NES). As these disorders may significantly affect outcome, adequate assessment and treatment of the full range of eating disorders is critical in the management of obese patients.

This chapter describes the features of disordered eating that are common in obesity, as well as the psychopathology associated with eating disorders in obese individuals. It concludes with practical guidelines for identifying, assessing and treating obese individuals with disordered eating.

Binge eating and binge eating disorder

Definitions

Binge eating is characterized by eating, within a discrete time-period, more food than most others would consume in similar circumstances, this being accompanied by a sense of loss of control over eating (American Psychiatric Association, 1994). Many individuals also report losing control over eating even when they have not consumed an objectively large amount of food; such episodes are termed *subjective* (as opposed to *objective*) binge eating. Studies analysing recorded food intake have found that obese binge eaters report binge eating episodes that vary greatly in caloric content, ranging from a few hundred calories up to several thousand calories. A 'typical' binge recorded by a patient using a food diary is shown in Figure 20.1.

Binge eating disorder

When binge eating is sufficiently frequent and prolonged, BED may be diagnosed. BED was included in the appendix of DSM-IV (American Psychiatric Association, 1994) as an example of 'Eating Disorder Not Otherwise Specified' (ED-NOS), following the DSM-IV field trials (Spitzer *et al.*, 1992). According to DSM-IV criteria (Table 20.1), BED is characterized by a pattern of binge eating that is regular, sustained and accompanied by evidence of marked distress caused by the binges. Crucially, BED is not associated with the use of inappropriate compensatory behaviour such as self-induced vomiting, laxative or diuretic misuse, or excessive exercise – which would instead suggest a diagnosis of bulimia nervosa (BN) (see Table 20.2 for a comparison of eating disorders).

Table 20.1 DSM-IV criteria for diagnosing BED (American Psychiatric Association, 1994)

BED is characterized by a pattern of binge eating that is:
• regular (an average of two or more episodes per week)
• sustained (episodes for at least six months)
• causing marked distress, with at least three of the following:
(i) eating very rapidly
(ii) eating until uncomfortably full
(iii) eating large amounts of food when not physically hungry
(iv) eating alone due to embarrassment at the amount consumed
(v) feeling disgusted or guilty after overeating
• *not* accompanied by regular inappropriate compensatory behaviours such as self-induced vomiting, laxative misuse or excessive exercise.

Obesity: Science to Practice   Edited by Gareth Williams and Gema Frühbeck
© 2009 John Wiley & Sons, Ltd

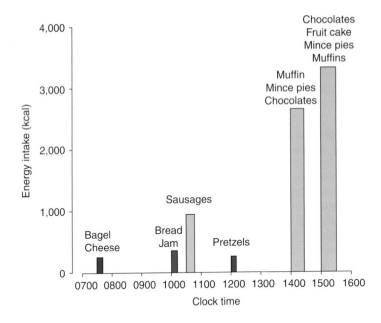

Self-monitoring Record

Day: Saturday   Date: 01/04/07

Time	Food and drink consumed	Place	Binge (*)	Calories	Comments
7.30 am	1 bagel	Kitchen		155	Relaxed
	cheese			77	
	1 cup of tea			10	
10.00 am	2 pieces of bread	Car		154	Hungry – glad I took this snack with me
	Jam			100	
	1 apple juice			105	
10.30 am	5 sausages	Car	*	950	Went to buy fried fish and sausages for dinner. Felt it was all too much. Bought 10 sausages but scoffed 5 in the car on the way home.
12.00	Half a cup of pretzels	Kitchen		240	Feeling vulnerable – pretzel packet on kitchen table
2.00 pm	1 muffin	Shopping centre	**	240	Can't get food out of my mind while shopping. Really battling with my "bingeing demons". Felt as though I'd totally lost control. Thought to myself "I've blown it so I may as well blow it some more".
	4 mince pies			1712	
	10 chocolates			678	
3.00 pm	1 box chocolates	Lounge room	***	1600	Don't even want to think about calories! Out of control. Feeling rushed, bloated, anxious.
	1 fruit cake (small)			540	
	1 muffin			240	
	2 mince pies			860	
					Had planned to go for a walk, but as a result of this binge I didn't go.

Figure 20.1 Binge eating disorder. Amounts of food, and the calculated energy content, consumed during a typical day by a subject with BED. Energy intake is shown in the upper panel, and the subject's food diary in the lower panel. The subject scored each binge from * to ***.

Table 20.2   Behavioural and cognitive features of BN, BED and EDNOS.

	Bulimia nervosa	Binge eating disorder	Eating disorder – not otherwise specified
Binge eating	Recurrent episodes of binge eating. On average, occurring at least twice a week for three months	Recurrent episodes of binge eating. On average, occurring at least twice a week for six months	Binge eating may occur but at a frequency of less than twice a week for a duration of less than three months
Compensatory behaviours	Inappropriate compensatory behaviours occur, on average, at least twice a week for three months	Compensatory behaviours are rarely used	Compensatory behaviours may occur, but less frequently than in BN
Eating pattern outside of binge eating episodes	Eating between episodes of binge eating tends to be highly restrictive	No restriction of dietary intake between episodes of binge eating	Eating behaviour between binge eating episodes may vary, alternating between overeating and restrictive eating
Weight and shape concerns	Self-evaluation strongly influenced by body shape and weight	Self-evaluation strongly influenced by body shape and weight	Self-evaluation strongly influenced by body shape and weight

Prevalence

Binge eating in obese subjects was first described almost 50 years ago by Stunkard (1959), and much evidence suggests that it is a relatively common and serious problem. Data from multi-site population-based studies and obesity treatment centres indicate that various degrees of binge eating are reported by 20–50% of obese individuals who are actively seeking treatment (Yanovski, 1999). However, most of these studies relied on self-reported measures of binge eating and did not use standardized interview methods based on the DSM-IV diagnostic criteria; accordingly, the true prevalence may have been overestimated. Community-based studies of the prevalence of binge eating among obese individuals who are not seeking treatment yield much lower estimates, ranging from 5 to 9% (Yanovski, 1999).

BED, as strictly defined by the DSM-IV criteria, is strongly associated with obesity. Several studies have reported BED rates as high as 30% among obese women presenting for weight loss treatment (e.g. Lapidoth, Ghaderi and Norring, 2006) and up to 49% of bariatric surgery candidates (Allison *et al.*, 2006).

Estimated prevalence rates of BED among various samples of obese individuals range from 1% to 19% (Yanovski, 1999; Allison *et al.*, 2006).

BED often occurs in males and frequently affects middle-aged individuals – in contrast to BN.

Aetiology

Two theoretical frameworks – dietary restraint and affect regulation - have been proposed to account for the aetiology and maintenance of recurrent binge eating in adults. These two broad mechanisms may be complementary rather than competing, and both may operate to varying degrees in individuals.

Restraint theory postulates that some dieting individuals set themselves rigid and inflexible dietary rules, but then tend to react to their own minor transgressions with an 'all or nothing' response, leading to binge eating. Strict dietary restraint is a critical factor in cognitive behavioural models advanced to explain how binge eating is maintained in BN, and most of these individuals are not overweight. However, obese individuals tend to binge eat in the context of general overeating, rather than against a background of strict dietary restraint (Cooper, Fairburn and Hawker, 2003). In addition, about half of obese subjects with BED report that they began binge eating before any attempts at dietary restraint (Abbott *et al.*, 1998).

Affect regulation theory suggests that individuals binge eat in an attempt to control negative mood states such as anger, sadness, anxiety, loneliness or boredom, or to 'block out' unpleasant thoughts (Masheb and Grilo, 2006). This tendency is often termed 'emotional eating.'

Clinical features

Binge eating tends to be a secretive behaviour accompanied by feelings of shame and disgust. Because of this, there are often few warning signs that are discernable to health professionals. In many obese subjects, even significant binge eating is not clinically obvious and will remain undetected unless diagnostic behaviours and attitudes are specifically sought. Some of these behaviours and attitudes are listed in Table 20.3.

Other features in the patient's history may also raise the possibility of BED and should prompt further detailed enquiry. Compared with obese individuals without BED, those with the disorder often report an earlier onset of obesity, a higher maximum lifetime weight and a history of more frequent weight fluctuations (Yanovski et al., 1993). Obese subjects with BED have also been found to consume significantly more energy than obese non-binge eaters during both binges and regular meals, and as a result gain significantly more weight than obese non-binge eaters over time (Mitchell et al., 1998). Also, as discussed below, psychological and psychiatric problems are more common in obese subjects with BED.

Table 20.3 Indicators of possible binge eating and/or eating disorder.

- Rapid weight gain or repeated weight fluctuations
- Patient reports a sense of being 'out of control' or a 'loss of control' over eating
- Hoarding or hiding food
- Eating in secret
- Chaotic eating patterns
- Attempts to manage emotional states such as stress, depression or frustration by eating (patients may talk about 'comfort eating')
- Feeling disgusted or guilty after overeating
- Patient cannot tell when to stop eating, and often eats until he/she feels uncomfortably full
- Avoidance of certain types of foods because patients feel that eating these foods may 'trigger' a loss of control over eating
- Avoidance of social situations that involve food
- Extreme distress about and/or preoccupation with issues to do with weight, shape or eating
- Patient reports taking laxatives, diuretics or other medications to control their weight
- Patient reports self-induced vomiting

Night eating syndrome

NES was originally described in 1955 by Stunkard and colleagues (Stunkard, Grace and Wolff, 1955). Like BED, NES was included in the appendix of DSM-IV as an example of ED-NOS. The central feature of NES is an abnormal circadian pattern of eating, which includes 'evening hyperphagia' (i.e. consuming over 25% of daily energy intake after the evening meal), and/or eating during the night for half of the time spent awake. Accompanying features include morning anorexia and delayed intake of the first daily meal, although these are not essential to the diagnosis of NES.

In community-based samples, NES occurs in approximately 1.5% of unselected individuals. Its prevalence is positively associated with obesity: NES has been estimated to occur in 9–15% of individuals presenting for weight loss treatment and in 8–42% of those being assessed for bariatric surgery (Rand, Macgregor and Stunkard, 1997).

The aetiology of NES is unexplained, but it has been suggested that its onset is likely to be associated with stress and/or depression (Allison et al., 2005).

Psychopathology associated with BED and NES in obese individuals

A growing mass of evidence suggests that obese individuals with BED or NES carry greater psychological and psychiatric burdens than do unaffected obese individuals. Obese subjects with BED are significantly more likely to report current depressive symptoms or a life-time history of major depression, anxiety or personality disorders. They also display lower self-esteem, more extreme concerns about shape and weight, greater body dissatisfaction, and greater impairment in work and social functioning than those without binge eating (Yanovski et al., 1993). Among obese binge-eaters, a higher frequency of binge eating appears to be associated with more severe psychopathology (Latner et al., 2007).

Obese individuals with NES have also been found to exhibit higher levels of depression and poorer self-esteem than unaffected subjects, and are more likely to report a history of major depressive disorder, anxiety or substance abuse or dependence (Allison et al., 2005).

Body dissatisfaction and preoccupation with weight and shape

'Body dissatisfaction' refers to a spectrum of negative thoughts and feelings about one's body shape and weight. Among obese people, as in the general population, body dissatisfaction spans a continuum ranging from mild feelings of unattractiveness to an extreme preoccupation with physical appearance that impairs functioning.

Overall, body dissatisfaction impairs the quality of life of a substantial proportion of obese individuals. Studies have consistently demonstrated that, compared with healthy-weight subjects, obese people are significantly more dissatisfied, embarrassed by and preoccupied with their physical appearance, and also avoid more social situations because of their appearance (e.g. Sarwer, Wadden and Foster, 1998). Excessive weight per se does not appear to be the sole determinant of body dissatisfaction, as studies of obese populations show no significant relationship between BMI and dissatisfaction scores (Sarwer, Wadden and Foster, 1998). Other cognitive factors, such as the importance of weight and shape for self-evaluation or the degree of preoccupation with weight and shape, probably modulate the influence of weight on body dissatisfaction.

Among obese individuals, body dissatisfaction appears to occur most often in those with childhood-onset obesity, who have faced adverse teasing about their weight and shape during childhood. Overall, obese women show greater body dissatisfaction than obese men (Grilo et al., 1994). Body dissatisfaction has been found to be significantly associated with increased levels of self-reported depressive symptoms, and decreased levels of self-esteem in obese individuals (Sarwer, Wadden and Foster, 1998; Grilo et al., 1994).

Distinct from body dissatisfaction is the concept of 'overvaluation' of weight or shape, that is, the undue influence of body weight or shape on self-esteem (American Psychiatric Association, 1994). Individuals who overvalue shape and weight view these features as the primary indicators of their self-worth. The overvaluation of, and resulting preoccupation with, weight or shape is a diagnostic criterion for both anorexia nervosa and bulimia nervosa; this feature is often prominent among individuals with BED, and it has been argued that it should also be included as a diagnostic criterion for BED (Hrabosky et al., 2007).

Assessment and treatment of eating disorders in obese individuals

Assessment

Ideally, a structured psychological evaluation should be undertaken at the beginning of treatment for obesity in order to identify disorders in eating attitudes and behaviours and to guide therapeutic strategy. Investigator-based interviews using the tools described below are the most rigorous way to assess complex behaviours such as binge eating. These require expert training to be administered and interpreted and are beyond the scope of many obesity clinics. Practical guidelines to help identify individuals at risk of clinically-significant eating disorders, and who would therefore benefit from referral to a clinical psychologist, are set out above in Table 20.3.

The Eating Disorders Examination (EDE), a semi-structured investigator-based interview, is generally recognized as the 'gold standard' for assessing eating disorders and associated psychopathology (Fairburn and Cooper, 1993). The EDE assesses the different forms of binge eating as well as cognitive, affective and behavioural symptoms of eating disorders, including concerns about weight, shape and eating. A self-reported version of the EDE, the EDE-Q (Fairburn and Beglin, 1994), with 36 questions, takes 20 minutes to complete.

Body dissatisfaction can be specifically measured with various widely used, well-validated self-report measures, including the Multidimensional Body-Self Relations Questionnaire (MBSRQ) (Cash, 1994) and the Body Shape Questionnaire (BSQ) (Cooper et al., 1987).

Symptoms of NES can be evaluated using the Night Eating Questionnaire (NEQ) (Marshall et al., 2004), a self-reported inventory that assesses hunger and craving patterns, proportion of daily energy intake ingested after the evening meal, insomnia and awakenings, nocturnal food cravings and consumption, and mood.

Treatment of BED

There is substantial evidence that cognitive-behavioural therapy (CBT) – the best evaluated of the evidence-based treatments for bulimia nervosa – is also effective in BED (Wonderlich et al., 2003). However, adequate weight loss cannot always be achieved for binge eating by CBT alone (Gladis et al., 1998); therefore, CBT to treat BED in obese individuals should be used

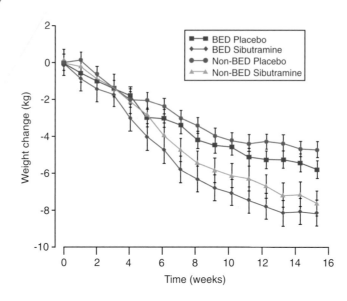

Figure 20.2 Weight loss during sibutramine treatment is comparable between obese subjects with BED and matched subjects who did not have BED. From J.C. Appolinario *et al.* (2003) with permission of the editor of *Archives of General Psychiatry*.

to supplement the general obesity management programmes. As previously mentioned, strict dietary restraint is a major trigger for binge eating in bulimia nervosa, but this does not appear to apply in most cases of BED; indeed, conventional behavioural weight-loss programmes (BWL) that aim for moderate caloric restriction may ameliorate binge eating in obese patients (Gladis *et al.*, 1998). Moreover, obese binge-eaters appear to lose as much weight as non-binge eaters in response to standard BWL, although there is some evidence that obese binge-eaters are more likely than their counterparts without binge eating to terminate BWL prematurely, and to regain the weight lost in treatment (Gladis *et al.*, 1998). A promising approach to the treatment of BED in obese patients is to combine elements of CBT, specifically to target the eating disorder and address body dissatisfaction, together with BWL based on moderate caloric restriction and increased physical activity as a general weight-reducing strategy (Gladis *et al.*, 1998).

Pharmacotherapy and surgery for eating disorders in obesity

Studies are currently ongoing to determine the effects of anti-obesity drugs and other medications, such as antidepressants, on both binge eating and weight loss in obese binge eaters (Appolinario *et al.*, 2003; Baur, Fischer and Keller, 2006) Appolinario *et al.* (2003) reported that weight loss during sibutramine treatment was comparable in obese subjects with BED and in those who did not have BED (Figure 20.2). Most comparisons between CBT and/or BWL and CBT and/or BWL combined with medication (usually anti-depressants) have shown that CBT is superior to drug treatment alone, and that medication does not add to the efficacy of BWL or CBT in reducing the frequency of binge eating (Gladis *et al.*, 1998; Baur, Fischer and Keller, 2006). Antidepressants may enhance weight loss beyond the effects of CBT and BWL (Gladis *et al.*, 1998).

Bariatric surgery for obese binge eaters has also yielded mixed results. Some studies report less weight loss in those with binge eating, whereas others find that regular binge eating before the operation does not predict a poor outcome for bariatric surgery (Sarwer, Wadden and Fabricatore, 2005; Herpertz *et al.*, 2004).

Treatment of NES

Very little research has focused specifically on treatment of NES, although anecdotal reports and some recent research suggest that selective serotonin reuptake inhibitors (SSRIs) may be helpful due to their favourable effects on disturbances in mood and sleep (O'Reardon *et al.*, 2006).

References

Abbott, D.W., de Zwaan, M., Mussell, M.P. *et al.* (1998) Onset of binge eating and dieting in overweight women: implications for etiology, associated features and treatment. *Journal of Psychosomatic Research*, **44**, 367–74.

Allison, K.C., Grilo, C.M., Masheb, R.M. and Stunkard, A.J. (2005) Binge eating disorder and night eating syndrome: a comparative study of disordered eating. *Journal of Consulting and Clinical Psychology*, **73** (6), 1107–15.

Allison, K.C., Wadden, T.A., Sarwer, D.B. *et al.* (2006) Night eating syndrome and binge eating disorder among persons seeking bariatric surgery: prevalence and related features. *Surgery for Obesity and Related Issues*, **2** (2), 153–8.

American Psychiatric Association (1994) *Diagnostic and Statistical Manual of Mental Disorders*, 4th edn (DSM-IV), American Psychiatric Association, Washington DC.

Appolinario, J.C., Bacaltchuk, J., Sichieri, R. *et al.* (2003) A randomized, double-blind, placebo-controlled study of sibutramine in the treatment of binge eating disorder. *Archives of General Psychiatry*, **60**, 1109–16.

Baur, C., Fischer, A. and Keller, U. (2006) Effect of sibutramine and of cognitive-behavioural weight loss therapy in obesity and subclinical binge eating disorder. *Diabetes, Obesity and Metabolism*, **8**, 289–95.

Cash, T.F. (1994) *The Multidimensional Body-Self Relations Questionnaire Users' Manual*, Old Dominion University, Norfolk VA.

Cooper, P.J., Taylor, M.J., Cooper, Z. and Fairburn, C.G. (1987) The development and validation of the Body Shape Questionnaire. *International Journal of Eating Disorders*, **6**, 485–94.

Cooper, Z., Fairburn, C.G. and Hawker, D.M. (2003) *Cognitive-Behavioural Treatment of Obesity: A Clinician's Guide*, The Guilford Press, New York.

Fairburn, C.G. and Beglin, S.J. (1994) The assessment of eating disorders: interview or self-report questionnaire? *International Journal of Eating Disorders*, **16**, 363–70.

Gladis, M.M., Wadden, T.A., Vogt, R.A. *et al.* (1998) Behavioral treatment of obese binge eaters: Do they need different care? *Journal of Psychosomatic Research*, **44**, 375–84.

Grilo, C.M., Wilfley, D.E., Brownell, K.D. and Rodin, J. (1994) Teasing, body image, and self-esteem in a clinical sample of obese women. *Addictive Behaviours*, **19**, 443–50.

Herpertz, S., Kielmann, R., Wolf, A.M. *et al.* (2004) Do psychosocial variables predict weight loss or mental health after obesity surgery? A systematic review. *Obesity Research*, **12** (10), 1554–69.

Hrabosky, J.I., Masheb, R.M., White, M.A. and Grilo, C.M. (2007) Overvaluation of shape and weight in binge eating disorder. *Journal of Consulting & Clinical Psychology.*, **75** (1), 175–80.

Fairburn, C.G. and Cooper, Z. (1993) The eating disorder examination, in *Binge Eating: Nature, Assessment and Treatment* 12th edn, (eds C.G. Fairburn and G.T. Wilson), Guilford Press, New York, pp. 317–60.

Lapidoth, J., Ghaderi, A. and Norring, C. (2006) Eating disorders and disordered eating among patients seeking non-surgical weight-loss treatment in Sweden. *Eating Behaviors*, **7**, 15–26.

Latner, J.D., Hildebrandt, T., Rosewall, J.K. *et al.* (2007) Loss of control over eating reflects eating disturbances and general psychopathology. *Behaviour Research and Therapy*, **45** (9), 2203–11.

Marshall, A.M., Allison, K.C., O'Reardon, J.P. *et al.* (2004) Night eating syndrome among nonobese persons. *International Journal of Eating Disorders*, **35**, 217–22.

Masheb, R.M. and Grilo, C.M. (2006) Emotional overeating and its associations with eating disorder psychopathology among overweight patients with binge eating disorder. *International Journal of Eating Disorders*, **39**, 141–6.

Mitchell, J.E., Crow, S., Peterson, C.B. *et al.* (1998) Feeding laboratory studies in patients with eating disorders: a review. *International Journal of Eating Disorders*, **24**, 115–24.

O'Reardon, J.P., Allison, K.C., Martino, N.S. *et al.* (2006) A randomized placebo-controlled trial of sertraline in the treatment of the night eating syndrome. *American Journal of Psychiatry*, **163** (5), 893–8.

Rand, C.S., Macgregor, M.D. and Stunkard, A.J. (1997) The night eating syndrome in the general population and amongst post-operative obesity surgery patients. *International Journal of Eating Disorders*, **22**, 65–9.

Sarwer, D.B., Wadden, T.A. and Fabricatore, A.N. (2005) Psychosocial and behavioral aspects of bariatric surgery. *Obesity Research*, **13** (4), 639–48.

Sarwer, D.B., Wadden, T.A. and Foster, G.D. (1998) Assessment of body image dissatisfaction in obese women: specificity, severity, and clinical significance. *Journal of Consulting and Clinical Psychology*, **66**, 651–4.

Spitzer, R.L., Devlin, M., Walsh, B.T. *et al.* (1992) Binge eating disorder: a multi-site field trial of the diagnostic criteria. *International Journal of Eating Disorders*, **11**, 191–203.

Stunkard, A.J. (1959) Eating patterns and obesity. *Psychiatry Quarterly*, **33**, 284–92.

Stunkard, A.J., Grace, W.J. and Wolff, H.G. (1955) The night-eating syndrome: A pattern of food intake among certain obese patients. *American Journal of Medicine*, **19**, 78–86.

Wonderlich, S.A., de Zwaan, M., Mitchell, J.E. *et al.* (2003) Psychological and dietary treatments of binge eating disorder: conceptual implications. *International Journal of Eating Disorders*, **34**, S58–63.

Yanovski, S.Z. (1999) Diagnosis and prevalence of eating disorders in obesity, in *Progress in Obesity Research: 8*, (eds B. Guy-Grand and G. Ailhaud), John Libby & Co., London, pp. 229–36.

Yanovski, S.Z., Nelson, J.E., Dubbert, B.K. and Spitzer, R.L. (1993) Association of binge eating disorder and psychiatric comorbidity in obese subjects. *American Journal of Psychiatry*, **150**, 1472–79.

Obesity in Childhood

Key points

- Obesity is spreading rapidly among children worldwide, affecting 10–30% of those in developed countries.

- In childhood, obesity is generally defined as a BMI that exceeds the 95th centile of the age- and gender-matched population, and overweight as a BMI above the 85th centile.

- Most cases are due to an obesogenic lifestyle, with an excessive energy intake (energy-dense foods and sweetened drinks often contribute) and/or decreased physical activity. Time spent watching television is related to the risk of obesity, apparently because of associated over-eating.

- Rare causes of childhood obesity include endocrine disorders such as Cushing syndrome and hypothyroidism, and obesogenic medication including glucocorticoids, antidiabetic drugs and antiepileptic agents. Numerous inherited syndromes are characterized by childhood obesity, the most common being Prader-Willi syndrome (with muscular hypotonia, hyperphagia and obesity, short stature and mental retardation). Monogenic causes of obesity (usually morbid and presenting in childhood) include mutations of leptin, the leptin receptor and the melanocortin-4 receptor (MC4-R).

- Type 2 diabetes is becoming more common among children, because of the spread of obesity, with a 10-fold increase in incidence in a decade in some centres. Asian and Black children, and those with a positive family history of type 2 diabetes, are at increased risk. The risks of cardiovascular disease, diabetic retinopathy and nephropathy are high, and features of the metabolic syndrome (dyslipidaemia, hypertension and fatty liver) are often present. Polycystic ovarian syndrome (PCOS), obstructive sleep apnoea and obesity-related glomerulopathy (which can lead to renal failure) are recognized complications.

- Investigation aims to identify the cause of obesity, determine its severity and associated health risks, and guide management. BMI and growth must be monitored, together with blood pressure; screening for hypothyroidism, hyperglycaemia, dyslipidaemia and liver dysfunction should be performed.

- Lifestyle intervention is the cornerstone of management, with healthy eating (three meals per day, avoiding snacking and sweetened drinks) and encouraging physical exercise to replace sedentary behaviours. Positive involvement of the parents may improve the outcome.

- Pharmacotherapy can be considered to supplement lifestyle measures, if these have proved inadequate after 6–12 months. Orlistat (a gut lipase inhibitor) and sibutramine (a centrally-acting appetite suppressant) are both effective in children and appear relatively safe, although their long-term efficacy and safety are unknown. Orlistat causes steatorrhoea and could impair fat-soluble vitamin absorption; sibutramine has sympathomimetic side effects including hypertension. Bariatric surgery (e.g. laparoscopic gastric banding) is increasingly used to treat obesity in adolescents.

- Type 2 diabetes is treated by lifestyle modification and weight reduction in the first instance, with metformin as first-line therapy; insulin treatment may be required. Hypertension, dyslipidaemia, fatty liver and PCOS also improve with weight loss.

- Prevention of childhood obesity is an important public health priority. Measures include breastfeeding, school- and family-based interventions to improve diet and encourage physical activity, and restricting advertising (especially of energy-dense foods and drinks) to children.

Chapter 21　Obesity in Childhood

Julian Shield and Carolyn Summerbell

Childhood obesity is a rapidly increasing problem in many countries and is arguably the most serious aspect of the global spread of the disease. In many developed countries, between 10% and 30% of children are overweight to an extent that will lead to significant morbidity in adult life, and ultimately to a shortened life expectancy. Type 2 diabetes, until recently regarded as a disease of the middle-aged or elderly, now affects ever more adolescents and children as young as 10 years of age. Obesity in children and adolescents requires careful investigation and assessment, to identify endocrine and other causes, as well as specific syndromes and the monogenic forms of obesity that have recently been characterized. The management of childhood obesity poses many challenges but can potentially be rewarded by preventing obesity from continuing into adult life, thus reducing the risks of morbidity and premature death.

This chapter reviews the ways of defining obesity in children and adolescents, the causes and consequences of childhood obesity, and its investigation, management and prevention. The epidemiology of obesity is discussed further in Chapter 2, while preventative strategies are covered in greater detail in Chapter 22.

Defining obesity in children

Childhood development is a dynamic process that differs markedly between boys and girls, is heavily influenced by the onset of puberty, and also shows considerable ethnic and socio-economic variation. This makes it particularly difficult to derive a robust and reproducible definition of obesity in childhood, and especially one that can be used by clinicians to identify children who require evaluation and treatment. The main anthropometric measures currently used to define obesity and overweight, and to identify increased cardiovascular and metabolic risk, are discussed below.

Body mass index (BMI)

The continuing changes in body weight and build throughout childhood mean that overweight and obesity cannot be defined by the static BMI thresholds that are used by adults aged 18 years or older (overweight = BMI 25–29.9 kg/m²; obese = BMI ≥30 kg/m²). Instead, the child's BMI is compared with the distribution of BMI in a reference population of the same age and sex. Conventionally, the reference data are expressed as percentiles: the 50th percentile represents the mean value for that age and sex, while the 85th and 95th centiles respectively contain the highest 15% and 5% of values in the reference population (Reilly, 2005; Network SI-CG, 2003; Speiser et al., 2005). At present, the 85th percentile is used in the UK as the threshold for overweight (equivalent to 'at risk of overweight' in the USA), while a BMI above the 95th percentile represents obesity (Figure 21.1). An obvious anomaly when using population-based reference data is that the general population is becoming heavier as obesity spreads, so that the BMI levels defining the 85th and 95th percentiles will increase year by year. One solution is to use historical reference data from when childhood obesity was still relatively rare; in the UK, BMI charts are derived from data collected in 1990 (Cole, Freeman and Preece, 1995), and will continue to be used for the foreseeable future.

For research purposes, BMI and changes in BMI are often reported as standard deviation scores (SDS) or 'z' scores, that is the number of standard deviations (SD) above or below the age- and gender-matched population mean at which the individual's BMI lies. The z-score is

Obesity: Science to Practice　Edited by Gareth Williams and Gema Frühbeck
© 2009 John Wiley & Sons, Ltd

calculated as (*x*-mean)/SD, where *x* is the case value; a *z*-score of 3.0, that is 3 standard deviations above the mean, equates to the 99.8th percentile.

An 'overweight' or 'obese' BMI in a child may be associated with adverse health outcomes during childhood such as type 2 diabetes, and there is sound evidence that childhood obesity (as defined by BMI) tracks into adulthood (Freedman *et al.*, 2005), and that a BMI above the 85th percentile increases cardiovascular risk in adult life (Freedman *et al.*, 2004; Freedman *et al.*, 1999). These BMI thresholds, mostly based on national data, are therefore used to guide clinical decisions about investigation and management of individual children.

International reference data are also available, derived from six large national cross-sectional studies of childhood growth in Brazil, the UK, Hong Kong, the Netherlands, Singapore and the USA (Cole *et al.*, 2000). For each of the surveys, centile curves were constructed that, at age

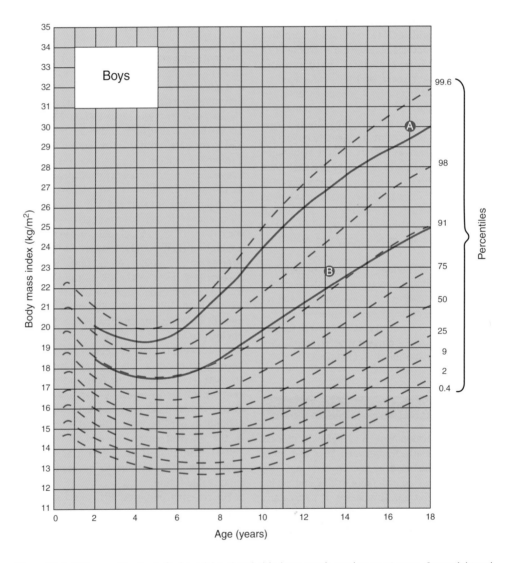

Figure 21.1 BMI percentile charts for boys (above) and girls (next page), aged up to 18 years. Overweight and obesity are defined as a BMI that exceeds the 85th and 95th percentiles, respectively, for the appropriate age and gender. These charts are in use in the UK, based on data collected in 1990. Some BMI percentile charts in clinical use also show the recently-defined thresholds for overweight (B) and obesity (A) that are illustrated in Figure 21.2.

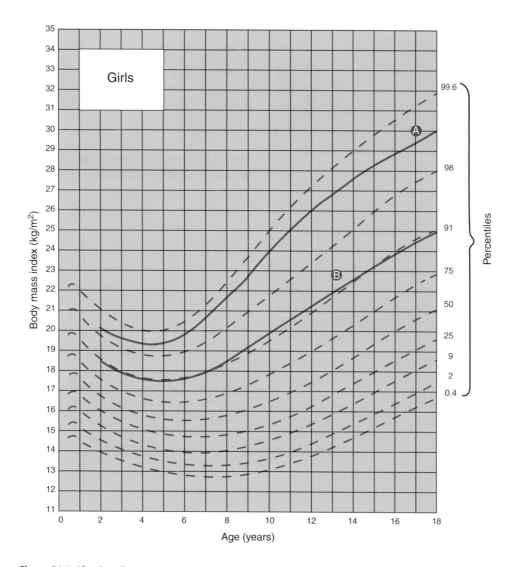

Figure 21.1 (*Continued*)

18 years, met the BMI values of 25 and 30 kg/m² that respectively define overweight and obesity in adult life. The resulting curves were averaged to produce age- and sex-specific cut-off points for overweight and obesity from early childhood to adult life (Figure 21.2). These composite international charts are intended primarily for epidemiological use in comparing obesity prevalence between countries, rather than for clinical management. Compared with the UK standard reference charts (Figure 21.1), the international data have lower sensitivity and considerably underestimate obesity, especially in boys (Reilly, 2005).

Waist circumference

The importance of abdominal and visceral adiposity in determining metabolic and cardio-vascular risk in adults is described in Chapter 9. There is evidence that visceral obesity in children also confers increased cardiovascular risk (Maffeis *et al.*, 2001; Janssen *et al.*, 2005; McCarthy, 2006). Waist circumference is a simple and useful measurement that is correlated with intra-abdominal fat mass (see Chapter 3), and paediatric cut-off values that indicate increased cardio-metabolic risk are now available for various childhood populations, including the UK (McCarthy, Jarrett and

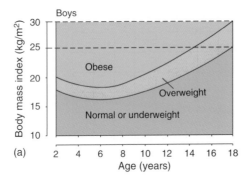

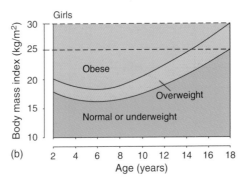

Figure 21.2 BMI cut-off curves defining overweight and obesity for (a) boys and (b) girls. The cut-off curves are constructed so as to coincide with the BMI values of 30 kg/m² (obesity) and 25 kg/m² (overweight) at age 18 years, the age from which the adult BMI thresholds apply. From Cole *et al.* (2000).

Crawley, 2001), Australia (Eisenmann, 2005) and USA (Fernandez *et al.*, 2004). These can be used to define metabolic risk from ages 10 to 16 years, based on new guidelines from the International Diabetes Federation (Zimmet *et al.*, 2007).

Body fat mass

A high BMI can be due to increased lean mass or bone rather than fat – which alone determines the comorbidities associated with obesity. As discussed in Chapter 3, specific measurements of body fat can be useful in monitoring risk and response to treatment; these can now be made using widely available, accurate and relatively cost-effective methods such as bio-impedance, DEXA scanning and air-displacement plethysmography. Body fat reference curves for boys and girls have recently been generated using bioimpedance, and validated against DEXA

and plethysmography (McCarthy *et al.*, 2006; Cowell *et al.*, 1997; Pietrobelli *et al.*, 2003; Pietrobelli *et al.*, 2004). These span the pubertal age-range, and demonstrate clearly the striking sexual dimorphism in fat deposition, with girls having 60% more body fat by 18 years of age (McCarthy *et al.*, 2006).

Aetiology of childhood obesity

The vast majority of childhood obesity is due, as in adults, to lifestyle factors that result in an excess of energy intake over expenditure. Increasingly, lifestyle-related obesity causes severe and accelerated weight gain in children (Figure 21.3).

There are myriad other putative causes of childhood obesity, as described below, but known diagnoses account for <5% of cases in routine clinical practice. Figure 21.4 shows the relative frequencies of the causes identified at a tertiary referral centre in Bristol, UK. This probably overstates the general population prevalences of the endocrine, syndromic and monogenic causes of obesity, most of which are extremely rare. Nonetheless, such cases are encountered in a non-specialist setting and deserve consideration because they may require specific treatments that can sometimes greatly improve or even cure obesity. Lifestyle-related obesity, although overwhelmingly common, is a diagnosis of exclusion; systematic assessment and investigation are therefore crucial.

It should be borne in mind that a significant proportion of children referred to specialist obesity clinics have significant, additional learning or physical handicaps (Drake *et al.*, 2001) and that within this group there are likely to be a number of children with as yet unrecognized genetic or syndromic obesity.

Lifestyle-related obesity

Chapter 8 considers the general impact of the 'obesogenic' environment, and its interplay with the many genes that determine the inherited susceptibility to obesity. Table 21.1 shows some components of eating behaviour and physical activity that have emerged from a systematic review as important contributors to childhood overweight and obesity (Brown, Kelly and Summerbell, 2007). Both dietary factors

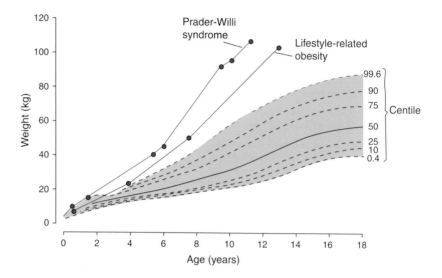

Figure 21.3 Progressive weight gain throughout childhood in a girl with lifestyle-related obesity. By age 13 years, she weighed 105 kg and had a BMI of 38 kg/m² (99.8th percentile). This pattern is similar to that seen in some inherited obesity syndromes; for comparison, the weight curve of a girl with Prader-Willi syndrome is also shown.

(notably overconsumption of energy-dense foods and drinks) and the replacement of physical activity by sedentary pursuits appear to be important, but to varying degrees in different populations.

Dietary factors

Perhaps surprisingly, self-reported energy intake in the USA and UK appears to have changed little (or even fallen) during the last 20 years,

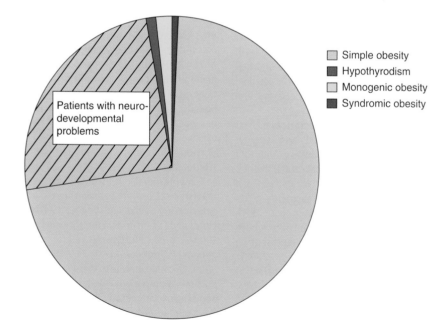

Figure 21.4 Frequency of identified causes of obesity referred to the Bristol Children's Hospital, UK, a tertiary referral centre. Note that one-third of those with no known cause have neurodevelopmental problems, which may point to an underlying diagnosis.

Table 21.1 Components of diet and physical activity that are currently considered to be important determinants of overweight and obesity in childhood.

Evidence	Decreases risk of overweight and obesity	Increases risk of overweight and obesity
Convincing	Long-term increase in total physical activity	
Probable	Breast-feeding (shown to prevent obesity in children up to 5 years of age)	Frequent, large portions of energy-dense foods
	Diets rich in foods with low energy density (wholegrain cereals and cereal products; foods rich in non-starch polysaccharides and dietary fibre)	Sugary drinks

while the current obesity epidemic has been gaining momentum in children (Rennie, Johnson and Jebb, 2005). This impression may be erroneous, because overweight people in general fail to recognize their total energy intake and systematically under-report what they eat ((Rennie *et al.*, 2005); see Chapters 3 and 8).

The quality, and especially the energy density, of food eaten by children has undoubtedly changed during this period, in ways that tend to encourage overconsumption. Increasing consumption of energy-dense foods, rich in sugars and/or fats, is likely to play an important role. Bulky foods with a low energy density (e.g. whole-grain cereals, products rich in non-starch polysaccharides and fibre, pasta, fruit and vegetables) tend to satiate faster than energy-dense foods, so that the latter may be over-eaten at meal times or at snacks between meals. Indeed, energy-dense diets can undermine normal appetite regulation in humans, a process termed 'passive overconsumption' (Green, Burley and Blundell, 1994).

In the USA, children's consumption of fast foods, mostly highly-processed and energy-dense, has risen threefold during the last 20 years (Rennie, Johnson and Jebb, 2005; Nielsen, Siega-Riz and Popkin, 2002). Many fast-food outlets actively encourage overeating by offering bigger portions for little extra cost, which may appeal especially to lower-income groups because these are perceived as representing better value for money (McConahy *et al.*, 2002).

Dramatic changes in the consumption of soft drinks may also contribute. Children have abandoned milk in favour of sugar-sweetened fizzy drinks and fruit juices (Nielsen and Popkin, 2004). These beverages have little nutritional value but a high energy content, notably those sweetened with high-fructose corn syrup (Bray, Nielsen and Popkin, 2004), and constitute an additional and often unrecognized source of energy intake.

Interestingly, children who were breast-fed show a reduced risk of obesity that extends at least beyond 4 years of age; possible mechanisms include better self-regulation of energy intake and favourable metabolic programming in early life (Mayer-Davis *et al.*, 2006; Gillman *et al.*, 2006; Dewey, 2003). The promotion of breast-feeding and the avoidance of infant formula foods (which make it easy to overnourish babies) is the basis for various public-health campaigns to prevent obesity (see Chapter 22).

Physical activity

Physical activity declines markedly through childhood, especially among girls (Riddoch *et al.*, 2004), but the cross-sectional nature of many of the studies makes it difficult to determine how much this contributes to increasing obesity. This trend to reduced physical activity has been accentuated by falls in the provision of physical education in schools, and in the proportion of children who walk or cycle to school (McDonald, 2007).

Some observational studies have reported an inverse relationship between levels of physical activity and overweight or obesity status during childhood (Levin *et al.*, 2003; Stevens *et al.*, 2007; Treuth *et al.*, 2007). The relationship appears generally stronger in studies published since 2000, possibly because these have had greater statistical power, with larger samples and better adjustment for confounders, and have employed more precise measures of diet and physical activity (e.g. movement recorders) rather than self-reported diaries (see Chapter 3).

Television viewing has been implicated as a prime sedentary behaviour that contributes

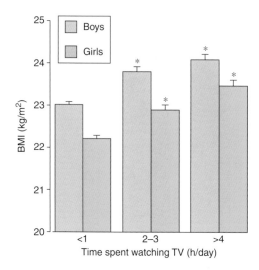

Figure 21.5 Relationship between BMI and time spent watching television, in American adolescents aged 14–18 years. *: $p < 0.05$ versus gender-matched groups watching <1 h/day. From Eisenmann *et al.* (2002) *Obesity Research* 10: 379–85.

to obesity in childhood and adolescence (see Chapter 8). Recently, the European Youth Heart Study (Rennie, Johnson and Jebb, 2005) confirmed that the time spent watching television was related to the prevalence of obesity among children aged 9–10 and 15–16 years (Figure 21.5). However, this was not explained simply by physical inactivity whilst watching television, because there was no significant relationship with total daily physical activity levels (Ekelund *et al.*, 2006). An associated increase in food intake is apparently responsible: children watching television are exposed to high-pressure advertising for energy-dense food and drinks, and some snack continuously while viewing (Rennie, Johnson and Jebb, 2005).

Other factors

Socio-economic status is important in determining the risk of obesity in childhood. In wealthy societies, obesity is common among children of the affluent, but becomes ever more prevalent as socio-economic status declines (Stamatakis *et al.*, 2005). Moreover, parental obesity – which is itself inversely related to socio-economic status – is also a risk factor for obesity in children (Zaninotto *et al.*, 2006).

As discussed in Chapter 2, obesity appears to be particularly prevalent in certain racial groups (e.g. Asians, and Black, Hispanic and Native Americans), and children in these populations also appear to be at increased risk (Ogden *et al.*, 2002; Wardle *et al.*, 2006).

Intriguingly, sleep disturbance may be a determinant of childhood obesity. Recent studies suggest that a short duration of sleep increases obesity risk in children under 10 years of age (Chaput, Brunet and Tremblay, 2006; Reilly *et al.*, 2005); this may be explained by elevated circulating levels of the orexigenic gut peptide, ghrelin (Taheri, 2006).

Endocrine disorders

Endocrine disorders include Cushing syndrome, hypothyroidism, hypopituitarism and growth hormone deficiency; in post-pubertal girls, obesity may be associated with the polycystic ovarian syndrome (PCOS) (see Chapters 8 and 13). All these conditions are rare except PCOS, which is being increasingly recognized in obese, adolescent females (Hassan and Gordon, 2007).

Cushing syndrome may present with delayed or arrested growth in a child with central obesity; the classical adult features – rounded 'moon face', 'buffalo hump', purplish-red cutaneous striae and proximal myopathy – may be more or less apparent (Figure 21.6). Blood pressure is often raised and hypokalaemia may occur. Causes include corticotroph pituitary adenomas, adrenocortical tumours and glucocorticoid therapy.

Hypothyroidism may also cause growth delay or arrest with obesity, and other manifestations may not be obvious (Figure 21.7). Hypothalamic damage resulting from tumours such as a craniopharyngioma or cranial radiotherapy can cause hyperphagia and obesity, especially if the ventromedial hypothalamus is involved, and typically worsens when corticosteroid replacement therapy is started (Figure 21.8).

Drug-induced obesity

Several drugs used to treat childhood illnesses can induce weight gain (see Chapter 8). In addition to glucocorticoids, these include anti-epileptic drugs (valproate, phenytoin, gabapentin), anti-psychotic agents (clozapine, olanzepine), insulin and oral hypoglycaemic drugs (sulphonyureas, thiazolidinediones).

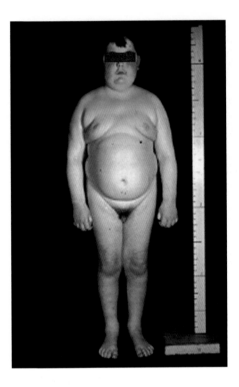

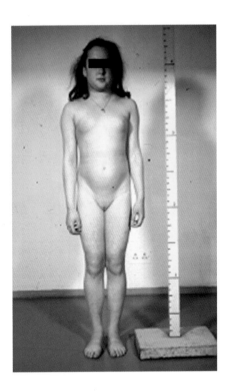

Figure 21.6 Cushing syndrome in a 14-year old boy. The patient had a rounded plethoric face, marked truncal obesity and hypertension. Image reproduced courtesy of the late Professor Graham F. Joplin, Royal Postgraduate Medical School, London.

Genetic syndromes that include obesity

Numerous inherited syndromes that become manifest during infancy and childhood have a phenotype that includes obesity. Some of the more common conditions are shown in Table 21.3 (on page 525).

Prader-Willi syndrome (PWS)

PWS (OMIM 176 270) is probably the most frequently recognized syndrome of childhood obesity. It is characterized by diminished fetal activity, poor feeding during the first year of life, pronounced muscular hypotonia and mental retardation. Hyperphagia appears between the ages of 12 and 18 months and children become obese, with short stature and typically small hands and feet (Figure 21.9). Hypogonadotrophic hypogonadism is also a feature in males (Whittington *et al.*, 2002).

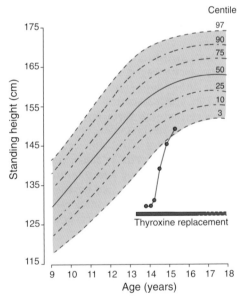

Figure 21.7 Hypothyroidism in a 13-year old girl (upper panel). The patient presented with weight gain (but not obesity in this case) and growth arrest. Note the rapid increase in height after starting thyroxine replacement (lower panel). Image reproduced courtesy of the late Professor Graham F. Joplin, Royal Postgraduate Medical School, London.

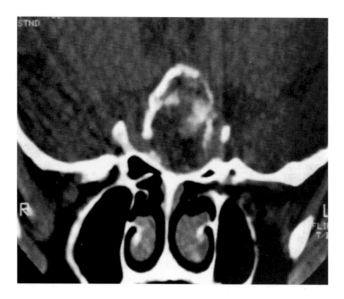

Figure 21.8 Craniopharyngioma in a 40-year old man, showing the characteristic supra-sellar calcification. During childhood, the patient had developed hyperphagia and obesity, which became more pronounced when cortisol replacement therapy was started. Image reproduced courtesy of Professor Gareth Williams, University of Bristol, UK.

PWS is a contiguous gene syndrome resulting from deletions of paternal copies of the imprinted SNRPN and necidin genes, or due to maternal uniparental disomy on the long arm of chromosome 15 (15q11.2–q12). Many of the phenotypic abnormalities remain unexplained. Intriguingly, levels of the fatty acid transporter, FAT (also known as CD36), which is encoded by a remote gene on chromosome 7q, were found to be reduced in subjects with PWS. FAT is involved in the cellular uptake of free fatty acids and is integral to normal fatty acid metabolism (see Chapter 4); its down-regulation could therefore contribute to abnormalities in lipid and carbohydrate handling (Webb *et al.*, 2006). There is evidence that levels of ghrelin are raised and fail to show the normal suppression after eating; this might contribute to hyperphagia (Cummings, 2006).

The Prader-Willi phenotype of fragile X syndrome (OMIM 300624)

Fragile X mental retardation is characterized by moderate to severe mental retardation, macroorchidism and distinct facial features, including a long face, large ears, and prominent jaw. In most cases, the disorder is caused by the unstable expansion of a CGG repeat in the FMR1 gene

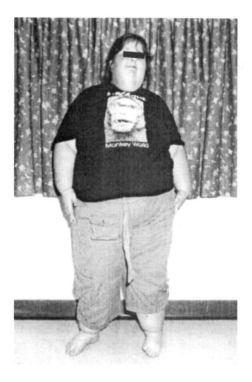

Figure 21.9 Child with obesity secondary to Prader-Willi Syndrome. Note the small hands and feet and central adiposity. Parental permission was granted to publish this image.

and abnormal methylation, which results in suppression of FMR1 transcription and decreased protein levels in the brain (Devys *et al.*, 1993). A phenotype associated with significant truncal obesity, delayed or incomplete puberty, autism and obsessive-compulsive behaviour without short stature and variable neonatal hypotonia has been termed *Fragile X with PWS phenotype*. CYFIP mRNA levels were recently shown to be reduced in these cases (Nowicki *et al.*, 2007); CYFIP is a protein that interacts with FMR1 protein and maps to 15q11–13.

Albright's hereditary osteodystrophy (OMIM 103580)

In 1942, Albright described three patients with short stature, obesity, rounded face, short neck and shortened metacarpals who had hypocalcaemia and hyperphosphataemia. A phenotypically similar syndrome is that of pseudohypoparathroidism with normal calcium metabolism. These conditions are caused by mutations, including imprinting defects, in the GNAS1 gene on chromosome 20. Only maternally inherited mutations lead to resistance to hormone action (Mantovani and Spada, 2006).

Monogenic obesity syndromes

Since the late 1990s, systematic studies have been undertaken in human obesity of various peripheral and CNS signals that are known to regulate energy homeostasis in lower mammals. These have led to the identification of several single-gene defects that cause severe obesity, mostly appearing during early childhood – thus proving the concept that these signals also operate, to some degree, in humans (Figure 21.10).

The known disorders are rare and are overwhelmed by lifestyle-related obesity, which is increasingly responsible for early-onset weight gain (Figure 21.3). In total, however, they may account for around 5% of cases of morbid obesity presenting in childhood, with polymorphisms of the melanocortin-4 receptor (MC4-R) accounting for perhaps 6% of selected cohorts (Farooqi and O'Rahilly, 2006). Moreover, the large number of obese children who also have learning difficulties but who do not conform to any known syndrome (Ells *et al.*, 2006) may imply that further single-gene disorders, affecting

energy homeostasis and neurocognitive function, are yet to be identified.

Leptin and leptin receptor mutations

As described in Chapter 4, leptin is a 16-kDa protein secreted by adipose tissue that, in rodents, acts centrally to decrease feeding and increase sympathetically-mediated thermogenesis. Leptin therefore has the properties of a homeostatic signal that acts to indicate and maintain fat mass (Figure 21.10). Mice homozygous for *ob* mutations that prevent the expression of bioactive leptin show hyperphagia, decreased energy expenditure and severe obesity, with marked insulin resistance that leads to type 2 diabetes. Administering exogenous leptin reverses hyperphagia, obesity and diabetes.

In humans, homozygosity for various mutations in the leptin gene *LEP* (OMIM 164160) has been described in a few families with a phenotype of hyperphagia soon after weaning and rapidly-progressing obesity from infancy (Montague *et al.*, 1997) (see Figure 21.11). Other features include insulin resistance, dyslipidaemia, hypogonadotrophic hypogonadism and immune abnormalities, notably reduced circulating CD4 +ve T cells and impaired T cell proliferation and cytokine release (Farooqi *et al.*, 2002). Administration of recombinant leptin rapidly reduces hyperphagia and body weight – in marked contrast to lifestyle-related obesity, in which leptin therapy is ineffective – and also corrects the other phenotypic abnormalities ((Farooqi *et al.*, 2002); see Figure 21.11).

In rodents, homozygosity for mutations that disable the leptin receptor (e.g. *db/db* mice, *fa/fa* and *cp/cp* rats) also causes hyperphagia, obesity and severe insulin resistance, sometimes with diabetes (*db/db* mice) or dyslipidaemia (*fa/fa* and *cp/cp* rats). Humans homozygous for mutations of the leptin receptor (*LEP-R*; OMIM 601007) similarly display hyperphagia and early-onset obesity with secondary hypothyroidism and hypogonadotrophic hypogonadism (Clement *et al.*, 1998).

Melanocortin axis mutations

In rodents, hypothalamic neurones expressing pro-opiomelanocortin (POMC) are an important effector of leptin's central actions: they are stimulated by leptin to release α-MSH, which acts via melanocortin-3 and -4 receptors (MC3-R,

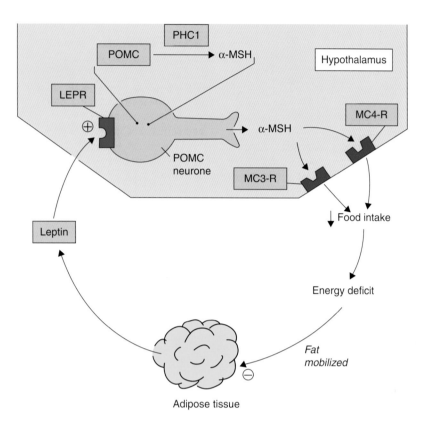

Figure 21.10 The melanocortin neuronal pathway in the hypothalamus through which leptin regulates body fat mass and weight, showing the principal sites of mutations that can give rise to obesity in humans. α-MSH: α-melanocyte stimulating hormone; PHC1: prohormone convertase-1; POMC: proopiomelanocortin; MC3-R, MC4-R: melanocortin-3 and -4 receptors; LEPR: leptin receptor.

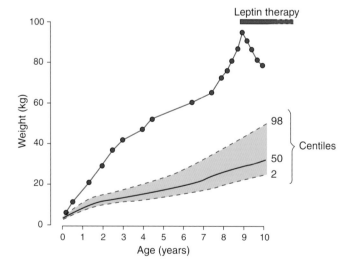

Figure 21.11 Weight gain in a girl with congenital leptin deficiency, showing severe obesity with onset in the first months of life. Weight fell rapidly during treatment with recombinant human leptin, due almost entirely to loss of fat mass. From Farooqi *et al.* (1999) *New England Journal of Medicine* 341: 879–84.

MC4-R) to inhibit feeding, increase energy expenditure and thus decrease body fat and weight (Figure 21.10). In the yellow obese (A^y) mouse, genetic overexpression of the agouti protein, an endogenous antagonist of the melanocortin receptors, leads to hyperphagia and obesity.

Several mutations of the melanocortin axis have been identified in humans as causes of early-onset obesity (Figure 21.10). Affected genes include POMC itself (the precursor of α-MSH; OMIM 609734), prohormone convertase-1 (the enzyme that cleaves POMC to yield α-MSH; OMIM 162150), and both the MC3-R and MC4-R (OMIM 155540 and 155441, respectively). Common features are again hyperphagia and severe, early-onset obesity, often appearing before the age of 5 years of age. MC4-R mutations are the most common monogenic cause of obesity yet identified; hyperphagia is less marked than in other monogenic obesity syndromes, while linear growth is accelerated and lean body mass and bone mineral density are enhanced (Farooqi et al., 2003).

Neuronal tyrosine kinase receptor B mutations (OMIM 600456) are rare but of particular interest because the index child had global developmental delay with specific defects in speech and language (Yeo et al., 2004) – which points to the involvement of this receptor in a wide range of cellular functions.

Consequences of childhood obesity

Many of the metabolic and cardiovascular complications of obesity are already manifest during childhood, and are intimately linked to the presence of insulin resistance, hyperinsulinaemia, and abnormal carbohydrate and lipid metabolism (Weiss and Caprio, 2005). In addition, the endocrine and other sequelae of obesity also affect children.

Type 2 diabetes

This remains rare but its incidence is rising and the disease is set to become the most important consequence of childhood obesity worldwide. The mechanisms by which obesity induces insulin resistance and leads to impaired glucose tolerance (IGT) and ultimately type 2 diabetes are described in Chapter 10. The true prevalence of IGT among obese children is unknown, but the proportion of children and adolescents attending specialist obesity clinics who are found on screening to have IGT ranges between 10% or less in the UK and mainland Europe (Sabin et al., 2005; Invitti et al., 2006) to 25% in the USA (Sinha et al., 2002).

As discussed in Chapter 2, there is now good evidence that type 2 diabetes is spreading globally among children (Pinhas-Hamiel and Zeitler, 2005). In the USA, various centres have recorded dramatic increases in the number of children diagnosed with type 2 diabetes; a 10-fold increase was reported from one centre in New York from 1990 to 2000 with 50% of all new cases of diabetes having type 2 (Grinstein et al., 2003). Obesity-driven type 2 diabetes is predicted to become the most common form of newly-diagnosed diabetes in American adolescents by 2015. In Europe, type 2 diabetes remains a rare disease in children, with annual incidences ranging from 0.25 cases per 100 000 children in Austria (Rami et al., 2003) to 0.53 per 100 000 in the UK (Haines et al., 2007), but is steadily becoming more common in several countries. In the UK, the incidence is increased between threefold and 11-fold in southern Asian and Black children respectively, as compared with the white population; type 2 diabetes is strongly associated with a family history of the disease, and overweight or obesity are omnipresent (Haines et al., 2007). Asia also faces a growing threat from the disease: in the last 20 years, Japan has seen a rise in annual incidence from 1.73 per 100 000 to 2.76 per 100 000, and evidence is emerging of marked increases in urban south Asia, Singapore and Taiwan – where the estimated annual incidence is now 6.5 per 100 000 children (Wei et al., 2003).

The emergence of type 2 diabetes in adolescents has important implications for the patient's health, the family and healthcare resources. Early signs of cardiovascular disease are already present in many cases (Gungor et al., 2005; Ettinger et al., 2005; see below), while several studies suggest an accelerated risk of both diabetic nephropathy (Svensson et al., 2003) and retinopathy (Yoshida et al., 2001), as compared with children with type 1 diabetes. Moreover, psychological health (Katz et al., 2005) and compliance with treatment (Kawahara et al., 1994) are often poor in these children. The few available longitudinal data are worrying: of 79 Canadian children reviewed up to 15 years after the diagnosis of type 2 diabetes, 9% had died and 6% were undergoing dialysis (Dean and Flett, 2002). The management of type 2 diabetes is discussed in Section 21.5.5.1 later in this chapter.

Cardiovascular disease

Obesity confers cardiovascular risk independently of that associated with diabetes (Chapter 12) and this is already apparent in non-diabetic, obese children. Compared with normal-weight controls, normotensive obese children (mean age, 12 years) had significantly higher arterial wall stiffness and evidence of endothelial dysfunction – two markers of increased risk of atheroma and myocardial infarction (Tounian *et al.*, 2001). The thickness of the intima-media in the carotid artery (another predictor of myocardial infarction and of stroke) in adult life is directly related to childhood BMI, irrespective of adult BMI (Freedman *et al.*, 2004; Raitakari *et al.*, 2003). Furthermore, childhood obesity and its attendant abnormalities (raised low-density lipoprotein (LDL)-cholesterol, systolic hypertension) were associated with a higher density of atheromatous plaques in the coronary arteries of children and adolescents studied *post mortem* (Berenson *et al.*, 1998). Other studies have demonstrated an association between obesity during adolescence and increased left-ventricular mass in adults (Li *et al.*, 2004; see Chapter 12).

Many obese children show features of the metabolic syndrome, the reported prevalence varying according to the diagnostic criteria used (see Chapter 10). For example, the USA Adult Treatment Panel III (ATP-III) criteria comprise at least three of: fasting hyperglycaemia, abdominal obesity, dyslipidaemia (reduced high-density lipoprotein (HDL) and/or raised triglycerides) and hypertension (EPDETHBCA, 2001). By this definition, the metabolic syndrome was present in 29% of obese adolescents (BMI ≥95th percentile) enrolled in the NHANES cohort between 1988 and 1994; by 1999–2000, the proportion had risen to 32% (Cook *et al.*, 2003; Duncan *et al.*, 2004). Other studies, using different criteria, report prevalences of 25–33% among children referred to secondary-care obesity clinics (Sabin, Crowne and Shield, 2003; Viner *et al.*, 2005) and up to 50% in cohorts of severely obese children with a BMI SDS score of over +2.5 (Weiss *et al.*, 2004). Recently, the International Diabetes Federation has produced a consensus definition for the metabolic syndrome in children aged 10 to 16 years, comprising abdominal obesity (defined by waist circumference ≥90th percentile) with two or more of the following components: (elevated triglycerides, low HDL-cholesterol, hypertension and hyperglycaemia (Zimmet *et al.*, 2007).

Consistent with the rapid spread of obesity in the USA, a recent report from the NHANES-III survey found that 18% of unselected 12–16 year olds in the general population had three or four components of the metabolic syndrome, and that these co-segregated with raised BMI and waist circumference (Liu, Wade and Tan, 2007).

Fatty liver disease

Non-alcoholic fatty liver disease (NAFLD) frequently accompanies obesity in adults and is considered by some as a core feature of the metabolic syndrome (Burgert *et al.*, 2006; see Chapter 11). NAFLD was first reported in children in the early 1980s (Moran *et al.*, 1983), and many subsequent reports have confirmed the association and – as in adults – provide clear evidence that the early lesion (fatty infiltration) can progress through steatohepatitis to cirrhosis (Wieckowska and Feldstein, 2005; Marion, Baker and Dhawan, 2004). The condition is closely linked with visceral obesity and insulin resistance and is more common in boys. The classical feature is of raised liver enzymes, and the diagnosis is confirmed by CT or MR imaging of the liver (see Chapter 11). Treatment in children is discussed below.

Growth and sexual development

The hyperinsulinaemia and insulin resistance associated with obesity lead to decreased levels of insulin-like growth factor-1 (IGF-1) binding proteins-1 and -2 (IGFBP-1 and -2), and of sex-hormone binding globulin (SHBG), thus increasing the free circulating levels of free IGF-1 and of androgens, respectively. Increased IGF-1 bioavailability leads to increased linear growth, explaining the usual finding that obese children are relatively tall (Freemark, 2005).

Excess free androgens may induce early sexual hair development (premature adrenarche) in both boys and girls, while the enhanced conversion of androgens to oestrogens by the aromatase in adipose tissue has been implicated in early breast development in girls and gynaecomastia in boys – the latter complaint, often very distressing, being increasingly common in referrals to endocrine clinics (Slyper, 1998).

Overweight children are more liable to enter puberty early (Dunger, Ahmed and Ong, 2005); however, even though the prevalence of obesity among girls has increased markedly during the last 40 years (Viner, 2002), the mean age at first menstruation (menarche) does not appear to be falling.

Respiratory complications

Adult obesity is associated with the obstructive sleep apnoea (OSA) syndrome, characterized by episodic obstruction of the upper airway, leading to blood oxygen desaturation and repeated arousals; disruption of valuable REM sleep results in daytime lethargy and somnolence (see Chapter 13). OSA is now being increasingly recognized among obese children (Verhulst *et al.*, 2007a; Wing *et al.*, 2003). This is a potentially serious condition with evidence of increased left ventricular hypertrophy, pulmonary hypertension and risk of metabolic syndrome independent of BMI (Amin *et al.*, 2002; Marcus, 2000; Verhulst *et al.*, 2007b). Also, reduced sleeping time during childhood may be an additional risk factor for obesity – possibly through increased levels of the appetite-stimulating peptide, ghrelin – thus potentially causing a vicious circle of worsening obesity and sleep deprivation (Reilly *et al.*, 2005).

Obesity has also been associated with an increased risk of developing childhood asthma in some studies (Schaub and von Mutius, 2005), but not others (Ford, 2005).

Renal complications

Morbid obesity is recognized as a risk factor for increased glomerular size (glomerulomegaly) and focal glomerulosclerosis (de Jong *et al.*, 2002). This obesity-related glomerulopathy (ORG) is suggested to lead to progressive renal impairment and the eventual requirement for renal replacement therapy (Srivastava, 2006). A 10-fold increase in the numbers of patients with biopsy-proven ORG, including children as young as 8 years, was reported in the USA between 1986 and 1990 and 1996–2000; increased awareness and ascertainment may contribute, but this condition may now be reaching epidemic proportions (Kambham *et al.*, 2001; Adelman *et al.*, 2001).

Other complications

Musculoskeletal disorders related to obesity include slippage of the femoral epiphysis (Poussa, Schlenzka and Yrjonen, 2003) and possibly an increased risk of traumatic injury (Bazelmans *et al.*, 2004). This is an under-researched area and further in-depth studies are warranted.

Benign intracranial hypertension, with intractable headaches in a minority of cases, is also described (Kesler and Fattal-Valevski, 2002).

The risk of certain cancers is known to be increased by obesity in adult life (see Chapter 13). There is little direct information relating childhood obesity to cancer risk in adult life; one retrospective study has reported an increased prevalence of colon cancer 55 years later in men who had been obese during adolescence (Must *et al.*, 1992).

The psychological impact of obesity can begin in childhood, and many obese children and adolescents report dissatisfaction with their bodies and poor self-esteem (Ricciardelli and McCabe, 2001; see Chapter 14). The true prevalence and gravity of psychological burden may be hard to determine in children. It may be overestimated in those attending obesity clinics (Friedman and Brownell, 1995) – a highly-selected group whose desire to seek professional help may be partly motivated by psychological distress – whereas others may conceal the true extent of their unhappiness. Wardle and Cooke have highlighted the need to discover why some obese children appear relatively unaffected by the adverse social consequences of obesity, and how the attitudes of health professionals and children impact on clinical management of obesity (Wardle and Cooke, 2005).

Investigation and assessment

The aims are to identify the rare secondary and genetic causes of obesity, which may have different prognoses and require specific treatment; to determine the relative contributions of lifestyle factors to overweight; and to assess risk and the need for treatment. Most cases are due to lifestyle-related obesity, but rare causes must always be borne in mind; some important diagnostic features are shown in Table 21.2 and described below.

History

A detailed personal and family history should be taken, starting with the neonatal period. Early feeding and development are important. Poor feeding and hypotonia during the first year of life is suggestive of PWS, while visual and auditory defects, often with developmental delay, are frequently associated with genetic obesity syndromes.

Table 21.2 Inherited syndromes, other than Prader-Willi syndrome, that are associated with obesity in childhood.

Syndrome and OMIM No	Frequency	Gene or mechanism	Salient clinical features
Fragile X 300624	1:4000 males	98% due to expansion of a CGG tri-nucleotide repeat in the FMR1 gene (>200)	Moderate to severe mental retardation, macroorchidism, large ears, macrocephaly, behavioural problems such as autism
Bardet-Biedl 209900	<1:100000	Autosomal recessive linked to nine loci so far on different chromosomes	Hypogonadism, polydactyly, renal abnormalities, rod-cone dystrophy, learning difficulties
Alström 203800	Unknown but rare	Autosomal recessive mutations in gene ALMS1	Cardiomyopathy, rod-cone dystrophy, sensory hearing loss, hypogonadism, hypothyroidism, type 2 diabetes, renal and liver abnormalities, some developmental delay
Albright's Hereditary Osteodystrophy 103580	Relatively common	Autosomal dominant, caused by mutation in the G-protein, alpha-stimulating 1 gene (GNAS1); tissue-specific imprinting causing more severe manifestations in maternally transmitted cases	Short metacarpals and metatarsals (fourth and fifth digit), short stature, ectopic calcification, round facies, hypocalcaemia, hypothyroidism, mental retardation
Cohen 216550	Rare (except in Finland)	Autosomal recessive, mutation in COH1 gene in some patients	Mental retardation, microcephaly, short stature retinochoroidal dystrophy, prominent upper central incisors with characteristic facies, neutropenia
Borjeson-Forssman-Lehmann 301900	Rare	PHF6 gene on X chromosome	Severe mental retardation (IQ 10–40), hypotonia, short stature, microcephaly, post-pubertal gynecomastia, small penis and testes or cryptorcidism
MOMO 157890	Rare	Autosomal dominant	Overgrowth syndrome characterized by macrocrania, obesity, ocular abnormalities (retinal coloboma and nystagmus), downward slant of the palpebral fissures, mental retardation, and delayed bone maturation
MEHMO 300148	Rare	X-linked mitochondrial disorder	Mental retardation, epileptic seizures, hypogonadism and hypogenitalism, microcephaly, early death
Clark-Baraitser (tall stature) 300602, or Atkin-Flaitz (short stature) 300431	Rare	X-linked	Macroorchidism, mental retardation, seizures, central incisor gap, microdontia, macrocephaly, coarse facial features, tapered fingers with short, broad hands
Coloboma-Obesity-Hypogenitalism-Mental Retardation 601794	Rare	Autosomal dominant	Retinal coloboma, microphthalmia, cataracts, hypogonadism, cryptorchidism gynecomastia, mild mental retardation

The age at onset and time-course of obesity may provide useful clues, because early-onset obesity (before 5 years, and especially before 2 years) is more likely to have a genetic cause. Hyperphagia and lack of normal satiety after meals is characteristic of many inherited obesity syndromes, and also of hypothalamic damage from tumours, irradiation or surgery. Previous and current drugs must be checked for possible causes of weight gain, and the family history taken for consanguinity, morbid obesity and type 2 diabetes.

Lifestyle factors should be carefully explored, to assess their contribution to weight gain and to open discussion about eventual management to reduce and stabilize weight. A diary is useful to record the following, perhaps for 2–4 weeks before treatment starts:

- number and timing of regular meals;
- details of snacks and energy-dense food;
- consumption of soft drinks;
- physical activity, both background and formal exercise;
- sedentary activities, such as watching TV and playing computer games.

Examination

Anthropometry and general examination

Height, weight and ideally BMI should be plotted on percentile charts (see Figure 21.1). The child's height should be related to the predicted, final mid-parental corrected height, which can be estimated as the paternal and maternal height (in cm) divided by 2, plus 7 cm in boys and minus 7 cm in girls. Children with lifestyle-related obesity are generally relatively tall, whereas those who are disproportionately short, especially by comparison with parental heights, should be considered for investigation of conditions such as hypothyroidism, Cushing syndrome or growth hormone deficiency. Serial plots of height, weight and BMI may also highlight an emerging mismatch between obesity and longitudinal growth.

As mentioned above, waist circumference is increasingly used to assess central adiposity. Body fat mass and lean mass can be measured easily and non-invasively by bioimpedance, and related to published percentile ranges (McCarthy *et al.*, 2006); serial measurements of fat and lean mass can be useful in monitoring the progress of obesity treatment, but may be difficult to interpret in children especially around puberty.

Blood pressure should always be measured, to determine cardiovascular risk and as a pointer to Cushing syndrome.

Stage of puberty

Formal staging of pubertal development is essential when assessing obesity. Delayed puberty is a feature of several genetic obesity syndromes, while premature adrenarche (sexual and axillary hair growth), early breast development or gynaeconastia are quite frequent in lifestyle-related obesity.

Other features

Hirsutism may indicate premature adrenarche and is a feature of PCOS. Acanthosis nigricans (Figure 21.12) should be sought on the neck,

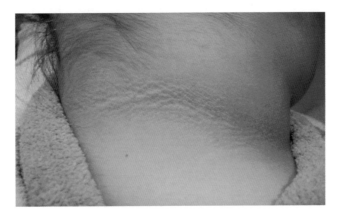

Figure 21.12 Acanthosis nigricans on the neck of a child with extreme obesity, insulin resistance and hyperinsulinaemia. This can also be seen in the axillae, groins and sometimes over the knuckles of the hand (see Figure 13.7).

axillae, groins and knuckles and is more easily seen in dark-skinned people; it is strongly associated with insulin resistance, and its presence warrants the assessment of glucose tolerance. Features of Cushing syndrome include cutaneous striae, facial plethora and thin skin, characteristically in a short child with truncal obesity and a moon face.

Fundoscopy and visual field testing should be performed, to seek evidence of papilloedema (intracranial tumours, benign intracranial hypertension), optic nerve compression (pituitary or hypothalamic tumours) or specific retinal lesions such as diabetic retinopathy and the pigmented retinopathy of Bardet-Biedl syndrome.

Further investigations

Thyroid and liver function tests, fasting blood glucose and lipids should be measured routinely. Fasting glucose may be normal in some patients with diabetes and by definition cannot detect IGT (Wiegland et al., 2004). A formal glucose tolerance test, although longer and more invasive, is required to diagnose such cases and is advised for children at increased risk of glucose intolerance (Reinehr, 2005; Table 21.3).

Appropriate endocrine and cytogenetic tests are needed to diagnose the rarer causes of childhood obesity (see Table 21.2). Advice about testing for suspected monogenic causes of obesity can be obtained from

Table 21.3 Risk factors for type 2 diabetes, which indicate the need for a formal oral glucose tolerance test in obese children over 10 years old.

Features indicating or accompanying insulin resistance

- Acanthosis nigricans

- Polycystic ovarian disease

- Dyslipidaemia

A close (first or second degree) family history of type 2 diabetes

High-risk ethnic groups

- African, or African-Americans

- Hispanic-American

- South Asian

Extreme obesity

national centres, such as the MRC Centre for Obesity and Related Metabolic Diseases in Cambridge, UK.

Treatment of childhood obesity

Rationale and targets

Many arguments support the need to treat obese children. First, obesity in childhood generally tracks into adult life. This is illustrated by a recent report from the North American Bogalusa study: 65% of children with a BMI ≥95th centile, and 85% of those ≥99th percentile, went on to have an adult BMI of ≥35 kg/m² (Freedman et al., 2007). Second, adolescent obesity apparently predicts premature death in adulthood (Engeland et al., 2003), and signs of organ damage may already be manifest in obese children. In addition, there is evidence that interventions in childhood may be more successful, beneficial and cost-effective than in adult life (Speiser et al., 2005; Epstein et al., 1995).

Treatment targets differ from those in adults, because of the dynamic nature of growth in childhood. In children with normal linear growth, simply maintaining weight will progressively lower BMI and may improve the outcome (see Figure 21.13. For example, Weiss et al. (2005) showed that the progression from IGT to overt diabetes over a 20-month period in 13-year old obese children depended on whether weight increased or was maintained during that time. Reinehr and Andler demonstrated that a fall in BMI SDS of ≥0.5 is required to lower blood pressure (by 11 (SD 15) mm Hg systolic) and improve lipid profiles and insulin sensitivity (Reinehr and Andler, 2004). Consistent with this, a fall in BMI SDS of 0.5–0.6 is needed to be certain of reducing body fat, suggesting that the improvement in metabolic and cardiovascular risk factors is related to reduced adiposity (Hunt et al., 2007) (Figure 21.14).

Lifestyle interventions

As in adults, the foundation of obesity management is lifestyle modification through promoting exercise and healthy eating. In practice, these changes can be extremely difficult to implement, and there is little solid evidence to prove that specific interventions are

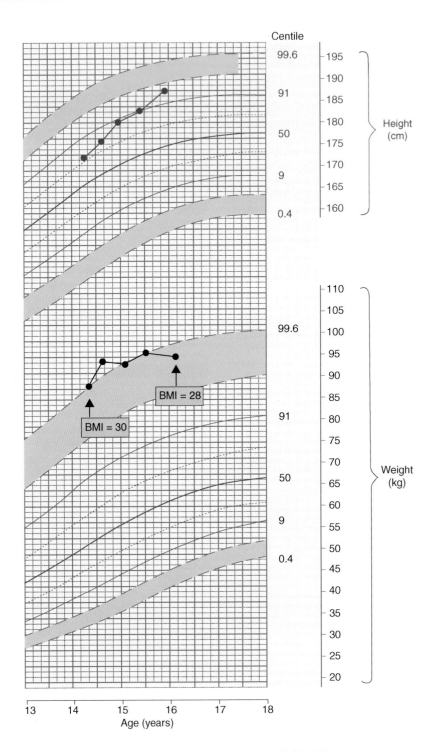

Figure 21.13 Stabilization of weight during active growth leads to a fall in BMI.

effective; indeed, a recent Cochrane review (albeit dominated by studies of American children aged 7–12 years) has highlighted the lack of sufficiently rigorous studies on which to base robust recommendations (Summerbell *et al.*, 2003).

'Positive parenting' and the active involvement of parents can increase the success of measures

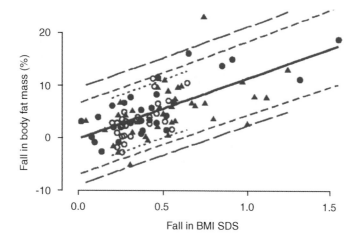

Figure 21.14 Linear relationship between fall in fat mass and BMI during weight loss in obese children. Pairs of results which were less than 0.5 years apart, between 0.5 and 1 year apart and more than 1 year apart are shown, respectively, as open circles, closed circles and triangles. The solid black line indicates the predicted values and approximate 95% prediction intervals (PIs)* for the three respective subgroups are shown with dotted, short-dashed and long-dashed lines. From Hunt *et al.* (2007) *Archives of Disease in Childhood* 92: 399–403.

to manage and prevent obesity in their children (Steinbeck, 2005; McLean *et al.*, 2003). Giving parents the primary responsibility for changing behaviour in the child – and ideally in the family as a whole – may confer additional benefits. Conversely, parents who lack insight or are indifferent to their child's obesity (and often their own) can undermine such efforts (Jeffery *et al.*, 2005). This highlights the need to educate the general population about the dangers of childhood obesity (Crawford *et al.*, 2006; see also Chapter 22).

It has been suggested that enforcing 'dieting' in children may increase the risk of them (especially girls) developing eating disorders. However, several studies have found no such association, and clinically significant eating disorders remain rare in comparison with obesity. The risks of the approaches described here are judged acceptable, although individual patients should be monitored for signs of eating disorders.

Some approaches that have proved effective in particular settings are described below, with the caveat they may not necessarily succeed elsewhere or in different age groups.

Healthy eating

Basic measures include encouraging three meals per day with no snacking between meals. Meals should be based on a healthy balance of nutrients, aiming to reduce dietary fat and sugar intakes. Many countries have produced national dietary guidelines, as illustrated in Table 21.4 and Figure 21.15.

Simple dietary manipulation, such as the 'traffic light' diet, can be successful. This scheme, combined with behavioural therapy and increased physical activity, was used by Epstein *et al.* (1998), who found that over 10 years, one-third of children were no longer obese, and a further one-third had reduced their excess weight by ≥20%. Further longitudinal studies are required to determine whether this approach will translate successfully to other sites (Steinbeck, 2005); two studies are currently running in the UK to evaluate a modified 'traffic light' scheme in combination with other lifestyle interventions (Stewart *et al.*, 2005; Edwards *et al.*, 2006).

Other approaches tried include moderate dietary restriction in the setting of a 6-week residential programme that also included daily skill-based, enjoyable physical activity and group-based education (Gately *et al.*, 2005). During the stay, children lost an average of 6 kg (BMI SDS fall of 0.28), but this was not maintained after returning to their usual obesogenic environment.

Table 21.4 Proportion of different foods, suggested for a healthy diet: from the UKs 'Balance of Good Health' guidelines.

- 33% fruit and vegetables
- 33% bread, other cereals and potatoes
- 15% milk and dairy products
- 12% meat, fish and protein alternatives (nuts)
- 7% foods containing fat and refined sugar

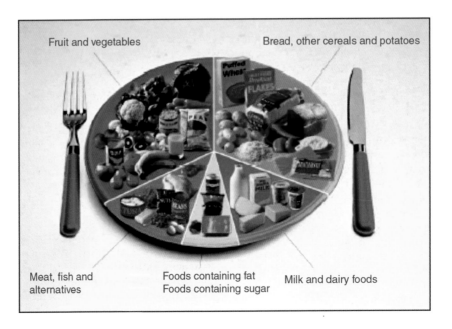

Fruit and vegetables

Bread, other cereals and potatoes

Meat, fish and alternatives

Foods containing fat
Foods containing sugar

Milk and dairy foods

Figure 21.15 A practical approach to teaching families the correct proportions of different foods. Taken from Food Standards Agency website: www.food.gov.uk.

Eliminating or reducing consumption of sugar-rich soft drinks is likely to be helpful, because these can significantly increase total daily energy intake (Ludwig, Peterson and Gortmaker, 2001). However, as with other lifestyle inter-ventions, any benefits are likely to decline after the end of the programme.

There is some evidence that low glycaemic index diets may be beneficial in obese adolescents (Ebbeling *et al.*, 2003). By contrast, very-low calorie diets are not advocated in childhood or adoles-cents, except under specialist care and in excep-tional circumstances, such as those with serious obesity-related comorbidities (Steinbeck, 2005).

Physical activity

There are two complementary goals, reducing sed-entary behaviours and encouraging more physi-cal exercise. Decreasing sedentary behaviour, notably television viewing, is vital because it is associated with improved overall physical activity levels and a reduction in the intake of snacks and fat (Epstein *et al.*, 2000; Goldfield *et al.*, 2006). There are few data on the efficacy of direct attempts to enhance physical activ-ity in childhood, although some studies show significant (but modest) reductions in body fat and increased lean mass (Carrel *et al.*, 2005; DeStefano *et al.*, 2000). Even if not

effective alone, increasing physical activity is a valuable adjunct to reducing sedentary behaviours and healthy eating, and can also help to prevent the comorbidities of obesity, notably type 2 diabetes and cardiovascular disease (see Chapter 22).

Exercise is important in enhancing insulin action and sensitivity. It increases several intra-cellular events mediated by AMP kinase such as fatty acid oxidation (Winder and Hardie, 1996; Hardie, 2004), while reducing malonyl CoA lev-els (a potent endogenous inhibitor of carnitine palmitoyltransferase-I (CPT-I), a fatty acid transporter localized in the outer mitochondrial membrane) (Kuhl *et al.*, 2006) and increasing basal glucose uptake into muscles (Hayashi *et al.*, 2000). It also enhances mitochondrial biogenesis (i.e. the increase in mitochondria seen in muscle after regular exercise), thus improving fuel utilization (Hood, 2001).

Pharmacotherapy

Anti-obesity drugs may be appropriate for some children, although – as in adults – the available drugs achieve relatively modest improvements in body composition and there are insufficient long-term safety or efficacy data. The latter point is of particular importance in children, who could potentially face decades of treatment.

All these drugs aim to supplement, not replace, lifestyle modification. Indications, treatment targets and the duration of treatment in children all remain vague. Pharmacotherapy could be considered when inadequate progress has been made with a well-supported lifestyle programme after 6–12 months – even though these drugs are relatively ineffective if lifestyle is not improved (see Chapter 17).

Orlistat or sibutramine can be chosen, according to their specific side effect profiles; orlistat is best avoided if fat intake remains high, and sibutramine avoided in the presence of refractory hypertension (see Chapter 14). Drug treatment should be stopped if there is no improvement (e.g. a fall in SDS of 0.5 or more) after 6–12 months. The other drug could then be tried if appropriate, although the main cause of failure is probably the inability to make the necessary lifestyle changes. There are currently no data or guidelines on how long treatment should be continued.

Orlistat

Orlistat inhibits pancreatic and gut lipases, thus preventing the absorption of dietary triglyceride. It acts only in the gut lumen, and it's side effects (fatty diarrhoea and occasionally faecal incontinence) relate to the undigested fat that remains in the intestine. Long-term use may also impair fat-soluble vitamin absorption, and we recommend that a vitamin supplement should be taken at bedtime. In adolescents, a randomized controlled trial has shown that orlistat achieved slightly but significantly greater weight loss than lifestyle modification alone; with orlistat, 27% of subjects lost ≥5% of BMI after one year, as compared with 16% of those given lifestyle advice only (Chanoine et al., 2005).

In the USA, orlistat is licensed for use in children over 12 years of age. The dosage recommended for children is 120 mg thrice-daily. A 6-month trial is reasonable for assessing the response to treatment; an inadequate response probably reflects poor compliance with the recommended low-fat diet, or overweight that is sustained particularly by high carbohydrate intake (e.g. from sweetened drinks).

Sibutramine

Sibutramine, a non-selective inhibitor of the neuronal reuptake of serotonin and noradrenaline (and also of dopamine), is a central appetite suppressant. Sibutramine's central sympathonimetic effects cause tachycardia and occasionally an increase in blood pressure; cardio-vascular status must therefore be carefully monitored.

In combination with dietary restriction and a family-based behavioural programme, one year of sibutramine treatment reduced BMI in obese adolescents by 3 kg/m^2, whereas untreated subjects showed no significant change (Berkowitz et al., 2006). The dosage used for adolescents aged 12–16 years in this trial was 10–15 mg once daily.

Rimonabant

Rimonabant, a cannabinoid receptor 1 (CB1) antagonist, acts centrally to reduce food intake and body weight. In adults, its efficacy is comparable to that of orlistat and sibutramine, but it is not yet licensed for use in children. Side effects include depression, which can occasionally be severe; concerns about a potential risk of suicide have delayed licensing approval in the USA and have now led to withdrawal of its licensing approval in Europe.

Other drugs

Metformin, a biguanide long used to treat type 2 diabetes in adults, is now first-line oral drug therapy for the disease in children and adolescents (see below). It can also improve insulin sensitivity and restore ovulation in PCOS (Driscoll 2003). It acts primarily by inhibiting gluconeogenesis in the liver, thus decreasing hepatic glucose production. It may also have a mild anorectic effect, possibly related to its gastrointestinal side effects of nausea, abdominal discomfort and diarrhoea. Two small, short-term trials have demonstrated a modest reduction in weight and SDS compared with placebo (Freemark and Bursey, 2001; Kay et al., 2001), but there are no data on long-term efficacy or duration of treatment in children. The dosage suggested for type 2 diabetes and PCOS in children and adolescents is 500 mg twice daily, which can be increased to thrice daily if necessary.

Topiramate is an anti-convulsant, which has been shown to cause weight loss. It has significant side effects (see Chapter 17) and should not be used specifically as an anti-obesity drug. However, it may be useful in obese children who also have epilepsy as a substitute for other anti-epileptic drugs, such as valproate and car-bamazepine that cause weight gain.

Bariatric surgery

The various procedures, and their indications and outcomes in adults, are described in Chapter 18. In the USA and certain other countries, bariatric surgery is also being used to treat severe obesity in a small but increasing number of adolescents (Davis *et al.*, 2006), and there is evidence of its benefits in highly-selected cases, especially those with comorbidities (Apovian *et al.*, 2005). The optimal procedure for adolescents is still debated; laparoscopic gastric banding, with its low complication rate, may have advantages over more invasive procedures such as gastric bypass with a Roux-en-Y or biliopancreatic bypass (Horgan *et al.*, 2005; Abu-Abeid *et al.*, 2003; Dolan and Fielding, 2004).

Current indications and contraindications for bariatric surgery in adolescents are shown in Table 21.5.

Treatment of comorbidities

Type 2 diabetes

Lifestyle modification is important and should be the mainstay of initial therapy. However,

Table 21.5 Criteria for considering adolescents for bariatric surgery.

Severe obesity

- BMI $\geq$40 kg/m^2 with one serious comorbidity (type 2 diabetes, sleep apnoea, complicated hypertension or benign intracranial hypertension) *or*
- BMI $\geq$50 kg/m^2 with less serious comorbidities
- BMI 35–40 kg/m^2 and life-threatening comorbidities should be considered on a case-by-case basis

Previous failure of non-surgical treatments
Absence of the following exclusion criteria

- Patient has not yet reached puberty (Tanner stage IV)
- Patient has not attained 95% of adult height, according to estimates of bone age (from an X-ray of the left hand and wrist)
- Pregnant females, or those planning pregnancy within two years of surgery

---

there are currently no data on its efficacy in the treatment of type 2 diabetes in adolescence.

The American Diabetes Association's recommendation for first-line drug therapy is metformin, which has the advantage of also reducing appetite and perhaps weight (see above) (Gahagan and Silverstein, 2003). There is no information on the long-term efficacy or safety of sulphonylureas or thiazolidinediones in childhood type 2 diabetes. An ongoing study in the USA entitled 'Treatment Options for Type 2 Diabetes in Adolescents and Youth' (TODAY) is comparing metformin and rosiglitazone versus metformin and intensive lifestyle changes, with the primary outcome being the time taken to reach poor glycaemic control (HbA$_{1c}$ >8%), in 800 patients aged 10–17 years (Zeitler *et al.*, 2007).

Insulin therapy is recommended for patients presenting with type 2 diabetes and a fasting plasma glucose of >13.9 mmol/l or ketoacidosis (Gahagan and Silverstein, 2003), which is a remarkably common finding at initial diagnosis in adolescence (Haines *et al.*, 2007). Once metabolic control has been achieved it may be possible to reduce or stop insulin therapy in favour of lifestyle changes and/or metformin therapy.

In adults, bariatric surgery can achieve major weight loss and can reverse established type 2 diabetes in 75% or more of cases, with biliopancreatic diversion being particularly effective (see Chapter 18). There are no outcome data for surgery in terms of secondary morbidities in adolescence, but weight loss is impressive as are improvements in insulin resistance and dyslipidaemia (Lawson *et al.*, 2006; Shield *et al.*, 2007).

As previously mentioned, micro- and macrovascular complications may progress more rapidly than in children with type 1 diabetes, and young patients with type 2 diabetes require careful, frequent and long-term monitoring.

Other comorbidities

Hypertension and dyslipidaemia can resolve with weight loss. If hypertension persists, the use of an ACE inhibitor is recommended (Gahagan and Silverstein, 2003). The treatment of dyslipidaemia remains uncertain, because there are few data on the efficacy of the standard drugs used in adult practice such as the statins.

Fatty liver can also improve after weight loss – which should not exceed 0.5 kg per week, because of the risk of aggravating the inflammation that underlies progressive liver damage (Marion, Baker and Dhawan, 2004). Alter-native therapies for obesity-related liver disease currently under study include metformin (Schwimmer *et al.*, 2005) and vitamin E (Festi *et al.*, 2004).

Some features of PCOS improve with weight loss and the condition can be treated with metformin, which can induce ovulation without major weight loss (see Chapter 13). Adjunctive therapies include anti-androgen therapy using cyproterone acetate in the form of a contraceptive pill combined with ethinyloestradiol, and possibly topical eflornithine to remove facial hair.

Prevention of childhood obesity

The prevention of obesity and the development of its comorbidities (especially type 2 diabetes) is discussed in detail in Chapter 22. An urgent priority is to identify and implement effective primary prevention strategies (i.e. to stop normal-weight subjects from becoming overweight), although it is still not clear whether these should target whole populations or specific socio-economic, racial or vulnerable groups that are at increased risk (Ells *et al.*, 2005; Mulvihill and Quigley, 2003).

Early-life interventions, during the perinatal period, can provide a powerful opportunity to access and influence an at-risk population. Maternal obesity apparently contributes to the child's later risk of obesity (Whitaker, 2004; Li *et al.*, 2005), and education during pregnancy and after birth – and ideally before conception – can potentially improve both maternal weight and the child's nutrition. One encouraging initiative is the promotion of breast-feeding, which helps to prevent overnutrition of the baby and protects against obesity into childhood (Mayer-Davis *et al.*, 2006; Gillman *et al.*, 2006).

School-based interventions are theoretically attractive, because school children are a 'captive' population and intervention could potentially be applied to all children. Many initiatives have sprung up, often without any robust evaluation of clinical outcome or cost-effectiveness. Restricted targeting of a single obesogenic factor (e.g. consumption of sugar-rich soft drinks) generally produces only modest or no benefit (Reilly *et al.*, 2006; Reilly and McDowell, 2003). Multi-faceted interventions that address both nutrition and exercise (increasing activity while reducing sedentary pursuits) appear to be more effective in changing behaviour (Ells *et al.*, 2005; Lister-Sharp *et al.*, 1999). However, even these may still not achieve the core aim of reducing the prevalence of obesity (Budd and Volpe, 2006).

Family-based interventions should help to break through the complex and interdependent factors that create an obesogenic environment from which the obese child may struggle to escape (Davison and Birch, 2001; Davison and Birch, 2002). 'Interested but healthy' families are relatively easy to recruit to these initiatives, whereas families with obese children and parents, and whose habits need to be changed, are often resistant (Danielzik *et al.*, 2005). So far, family-based interventions have had little lasting impact, although using parents as agents of change may help obese children to lose weight (NHS.CRD, 2002).

Governmental and societal interventions may be needed to legislate for a healthier environment for children. It is estimated that young people in Western countries see 40 000 advertisements each year, of which half are for food and especially sugared cereals and energy-dense snacks; significantly, children under 8 years of age are unable to distinguish truth from advertising hyperbole (Strasburger, 2006). The example of Sweden – which has banned all advertising directed at children under 12 years of age – should be followed worldwide. Concerted action at local and governmental levels may also be required to encourage physical activity in and out of school, by investing in recreational facilities and urban design that encourages safe active transport by walking and cycling.

Children are much more likely to respond positively to role-modelling and rewards when these are promoted by people close to their own age, and such peer-led educational programmes should be encouraged in schools and the media (Horne *et al.*, 2004).

The usefulness of intervention for preventing overweight and obesity in children aged 2–5 years, school-aged children and the family setting has recently been reviewed by the UK National Institute for Clinical Effectiveness (NICE) and by a systematic Cochrane review (NICE 2008; Summerbell *et al.*, 2005). The results, summarized in Tables 21.6 and 21.7, indicate that there is still a long way to go in the effective prevention of childhood obesity.

Table 21.6 Interventions for the prevention of overweight and obesity in school children, and their outcomes; from Danielzik *et al.*, 2005.

Weight outcomes

1 The evidence of effectiveness of multi-component school-based interventions is equivocal

2 School-based physical activity interventions (promoting physical activity, reducing television viewing) may help children to maintain a healthy weight

3 There is limited evidence (from one UK-based study) to suggest that interventions to reduce consumption of carbonated drinks containing sugar may help to reduce the prevalence of overweight and obesity

Diet and physical activity outcomes

4 Some evidence suggests that school-based, multi-component interventions addressing various aspects of diet and/or activity in the school – including the school environment (a 'whole-school approach') – are effective in improving physical activity and dietary behaviour, at least while the intervention is in place

5 Some evidence suggests that short-term and long-term school-based interventions to improve children's dietary intake may be effective, at least while the intervention is in place. This includes interventions aiming to increase fruit and vegetable intake, improve school lunches and/or promote water consumption

6 UK-based evidence suggests that school children with the lowest fruit and vegetable intake at baseline may benefit the most from school-based dietary interventions

7 Some evidence from multi-component interventions suggests that short-term and long-term school-based physical-activity-focused interventions may be effective, at least while the intervention is in place

Table 21.7 Interventions for the prevention of overweight and obesity in children aged 2–5 and family-based interventions, and their outcomes.

Weight outcomes

1 There is some, though limited, evidence that interventions focusing on the prevention of obesity by improving diet and activity have a small but important impact on body weight that may aid weight maintenance

2 Improvements in the food service to pre-school children can result in reductions in dietary intakes of fat and improved weight outcomes

3 No family studies were identified among children under 5 years of age

4 Family-based interventions that target improved weight maintenance in children and adults, focusing on diet and activity, can be effective, at least for the duration of the intervention

5 The effectiveness of interventions tends to be associated with the number of behaviour-change techniques taught to both parents and children

6 It remains unclear whether the age of the child influences the effectiveness of family-based interventions compared with individual interventions

Diet and physical activity outcomes

7 Interventions that do not lead to significant, positive trends in weight maintenance may still produce significant, positive trends in diet and physical activity behaviours

8 There is some evidence that interventions that do not focus on preventing obesity but aim to bring about modest changes in dietary and physical activity behaviour are unlikely to demonstrate an impact on body weight

Table 21.7 *(Continued)*

9 There is evidence for small but important beneficial effects of interventions that aim to improve dietary intake (such as videos, interactive demonstrations and changing food provision at nursery school), as long as these interventions do not focus solely on nutrition education

10 The provision of regular meals in a supportive environment free from distractions may improve dietary intake

11 There is limited evidence that structured physical activity programmes in nurseries can increase physical activity levels

12 Interventions that involve parents in a significant way may be particularly effective; they can increase parents' active playing with their children, and improve a child's dietary intake

From (NHS.CRD, 2002).

References

Abu-Abeid, S., Gavert, N., Klausner, J.M. and Szold, A. (2003) Bariatric surgery in adolescence. *Journal of Pediatric Surgery*, **38** (9), 1379–82.

Adelman, R.D., Restaino, I.G., Alon, U.S. and Blowey, D.L. (2001) Proteinuria and focal segmental glomerulosclerosis in severely obese adolescents. *The Journal of Pediatrics*, **138** (4), 481–5.

Amin, R.S., Kimball, T.R., Bean, J.A. *et al.* (2002) Left ventricular hypertrophy and abnormal ventricular geometry in children and adolescents with obstructive sleep apnea. *American Journal of Respiratory and Critical Care Medicine*, **165** (10), 1395–9.

Apovian, C.M., Baker, C., Ludwig, D.S. *et al.* (2005) Best practice guidelines in pediatric/adolescent weight loss surgery. *Obesity Research*, **13** (2), 274–82.

Bazelmans, C., Coppieters, Y., Godin, I. *et al.* (2004) Is obesity associated with injuries among young people? *European Journal of Epidemiology*, **19** (11), 1037–42.

Berenson, G.S., Srinivasan, S.R., Bao, W. *et al.* (1998) Association between multiple cardiovascular risk factors and atherosclerosis in children and young adults. The Bogalusa Heart Study. *The New England Journal of Medicine*, **338** (23), 1650–6.

Berkowitz, R.I., Fujioka, K., Daniels, S.R. *et al.* (2006) Effects of sibutramine treatment in obese adolescents: a randomized trial. *Annals of Internal Medicine*, **145** (2), 81–90.

Bray, G.A., Nielsen, S.J. and Popkin, B.M. (2004) Consumption of high-fructose corn syrup in beverages may play a role in the epidemic of obesity. *The American Journal of Clinical Nutrition*, **79** (4), 537–43.

Brown, T., Kelly, S. and Summerbell, C. (2007) Prevention of obesity: a review of interventions. *Obesity Reviews*, **8** (Suppl 1), 127–30.

Budd, G.M. and Volpe, S.L. (2006) School-based obesity prevention: research, challenges, and recommendations. *Journal of School Health*, **76** (10), 485–95.

Burgert, T.S., Taksali, S.E., Dziura, J. *et al.* (2006) Alanine aminotransferase levels and fatty liver in childhood obesity: associations with insulin resistance, adiponectin, and visceral fat. *The Journal of Clinical Endocrinology and Metabolism*, **91** (11), 4287–94.

Carrel, A.L., Clark, R.R., Peterson, S.E. *et al.* (2005) Improvement of fitness, body composition, and insulin sensitivity in overweight children in a school-based exercise program: a randomized, controlled study. *Archives of Pediatrics & Adolescent Medicine*, **159** (10), 963–8.

Chanoine, J.P., Hampl, S., Jensen, C. *et al.* (2005) Effect of orlistat on weight and body composition in obese adolescents: a randomized controlled trial. *The Journal of the American Medical Association*, **293** (23), 2873–83.

Chaput, J.P., Brunet, M. and Tremblay, A. (2006) Relationship between short sleeping hours and childhood overweight/obesity: results from the 'Quebec en Forme' Project. *International Journal of Obesity (London)*, **30** (7), 1080–5.

Clement, K., Vaisse, C., Lahlou, N. *et al.* (1998) A mutation in the human leptin receptor gene causes obesity and pituitary dysfunction. *Nature*, **392** (6674), 398–401.

Cole, T.J., Bellizzi, M.C., Flegal, K.M. and Dietz, W.H. (2000) Establishing a standard definition for child overweight and obesity worldwide: international survey. *British Medical Journal*, **320** (7244), 1240–3.

Cole, T.J., Freeman, J.V. and Preece, M.A. (1995) Body mass index reference curves for the UK, 1990. *Archives of Disease in Childhood*, **73** (1), 25–9.

Cook, S., Weitzman, M., Auinger, P. *et al.* (2003) Prevalence of a metabolic syndrome phenotype in adolescents: findings from the third National Health and Nutrition Examination Survey, 1988–1994. *Archives of Pediatrics and Adolescent Medicine*, **157** (8), 821–7.

Cowell, C.T., Briody, J., Lloyd-Jones, S. *et al.* (1997) Fat distribution in children and adolescents – the influence of sex and hormones. *Hormone Research*, **48** (Suppl 5), 93–100.

Crawford, D., Timperio, A., Telford, A. and Salmon, J. (2006) Parental concerns about childhood obesity and the strategies employed to prevent unhealthy weight gain in children. *Public Health Nutrition*, **9** (7), 889–95.

Cummings, D.E. (2006) Ghrelin and the short- and long-term regulation of appetite and body weight. *Physiology & Behavior*, **89** (1), 71–84.

Danielzik, S., Pust, S., Landsberg, B. and Muller, M.J. (2005) First lessons from the Kiel Obesity Prevention Study (KOPS). *International Journal of Obesity (London)*, **29** (Suppl 2), S78–83.

Davis, M.M., Slish, K., Chao, C. and Cabana, M.D. (2006) National trends in bariatric surgery, 1996–2002. *Archives of Surgery*, **141** (1), 71–4; discussion 75.

Davison, K.K. and Birch, L.L. (2001) Childhood over-weight: a contextual model and recommendations for future research. *Obesity Reviews*, **2** (3), 159–71.

Davison, K.K. and Birch, L.L. (2002) Obesigenic families: parents' physical activity and dietary intake patterns predict girls' risk of overweight. *International Journal of Obesity and Related Metabolic Disorders*, **26** (9), 1186–93.

de Jong, P.E., Verhave, J.C., Pinto-Sietsma, S.J. and Hillege, H.L. (2002) Obesity and target organ damage: the kidney. *International Journal of Obesity and Related Metabolic Disorders*, **26** (Suppl 4), S21–4.

Dean, H. and Flett, B. (2002) Natural history of type 2 diabetes diagnosed in childhood: long term follow up in young adult years (abstract). *Diabetes*, **51**, A24.

DeStefano, R.A., Caprio, S., Fahey, J.T. *et al.* (2000) Changes in body composition after a 12-wk aerobic exercise program in obese boys. *Pediatric Diabetes*, **1** (2), 61–5.

Devys, D., Lutz, Y., Rouyer, N. *et al.* (1993) The FMR-1 protein is cytoplasmic, most abundant in neurons and appears normal in carriers of a fragile X premutation. *Nature Genetics*, **4** (4), 335–40.

Dewey, K.G. (2003) Is breastfeeding protective against child obesity? *Journal of Human Lactation*, **19** (1), 9–18.

Dolan, K. and Fielding, G. (2004) A comparison of laparoscopic adjustable gastric banding in adolescents and adults. *Surgical Endoscopy*, **18** (1), 45–7.

Drake, A.J., Greenhalgh, L., Newbury-Ecob, R. *et al.* (2001) Pancreatic dysfunction in severe obesity. *Archives of Disease in Childhood*, **84** (3), 261–2.

Driscoll, D.A. (2003) Polycystic ovary syndrome in adolescence. *Annals of the New York Academy of Sciences*, **997**, 49–55.

Duncan, G.E., Li, S.M. and Zhou, X.H. (2004) Prevalence and trends of a metabolic syndrome phenotype among U.S. Adolescents, 1999–2000. *Diabetes Care*, **27**, 2438–43.

Dunger, D.B., Ahmed, M.L. and Ong, K.K. (2005) Effects of obesity on growth and puberty. *Best Practice & Research. Clinical Endocrinology & Metabolism*, **19** (3), 375–90.

Ebbeling, C.B., Leidig, M.M., Sinclair, K.B. *et al.* (2003) A reduced-glycemic load diet in the treatment of adolescent obesity. *Archives of Pediatrics & Adolescent Medicine*, **157** (8), 773–9.

Edwards, C., Nicholls, D., Croker, H. *et al.* (2006) Family-based behavioural treatment of obesity: acceptability and effectiveness in the UK. *European Journal of Clinical Nutrition*, **60** (5), 587–92.

Eisenmann, J.C. (2005) Waist circumference percentiles for 7- to 15-year-old Australian children. *Acta Paediatrica*, **94** (9), 1182–5.

Eisenmann *et al.* (2002) Physical activity, TV viewing and weight in U.S. Youth:1999 Youth Risk Behaviour Study. Eisenmann JC, Bartee RT Wang MQ. *Obesity Research*, **10**, 379–85.

Ekelund, U., Brage, S., Froberg, K. *et al.* (2006) TV viewing and physical activity are independently associated with metabolic risk in children: the European Youth Heart Study. *PLoS Medicine*, **3** (12), e488.

Ells, L.J., Campbell, K., Lidstone, J. *et al.* (2005) Prevention of childhood obesity. *Best Practice & Research. Clinical Endocrinology & Metabolism*, **19** (3), 441–54.

Ells, L.J., Lang, R., Shield, J.P. *et al.* (2006) Obesity and disability – a short review. *Obesity Reviews*, **7** (4), 341–5.

Engeland, A., Bjorge, T., Sogaard, A.J. and Tverdal, A. (2003) Body mass index in adolescence in relation to total mortality: 32-year follow-up of 227,000 Norwegian boys and girls. *American Journal of Epidemiology*, **157** (6), 517–23.

Expert Panel on Detection, Evaluation and Treatment of High Blood Cholesterol in Adults (2001) Executive summary on the third report on The National Cholesterol Education Program (NCEP) Expert Panel on Detection, Evaluation and Treatment of High Blood Cholesterol in Adults (Adult Treatment Panel III). *The Journal of the American Medical Association*, **285** 2486–97.

Epstein, L.H., Myers, M.D., Raynor, H.A. and Saelens, B.E. (1998) Treatment of pediatric obesity. *Pediatrics*, **101** (3 Pt 2), 554–70.

Epstein, L.H., Paluch, R.A., Gordy, C.C. and Dorn, J. (2000) Decreasing sedentary behaviors in treating pediatric obesity. *Archives of Pediatrics & Adolescent Medicine*, **154** (3), 220–6.

Epstein, L.H., Valoski, A.M., Kalarchian, M.A. and McCurley, J. (1995) Do children lose and maintain weight easier than adults: a comparison of child and parent weight changes from six months to ten years. *Obesity Research*, **3** (5), 411–7.

Ettinger, L.M., Freeman, K., DiMartino-Nardi, J.R. and Flynn, J.T. (2005) Microalbuminuria and abnormal ambulatory blood pressure in adolescents with type 2 diabetes mellitus. *The Journal of Pediatrics*, **147** (1), 67–73.

Farooqi, S. *et al.* (1999) Effects of recombinant leptin therapy in a child with congenital leptin deficiency. *New England Journal of Medicine*, **341**, 879–84.

Farooqi, S. and O'Rahilly, S. (2006) Genetics of obesity in humans. *Endocrine Reviews*, **27** (7), 710–8.

Farooqi, I.S., Keogh, J.M., Yeo, G.S. (2003) Clinical spectrum of obesity and mutations in the melanocortin 4 receptor gene. *The New England Journal of Medicine*, **348** (12), 1085–95.

Farooqi, I.S., Matarese, G., Lord, G.M. *et al.* (2002) Beneficial effects of leptin on obesity, T cell hyporesponsiveness, and neuroendocrine/metabolic dysfunction of human congenital leptin deficiency. *The Journal of Clinical Investigation*, **110** (8), 1093–103.

Fernandez, J.R., Redden, D.T., Pietrobelli, A. and Allison, D.B. (2004) Waist circumference percentiles in nationally representative samples of African-American, European-American, and Mexican-American children and adolescents. *The Journal of Pediatrics*, **145** (4), 439–44.

Festi, D., Colecchia, A., Sacco, T. *et al.* (2004) Hepatic steatosis in obese patients: clinical aspects and prognostic significance. *Obesity Reviews*, **5** (1), 27–42.

Ford, E.S. (2005) The epidemiology of obesity and asthma. *The Journal of Allergy and Clinical Immunology*, **115**, 897–909.

Freedman, D.S., Dietz, W.H., Srinivasan, S.R. and Berenson, G.S. (1999) The relation of overweight to cardiovascular risk factors among children and adolescents: the Bogalusa Heart Study. *Pediatrics*, **103** (6 Pt 1), 1175–82.

Freedman, D.S., Dietz, W.H., Tang, R. *et al.* (2004) The relation of obesity throughout life to carotid intima-media thickness in adulthood: the Bogalusa Heart Study. *International Journal of Obesity and Related Metabolic Disorders*, **28** (1), 159–66.

Freedman, D.S., Khan, L.K., Serdula, M.K. *et al.* (2005) Racial differences in the tracking of childhood BMI to adulthood. *Obesity Research*, **13** (5), 928–35.

Freedman, D.S., Mei, Z., Srinivasan, S.R. *et al.* (2007) Cardiovascular risk factors and excess adiposity among overweight children and adolescents: the Bogalusa Heart Study. *The Journal of Pediatrics*, **150** (1), 12–7; e2.

Freemark, M. (2005) Metabolic consequences of obesity and their management, in *Clinical Pediatric Endocrinology*, 5th edn (eds C. Brook, P. Clayton and R. Brown), Blackwell Publishing Ltd, Oxford.

Freemark, M. and Bursey, D. (2001) The effects of metformin on body mass index and glucose tolerance in obese adolescents with fasting hyperinsulinemia and a family history of type 2 diabetes. *Pediatrics*, **107** (4), E55.

Friedman, M.A. and Brownell, K.D. (1995) Psychological correlates of obesity: moving to the next research generation. *Psychological Bulletin*, **117** (1), 3–20.

Gahagan, S. and Silverstein, J. (2003) Prevention and treatment of type 2 diabetes mellitus in children, with special emphasis on American Indian and Alaska Native children. American Academy of Pediatrics Committee on Native American Child Health. *Pediatrics*, **112** (4), e328.

Gately, P.J., Cooke, C.B., Barth, J.H. *et al.* (2005) Children's residential weight-loss programs can work: a prospective cohort study of short-term outcomes for overweight and obese children. *Pediatrics*, **116** (1), 73–7.

Gillman, M.W., Rifas-Shiman, S.L., Berkey, C.S. *et al.* (2006) Breast-feeding and overweight in adolescence. *Epidemiology*, **17** (1), 112–14.

Goldfield, G.S., Mallory, R., Parker, T. *et al.* (2006) Effects of open-loop feedback on physical activity and television viewing in overweight and obese children: a randomized, controlled trial. *Pediatrics*, **118** (1), e157–66.

Green, S.M., Burley, V.J. and Blundell, J.E. (1994) Effect of fat- and sucrose-containing foods on the size of eating episodes and energy intake in lean males: potential for causing overconsumption. *European Journal of Clinical Nutrition*, **48** (8), 547–55.

Grinstein, G., Muzumdar, R., Aponte, L. *et al.* (2003) Presentation and 5-year follow-up of type 2 diabetes mellitus in African-American and Caribbean-Hispanic adolescents. *Hormone Research*, **60** (3), 121–6.

Gungor, N., Thompson, T., Sutton-Tyrrell, K. *et al.* (2005) Early signs of cardiovascular disease in youth with obesity and type 2 diabetes. *Diabetes Care*, **28** (5), 1219–21.

Haines, L., Wan, K.C., Lynn, R. *et al.* (2007) Rising incidence of type 2 diabetes in children in the U.K. *Diabetes Care*, **30** (5), 1097–1101.

Hardie, D.G. (2004) AMP-activated protein kinase: a key system mediating metabolic responses to exercise. *Medicine and Science in Sports and Exercise*, **36** (1), 28–34.

Hassan, A. and Gordon, C.M. (2007) Polycystic ovary syndrome update in adolescence. *Current Opinion in Pediatrics*, **19** (4), 389–97.

Hayashi, T., Hirshman, M.F., Fujii, N. *et al.* (2000) Metabolic stress and altered glucose transport: activation of AMP-activated protein kinase as a unifying coupling mechanism. *Diabetes*, **49** (4), 527–31.

Hood, D.A. (2001) Invited review: contractile activity-induced mitochondrial biogenesis in skeletal muscle. *Journal of Applied Physiology*, **90** (3), 1137–57.

Horgan, S., Holterman, M.J., Jacobsen, G.R. *et al.* (2005) Laparoscopic adjustable gastric banding for the treatment of adolescent morbid obesity in the United States: a safe alternative to gastric bypass. *Journal of Pediatric Surgery*, **40** (1), 86–90; discussion 90–91.

Horne, P.J., Tapper, K., Lowe, C.F. *et al.* (2004) Increasing children's fruit and vegetable consumption: a peer-modelling and rewards-based intervention. *European Journal of Clinical Nutrition*, **58** (12), 1649–60.

Hunt, L.P., Ford, A., Sabin, M.A. *et al.* (2007) Clinical measures of adiposity and percentage fat loss: which measure most accurately reflects fat loss and what should we aim for? *Archives of Disease in Childhood*, **92**, 399–403.

Invitti, C., Gilardini, L., Pontiggia, B. *et al.* (2006) Period prevalence of abnormal glucose tolerance and cardiovascular risk factors among obese children attending an obesity centre in Italy. *Nutrition, Metabolism, and Cardiovascular Diseases*, **16** (4), 256–62.

Janssen, I., Katzmarzyk, P.T., Srinivasan, S.R. *et al.* (2005) Combined influence of body mass index and waist circumference on coronary artery disease risk factors among children and adolescents. *Pediatrics*, **115** (6), 1623–30.

Jeffery, A.N., Voss, L.D., Metcalf, B.S. *et al.* (2005) Parents' awareness of overweight in themselves and their children: cross sectional study within a cohort (EarlyBird 21). *British Medical Journal*, **330** (7481), 23–4.

Kambham, N., Markowitz, G.S., Valeri, A.M. *et al.* (2001) Obesity-related glomerulopathy: an emerging epidemic. *Kidney International*, **59** (4), 1498–509.

Katz, L.S.S., Abraham, M., Murphy, K.M. *et al.* (2005) Neuropsychiatric disorders at the presentation of type 2 diabetes mellitus in children. *Pediatric Diabetes*, **6**, 79–83.

Kawahara, R., Amemiya, T., Yoshino, M. *et al.* (1994) Dropout of young non-insulin-dependent diabetics from diabetic care. *Diabetes Research and Clinical Practice*, **24** (3), 181–5.

Kay, J.P., Alemzadeh, R., Langley, G. *et al.* (2001) Beneficial effects of metformin in normoglycemic morbidly obese adolescents. *Metabolism: Clinical and Experimental*, **50** (12), 1457–61.

Kesler, A. and Fattal-Valevski, A. (2002) Idiopathic intracranial hypertension in the pediatric population. *Journal of Child Neurology*, **17** (10), 745–8.

Kuhl, J.E., Ruderman, N.B., Musi, N. *et al.* (2006) Exercise training decreases the concentration of malonyl CoA and increases the expression and activity of malonyl CoA decarboxylase in human muscle. *American Journal of Physiology. Endocrinology and Metabolism*, **290**, E1296–1303.

Lawson, M.L., Kirk, S., Mitchell, T. *et al.* (2006) One-year outcomes of Roux-en-Y gastric bypass for morbidly obese adolescents: a multicenter study from the Pediatric Bariatric Study Group. *Journal of Pediatric Surgery*, **41** (1), 137–43.

Levin, S., Lowry, R., Brown, D.R. and Dietz, W.H. (2003) Physical activity and body mass index among US adolescents: youth risk behavior survey, 1999. *Archives of Pediatrics & Adolescent Medicine*, **157** (8), 816–20.

Li, C., Kaur, H., Choi, W.S. *et al.* (2005) Additive interactions of maternal prepregnancy BMI and breast-feeding on childhood overweight. *Obesity Research*, **13** (2), 362–71.

Li, X., Li, S., Ulusoy, E., Chen, W. *et al.* (2004) Childhood adiposity as a predictor of cardiac mass in adulthood: the Bogalusa Heart Study. *Circulation*, **110** (22), 3488–532.

Lister-Sharp, D., Chapman, S., Stewart-Brown, S. and Sowden, A. (1999) Health promoting schools and health promotion in schools: two systematic reviews. *Health Technology Assessment*, **3** (22), 1–207.

Liu, J., Wade, T.J. and Tan, H. (2007) Cardiovascular risk factors and anthropometric measurements of adolescent body composition: a cross-sectional analysis of the Third National Health and Nutrition Examination Survey. *International Journal of Obesity (London)*, **31** (1), 59–64.

Ludwig, D.S., Peterson, K.E. and Gortmaker, S.L. (2001) Relation between consumption of sugar-sweetened drinks and childhood obesity: a prospective, observational analysis. *Lancet*, **357** (9255), 505–8.

Maffeis, C., Pietrobelli, A., Grezzani, A. *et al.* (2001) Waist circumference and cardiovascular risk factors in prepubertal children. *Obesity Research*, **9** (3), 179–87.

Mantovani, G. and Spada, A. (2006) Mutations in the Gs alpha gene causing hormone resistance. *Best Practice & Research. Clinical Endocrinology & Metabolism*, **20** (4), 501–13.

Marcus, C.L. (2000) Sleep-disordered breathing in children. *Current Opinion in Pediatrics*, **12** (3), 208–12.

Marion, A.W., Baker, A.J. and Dhawan, A. (2004) Fatty liver disease in children. *Archives of Disease in Childhood*, **89** (7), 648–52.

Mayer-Davis, E.J., Rifas-Shiman, S.L., Zhou, L. *et al.* (2006) Breast-feeding and risk for childhood obesity: does maternal diabetes or obesity status matter? *Diabetes Care*, **29** (10), 2231–7.

McCarthy, H.D. (2006) Body fat measurements in children as predictors for the metabolic syndrome: focus on waist circumference. *Proceedings of the Nutrition Society*, **65** (4), 385–92.

McCarthy, H.D., Cole, T.J., Fry, T. *et al.* (2006) Body fat reference curves for children. *International Journal of Obesity (London)*, **30** (4), 598–602.

McCarthy, H.D., Jarrett, K.V. and Crawley, H.F. (2001) The development of waist circumference percentiles in British children aged 5–16.9 years. *European Journal of Clinical Nutrition*, **55** (10), 902–7.

McConahy, K.L., Smiciklas-Wright, H., Birch, L.L. *et al.* (2002) Food portions are positively related to energy intake and body weight in early childhood. *The Journal of Pediatrics*, **140** (3), 340–7.

McDonald, N.C. (2007) Active transportation to school: trends among U.S. schoolchildren, 1969–2001. *American Journal of Preventive Medicine*, **32** (6), 509–16.

McLean, N., Griffin, S., Toney, K. and Hardeman, W. (2003) Family involvement in weight control, weight maintenance and weight-loss interventions: a systematic review of randomised trials. *International Journal of Obesity and Related Metabolic Disorders*, **27** (9), 987–1005.

Montague, C.T., Farooqi, I.S., Whitehead, J.P. *et al.* (1997) Congenital leptin deficiency is associated with severe early-onset obesity in humans. *Nature*, **387** (6636), 903–8.

Moran, J.R., Ghishan, F.K., Halter, S.A. and Greene, H.L. (1983) Steatohepatitis in obese children: a cause of chronic liver dysfunction. *The American Journal of Gastroenterology*, **78** (6), 374–7.

Mulvihill, C. and Quigley, R. (2003) The management of obesity and overweight: An analysis of reviews of diet, physical activity and behavioural approaches. *Health Development Agency October*, www.hda-online.org.uk.

Must, A., Jacques, P.F., Dallal, G.E. *et al.* (1992) Long-term morbidity and mortality of overweight adolescents. A follow-up of the Harvard Growth Study of 1922 to 1935. *The New England Journal of Medicine*, **327** (19), 1350–5.

Network SI-CG. Obesity in children and young people: a national clinical guideline. See www.sign.ac.uk 2003; Guideline 69, (last accessed 14 July 2008).

NHS.CRD (2002) The prevention and treatment of childhood obesity. *Effective Health Care*, 7.

NICE Consultation on Obesity http://www.nice.org.uk/page.aspx?o=296553 (last accessed 14 July 2008).

Nielsen, S.J. and Popkin, B.M. (2004) Changes in beverage intake between 1977 and 2001. *American Journal of Preventive Medicine*, **27** (3), 205–10.

Nielsen, S.J., Siega-Riz, A.M. and Popkin, B.M. (2002) Trends in food locations and sources among adolescents and young adults. *Preventive Medicine*, **35** (2), 107–13.

Nowicki, S.T., Tassone, F., Ono, M.Y. *et al.* (2007) The Prader-Willi phenotype of fragile X syndrome. *Journal of Developmental and Behavioral Pediatrics*, **28** (2), 133–8.

Ogden, C.L., Flegal, K.M., Carroll, M.D. and Johnson, C.L. (2002) Prevalence and trends in overweight among US children and adolescents, 1999–2000. *The Journal of the American Medical Association*, **288** (14), 1728–32.

Pietrobelli, A., Andreoli, A., Cervelli, V. *et al.* (2003) Predicting fat-free mass in children using bioimpedance analysis. *Acta Diabetologica*, **40** (Suppl 1), S212–5.

Pietrobelli, A., Rubiano, F., St-Onge, M.P. and Heymsfield, S.B. (2004) New bioimpedance analysis system: improved phenotyping with whole-body analysis. *European Journal of Clinical Nutrition*, **58** (11), 1479–84.

Pinhas-Hamiel, O. and Zeitler, P. (2005) The global spread of type 2 diabetes mellitus in children and adolescents. *The Journal of Pediatrics*, **146** (5), 693–700.

Poussa, M., Schlenzka, D. and Yrjonen, T. (2003) Body mass index and slipped capital femoral epiphysis. *Journal of Pediatric Orthopaedics – Part B*, **12** (6), 369–71.

Raitakari, O.T., Juonala, M., Kahonen, M. *et al.* (2003) Cardiovascular risk factors in childhood and carotid artery intima-media thickness in adulthood: the Cardiovascular Risk in Young Finns Study. *The Journal of the American Medical Association*, **290** (17), 2277–83.

Rami, B., Schober, E., Nachbauer, E. and Waldhor, T. (2003) Type 2 diabetes mellitus is rare but not absent in children under 15 years of age in Austria. *European Journal of Pediatrics*, **162** (12), 850–2.

Reilly, J.J. (2005) Descriptive epidemiology and health consequences of childhood obesity. *Best Practice & Research. Clinical Endocrinology & Metabolism*, **19** (3), 327–41.

Reilly, J.J., Armstrong, J., Dorosty *et al.* (2005) Early life risk factors for obesity in childhood: cohort study. *British Medical Journal*, **330** (7504), 1357.

Reilly, J.J., Kelly, L., Montgomery, C. *et al.* (2006) Physical activity to prevent obesity in young children: cluster randomised controlled trial. *British Medical Journal*, **333** (7577), 1041.

Reilly, J.J. and McDowell, Z.C. (2003) Physical activity interventions in the prevention and treatment of paediatric obesity: systematic review and critical appraisal. *Proceedings of the Nutrition Society*, **62** (3), 611–9.

Reinehr, T. (2005) Clinical presentation of type 2 diabetes mellitus in children and adolescents. *International Journal of Obesity (London)*, **29** (Suppl 2), S105–110.

Reinehr, T. and Andler, W. (2004) Changes in the atherogenic risk factor profile according to degree of weight loss. *Archives of Disease in Childhood*, **89** (5), 419–22.

Rennie, K.L., Jebb, S.A., Wright, A. and Coward, W.A. (2005) Secular trends in under-reporting in young people. *The British Journal of Nutrition*, **93** (2), 241–7.

Rennie, K.L., Johnson, L. and Jebb, S.A. (2005) Behavioural determinants of obesity. *Best Practice & Research. Clinical Endocrinology & Metabolism*, **19** (3), 343–58.

Ricciardelli, L.A. and McCabe, M.P. (2001) Children's body image concerns and eating disturbance: a review of the literature. *Clinical Psychology Review*, **21** (3), 325–44.

Riddoch, C.J., Bo Andersen, L., Wedderkopp, N. *et al.* (2004) Physical activity levels and patterns of 9- and 15-yr-old European children. *Medicine and Science in Sports and Exercise*, **36** (1), 86–92.

Sabin, M.A., Crowne, E.C. and Shield, J.P.H. (2003) Cardiovascular risk factors in obese children and their association with insulin resistance. *Journal of Endocrinology (Endocrine Abstracts)*, **5**, 92.

Sabin, M.A., Ford, A.L., Holly, J.M. *et al.* (2005) Characterisation of morbidity in a UK, hospital-based, obesity clinic. *Archives of Disease in Childhood*, **91**, 126–30.

Schaub, B. and von Mutius, E. (2005) Obesity and asthma, what are the links? *Current Opinion in Allergy & Clinical Immunology*, **5**, 185–93.

Schwimmer, J.B., Middleton, M.S., Deutsch, R. and Lavine, J.E. (2005) A phase 2 clinical trial of metformin as a treatment for non-diabetic paediatric non-alcoholic steatohepatitis. *Alimentary Pharmacology & Therapeutics*, **21** (7), 871–9.

Shield, J.P., Crowne, E.C. and Morgan, J.D. (2007) Is there a place for bariatric surgery in childhood obesity? *Archives of Disease in Childhood*. **93**, 369–72

Sinha, R., Fisch, G., Teague, B. *et al.* (2002) Prevalence of impaired glucose tolerance among children and adolescents with marked obesity. *The New England Journal of Medicine*, **346** (11), 802–10.

Slyper, A.H. (1998) Childhood obesity, adipose tissue distribution, and the pediatric practitioner. *Pediatrics*, **102** (1), e4.

Speiser, P.W., Rudolf, M.C., Anhalt, H. *et al.* (2005) Childhood obesity. *The Journal of Clinical Endocrinology and Metabolism*, **90** (3), 1871–87.

Srivastava, T. (2006) Nondiabetic consequences of obesity on kidney. *Pediatric Nephrology*, **21** (4), 463–70.

Stamatakis, E., Primatesta, P., Chinn, S. *et al.* (2005) Overweight and obesity trends from 1974 to 2003 in English children: what is the role of socioeconomic factors? *Archives of Disease in Childhood*, **90** (10), 999–1004.

Steinbeck, K. (2005) Childhood obesity. Treatment options. *Best Practice & Research. Clinical Endocrinology & Metabolism*, **19** (3), 455–69.

Stevens, J., Murray, D.M., Baggett, C.D. *et al.* (2007) Objectively assessed associations between physical activity and body composition in middle-school girls: the Trial of Activity for Adolescent Girls. *American Journal of Epidemiology*, **166** (11), 1298–305.

Stewart, L., Houghton, J., Hughes, A.R. *et al.* (2005) Dietetic management of pediatric overweight: development and description of a practical and evidence-based behavioral approach. *Journal of the American Dietetic Association*, **105** (11), 1810–5.

Strasburger, V.C. (2006) Children, adolescents, and advertising. *Pediatrics*, **118** (6), 2563–9.

Summerbell, C.D., Ashton, V., Campbell, K.J. *et al.* (2003) Interventions for treating obesity in children. *Cochrane Database of Systematic Reviews* (3), CD001872.

Summerbell, C.D., Waters, E., Edmunds, L.D. *et al.* (2005) Interventions for preventing obesity in children. *Cochrane Database of Systematic Reviews*, (3), CD001871.

Svensson, M., Sundkvist, G., Arnqvist, H.J. *et al.* (2003) Signs of nephropathy may occur early in young adults with diabetes despite modern diabetes management: results from the nationwide population-based Diabetes Incidence Study in Sweden (DISS). *Diabetes Care*, **26** (10), 2903–9.

Taheri, S. (2006) The link between short sleep duration and obesity: we should recommend more sleep to prevent obesity. *Archives of Disease in Childhood*, **91** (11), 881–4.

Tounian, P., Aggoun, Y., Dubern, B. *et al.* (2001) Presence of increased stiffness of the common carotid artery and endothelial dysfunction in severely obese children: a prospective study. *Lancet*, **358** (9291), 1400–4.

Treuth, M.S., Catellier, D.J., Schmitz, K.H. *et al.* (2007) Weekend and weekday patterns of physical activity in overweight and normal-weight adolescent girls. *Obesity (Silver Spring)*, **15** (7), 1782–8.

Verhulst, S.L., Schrauwen, N., Haentjens *et al.* (2007a) Sleep-disordered breathing and the metabolic syndrome in overweight and obese children and adolescents. *The Journal of Pediatrics*, **150** (6), 608–12.

Verhulst, S.L., Schrauwen, N., Haentjens, D. *et al.* (2007b) Sleep-disordered breathing in overweight and obese children and adolescents: prevalence, characteristics and the role of fat distribution. *Archives of Disease in Childhood*, **92** (3), 205–8.

Viner, R. (2002) Splitting hairs. *Archives of Disease in Childhood*, **86** (1), 8–10.

Viner, R.M., Segal, T.Y., Lichtarowicz-Krynska, E. and Hindmarsh, P. (2005) Prevalence of the insulin resistance syndrome in obesity. *Archives of Disease in Childhood*, **90**, 10–4.

Wardle, J., Brodersen, N.H., Cole, T.J. *et al.* (2006) Development of adiposity in adolescence: five year longitudinal study of an ethnically and socioeconomically diverse sample of young people in Britain. *British Medical Journal*, **332** (7550), 1130–5.

Wardle, J. and Cooke, L. (2005) The impact of obesity on psychological well-being. *Best Practice & Research. Clinical Endocrinology & Metabolism*, **19** (3), 421–40.

Webb, T., Whittington, J., Holland, A.J. *et al.* (2006) CD36 expression and its relationship with obesity in blood cells from people with and without Prader-Willi syndrome. *Clinical Genetics*, **69** (1), 26–32.

Wei, J.N., Sung, F.C., Lin, C.C. *et al.* (2003) National surveillance for type 2 diabetes mellitus in Taiwanese children. *The Journal of the American Medical Association*, **290** (10), 1345–50.

Weiss, R. and Caprio, S. (2005) The metabolic consequences of childhood obesity. *Best Practice & Research. Clinical Endocrinology & Metabolism*, **19** (3), 405–19.

Weiss, R., Dziura, J., Burgert, T.S. *et al.* (2004) Obesity and the metabolic syndrome in children and adolescents. *The New England Journal of Medicine*, **350**, 2362–74.

Weiss, R., Taksali, S.E., Tamborlane, W.V. *et al.* (2005) Predictors of changes in glucose tolerance status in obese youth. *Diabetes Care*, **28** (4), 902–9.

Whitaker, R.C. (2004) Predicting preschooler obesity at birth: the role of maternal obesity in early pregnancy. *Pediatrics*, **114** (1), e29–36.

Whittington, J., Holland, A., Webb, T. *et al.* (2002) Relationship between clinical and genetic diagnosis of Prader-Willi syndrome. *Journal of Medical Genetics*, **39** (12), 926–32.

Wieckowska, A. and Feldstein, A.E. (2005) Nonalcoholic fatty liver disease in the pediatric population: a review. *Current Opinion in Pediatrics*, **17** (5), 636–41.

Wiegand, S., Maikowski, U., Blankenstein, O., *et al.* (2004) Type 2 diabetes and impaired glucose tolerance in European children and adolescents with obesity – a problem that is no longer restricted to minority groups. *European Journal of Endocrinology/ European Federation of Endocrine Societies*, **151** (2), 199–206.

Winder, W.W. and Hardie, D.G. (1996) Inactivation of acetyl-CoA carboxylase and activation of AMP-activated protein kinase in muscle during exercise. *The American Journal of Physiology*, **270** (2 Pt 1), E299–304.

Wing, Y.K., Hui, S.H., Pak, W.M. *et al.* (2003) A controlled study of sleep related disordered breathing in obese children. *Archives of Disease in Childhood*, **88** (12), 1043–7.

Yeo, G.S., Connie Hung, C.C., Rochford, J. *et al.* (2004) A de novo mutation affecting human TrkB associated with severe obesity and developmental delay. *Nature Neuroscience*, **7** (11), 1187–9.

Yoshida, Y., Hagura, R., Hara, Y. *et al.* (2001) Risk factors for the development of diabetic retinopathy in Japanese type 2 diabetic patients. *Diabetes Research and Clinical Practice*, **51** (3), 195–203.

Zaninotto, P.W., Stamatakis, H., Mindell, E. and Head, J. (2006) *Forecasting Obesity to 2010*, Department of Health, London.

Zeitler, P., Epstein, L., Grey, M. *et al.* (2007) Treatment options for type 2 diabetes in adolescents and youth: a study of the comparative efficacy of metformin alone or in combination with rosiglitazone or lifestyle intervention in adolescents with type 2 diabetes. *Pediatric Diabetes*, **8** (2), 74–87.

Zimmet, P., Alberti, G., Kaufman, F. *et al.* (2007) The metabolic syndrome in children and adolescents. *Lancet*, **369** (9579), 2059–61.

Prevention of Obesity

Key points

- Prevention of obesity comprises three stages: primary (to prevent normal-weight subjects from becoming overweight), secondary (to prevent overweight individuals from becoming obese) and tertiary (preventing obese subjects from developing the comorbidities of obesity).

- Many primary and secondary preventative strategies have failed to improve obesogenic behaviours and/or to reduce the prevalence of overweight or obesity. Successful measures are generally population-wide, multi-disciplinary, sustainable and able to address social, ethnic and cultural diversity, notably social and financial deprivation.

- Strategies targeting children at school have promoted healthy eating and/or increased exercise to replace sedentary play. Combined approaches, with school and parental support, are most likely to succeed, but any benefits are often transient.

- Pre-school children may benefit from certain strategies to promote a healthy lifestyle for the whole family. Breast-feeding reduces the risk of overweight and obesity by as much as 20% for up to 4 years of age, and should be actively encouraged.

- Obesity prevention strategies for adults have been tried in workplace and community settings. Successful measures are generally multi-faceted programmes that are sensitive to cultural and social priorities, but few have achieved lasting benefits.

- WHO expert committees have issued guidelines for obesity prevention that include promising but untried measures as well as others of proven benefit. These include a healthy diet (especially avoiding energy-dense snacks and drinks for children), promoting physically active transport and pursuits instead of sedentary pastimes, a better understanding of the health hazards of obesity, and restricting the advertising of snacks and drinks to children.

- Lifestyle improvement (healthy diet, increased exercise) can reduce by 40% or more the risks of subjects with impaired glucose tolerance (IGT) progressing to develop type 2 diabetes over several years. Weight loss may be relatively modest.

- The cost-effectiveness of obesity prevention strategies has not been adequately evaluated. Some have been shown to be cost-effective in their original setting, but this may not apply in different social or economic circumstances.

Chapter 22   Prevention of Obesity

Tim Lobstein

Once established, obesity is difficult to reverse and the treatment of its comorbidities is expensive and often unsuccessful. Prevention would therefore appear to be a better strategy, although the practical implementation of public health and health education approaches is also challenging.

Prevention should be distinguished from treatment, which is targeted at individuals with the aim of reducing or stabilizing weight, or in the case of growing children, of limiting weight gain so that overweight children grow into normal-weight adults. In the context of obesity, preventative strategies comprise three levels:

- primary prevention: aiming to prevent normal-weight individuals from becoming overweight;
- secondary prevention: aiming to prevent overweight individuals from becoming obese;
- tertiary prevention: aiming to prevent obese individuals from developing comorbidities.

Experience in the field of public health suggests that the most cost-effective initiatives are generally population-wide and based on an integrated, multidisciplinary, comprehensive and sustainable range of complementary actions that address the individual, community, environment and society at large. Providing information about healthy options is often ineffective unless there is a change to the context in which health behaviour occurs. This appears especially true for people with low incomes and who live in highly obesogenic environments. Health education strategies therefore need to be complemented with appropriate measures designed to improve health behaviour across the social spectrum, if inequalities in health are not to be widened. In particular, as stated by the Ottawa Charter (WHO, 1986), effective interventions need to tackle the broader determinants of health, including social exclusion and social cohesion, as well as environmental and demographic factors.

This chapter focuses mainly on primary and secondary measures to prevent weight gain. An important aspect of tertiary prevention, namely attempts to prevent the development of type 2 diabetes, will also be discussed. The evidence that preventative measures are clinically and financially effective will be critically reviewed, as will the role of expert opinion in areas where firm evidence is currently lacking. Finally, the importance of engaging policy-makers in implementing strategies to combat obesity will be emphasized.

Primary and secondary obesity prevention

These strategies, designed to prevent increases in body weight, exploit a wide variety of measures to promote 'healthy eating' and increased physical exercise, and may be targeted at individuals, families, schools or entire communities.

It is often difficult to evaluate the effectiveness of the measures, for several reasons. First, there can be practical problems in constructing control groups for particular interventions, including 'contamination' by behaviours acquired from the intervention group. Second, long-term follow-up of outcomes such as the prevalence and health impact of obesity can be difficult and expensive; many studies have opted instead for short-term surrogate end-points such as improvements in eating and/or exercise habits. Third, because of the great cultural and behavioural diversity between populations, an intervention shown to produce positive benefits in a specific setting may not prove effective when tried elsewhere. In addition to these challenges, it can be difficult to determine whether preventative measures are cost-effective. Partly because of these problems, many interventions have no firm evidence base and cannot be rigorously evaluated according to the conventional medical model.

Obesity: Science to Practice   Edited by Gareth Williams and Gema Frühbeck
© 2009 John Wiley & Sons, Ltd

In the following sections we describe some examples of interventions that have been tried, with varying effectiveness, in children and adults.

Interventions in children

The diversity of interventions to prevent obesity and/or to encourage healthy body weight in children in various settings is illustrated in Table 22.1. Each of these studies had an appropriate control group, which allowed statistical evaluation of outcomes that included direct measurements of body weight or adiposity. In addition, many controlled studies have been performed to evaluate the impact of various interventions on other outcomes (e.g. patterns of food consumption or physical activity) that are directly relevant to obesity, but without including measurements of adiposity; likely benefits can therefore be inferred but not proven. Some of these studies are shown in Table 22.2. The variety and imagination of the approaches used is striking, ranging from targeted counselling of individual overweight

Table 22.1   Examples of trials to prevent obesity in children.

Setting	Conclusion
Australia (*New South Wales*). Group education programme for families with overweight children.	After 6 months, half of overweight or obese children stabilized or reduced their BMI for age. Obese parents also lost weight (NSW, 2001).
Australia (*New South Wales*). School-based, multi-faceted nutrition programme.	High level of engagement; potential to include physical activity and healthy weight focus (NSWG, 2005).
Australia (*Perth*). School and home programme to increase opportunities for physical activity, for 11-year-old urban children.	Significantly better fitness levels in boys and girls initially, but no significant difference in physical activity at the end of the intervention (Burke *et al.*, 1998).
Chile. 6 month nutrition education and physical activity intervention for primary school children. Included education for parents.	Increased physical activity observed for both genders. Reduced adiposity for boys only (Kain *et al.*, 2004).
Crete. School-based health education prospective study for children aged 6 (through to age 12).	BMI improvements in intervention group compared with the control group; BMI rose in both groups during the study (Mamalakis *et al.*, 2000; Manios *et al.*, 2002).
Denmark. Family counselling, shopping and meal planning.	21 out of 25 children lost weight during a 2-year intervention (Nielsen and Gerlow, 2004).
France. School and non-school physical activity programme for adolescents.	Improved participation in activities compared with controls, especially for girls. Reduced sedentary behaviour. Little impact on proportion overweight after 6 months (Simon *et al.*, 2004).
Israel. Multidisciplinary dietary + behavioural + exercise intervention for obese children and adolescents.	The intervention decreased body weight and BMI and improved fitness, especially if the parents were not overweight (Eliakim *et al.*, 2002).
Japan. Family support for parental weight loss.	Children of overweight parents who became non-overweight also lost weight and improved CV risk factors. Children of parents who remained overweight did not improve (Kanda, Kamiyama and Kawaguchi, 2004).
Japan. Screening and treatment for overweight among elementary school children.	Older children and those most overweight showed reduced adiposity in both control and intervention groups, but intervention group showed greater degree of improvement (Yoshinaga *et al.*, 2004).

Setting	Conclusion
Singapore. Clinic-based session with pre-school children (age 3–6 years); dietetic interventions for the most overweight, and nurse-led counselling for moderate overweight.	After 1 year, 40% of the children were less obese, and 20% reached normal BMI (Ray, Lim and Ling, 1994).
Singapore. 'Trim and Fit' programme of school-based nutrition and physical activity; teacher training and Ministry of Education input.	Decrease in the prevalence of obesity from 16 to 14% over 8 years. Not rigorously evaluated or peer reviewed (Singapore Ministry of Health, 2002; Toh, Cutter and Chew, 2002).
Thailand. Exercise programme for kindergarten children, duration 30 weeks.	Both the exercise and control groups decreased adiposity; girls in the exercise group were less likely to gain weight than the controls (Mo-suwan *et al.*, 1998).
Thailand. School-based weight control programme.	Adiposity increased significantly less among children in the programme compared with controls (Mo-suwan, Junjana and Puetpaiboon, 1993).
USA. Native Americans. 'Pathways' school-based interventions on nutrition and physical activity.	Improved self-reported awareness and nutrition, but not validated by observed food intake. No improvements in activity levels or adiposity (Caballero *et al.*, 2003).
US–Mexico border. Elementary school-based cardiovascular health programme for low-income Spanish speakers.	Overweight increased, but less in participating than control schools. Greater community participation in forming and evaluating the programme was recommended (Coleman *et al.*, 2005).

children to population-wide measures to increase physical activity (Shephard, 2001; Matsudo *et al.*, 2002) or to reduce the fat content of French fries (WHO, 2004).

The findings highlight some important points. Certain strategies have achieved at least some success in particular settings, for example the improved fitness and reductions in BMI in overweight Israeli children and adolescents who received a multidisciplinary diet and exercise package (Eliakim *et al.*, 2002). By contrast, other interventions – such as the Pathways study in Native American children (Caballero *et al.*, 2003) – failed to improve outcomes, even though they may contain the same basic components as in successful trials elsewhere. This implies that factors specific to the study and setting are crucial, and that careful tailoring of interventions to the needs of the target population is critical to success. Different age-groups, ethnic populations and genders require different approaches (Lytle *et al.*, 2002).

Furthermore, education interventions can improve awareness and understanding of the risks of obesity, and of the benefits and practical measures of healthy living, but the knowledge may not be translated into changed behaviour, or a small change in behaviour may not be reflected

in a significant improvement in adiposity. Many school-based interventions show gains in children's nutritional understanding, sometimes accompanied by increased physical activity or improved diet, but few demonstrate significant effects on BMI or prevalence of overweight. Moreover, any benefits may not endure: very few studies in children last more than a year, and those with longer follow-up suggest that the initial advantages gained by the intervention are reduced over time. In Crete, lifestyle intervention among a group of schoolchildren reduced the relative risk of becoming overweight after six years by 18% as compared with controls, but this difference declined to 16% after a further four years (Kafatos, Manios and Moschandreas, 2005) (Figure 22.1).

Most reviews of controlled, school-based interventions conclude that combined, multiple approaches to obesity prevention – including education, food services and physical activity – are more likely to succeed than single-dimensional strategies. Effectiveness may be increased by linking school-based programmes to out-of-school actions, through the family and community, such as reductions in television viewing and greater participation in physical activities in the community.

Table 22.2   Examples of controlled trials in children that examined end-points relevant to obesity, but did not measure adiposity or weight.

Country	Intervention/policy	Comment and outcomes
Australia (Victoria)	WHO Collaborating Centre for Obesity Prevention (State of Victoria, 2008)	After-school activity programme plus healthier take-away food (hot chips) and community newsletter.
Brazil	'Agita São Paulo' Programme: promotion of physical activity (Matsudo et al., 2002)	Significant increase in physical activity measures; demonstration that broad-based approaches give positive results e.g. through the media, community and school/workforce.
Denmark	'6 a Day' programme (WHO, 2003a)	Three interventions: workplace free fruit scheme, school fruit snacks (parent aid) and catering initiatives at worksite restaurants.
Kazakhstan	Health promoting schools (HPSs) (Aimbetova, 2002)	From 1999 to 2002, the number of HPSs rose from 15 to 300. Guidelines have been formulated for the school project coordinators; each school has carried out a pre-implementation analysis and identified project priorities; workshops have been organized for regional and school coordinators.
Norway	Maternal leave (2 h per day) to promote breast-feeding (NBFA, 1995)	After the programme, 98% of women starting breast-feeding, and 90% were still breast-feeding at 3–4 months and 75% at 6 months.
Slovakia	'Baby Friendly Hospital' Initiative (Geckova, 2002)	Compared with 1980, the breast-feeding rate in 2000 increased at 1 month from 61 to 79%, and at 6 months from 6 to 30%.
United Kingdom	'Fighting Fat, Fighting Fit' TV campaign. (Wardle et al., 2001)	Good awareness, but poor recall of lifestyle message, especially among those with lower levels of education and in ethnic minority groups. Participation low, even among target groups.
United Kingdom	'Water is Cool in School'. Schools provide water coolers and free water bottles for every child (Carr, 2004)	This has helped to reduce disruptions to lessons and increases concentration.
United Kingdom	'Walking buses' (walkingbus.com, 2005)	Adults accompany children in a group walking to school along a set route, picking up additional 'passengers' at specific 'bus-stops' along the way.
USA	'1% or Less' social marketing programme (Reger et al., 1998)	Doubled the market share of low-fat and fat-free milk in several communities through intensive, 7-week advertising and public relations campaigns that cost as little as 22 cents per person.

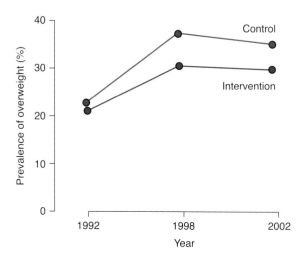

Figure 22.1 Impact of lifestyle intervention on the prevalence of overweight among schoolgirls in Crete. From Kafatos, Manios and Moschandreas (2005).

Physical activity

For increasing physical activity in school, reviews of controlled interventions suggest that the most effective initiatives involve children throughout the school day, including lunch and recesses, as well as physical education lessons. Activities that appear interesting and innovative to children (such as dance clubs, self-defence clubs and skills training) are particularly successful, as are interventions that aim to reduce television-viewing time (Robinson *et al.*, 2003; Dietz and Gortmaker, 2001). These behaviours can be long-lasting: individuals who participated in physical activities at school are more likely to be active in adulthood than those who did not (Tammelin *et al.*, 2003).

Healthy eating

A comprehensive school food policy should cover not only school meals, but also snacks brought to school, vending machines, snack bars and access to local shops during breaks. Introducing nutritional standards for school foods needs to be supported by measures to ensure that children then select the healthy options, for example by restricting choice, offering incentives and using a range of promotional marketing techniques. Breakfast clubs, which provide food when children arrive early at school, can improve dietary intake and health, as well as behaviour, social interactions, attendance and possibly concentration and learning (Shemilt

et al., 2004). They can also reach lower-income families and so address social inequalities.

Lytle *et al.* (2002) reviewed the limited success of many studies and suggested several ways to improve outcomes. These include an adequate duration of intervention, closer involvement of participants to prevent drop-out and ensuring that the experimental design can accommodate subjects from diverse cultural backgrounds. Actively involving members of the study population in designing the intervention may help to make programmes more responsive to the social and cultural environment. Also, as noted by Richter *et al.* (2000), the intervention must not contradict or undermine other messages being delivered by health-promotion campaigns.

Pre-school and family-based settings

Interventions designed to prevent obesity in children aged 1–5 years have included practical advice about healthy eating and promoting physical exercise, but there have been few reviews of these studies. Some interventions appear to improve nutrition knowledge, but the impact on eating behaviour and body weight has been poorly assessed and the results are inconsistent (Tedstone *et al.*, 1998a).

A focus group involving 19 healthcare professionals in the American Women, Infants and Child programme has provided insights into the barriers encountered when counselling parents of overweight children (St Jeor *et al.*, 2002).

Some mothers were preoccupied by daily life stresses, and ate 'comfort' foods to cope with their problems. Some also used food as a tool in parenting, for example to reward good behaviour. They had difficulty in setting limits with their children in relation to food, and lacked knowledge about children's normal development and eating behaviour. More problematically, some mothers were not committed to the sustained behavioural changes associated with a healthy lifestyle for the family and many did not believe that their overweight children were overweight, or that the problem was sufficiently serious compared with the other problems they faced.

The outcome of family interventions targeted at older children also appears equivocal, whereas those aiming to treat obesity in adolescents are only moderately successful (Haddock et al., 1994; McLean et al., 2003). The importance of involving parents in family-based treatments for overweight is uncertain: one study (Brownell, Kelman and Stunkard, 1983) reported that treating the mother and child separately was significantly more effective in reducing weight than treating them together or treating the child alone, whereas another found no such effect (McLean et al., 2003). Interventions that link school and home activities appear to influence knowledge, but not necessarily behaviour (Hopper et al., 1996). Overall, family-based interventions tend to demand more resources than school-based interventions.

Promotion of breast-feeding

Breast-feeding is widely accepted as providing a small but consistent benefit in protecting children from excessive weight gain, with the risk of obesity being reduced by as much as 20% for up to four years (Hawkins and Law, 2006; Singhal, 2007). The mechanisms are not fully understood, but Singhal suggests that formula feeding results in relative over-nutrition and faster growth. An association has been shown between faster growth in infancy and later obesity in both high- and low-income countries and for both faster weight gain and an increase in the length/weight ratio.

The process of persuading mothers to breast-feed should start during the ante-natal period, when small-group health education sessions can increase both the initiation and continuation of breast-feeding among women of all ethnic and income groups (Protheroe et al., 2003). However, health education delivered on a one-to-one basis may be more effective than group sessions for women, especially for those who have already chosen to bottle-feed (Fairbank et al., 2000). Ante- and post-natal peer-support groups can also help women to begin and continue breast-feeding, and these should be targeted at women on low incomes who wish to breast-feed (Stockley, 2000; Tedstone et al., 1998b).

Maternity ward practices that promote mother–infant contact and autonomy, such as 'rooming in' (keeping the baby next to the mother) and breast-feeding support, are effective in encouraging the initiation and continuation of breast-feeding (Sjöström and Stockley, 2000). The Baby Friendly Hospitals initiative promoted by UNICEF, which includes many of these measures (Table 22.3), has shown pronounced benefits on both the uptake and duration of breast-feeding (Merten, Dratva and Ackermann-Liebrich, 2005;

Table 22.3   Ten steps to successful breast-feeding; from UNICEF (2007).

Step 1:   Have a written breast-feeding policy that is routinely communicated to all healthcare staff.

Step 2:   Train all healthcare staff in the skills necessary to implement the breast-feeding policy.

Step 3:   Inform all pregnant women about the benefits and management of breast-feeding.

Step 4:   Help mothers initiate breast-feeding soon after birth.

Step 5:   Show mothers how to breast-feed and how to maintain lactation even if they are separated from their babies.

Step 6:   Give newborn infants no food or drink other than breast-milk, unless medically indicated.

Step 7:   Practise rooming-in, allowing mothers and infants to remain together 24 h a day.

Step 8:   Encourage breast-feeding on demand.

Step 9:   Give no artificial teats or dummies to breast-feeding infants.

Step 10: Foster the establishment of breast-feeding support groups and refer mothers to them on discharge from the hospital or clinic.

Cattaneo and Buzzetti, 2001). Conversely, enthusiasm for breast-feeding may be undermined by the physical hospital environment and by hospital routines such as feeding at set times, separating the mother and baby, the institutional use of infant formula foods, and by adverse attitudes and expectations of health professionals.

Screening for obesity in children

Guidelines for screening for obesity in childhood have developed from experience over the last two decades (Elster and Kuznets, 1994; Feldman and Beagan, 1994; Beatty and Sigmon, 1993) (Table 22.4). Some interventions among children found at risk of obesity during screening have been moderately successful in reducing obesity, notably in the Trim and Fit programme in Singapore (Toh *et al.*, 2002; Singapore Ministry of Health, 2002) (Figure 22.2). To succeed, such programmes may require a high level of commitment from children, schools and families; in 2007, the Singapore government announced the closure of the programme, blaming resistance from parents (Associated Press, 2007).

Overall, however, the value of screening programmes for childhood obesity remains controversial. Apparently healthy children may not be willing to present themselves for examination, whereas the early detection of obesity may create expectations without necessarily improving the prognosis (Farmer and Miller, 1983). Screening large numbers of children is expensive and can divert both staff and resources from other health-service activities. Indeed, screening children for obesity might only be valuable if children found to be at risk are prepared to have further assessments and make changes to achieve a healthy weight – and if effective assessment, interventions and follow-up are available and accessible (NHS, 2002).

Interventions in adults

A review of adult screening programmes by family doctors based on BMI measurements has concluded that clinicians should offer at-risk patients intensive counselling and behavioural interventions and that this could promote sustained weight loss (USPS, 2003). However, there was insufficient evidence that such interventions would benefit overweight, but non-obese, adults. The National Screening Committee of the UK's National Health Service has recommended that, pending further evidence, routine screening for obesity should not be offered to adults (NSC, 2006).

As with children, numerous interventions have been tried to prevent overweight and obesity and to promote healthy body weight among adults. The most common settings for controlled trials are institutions such as workplaces, where specific inputs (e.g. educational sessions, improved food services, physical activity sessions) and their outcomes can be adequately monitored and evaluated. Many studies have shown short-term improvements in eating and/or exercise

Table 22.4   Guidelines for screening for obesity in childhood.

Setting:

- Schools (including pre-schools) are the best place in countries where education is compulsory or where most children are in the education system.

Conditions:

- Children should be willing to present themselves for examination.
- Those found to be obese are ready to have further assessments and make changes to achieve a healthy weight.
- Facilities for further assessment or treatment are available in the community.
- Effective intervention and follow-up programmes are accessible and available for the identified children.
- Staff and financial resources are available for health-service activities.

Cautions:

- Screening for obesity may create expectations without improving the prognosis.
- Screened individuals and their families may feel a sense of failure that can reduce self-esteem and motivation.

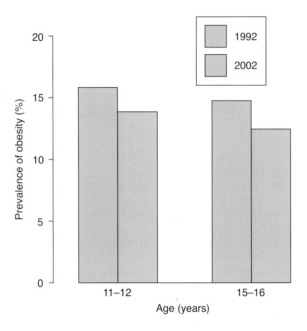

Figure 22.2 Impact of lifestyle improvement on the prevalence of obesity among children aged 11–12 and 15–16 years, who were found to be obese on screening in schools in Singapore. Data from the 'Trim and Fit' programme (Toh, Cutter and Chew, 2002).

habits, but the absence of long-term monitoring following most interventions makes it difficult to evaluate any lasting impact on obesity in the population at large.

Workplace settings

Strategies that target adults at their place of work have included nutritional education, aerobic or strength exercise (individually and in groups), training in behavioural techniques, provision of self-help materials, and specific dietary prescription.

Overall, there is little strong evidence of lasting benefits on overweight and obesity. The available literature supports interventions that combine instruction in healthier eating with a structured approach to increasing physical activity in the workplace (Katz *et al.*, 2005).

Involvement by employees and employers in the planning and implementation stages of interventions can be valuable. Ideally, the employer should be committed to the value and aims of workplace interventions. Demonstrating the cost-effectiveness of programmes (e.g. with reduced absenteeism because of sickness) may increase employers' interest,

and encourage their visible and enthusiastic support and involvement to motivate the entire workforce.

Community settings

Community-based actions to prevent obesity have included seminars, mailed educational packages and mass-media campaigns. A recent review concluded that, as with workplace interventions, there was no conclusive evidence that community-based interventions were effective (Mulvihill and Quigley, 2003); the authors recommended that education programmes linked with financial incentives should be further investigated.

Some more imaginative approaches are being evaluated. These include improved information and access to healthier food options (e.g. through major stores and local shops, food co-operatives, community cafés and home-produce clubs) and innovative health-promotion activities to improve knowledge and skills, such as shopping tours and cook-and-eat classes. Physical activity is being encouraged by providing better and safer walking and cycling routes, and voucher schemes for local swimming pools and other recreational facilities. Using community centres and churches as a setting for health education may also have a positive impact on healthy eating.

Supermarket promotions appear to be effective in improving consumption of healthy food, at least in the short term, particularly if accompanied by eye-catching labelling and helpful nutritional information (Lobstein, Landon and Lincoln, 2007).

Mass-media campaigns, commonly used by government agencies to promote health, have included dietary and physical activity messages. A study of a mass campaign undertaken by the BBC in the UK in January 1999 ('Fighting Fat, Fighting Fit') showed that awareness levels among all social groups was high, but that registration for further involvement and active participation were disappointingly low (Wardle *et al.*, 2001).

There is a lack of good evidence on the effective promotion of sustained changes in physical activity (Jackson *et al.*, 2005). Targeted programmes with tailored advice can change travel behaviour among motivated subgroups, and associated actions, such as subsidizing commuters to walk or cycle, may also be effective (Ogilvie *et al.*, 2004). Posters and banners encouraging the use of stairs rather than escalators can have a small, positive effect (Kahn *et al.*, 2002; Bungum, Meacham and Truax, 2007).

Untested interventions

Numerous interventions have been introduced with the intention of combating obesity, but which may not be structured to allow formal, controlled statistical evaluation. These initiatives can be valuable in driving change outside the traditional 'evidence-based' approach, and by showing what is practically feasible and achievable in a real-life setting. Examples include health-promotion efforts in the workplace, such as 'warm-ups' and 'workouts', supermarket-based health education leaflets, catering awards for healthy menus, and the provision of cycleways and walkways or subsidized sports facilities. Unhealthy eating has been targeted by, for example, setting nutritional standards for schools, hospitals and institutions; imposing sales taxes on sweet or fatty foods; formulating foods to reduce obesogenic nutrients or cosmetic additives; and by restricting the advertising of unhealthy foods. Government actions to promote healthy choices through 'social marketing', such as promoting 'five-a-day' fruit and vegetable consumption and running

advertising campaigns to reduce salt intake, may also be adapted to encourage lifestyle changes that will reduce the risk of obesity.

These largely untested interventions are introduced without evidence of effectiveness and on the assumption that, on balance, they will reduce the overall risk of ill-health. Some untested community interventions – for example the removal of vending machines selling soft drinks in schools – are a response to public (e.g. parental) pressure applied to the legislature or local authorities, schools or businesses. As a result, many initiatives are brought in piecemeal, without adequate funding, and may be poorly evaluated scientifically. Nevertheless, they may still reflect what is politically achievable.

Finally, success in one context may not necessarily transfer to another. 'Walking buses' (collecting children *en route* to walk to school) may be irrelevant if most children already walk or cycle to school, whereas television advertising controls may not be enforceable on commercial channels that broadcast from other countries. However, success in a community can spread to a much wider context: the Agito São Paulo movement – a broad-based strategy promoting physical activity, which involved schools, communities, workplaces and the media (Matsudo *et al.*, 2002) – has expanded progressively into Agito Brasil, Agito América and ultimately to Agito Mundo.

Recommendations of WHO expert groups

Policies are informed by expert opinion as well as evidence reviews. Expert opinion can consider target groups, settings and approaches that are not amenable to controlled trials but which, on the basis of other forms of evidence, may prove useful in controlling the obesity epidemic. The World Health Organization (WHO) has published reports of three expert committees, whose recommendations build on and extend the evidence already reviewed.

The first WHO Expert Meeting on obesity, convened in 1997 (WHO, 2000), described strategies for preventing and treating obesity in different health-service systems. The report urges national governments to commit themselves to controlling obesity and particularly to implementing food-based dietary guidelines. Responsibility for action should be shared between sectors, notably government, consumers, commerce and the media. This report led to an influential paper on preventing obesity

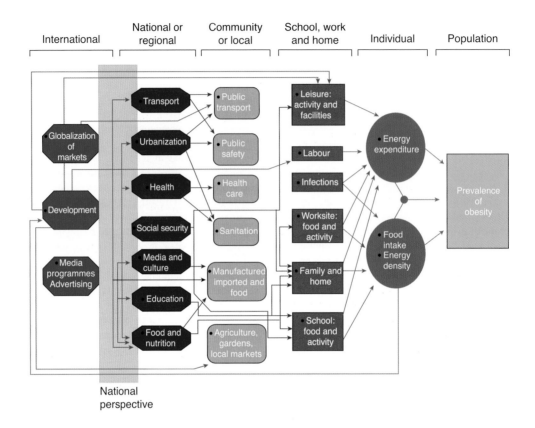

Figure 22.3 The 'causal web of obesity' proposed by the International Obesity Task Force (IOTF). The risk of obesity depends not only on individual susceptibility but also on family, community, national and international forces, which in turn influence factors such as food pricing and availability, work and the built environment.

(Kumanyika *et al.*, 2002), which emphasized the many complex interactions of factors that must be considered (Figure 22.3).

A second WHO consultation on diet, physical activity and the prevention of chronic disease took place in 2002 (WHO, 2003b). This emphasized recommendations for healthy eating, especially in children, and the promotion of high intakes of fruit and vegetables over energy-dense Westernized foods. The importance of physical activity was also emphasized.

The most recent consultation, held in Kobe, Japan in 2005, focused specifically on childhood obesity (WHO, 2008) and the interventions required at all levels – from local to international – to combat it.

The recommendations of the three reports can be summarized under the following six headings.

Public health campaigns

Key features of successful campaigns included:

- Adequate duration and persistency: programmes may take 10 years or more to show signs of success.
- A staged approach: this may be needed to help awareness to lead to motivation, experimentation and a sustained change in behaviour.
- Education to encourage changes to be made through participant choice, supported by consistent health messages from the media, health professionals and industry.
- Publicity and pressure from health advocacy organizations and experts to influence policy-makers and participants (as has proved effective in anti-smoking campaigns).
- Legislative action to support educational campaigns (as with seat-belt use and drink-driving).

Diet

Key dietary recommendations include:

- Consumption of plentiful fruit and vegetables should be encouraged, and traditional diets that promote this should be protected.
- Consumption of energy-dense, micronutrient-poor foods, notably snacks and soft drinks, should be restricted.

Physical activity

Key physical activity recommendations include:

- One hour each day of moderate-intensity activity, which may be undertaken in several short bouts, is recommended.
- Sedentary activity such as television viewing and video games should be discouraged.
- The environment should be modified to enhance opportunities for physical activity; examples include urban design to provide walkways and cycle paths.

Children and parents

Key features in this area include:

- Exclusive breast-feeding should be promoted, and the use of sugars in formula infant feeds avoided, allowing infants to regulate their own energy intake.
- Growth of infants should be monitored to prevent excessive weight gain and reduce the subsequent risk of obesity. At particular risk are preterm and low birth-weight babies.
- Parents should be encouraged to interact with their children, especially in infancy, to promote active play and development.
- Young children should not be exposed to aggressive marketing for energy-dense foods and drinks.
- Older children should be encouraged to follow an active lifestyle, with a healthy diet, restricted intake of energy-dense products and physical exercise replacing sedentary pursuits.
- Parents should be educated to understand that overweight and obesity in children do not represent good health.
- Health services should routinely monitor and advise women about a healthy lifestyle for themselves and their children, using opportunities in clinical, community and school settings.

Schools

Key recommendations for schools include:

- Nurseries and kindergartens should avoid the unnecessary restriction of physical activity during the growing years.
- A comprehensive approach to promote healthy eating and exercise is recommended, including children, parents and staff, and covering lessons, physical activities and food services.
- High nutritional standards should be set for all food in schools, including snacks and soft drinks as well as meals.
- Daily physical activity, using programmes designed to appeal to children, is recommended for all grades.
- Teachers may need additional training in health promotion, and to prevent stigmatization or bullying of obese children.
- Schools need to be financially independent, to avoid pressure from commercial interests such as snack and soft-drinks manufacturers to accept product marketing.

Governmental action

Key recommendations in this area include:

- Availability and affordability of fruit and vegetables should be improved, especially for low-income and disadvantaged groups.
- Full implementation is recommended of the WHO–UNICEF Code of Marketing of Breast Milk Substitutes (in order to discourage their use in favour of breast-feeding).
- An International Code on Marketing of Food and Beverage Products should be established and enforced by an international monitoring agency that reports to the WHO and United Nations. This should cover printed and electronic media, and aim to restrict marketing and formulation strategies designed to attract children to energy-dense foods and drinks.
- Incentives given to commercial concerns such as food or agricultural enterprises should include the impact on health.
- Political donations from food companies should be restricted or banned.

- Local and national resources should be built up to support public health initiatives. Activities and policies should be monitored by a separate agency, perhaps an 'obesity observatory'.

The implementation of all these recommendations raises numerous issues. Measures to reduce the prevalence of obesity must emphasize healthy behaviours and activities rather than idealized weight or appearance. Furthermore, care must be taken to ensure that obesity prevention programmes do not induce unhealthy slimming practices, which could theoretically lead to the development of clinical eating disorders or encourage risky behaviours such as smoking to control weight. There is little evidence that treatments of obesity can induce eating disorders, but there is a hypothetical risk that programmes focusing on dietary restriction may cause anxiety and disrupt eating patterns in vulnerable children, which may in turn trigger a clinical disorder (see Chapter 20).

Caveats also apply when encouraging increased physical activity. Children may have many reasons for not participating in sports activities, including embarrassment in changing facilities, fear of ridicule or failure, and discomfort from sweating or breathlessness. Schools may also need to consider their responsibilities for safety and the prevention of accidental injuries. Training for staff may also be valuable in helping to promote and provide physical activities, and to recognize and prevent discriminatory behaviours.

Extending the evidence base through future studies

The WHO Kobe consultation on childhood obesity (WHO, 2005) made several recommendations to improve the evidence base on obesity prevention strategies and to inform policy-making including:

- All interventions should include evaluation of outcomes and costs. Evaluation can include the impact on other parties (e.g. parents and siblings) and should take account of other factors such as social marketing, policy changes and individual health promotion.
- Interventions using control groups should describe explicitly what the 'normal' controls

actually experience, especially where usual practices are changing.
- More interventions are needed to address the needs of specific sub-populations, including low-income groups, immigrants and other ethnic and cultural groups.
- Extended programmes are needed to evaluate long-term outcomes, including changes in knowledge and attitudes, behaviours (diet and exercise), adiposity and comorbidities.
- More sophisticated evaluations, including prospective meta-analyses, should be considered.
- An international agency should be established to encourage networking of community-based interventions and to support evaluations and analysis of cost-effectiveness.
- Commercial interests should not fund or evaluate research into obesity. Moreover, previous programmes funded by industry should be examined to determine whether they have introduced bias into the evidence base.

Tertiary prevention

The impact of lifestyle changes, pharmacotherapy and bariatric surgery on obesity and its comorbidities are discussed elsewhere in this book.

Tertiary prevention – that is, prevention of the complications of obesity in subjects who are already overweight or obese – has met with some success. The main target has been to prevent the development of type 2 diabetes, which has now become one of the most important threats to global health (see Chapters 2 and 9). To date, studies have focused on individuals found on screening to have impaired glucose tolerance (IGT) and therefore a substantial risk (perhaps 50% over five years) of progressing to type 2 diabetes. Most individuals with IGT are overweight or obese, as defined by criteria of adiposity that are appropriate to their ethnic group (see Chapter 9). These studies can therefore test the hypothesis that lifestyle modification can prevent overweight and obese people from developing diabetes.

The target populations have ranged from large-scale populations to small communities. An early study of Australian aborigines (O'Dea, 1984) showed an increased risk of diabetes among those living in urban areas, with improved glucose tolerance when they resumed their traditional lifestyle.

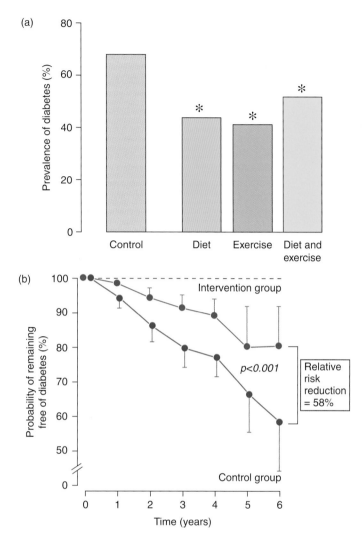

Figure 22.4 Lifestyle intervention to improve diet and/or exercise can significantly decrease the risk of developing diabetes among individuals with impaired glucose tolerance (IGT). Data from (a) the Da Qing study of adults from Northern China (Pan *et al.*, 1997) and (b) the Finnish Diabetes Prevention Study (Tuomilehto *et al.*, 2001). * = $p < 0.05$.

The Da Qing Diabetes study, conducted in Northern China between 1986 and 1992, followed up nearly 600 subjects with IGT, identified by screening almost 110 000 men and women (Pan *et al.*, 1997). Subjects were randomized to receive active management of diet, increased exercise or both, or no intervention. Among untreated controls, the cumulative incidence of diabetes after six years was 68%, but was significantly lower in each of the active management groups, representing a relative risk reduction of 32–40% (Figure 22.4a). These reductions in risk were

similar in individuals with a BMI either below or above 25 kg/m² , who made up 39 and 61% of the population, respectively.

In the Finnish Diabetes Prevention Programme, the impact of relatively modest lifestyle changes (avoiding fatty foods, taking regular exercise) was evaluated in 522 subjects with IGT (Tuomilehto *et al.*, 2001). Again, the cumulative incidence of diabetes was consistently lower in the intervention group than in untreated controls, being respectively 11 and 23% after four years, representing a relative risk reduction of almost 60% (Figure 22.4b).

Interestingly, the impact on body weight in the intervention group was greatest in the first year (a loss of 4.2 kg in the intervention group and 0.8 kg in the control group), with more modest differences in subsequent years.

Broadly similar findings emerged from the large US Diabetes Prevention Program. Weight loss was found to be more effective than the standard pharmacological treatment, metformin, in reducing the incidence of diabetes among patients with IGT (DPPRG, 2002).

These results indicate that changes in diet and physical activity can be introduced and sustained in diverse populations in the setting of a clinical trial. The challenge is to find methods for achieving similar sustained behavioural change through public health approaches in the community.

Cost-effectiveness of obesity prevention strategies

Cost is a primary concern to policy-makers and public-health managers but has been largely neglected in the evaluation of obesity prevention programmes. A recent review of workplace and community interventions noted that only two eligible studies of the former provided any analysis of cost-effectiveness (Katz et al., 2005). Only one study on the prevention of childhood obesity – the US Planet Health Program – has considered the costs of the intervention (Wang et al., 2003). This estimated that the intervention cost $14 per student per year; overall, the $34 000 invested was expected to save $16 000 in medical care costs and to recover $25 000 from lost productivity, thus yielding a net saving of around $7000. In this setting, this intervention was clearly cost-effective, but this favourable outcome does not necessarily apply to other populations, interventions or medical pricing systems.

Analyses undertaken in Australia (DHS, 2006; Haby et al., 2006) on the cost-effectiveness of various interventions in childhood obesity have compared costs incurred by the state with the estimated number of healthy years of life that would be saved (measured in Disability-Adjusted Life Years (DALYs)). The findings indicate that strategies such as controlling advertising to children, and educational programmes focusing on avoiding energy-dense foods and drinks and reducing television watching, bring greater cost-benefits than some schemes aiming to promote physical activity (see Table 22.5). Nonetheless, strategies

Table 22.5 Estimated health gains and public costs for different child obesity interventions, using economic modelling from Australian data. Note the huge variations in cost-effectiveness. Adapted from Haby et al. (2006) and DHS (2006).

Intervention	Population health gain (DALYs saved)	Average gross cost per DALY saved (Australian dollars)
Active after-school community programme	450	>80 000
Walking School Bus schemes	30	>70 000
TravelSMART active transport scheme	50	>25 000
Multi-faceted school-based without active PE	1600	>15 000
Orlistat therapy for obese adolescents	450	>14 000
GP-delivered family programme for overweight children	510	>12 000
Surgical gastric banding for obese adolescents	12 000	>10 000
Multi-faceted school-based including active PE	8000	>5000
Health education to reduce TV viewing	8600	>5000
Family-based programme targeting overweight children	2700	>3000
School programme targeting overweight children	360	>1500
Health education to cut soft drink consumption	5300	>500
Reduction of TV advertising to children	37 000	<10

DALY = Disability-adjusted life year.

to increase physical exercise may well confer other health benefits, such as cardiovascular fitness (see Chapter 16).

Rigorous economic analyses are still in their infancy, but will be essential to convince policy-makers to tackle obesity prevention with the determination that it demands.

Investing in health

It has been suggested that health-promoting strategies should be considered as investments rather than medical interventions. In health promotion, the return on investment can be measured as expected health gains and other desired outcomes, while risk equates with the consistency and likely effectiveness of the intervention. Hawe and Shiell (1995) have described a package of interventions as an investment portfolio containing both 'safe', low-return schemes and 'risky' but potentially high-return gambles.

This approach has been further developed in the 'portfolio promise' table described by Swinburn and Gill (2004) and by Swinburn, Gill and Kumanyika (2005). In this approach, risk is displayed in two dimensions: population impact (ranging from low to high) and the certainty of achieving benefit (also ranging from low to high); the resulting investment 'promise' similarly ranges from least (low certainty, low impact) to most (high certainty, high impact). This is illustrated in Table 22.6. Thus, intensive interventions that consistently improve health behaviour within small groups or individuals might be classi-

fied as low-risk but the overall return might be modest because they have only a limited impact on the health status of the community as a whole.

The process of weighing up potential gains and risks should permit the adoption of a mixed portfolio that includes untried but promising strategies as well as interventions that are based on robust evidence. This approach clearly demands a range of accurate information about costs, likely effectiveness, depth and extent of impact, sustainability and acceptability.

Inequalities and health promotion

Obesity, like several other chronic conditions, is found more frequently among lower-income and less well-educated people; this is particularly true in developed economies and is most evident among women and children (Molarius *et al.*, 2000; Robertson, Lobstein and Knai, 2008). Social factors must be taken into account when planning obesity prevention strategies, because inequalities in health behaviour and health status can be widened by some classical educational approaches.

Health behaviours can be differentially affected by educational strategies in various ways: there may be unequal access to, or comprehension of, the messages being promoted, while the opportunity to put the recommended behaviour into effect may not be available to some. For example, certain products (e.g. healthy food, sports equipment) may be unaffordable or inaccessible for deprived populations, as may services

Table 22.6 A 'promise table', indicating how investments in health promotion approaches can be assessed for their potential promise ('return on investment'). Here, risk is assessed in two dimensions: the likelihood that the intervention will have the intended outcome, and the proportion of the population likely to benefit; from Swinburn, Gill and Kumanyika (2005), 'Obesity prevention: a proposed framework for translating evidence into action. *'Obesity Review'*, 6: 23–33, with kind permission.

Certainty of effectiveness[a]	Potential population impact[b]		
	Low	Moderate	High
High	Promising	Very promising	Most promising
Medium	Less promising	Promising	Very promising
Low	Least promising	Less promising	Promising

[a]Certainty of effectiveness is judged by the quality of the evidence, the strength of the programme logic, and the sensitivity and uncertainty parameters in the modelling of the population impact.
[b]Potential population impact takes into account efficacy (impact under ideal conditions), reach across sub-groups and uptake within those groups.

such as subsidized works canteens and leisure facilities. Other factors that can differentially affect behaviours include poor safety and security in the local environment, which can deter walking and cycling; inadequate shopping or cooking skills; and adverse psychological factors (poor self-esteem and self-image) that may also be aggravated by an unfavourable environment.

Policies that rely too heavily on education therefore run the risk of increasing the 'health gap' between rich and poor – or more accurately, the gradient in health status across socio-economic classes. This strengthens the argument that the mix of interventions needed to prevent obesity must include population-wide measures in addition to strategies that specifically aim to reduce inequalities.

Conclusions

Public health preventative strategies will be tested by obesity and its comorbidities – especially as the accelerating global spread of the disease could be taken to indicate that current measures are failing.

There are some grounds for optimism. Awareness is growing of the hazards of obesity, especially in children (Ebbeling, Pawlak and Ludwig, 2002), and the WHO has given its authority to simple and achievable recommendations that can be applied in many countries. Moreover, evidence is accumulating that relatively small changes in diet and physical activity can achieve and sustain health benefits for some years. Whether such small changes are achievable in the context of strongly obesogenic environments is open to question.

Ultimately, as the WHO recommendations imply, the success of obesity prevention strategies will depend critically on the support and commitment of policy-makers at governmental and international level. Public policy decisions are based on numerous factors, including economic and political considerations, and may not necessarily be swayed by even a powerful medical and scientific evidence base.

References

Aimbetova, G. (2002) A health boost for school children. World Health Organization, The European Network of Health Promoting Schools. *Network News 2002*, **7**, 50.

Associated Press (2007) Singapore to Scrap Anti-Obesity Program. *Washington Post*. See http://www.washingtonpost.com/wp-dyn/content/article/2007/03/20/AR2007032001145.html (accessed 17 December 2007).

Beatty, L.A. and Sigmon, F.L. Jr, (1993) Well child care, in *Essentials of Family Medicine* 2nd edn, (eds P.D. Sloane, L.M. Slatt and P. Curtis), Williams & Wilkins, Baltimore, pp. 131–9.

Brownell, K.D., Kelman, J.H. and Stunkard, A.J. (1983) Treatment of obese children with and without their mothers: changes in weight and blood pressure. *Pediatrics*, **71**, 515–23.

Bungum, T., Meacham, M. and Truax, N. (2007) The effects of signage and the physical environment on stair usage. *Journal of Physical Activity & Health*, **4**, 237–44.

Burke, V., Milligan, R.A., Thompson, C. *et al.* (1998) A controlled trial of health promotion programs in 11-year-olds using physical activity 'enrichment' for higher risk children. *The Journal of Pediatrics*, **132**, 840–8.

Caballero, B., Clay, T., Davis, S.M. *et al.*, Pathways Study Research Group (2003) Pathways: a school-based, randomized controlled trial for the prevention of obesity in American Indian schoolchildren. *The American Journal of Clinical Nutrition*, **78**, 1030–8.

Carr, S. (2004) Water in school is cool! *Health News for Schools*, **16**, 2.

Cattaneo, A. and Buzzetti, R. (2001) Effect on rates of breastfeeding of training for the Baby Friendly Hospital Initiative. *British Medical Journal (Clinical Research Edition)*, **323**, 1358–62.

Coleman, K.J., Tiller, C.L., Sanchez, J. *et al.* (2005) Prevention of the epidemic increase in child risk of overweight in low-income schools: the El Paso coordinated approach to child health. *Archives of Pediatrics & Adolescent Medicine*, **159**, 217–24.

DHS: Department of Human Services (2006) ACE-Obesity: Assessing Cost-Effectiveness of obesity interventions in children and adults: Summary of Results. Victorian Government, Melbourne, Published online at http://www.health.vic.gov.au/healthpromotion/downloads/ace_obesity.pdf (accessed 20 December 2007).

Dietz, W. and Gortmaker, S. (2001) Preventing obesity in children and adolescents. *Annual Review of Public Health*, **22**, 337–53.

DPPRG (Diabetes Prevention Program Research Group) (2002) Reduction in the incidence of type 2 diabetes with lifestyle intervention or metformin. *The New England Journal of Medicine*, **346**, 393–403.

Ebbeling, C.B., Pawlak, D.B. and Ludwig, D.S. (2002) Childhood obesity: public-health crisis, common sense cure. *Lancet*, **360**, 473–82.

Eliakim, A., Kaven, G., Berger, I. *et al.* (2002) The effect of a combined intervention on body mass index and fitness in obese children and adolescents – a clinical experience. *European Journal of Pediatrics*, **161**, 449–54.

Elster, A.B. and Kuznets, N.J. (1994) *AMA Guidelines for Adolescent Preventive Services (GAPS). Recommendations and Rationale*, American Medical Association, Illinois.

Fairbank, L., O'Meara, S., Renfrew, M.J. *et al.* (2000) A systematic review to evaluate the effectiveness of interventions to promote the initiation of breastfeeding. *Health Technology Assessment Programme*, **4**, 1–171.

Farmer, R.D.T. and Miller, D.L. (1983) *Lecture Notes on Epidemiology and Community Medicine*, 2nd edn, Blackwell Scientific Publications, Oxford.

Feldman, W. and Beagan, B.L. (1994) Screening for childhood obesity, in Canadian Task Force on the Periodic Health Examination, *Canadian Guide to Clinical Health Care*, Health Canada, Ottawa, pp. 334–44.

Geckova, A. (2002) Slovakia – a national case. Baby friendly hospitals in Europe. Conference on Reducing Social Inequalities in Health among Children and Young People, 9–10 December 2002. Copenhagen, Denmark.

Haby, M.M., Vos, T., Carter, R. *et al.* (2006) A new approach to assessing the health benefit from obesity interventions in children and adolescents: the assessing cost-effectiveness in obesity project. *International Journal of Obesity*, **30**, 1463–75.

Haddock, C.K., Shadish, W.R., Klesges, R.C. and Stein, R.J. (1994) Treatments for childhood and adolescent obesity. *Annals of Behavioral Medicine*, **16**, 235–44.

Hawe, P. and Shiell, A. (1995) Preserving innovation under increasing accountability pressures: the health promotion investment portfolio approach. *Health Promotion Journal of Australia*, **5**, 4–9.

Hawkins, S.S. and Law, C. (2006) A review of risk factors for overweight in preschool children: a policy perspective. *International Journal of Pediatric Obesity*, **1**, 195–209.

Hopper, C.A., Gruber, M.B., Munoz, K.D. and MacConnie, S.E. (1996) School-based cardiovascular exercise and nutrition programs with parent participation. *Journal of Health Education*, **27**, S32–9.

Jackson, N.W., Howes, F.S., Gupta, S. *et al.* (2005) Interventions implemented through sporting organisations for increasing participation in sport. Cochrane Library, at http://www.cochrane.org/reviews/en/ab004812.html (accessed 16 July 2008).

Kafatos, A., Manios, Y., Moschandreas, J. and Preventive Medicine & Nutrition Clinic University of Crete Research Team (2005) Health and nutrition education in primary schools of Crete: follow-up changes in body mass index and overweight status. *European Journal of Clinical Nutrition*, **59**, 1090–2.

Kahn, E.B., Ramsey, L.T., Brownson, R.C. *et al.* (2002) The effectiveness of interventions to increase physical activity, a systematic review. *American Journal of Preventive Medicine*, **22** (S4), 73–107.

Kain, J., Uauy, R., Vio, F. *et al.* (2004) School-based obesity prevention in Chilean primary school children: methodology and evaluation of a controlled study. *International Journal of Obesity*, **28** 483–93.

Kanda, A., Kamiyama, Y. and Kawaguchi, T. (2004) Association of reduction in parental overweight with reduction in children's overweight with a 3-year follow-up. *Preventive Medicine*, **39**, 369–72.

Katz, D.L., O'Connell, M., Yeh, M.C. *et al.* and Task Force on Community Preventive Services (2005) Public health strategies for preventing and controlling overweight and obesity in school and worksite settings: a report on recommendations of the Task Force on Community Preventive Services. *MMWR Recommendations Reports*, **54**, 1–12. See http://www.cdc.gov/mmwr/preview/mmwrhtml/rr5410a1.htm (accessed 20 December 2007).

Kumanyika, S., Jeffery, R.W., Morabia, A. *et al.* and Public Health Approaches to the Prevention of Obesity (PHAPO) Working Group of the International Obesity Task Force (IOTF) (2002) Obesity prevention: the case for action. *International Journal of Obesity*, **26**, 1–12.

Lobstein, T., Landon, J. and Lincoln, P. (2007) *Misconceptions and Misinformation: The Problems with Guideline Daily Amounts (GDAs). A Review of GDAs and their use for Signalling Nutritional Information on Food and Drink Labels*, National Heart Forum, London.

Lytle, L.A., Jacobs, D.R., Perry, C.L. and Klepp, K.-I. (2002) Achieving physiological change in school-based intervention trials: what makes a preventive intervention successful? *British Journal of Nutrition*, **88**, 219–21.

Mamalakis, G., Kafatos, A., Manios, Y. *et al.* (2000) Obesity indices in a cohort of primary school children in Crete: a six year prospective study. *International Journal of Obesity*, **24**, 765–71.

Manios, Y., Moschandreas, J., Hatzis, C. and Kafatos, A. (2002) Health and nutrition education in primary schools of Crete: changes in chronic disease risk factors following a 6-year intervention programme. *The British Journal of Nutrition*, **88**, 315–24.

Matsudo, V., Matsudo, S., Andrade, D. *et al.* (2002) Promotion of physical activity in a developing country: the Agita Sao Paulo experience. *Public Health Nutrition*, **5**, 253–61.

McLean, N., Griffin, S., Toney, K. and Hardeman, W. (2003) Family involvement in weight control, weight maintenance and weight-loss interventions: a systematic review of randomised trials. *International Journal of Obesity*, **27**, 987–1005.

Merten, S., Dratva, J. and Ackermann-Liebrich, U. (2005) Do baby-friendly hospitals influence breastfeeding duration on a national level? *Pediatrics*, **116**, 702–8.

Molarius, A., Seidell, J.C., Sans, S. et al. (2000) Educational level, relative body weight, and changes in their association over 10 years: an international perspective from the WHO MONICA Project. *American Journal of Public Health*, **90**, 1260–312.

Mo-suwan, L., Junjana, C. and Puetpaiboon, A. (1993) Increasing obesity in school children in a transitional society and the effect of the weight control program. *The Southeast Asian Journal of Tropical Medicine and, Public Health*, **24**, 590–4. Erratum in **25**, 224.

Mo-suwan, L., Pongprapai, S., Junjana, C. and Puetpaiboon, A. (1998) Effects of a controlled trial of a school-based exercise program on the obesity indexes of preschool children. *The American Journal of Clinical Nutrition*, **68**, 1006–11.

Mulvihill, C. and Quigley, R. (2003) *The Management of Obesity and Overweight: An Analysis of Reviews of Diet, Physical Activity and Behavioural Approaches*, 1st edn, Evidence Briefing, Health Development Agency, London.

National Screening Committee (2006) National Library for Health, National Health Service on-line. See http://www.library.nhs.uk/screening/ViewResource.aspx?resID=60330 (accessed 20 December 2007).

NBFA (National Breast Feeding Association) (1995) Cited in Case study of Norway. Briefing paper. Baby Milk Action, Cambridge. See http://www.babymilkaction.org/pages/uklaw.html#1 (accessed 20 November 2007).

New South Wales (2001) Nutrition Project Register. Reported in T. Gill, L. King, K. Webb. Best options for promoting healthy weight and preventing weight gain in NSW. New South Wales Department of Health, 2005, http://www.health.nsw.gov.au/pubs/2005/healthyweight.html (accessed 20 December 2007).

NHS Centre for Reviews and Dissemination (2002) The prevention and treatment of childhood obesity. *Effective Health Care Bulletin*, **7**, 1–12.

NSWG (New South Wales Government) (2005) Northern Rivers Area Health Services. Tooty Fruity Vegie project. See http://www.health.nsw.gov.au/public-health/health-promotion/settings/schools/case-studies/tooty-fruity.pdf (accessed 20 December 2007).

Nielsen, J. and Gerlow, J. (2004) Evaluering af projekt for familier med overvaegtige born. [Evalution of a project for families with overweight children] Udviklings- og Formidlingscenter for Born og Unge: Copenhagen.

O'Dea, K. (1984) Marked improvement in carbohydrate and lipid metabolism in diabetic Australian aborigines after temporary reversion to traditional lifestyle. *Diabetes*, **33**, 596–603.

Ogilvie, D., Egan, M., Hamilton, V. and Petticrew, M. (2004) Promoting walking and cycling as an alternative to using cars: systematic review. *British Medical Journal (Clinical Research Edition)*, **329**, 763.

Pan, X.R., Li, G.W., Hu, Y.H. et al. (1997) Effects of diet and exercise in preventing NIDDM in people with impaired glucose tolerance. The Da Qing IGT and Diabetes Study. *Diabetes Care*, **20**, 537–44.

Protheroe, L., Dyson, M., Renfrew, M.J. et al. (2003) The effectiveness of public health interventions to promote the initiation of breastfeeding: Evidence briefing. London, Health Development Agency, (http://www.publichealth.nice.org.uk/download.aspx?o=502585 (accessed 20 December 2007).

Ray, R., Lim, L.H. and Ling, S.L. (1994) Obesity in preschool children: an intervention programme in primary health care in Singapore. *Annals of the Academy of Medicine, Singapore*, **23**, 335–41.

Reger, B., Wootan, M.G., Booth-Butterfield, S. and Smith, H. (1998) 1% or less: a community-based nutrition campaign. *Public Health Reports*, **113**, 410–9.

Richter, K.P., Harris, K.J., Paine-Andrews, A. and Fawcett, S.B. (2000) Measuring the health environment for physical activity and nutrition among youth: a review of the literature and applications for community initiatives. *Preventive Medicine*, **31**, S98–111.

Robertson, A., Lobstein, T. and Knai, C. (2008) Obesity and socio-economic groups in Europe: Evidence review and implications for action. Report SANCO/2005/C4-NUTRITION-03 DG Sanco, European Commission, Brussels (in press).

Robinson, T.N., Killen, J.D., Kraemer, H.C. et al. (2003) Dance and reducing television viewing to prevent weight gain in African-American girls: the Stanford GEMS pilot study. *Ethnicity and Disease*, **13**, S65–77.

Shemilt, I., Harvey, I., Shepstone, L. et al. (2004) A national evaluation of school breakfast clubs: evidence from a cluster randomized controlled trial and an observational analysis. *Child Care Health and Development*, **30**, 413–27.

Shephard, R.J. (2001) Communicating Physical Activity and Health Messages: Science into Practice, A brief report on the CDC/Health Canada Whistler Conference of December 2001. University of Toronto, Toronto. See http://www.lin.ca/resource/html/whistler/Shepard%20Summary.pdf (accessed 20 December 2007).

Simon, C., Wagner, A., DiVita, C. et al. (2004) Intervention centred on adolescents' physical activity and sedentary behaviour (ICAPS): concept and 6-month results. *International Journal of Obesity*, **28**, S96–103.

Singapore Ministry of Health (2002) *The State of Health 2001: The Report of the Director of Medical Services Singapore*, Ministry of Health, Singapore, p. 35.

Singhal, A. (2007) Does breastfeeding protect from growth acceleration and later obesity? *Nestle Nutrition Workshop Series: Pediatric Program*, **60**, 15–25.

Sjöström, M. and Stockley, L. (2000) Toward Public Health Nutrition Strategies in the European Union to Implement Food Based Dietary Guidelines and to Enhance Healthier Lifestyles, Final report of the Eurodiet programme, Working Party 3. Heraklion, University of Crete, 2000. See http://eurodiet.med.uoc.gr/ (accessed 20 December 2007).

State of Victoria (2008) Be Active Eat Well. Web-page updated 10 January 2008. Department of Human Services, State of Victoria, Australia. See http://www.goforyourlife.vic.gov.au/hav/articles.nsf/pracpages/Be_Active_Eat_Well, (accessed 18 July 2008).

St Jeor, S.T., Perumean-Chaney, S., Sigman-Grant, M. *et al.* (2002) Family-based interventions for the treatment of childhood obesity. *Journal of the American Dietetic Association*, **102**, 640–4.

Stockley, L. (2000) Consolidation and updating the evidence base for the promotion of breastfeeding, Cardiff, Health of Wales Information Service, http://www.wales.nhs.uk/publications/bfeeding-evidencebase.pdf (accessed 20 December 2007).

Swinburn, B. and Gill, T. (2004) *'Best Investments' to Address Child Obesity: A Scoping Exercise*, Centre for Public Health Nutrition, Sydney and Deakin University, Melbourne.

Swinburn, B., Gill, T. and Kumanyika, S. (2005) Obesity prevention: a proposed framework for translating evidence into action. *Obesity Reviews*, **6**, 23–33.

Tammelin, T., Näyhä, S., Hills, A.P. and Järvelin, M.R. (2003) Adolescent participation in sports and adult physical activity. *American Journal of Preventive Medicine*, **24**, 22–8.

Tedstone, A., Aviles, M., Shetty, P. and Daniels, L. (1998a) Effectiveness of interventions to promote healthy eating in pre-school children aged 1 to 5 years: a review, in *Health Promotion Effectiveness Reviews 10*, Health Education Authority, London.

Tedstone, A., Dunce, N., Aviles, M. *et al.* (1998b) Effectiveness of interventions to promote healthy feeding in infants under one year of age: A review, in *Health Promotion Effectiveness Reviews 9*, Health Education Authority, London.

Toh, C.M., Cutter, J. and Chew, S.K. (2002) School based intervention has reduced obesity in Singapore. *British Medical Journal (Clinical Research Edition)*, **324**, 427.

Tuomilehto, J., Lindström, J., Eriksson, J.G. *et al.* and Finnish Diabetes Prevention Study Group (2001) Prevention of type 2 diabetes mellitus by changes in lifestyle among subjects with impaired glucose tolerance. *The New England Journal of Medicine*, **344**, 1343–50.

UNICEF (2007) The Baby Friendly Initiative. See http://www.babyfriendly.org.uk/page.asp?page=102 (accessed 18 December 2007).

USPS Task Force (United States Preventive Services Task Force) (2003) Screening for Obesity in Adults: Recommendations and Rationale. *Annals of Internal Medicine*, **139**, 130–2. See http://www.annals.org/cgi/content/full/139/11/930?linkType=FULL&journalCode=annintmed&resid=139/11/930 (accessed 20 December 2007).

walkingbus.com. (2005) www.walkingbus.com (accessed 20 December 2007).

Wang, L.Y., Yang, Q., Lowry, R. and Wechsler, H. (2003) Economic analysis of a school-based obesity prevention program. *Obesity Research*, **11**, 1313–24.

Wardle, J., Rapoport, L., Miles, A. et al. (2001) Mass education for obesity prevention: the penetration of the BBC's 'Fighting Fat, Fighting Fit' campaign. *Health Education Research*, **16**, 343–55.

WHO (1986) Ottawa Charter for Health Promotion. First International Conference on Health Promotion, Ottawa, 21 November 1986. WHO/HPR/HEP/95.1. See (accessed 18 July 2008).

WHO (2000) Obesity, preventing and managing the global epidemic, WHO Technical Report Series, 894. World Health Organization: Geneva.

WHO (2003a) Fruit and vegetable promotion initiative, Report of a meeting held in Geneva, 24–27 August 2003 (WHO/NMH/NPH/NNP/0308). World Health Organization: Geneva. See http://www.panalimentos.org/planut/downloads/F&V%20Geneva%20Aug%202003.pdf (accessed 20 December 2007).

WHO (2003b) Diet, nutrition and the prevention of chronic disease, WHO Technical Report Series, 916. World Health Organization: Geneva.

WHO (2004) Collaborating Centre for Obesity Prevention. SSOP Be Active Eat Well project. See http://www.deakin.edu.au/hbs/who-obesity/downloads/reports/baew-2004pr.php (accessed 20 December 2007).

WHO (2005) Expert Meeting on Childhood Obesity, WHO Centre for Health Development, Kobe, Japan, 20–24 June 2005. Report in preparation.

WHO (2008) Obesity in childhood: report of an expert committee, Kobe, Japan, June. World Health Organization, Geneva, in press.

Yoshinaga, M., Sameshima, K., Miyata, K. *et al.* (2004) Prevention of mildly overweight children from development of more overweight condition. *Preventive Medicine*, **38**, 172–4.

A Look to the Future

Chapter 23   A Look to the Future

Gareth Williams and Gema Frühbeck

These are exciting times for all those working in the field of obesity, with interest in the subject and the pace of discovery both greater than ever before. The next 5–10 years will be a critical period for consolidating and applying our knowledge, and especially for testing our collective ability to limit the spread and impact of obesity. In this brief epilogue, we offer some thoughts about how particular aspects of the landscape of obesity might have changed by the time the second edition of this book is published in a few years' time.

Trying to look into the future is always a risky business and this particular crystal ball is quite seriously flawed – all too clear in some places, but stubbornly opaque in others. Unfortunately, some of the safest bets are also the most pessimistic.

Obesity and its fellow-travellers: here to stay

There will be no prizes for predicting that the obesity 'pandemic' will continue to gain momentum across much of the planet. The big questions are how far the current estimates of the spread of obesity will be outstripped, and the extent to which the increasing prevalence of obesity will be translated into excess morbidity, premature death and social and economic damage. Many previous forecasts of the rise in obesity and consequent type 2 diabetes were initially dismissed as scare-mongering, but have eventually proved to be conservative and have had to be revised upwards. The rate of climb in the prevalence of obesity appears to be steepening in many parts of the world – for example, the UK is steadily catching up with the USA – which suggests that the Westernised lifestyle is becoming even more obesogenic. If this trend were to be extrapolated to countries such as China and India, some of the most worrying predictions about the impact of obesity over the next 20 years could turn out to be substantial underestimates. As these populations are particularly susceptible to the metabolic and cardiovascular complications of obesity, the eventual burden of diabetes and coronary-heart disease is likely to present huge medical, social and financial challenges that could ultimately hold up economic development in these regions.

A major concern that recurs throughout this book, and one that will undoubtedly occupy more space in future editions, is the rapid spread of obesity among young people. Obesity does not spare the child, and indeed now appears to have a predilection for this age-group. In the UK, school uniforms are now available up to a 40-inch (102-cm) waist, coincidentally the threshold in adults for substantially increased cardiovascular risk. Perhaps the most sinister feature of childhood obesity is the development of type 2 diabetes – which only 10 years ago would have been regarded as a medical curiosity. Now well established in certain populations and steadily taking hold elsewhere, childhood-onset type 2 diabetes has not been with us long enough for its natural history to declare itself. This will become clearer during the next decade; given the refractoriness of childhood obesity and the fact that cardiovascular risk markers are already evident in obese children, it is unlikely that diabetes in this setting will run a benign course. Indeed, the rise of early-onset obesity could eventually lead to the arrest or even reversal of the decline in premature cardiovascular deaths that has occurred in many developed countries. Microvascular complications will pose other potentially serious threats to obese children with type 2 diabetes – perhaps notably nephropathy in Asian populations, whose susceptibility to renal disease is generally increased. Overall, this will be one of the grimmest spaces to watch.

Obesity is already changing the epidemiology of several other diseases, and will continue to

Obesity: Science to Practice   Edited by Gareth Williams and Gema Frühbeck
© 2009 John Wiley & Sons, Ltd

do so. Fatty liver has long been recognised in association with human obesity (and, for the gastronomically affluent, in force-fed geese), but its significance as a cause of cirrhosis and liver failure has only recently been appreciated. How well (or not) the liver will stand up to childhood-onset obesity, especially in adolescents and young adults who also abuse alcohol, is another interesting question that may well become an important medical and economic issue in the next decade. Adenocarcinoma of the oesophagus is an example of a disease whose incidence is rising steadily, especially among younger adults, and the increase is in a large part attributable to the spread of obesity. If present disease associations prove to be robust, the coming years will see progressive increases in the prevalence of many solid and haematological malignancies that can also be laid at the door of obesity.

The mechanistic links between obesity and its comorbidities will continue to be a fertile area for research. Some time-honoured disease associations have already been given a new and intriguing twist, such as the possible involvement of leptin and other adipokines in causing conditions as diverse as osteoarthritis, liver damage and sleep apnoea. Perhaps some good might ultimately come from the spread of obesity: following up these unexpected leads could, in theory, lead to novel treatments for other diseases.

More secrets from fat?

Fat, previously dismissed by many as dull and unattractive blubber, is now recognised as a highly active, versatile and communicative tissue with many important physiological and pathological roles. It is proving to be a rich source of diverse molecules with regulatory actions that may influence almost every tissue in the body, and many more adipocyte products must still be awaiting discovery. Characterising these and exploring their effects will certainly provide more clues about how excess fat can contribute to so many diseases.

Indeed, of the current hot topics in obesity, research into the biology of adipose tissue shows no sign of cooling off and is likely to warm up even further. While this book was in proof, some accepted wisdom was challenged (if not destroyed) by fresh experimental approaches

to the origins, development and fate of adipocytes. Brown adipocytes now appear to derive from a precursor that also gives rise to myocytes and not to white adipocytes – although we also know that prolonged sympathetic stimulation can induce white adipocytes to acquire a brown phenotype. Novel experimental methods have also pushed our understanding of adipocyte turnover beyond the simple classical concepts of hyperplasia (increased number) and hypertrophy (increased size of adipocytes) as determinants of fat mass. Individual adipocytes apparently survive for an average of 10 years, but some that are generated in early life may be doomed to remain with us for much longer – perhaps until death do us part. Wider application of these techniques will undoubtedly enable us to understand better the plasticity of adipose tissue and how it adapts to changes in energy balance, including those related to anti-obesity therapies.

Other promising areas of great potential interest include the disentangling of the links that are emerging between adipose tissue and key physiological processes such as sleeping and ageing. For example, epidemiological, clinical and molecular studies are under way to explore the interactions between adipocyte biology and circadian clock gene activity in peripheral tissues, and their impact on energy homeostasis.

Application of the 'omic' technologies – to examine patterns of gene expression and the downstream processes of protein production and metabolic and cellular function in particular tissues – has drawn attention to several interesting new players that go beyond the traditional territory of the adipokines and that may be critical in modulating aspects of lipid and glucose metabolism. These include integral membrane proteins such as caveolins and aquaporins, osteokines (bone-derived factors such as osteopontin and osteocalcin) and specific fatty acids. Osteokines are now known to be expressed by adipocytes and may help to underpin the cross-talk between fat and bone that seems to influence essential processes in both these tissues, such as bone turnover and remodelling, and the control of fat mass and glucose metabolism. 'Free fatty acids' (FFA) can no longer be regarded as a single biochemical entity, because some have quite different metabolic effects: for example, polyunsaturated fatty acids seem to have little effect on insulin signalling, while omega-3 fatty acids may actually enhance it. Moreover, palmitoleate, a FFA released into the circulation by adipocytes, increases insulin sensitivity in liver and muscle and has recently been given the title of 'lipokine' in recognition of this action.

Energy balance and obesity: signals and noise

Research into the physiological mechanisms controlling food intake, energy expenditure and body fat mass has produced many notable discoveries during the last 20 years. The most celebrated is that of leptin, which in the initial rush of excitement was seen as the key to understanding and treating obesity. Leptin has undoubtedly helped to open up the field of adipocyte biology as well as solving many of the mysteries of certain genetically obese rodents, and has also cast some new light (even if dimmer than originally hoped) on human obesity. It now appears to have wider endocrine, reproductive, immune and other roles that may be physiologically more significant than its effects on energy balance. Numerous other candidate regulatory signals have also gone through similar cycles of rising then falling enthusiasm before the conclusion is reached that they, like so many others, are probably bit-players that make only a limited contribution to the everyday control of energy homeostasis.

Several dozen neurotransmitters and circulating hormones and metabolites are known to have experimental effects on food intake and overall energy balance. As with any field crowded with players, the obvious challenge is to identify those that are genuinely important, and this task is probably far from being completed. We have every confidence that new candidate signals will continue to be discovered in brain, fat, gut and other sources, such as liver and muscle. We also have no doubt that some of their properties will be exciting, and that attractive hypotheses will be constructed about their real-life roles and interactions with the known players. However, we suspect that an all-powerful ultimate controller of energy balance, able to over-ride all other regulatory systems, will never be found; indeed, we doubt that it exists. To us, the overwhelming impression is of numerous systems that are designed to come into play under particular circumstances to control specific aspects of feeding behaviour and energy balance, rather than a top-down hierarchy. It remains to be seen whether these parallel mechanisms have evolved to provide all-round protection of the energy stores that are essential to survive and reproduce, or whether some have become surplus to requirement and are now truly 'redundant'.

In humans, further layers of complexity are added by the numerous psychological, social and cultural factors that shape eating behaviour and physical activity. These are powerful influences that cannot be accurately modelled in experimental animals; they appear much more relevant to everyday life than the mechanistic factors operating in lower mammals and are certainly potent enough to disturb the long-term control of body fat and weight. We would suggest (somewhat heretically, given our research backgrounds) that research into the psychosocial determinants of human feeding behaviour may ultimately be more rewarding than the continuing excavation of regulatory pathways in rodents.

In purely energetic terms, obesity holds little mystery as it simply represents the excess of energy intake over expenditure. An alternative view is that obesity is the result of hugely variable and complicated interactions between an individual's genetic background and his or her immediate environment, all heavily influenced by innumerable social and cultural factors. Many of the details of these processes continue to elude us, although pragmatists could argue that we already know enough about why obesity develops to make reasonable attempts to treat and prevent the disease. Research into the causes of obesity will continue to unearth new pieces of the complex puzzle of energy balance and the many ways in which it can be disturbed. However, the full value of these discoveries will only be realised if they can be understood in the everyday context of human obesity and if the new knowledge can be usefully exploited in the global battle against the disease.

Managing obesity: must do better

The treatment and prevention of obesity remain the thorniest issues and the greatest unmet needs in obesity. Those in the front line of the weight-management clinic might be forgiven for arguing that, with the possible exception of bariatric surgery, little has moved on in the last 10 years or even the last quarter-century. Indeed, the vast majority of obese people worldwide are not managed at all, or have no access to specialist services for diagnosis and treatment.

Lifestyle modification can be effective, but succeeds most convincingly in the resource-intensive setting of clinical trials. Even then, the vast majority of obese subjects fail to respond adequately and those who do will mostly return to their previous ways and weight when expert supervision and support are relaxed or withdrawn. Weight-reducing diets continue to proliferate, a sure sign that none really works. Against the expectations – and prejudice – of many obesity experts, one heavily-marketed diet now appears as effective (i.e. not very) as other more intuitive strategies. A hard look at why dietary recommendations succeed or fail has been urgently needed for decades, and this is still the case. We are now better placed than ever before to explore the physiological, psychological and molecular genetic determinants of dietary 'compliance' and outcome. However, to do this effectively, we will need a large-scale, coordinated and dispassionate approach – a combination that has so far proved elusive.

Anti-obesity drugs may also have reached a watershed. When we first drafted this chapter in mid-2008, three agents were established in clinical practice (at least in Europe) that, if appropriately prescribed and monitored, appeared adequately effective and acceptably safe. The excitement of checking the proofs was enhanced by the sudden removal, in October 2008, of licensing approval throughout Europe for rimonabant. The balance was tipped by further confirmation of a significantly increased risk of major psychiatric disorder, including suicide risk – problems that had already been highlighted in earlier studies and that had persuaded the manufacturers to withdraw the drug from consideration for licensing in the USA (but not to discontinue its use in Europe). Neither orlistat nor sibutramine appears to be at risk of a similar sudden fall from grace, but all of these drugs fall short of the ideal – which may in any case lie beyond the reach of pharmacotherapy. With each of these drugs, only about one-third of patients can expect to lose 10% or more of initial weight and virtually none will shed all their excess weight. On stopping treatment, weight and presumably the burden of comorbidities will return in most cases towards pre-treatment levels in those patients (the majority) who have not succeeded in putting their own anti-obesity lifestyle measures into place.

For drugs that could theoretically be indicated for at least one-fifth of the population, some worryingly big questions remain unanswered, mostly because there are no adequate long-term data on efficacy, safety and cost-effectiveness. Is it justifiable to use these drugs for longer than a couple of years, especially in young people who could potentially face life-long treatment? If not, does a limited course of pharmacotherapy buy enough lasting benefits by reducing the risks of morbidity or premature death, or by improving quality of life? Some basic physiological and pharmacological issues also need to be resolved. Weight loss with all anti-obesity drugs flattens off after several months; is this due to physiological adaptation (such as the inappropriate activation of protective 'anti-starvation' responses) or simply to poor compliance? Indeed, could poor compliance explain why most patients fail to lose significant amounts of weight with all the drugs that have been tested? Adherence to treatment for some diseases that are widely seen as 'dangerous' is surprisingly low; for example, many type 1 diabetic patients, at risk of unpleasant hyperglycaemic symptoms and potentially life-threatening ketoacidotic coma, may deliberately omit insulin or take small and ineffective dosages. It seems reasonable to blame the lack of success of obesity management programmes on the patient's presumed inability to comply with lifestyle changes, but we can only do this if we can reject the hypothesis that anti-obesity drugs fail simply because they are not taken.

Bariatric surgery has now emerged from its indifferent and poorly-appreciated infancy and stands out as the only one-off treatment that can have lasting and potentially life-long effects, and that can reduce weight sufficiently to shift some of the most persistent burdens of obesity. The reversal of type 2 diabetes is an outstandingly important clinical outcome of bariatric surgery. This finding also suggests that it may be possible, at least early in the development of the disease, to rewind the clock of β-cell dysfunction – although end-stage β-cell fallout is irreversible and remains beyond rescue, even by bariatric surgery. The surgical procedures in current use are safer than their predecessors but are still not without risk. Moreover, benefits are not permanent in a sizeable minority of cases and as with anti-obesity drugs, it will be important to determine whether this long-term failure is due to physiological adaptation or to non-compliance. Some aspects of how certain bariatric operations work are still a mystery, raising the tantalising but perhaps far-fetched possibility that the key mechanisms could be mimicked by novel drugs or other non-surgical means.

The next decade should see better organisation and coordination of weight-management services, possibly with the emergence of a new clinical specialist to lead the multidisciplinary team that will be needed for the comprehensive management of obesity and its complications. If current forecasts prove accurate, the obesiologist can be assured of a long and busy working life.

Prevention: better than cure, but ...

Given the long list of complications that it causes and the poor record of success in treating it, obesity is *par excellence* a disease that needs to be prevented. Unfortunately, this proved an impossible challenge during the twentieth century, and the continuing spread of obesity now indicates that whichever preventative measures are in place are still inadequate.

Under study conditions, some preventative strategies can be made to work, but the overall effects are generally small and wane after the end of the intervention. Moreover, the outcomes are often critically dependent on the context of the study: an intervention that has been shown to work well in one population may be doomed to failure in another. It is not clear whether this is due to study-specific effects such as the enthusiasm and motivation of the study team, or to the social and cultural determinants of the test populations – but whatever the cause, the poor transferability of preventative measures is potentially a major obstacle to the global sharing of knowledge to prevent obesity.

The heart of the problem may lie in our failure to capture the public's imagination and to convey the full importance of the problem. We need to be much more skilful and probably street-wise in getting across public-health messages about obesity. Current exhortations about healthy living – essentially "eat less, exercise more" – are dull, predictable and unappealing, especially for the many for whom this would amount to a near-total lifestyle transplant. These messages pale into insignificance beside foods and drinks that are specifically designed to encourage overconsumption, or the instant gratification of screen-based entertainment – or indeed the slick and heavily resourced advertising campaigns for these products.

Much more needs to be done to develop, test and spread effective anti-obesity messages that are powerful and persuasive enough to compete head-to-head with the best that the obesogenic industries can roll out. Crucially, these must be tailored deliberately to target the populations most at risk, including young people, ethnic groups susceptible to obesity, and low-income families. Ultimately, finding practical solutions to the problems of obesity may come to rely as much on the skills of experts in advertising and marketing as on clever science and good clinical practice.

Whose problem is it anyway?

Obesity is at last being recognised as a major global health, social and economic problem – or is it? In the UK, parents are to be told if their children are excessively heavy, but only if the child agrees to be weighed at school (and the word 'obesity' will be carefully avoided so as not to cause offence). Obesity has at last crept into many medical school curricula, yet many doctors still do not regard obesity as a 'real' disease that needs active management. The advertising of energy-dense foods and drinks on children's television has been banned in Sweden, but not in the countries with the highest rates of childhood obesity.

These and many other inconsistencies, whether due to conflicts of interest or to a general reluctance to take decisive action, highlight the critical need for concerted and coordinated strategies against obesity. Much is already being done, but our current best is not good enough and new resources will have to be harnessed and exploited. This could demand some lateral thinking, if not a fundamental reappraisal of our approaches to dealing with obesity. The notion of a united front of clinicians and policy-makers may seem fanciful enough, but a truly successful line-up may need to bring in other players that are otherwise too powerful to defeat – namely, the industrial giants selling food and drink, cars and screen-based entertainment. Working with 'the enemy' would be a challenge for both sides, but could be the basis for an effective partnership that will at last begin to contain the global spread of obesity and its consequences.

Index